MEDICAL TERMINOLOGY

An Anatomy and Physiology Systems Approach

SECOND EDITION

Bonnie F. Fremgen, Ph.D.

Suzanne S. Frucht, Ph.D.

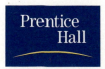

Upper Saddle River, New Jersey 07458

Library of Congress Cataloging-in-Publication Data

Fremgen, Bonnie F.

    Medical terminology : an anatomy and physiology systems approach / Bonnie F.
Fremgen, Sue Frucht.--2nd ed.

       p. cm.

    Includes bibliographical references and index.

    ISBN 0-13-031182-0

    1. Medicine--Terminology. I. Frucht, Sue. II. Title.

R123 .F697 2002

610′.1′4--dc21

2001046154

Publisher: Julie Levin Alexander
Acquisitions Editor: Mark Cohen
Senior Managing Editor: Marilyn C. Meserve
Assistant Editor: Melissa Kerian
Marketing Manager: David Hough
Director of Production and Manufacturing: Bruce Johnson
Managing Production Editor: Patrick Walsh
Manufacturing Manager: Ilene Sanford
Production Liaison: Julie Li
Production Editor: Amy Gehl
Media Development Editor: Sarah Hayday
Manager of Media Production: Amy Peltier
New Media Project Manager: Stephen J. Hartner
Creative Director: Cheryl Asherman
Cover Design Coordinator: Maria Guglielmo
Cover Designer: Kevin Kall
Composition: Carlisle Publishers Services
Printing and Binding: The Banta Company

> ### Dedication
>
> To my husband for his love
> and encouragement.
>
> *Bonnie Fremgen*
>
> To my husband, Rick, and my
> daughter, Kristin, for their
> love, support, and friendship.
>
> *Suzanne Frucht*

Notice: The authors and the publisher of this volume have taken care that the information and technical recommendations contained herein are based on research and expert consultation, and are accurate and compatible with the standards generally accepted at the time of publication. Nevertheless, as new information becomes available, changes in clinical and technical practices become necessary. The reader is advised to carefully consult manufacturers' instructions and information material for all supplies and equipment before use, and to consult with a health care professional as necessary. This advice is especially important when using new supplies or equipment for clinical purposes. The authors and publisher disclaim all responsibility for any liability, loss, injury, or damage incurred as a consequence, directly or indirectly, of the use and application of any of the contents of this volume.

Pearson Education, LTD.
Pearson Education Australia PTY, Limited
Pearson Education Singapore, Pte. Ltd.
Pearson Education North Asia Ltd.
Pearson Education Canada, Ltd.
Pearson Educación de Mexico, S.A. de C.V.
Pearson Education – Japan
Pearson Education Malaysia, Pte. Ltd.
Pearson Education, Upper Saddle River, New Jersey

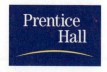

10 9 8 7 6 5 4 3 2 1

ISBN 0-13-031182-0

Classic and new features promote comprehension...

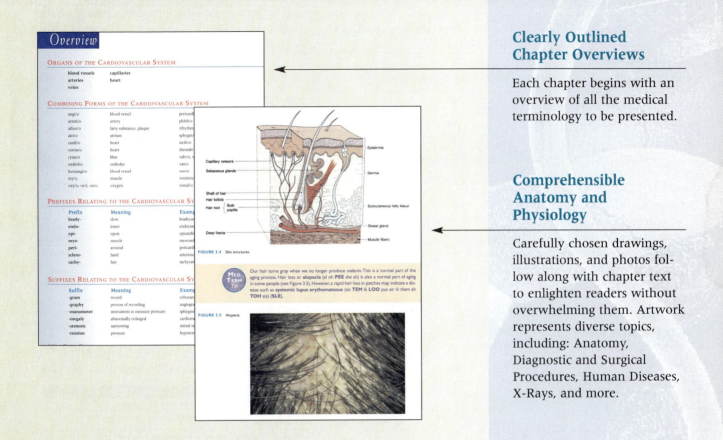

Clearly Outlined Chapter Overviews

Each chapter begins with an overview of all the medical terminology to be presented.

Comprehensible Anatomy and Physiology

Carefully chosen drawings, illustrations, and photos follow along with chapter text to enlighten readers without overwhelming them. Artwork represents diverse topics, including: Anatomy, Diagnostic and Surgical Procedures, Human Diseases, X-Rays, and more.

THEORY INTO PRACTICE: REAL WORLD APPLICATIONS

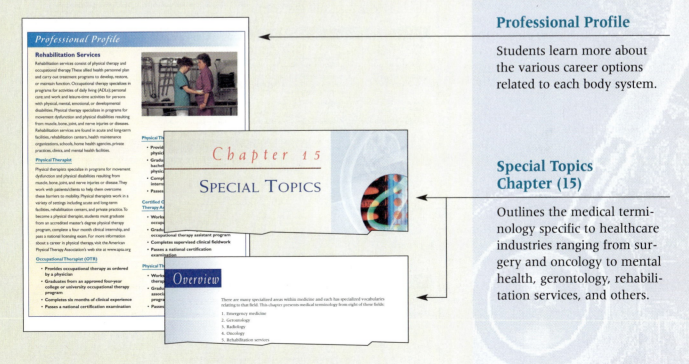

Professional Profile

Students learn more about the various career options related to each body system.

Special Topics Chapter (15)

Outlines the medical terminology specific to healthcare industries ranging from surgery and oncology to mental health, gerontology, rehabilitation services, and others.

CONSISTENT CHAPTER ORGANIZATION

Representing an individual body system, each chapter follows a consistent format to build student confidence and ensure clear understanding of the information presented.

Anatomy and Physiology

Details the A&P relating to the body system under discussion.

Word Building

Demonstrates how definitions can be reasoned out by translating individual word parts.

Med Term Tips

Engages students with useful tips for learning and comprehending medical terminology.

Vocabulary

Pathology

Diagnostic Procedures

Treatment Procedures

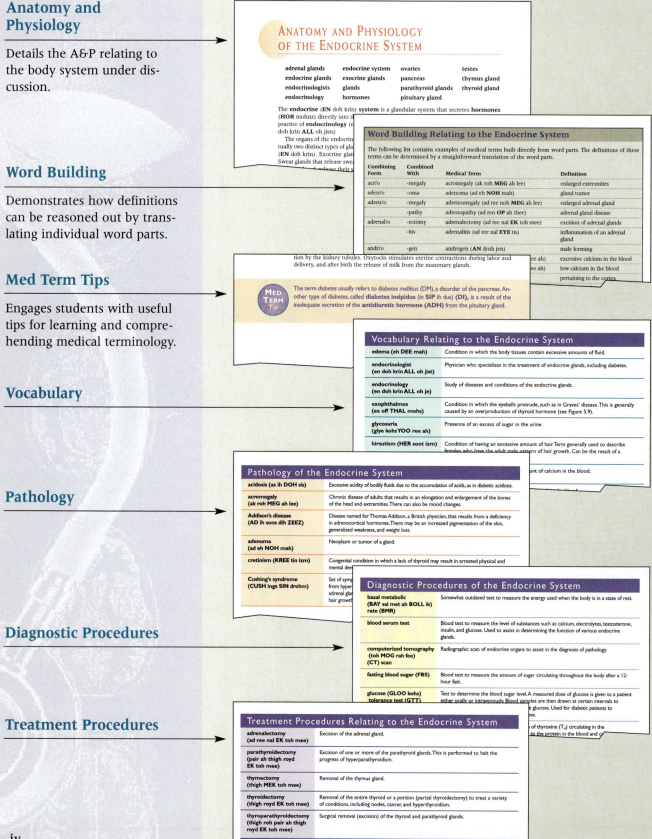

ANATOMY AND PHYSIOLOGY OF THE ENDOCRINE SYSTEM

adrenal glands	endocrine system	ovaries	testes
endocrine glands	exocrine glands	pancreas	thymus gland
endocrinologists	glands	parathyroid glands	thyroid gland
endocrinology	hormones	pituitary gland	

The **endocrine** (**EN** doh krin) **system** is a glandular system that secretes **hormones** (**HOR** mohnz) directly into t[...]
practice of **endocrinology** (e[...]
doh krin **ALL** oh jists)

The organs of the endocrin[...]
tually two distinct types of glan[...]
(**EN** doh krin). Exocrine glan[...]
Sweat glands that release swea[...]
[...]

Word Building Relating to the Endocrine System

The following list contains examples of medical terms built directly from word parts. The definitions of these terms can be determined by a straightforward translation of the word parts.

Combining Form	Combined With	Medical Term	Definition
acr/o	-megaly	acromegaly (ak roh **MEG** ah lee)	enlarged extremities
aden/o	-oma	adenoma (ad eh **NOH** mah)	gland tumor
adren/o	-megaly	adrenomegaly (ad ree noh **MEG** ah lee)	enlarged adrenal gland
	-pathy	adrenopathy (ad ren **OP** ah thee)	adrenal gland disease
adrenal/o	-ectomy	adrenalectomy (ad ree nal **EK** toh mee)	excision of adrenal glands
	-itis	adrenalitis (ad ree nal **EYE** tis)	inflammation of an adrenal gland
andr/o	-gen	androgen (**AN** druh jen)	male forming
		[...] ee ah)	excessive calcium in the blood
		[...] ee ah)	low calcium in the blood
			pertaining to the cortex

tion by the kidney tubules. Oxytocin stimulates uterine contractions during labor and delivery, and after birth the release of milk from the mammary glands.

MED TERM TIP — The term *diabetes* usually refers to diabetes mellitus (DM), a disorder of the pancreas. Another type of diabetes, called **diabetes insipidus** (in **SIP** ih dus) **(DI),** is a result of the inadequate secretion of the **antidiuretic hormone (ADH)** from the pituitary gland.

Vocabulary Relating to the Endocrine System

edema (eh **DEE** mah)	Condition in which the body tissues contain excessive amounts of fluid.
endocrinologist (en doh krin **ALL** oh jist)	Physician who specializes in the treatment of endocrine glands, including diabetes.
endocrinology (en doh krin **ALL** oh je)	Study of diseases and conditions of the endocrine glands.
exophthalmos (ex off **THAL** mohs)	Condition in which the eyeballs protrude, such as in Graves' disease. This is generally caused by an overproduction of thyroid hormone (see Figure 5.9).
glycosuria (glye kohs **YOO** ree ah)	Presence of an excess of sugar in the urine.
hirsutism (**HER** soot izm)	Condition of having an excessive amount of hair. Term generally used to describe females who have the adult male pattern of hair growth. Can be the result of a [...]

Pathology of the Endocrine System

acidosis (as ih **DOH** sis)	Excessive acidity of bodily fluids due to the accumulation of acids, as in diabetic acidosis.
acromegaly (ak roh **MEG** ah lee)	Chronic disease of adults that results in an elongation and enlargement of the bones of the head and extremities. There can also be mood changes.
Addison's disease (**AD** ih sons dih **ZEEZ**)	Disease named for Thomas Addison, a British physician, that results from a deficiency in adrenocortical hormones. There may be an increased pigmentation of the skin, generalized weakness, and weight loss.
adenoma (ad eh **NOH** mah)	Neoplasm or tumor of a gland.
cretinism (**KREE** tin izm)	Congenital condition in which a lack of thyroid may result in arrested physical and mental dev[...]
Cushing's syndrome (**CUSH** ings **SIN** drohm)	Set of symp[...] from hyper[...] adrenal glan[...] hair growth[...]

Diagnostic Procedures of the Endocrine System

basal metabolic rate (BMR) (**BAY** sal met ah **BOLL** ik)	Somewhat outdated test to measure the energy used when the body is in a state of rest.
blood serum test	Blood test to measure the level of substances such as calcium, electrolytes, testosterone, insulin, and glucose. Used to assist in determining the function of various endocrine glands.
computerized tomography (CT) scan (toh **MOG** rah fee)	Radiographic scan of endocrine organs to assist in the diagnosis of pathology.
fasting blood sugar (FBS)	Blood test to measure the amount of sugar circulating throughout the body after a 12-hour fast.
glucose tolerance test (GTT) (**GLOO** kohs)	Test to determine the blood sugar level. A measured dose of glucose is given to a patient either orally or intravenously. Blood samples are then drawn at certain intervals [...] glucose. Used for diabetic patients to [...]

Treatment Procedures Relating to the Endocrine System

adrenalectomy (ad ree nal **EK** toh mee)	Excision of the adrenal gland.
parathyroidectomy (pair ah thigh royd **EK** toh mee)	Excision of one or more of the parathyroid glands. This is performed to halt the progress of hyperparathyroidism.
thymectomy (thigh **MEK** toh mee)	Removal of the thymus gland.
thyroidectomy (thigh royd **EK** toh mee)	Removal of the entire thyroid or a portion (partial thyroidectomy) to treat a variety of conditions, including nodes, cancer, and hyperthyroidism.
thyroparathyroidectomy (thigh roh pair ah thigh royd **EK** toh mee)	Surgical removal (excision) of the thyroid and parathyroid glands.

DIVERSE END-OF-CHAPTER EXERCISES FACILITATE LEARNING

Case Study

DISCHARGE SUMMARY

Admitting Diagnosis: Difficulty breathing, hypertension, tachycardia

Final Diagnosis: CHF secondary to mitral valve prolapse

History of Present Illness: Patient was brought to the Emergency Room by her family because of SOB, tachycardia (a racing heart rate), and anxiety. Patient reports that she has experienced these symptoms for the past six months, brought on by exertion. The current episode began while she was cleaning house and is more severe than any previous episode. Upon admission in the ER, HR was 120 beats per minute and blood pressure was 180/110. The patient was cyanotic around the lips and nail beds and had severe edema in feet and lower legs. The results of an EKG and cardiac enzyme blood tests were normal. Medication improved the symptoms but she was admitted for observation and a complete cardiac workup for tachycardia, hypertension.

Summary of Hospital Course: Patient underwent a full battery of cardiac diagnostic tests. A prolapsed mitral valve was observed on an echocardiogram. A treadmill test had

to be stopped early due to onset of se—
breathing and cyanosis of the lips. Arterial
showed low oxygen, and supplemental oxy—
had to be used to resolve cyanosis. An
phy fail—
thrombo—
ting eder—
Lopress—
heart ra—
edema, —
pressure —
unless sh—

Disch—
infarction
angioplas—
placed o—
instructio—
gram. Sh—
pressor. —
a mitral v—

CRITICAL THINKING QUESTIONS

1. List the four medications this patient was given in the hospital and describe in your own words what condition each medication treats.

    a.

    b.

    c.

    d.

2. Two diagnostic tests conducted in the Emergency Room were normal. List them and describe each test in your own words. Because the results from these two tests were normal, a very serious heart condition could be ruled out. This is noted in the discharge plans. Identify the serious heart condition and describe it in your own words.

3. Expl—

4. Wh—
    diag—
    a. h—
    b. d—
    c. c—
    d. f—

5. The—
    pati—
    fails—
    surg—

6. Co—
    pro—

Chart Note Transcription

Chart Note

The chart note below contains ten phrases that can be reworded with a medical term that you learned in this chapter. Each phrase is identified with an underline. Determine the medical term and write your answers in the space provided.

Current Complaint: Patient is a 77-year-old male seen by the urologist with complaints of noca and difficulty with the release of semen from the urethra.[a]

Past History: Medical history revealed that the patient had failure of the testes to descend into the scrotum at birth,[b] which was repaired by surgical fixation of the testes. He had also undergone elective sterilization by removal of a segment of the vas deferens at the age of 41.

Signs and Symptoms: Patient states he first noted these symptoms about 5 years ago. They have become increasingly severe and now he is not able to sleep without waking up to urinate up to 20 times a night and difficulty completing the process of sexual relations.[c] Palpation of the prostate gland through the rectum revealed multiple round firm nodules in prostate gland. A needle biopsy was negative for slow-growing cancer that frequently affects males over 50 and a blood test for prostate cancer was normal.

Diagnosis: Non-cancerous enlargement of the prostate gland.

Treatment: Patient was scheduled for a surgical removal of prostate tissue through the urethra.[d]

1. _____
2. _____
3. _____
4. _____
5. _____
6. _____
7. _____
8. _____
9. _____
10. _____

Case Studies

These scenarios use critical thinking questions to help students connect the correct terminology to the information presented.

Chart Note Transcription Practice

Students read through a narrative patient scenario and replace descriptive information with the correct professional terminology.

Superior Study Tools

Look for eighteen double-sided pages of perforated flashcards bound right into every text.

Diverse End-of-Chapter Exercises

Review questions are presented in many different formats to promote comprehension and retention. **Answers** are found at the end of each chapter as well.

A. COMPLETE THE FOLLOWING STATEMENTS.

1. The study of the heart is called _____
2. The three layers of the heart are _____, _____, and _____
3. The impulse for the heartbeat (the pacemaker) originates in the _____
4. The artery that does not carry oxygenated blood is the _____
5. The four heart valves are _____, _____, _____, and _____
6. Three procedures that are used to correct heart and cardiovascular problems are _____, _____, and _____

B. STATE THE TERMS DESCRIBED USING THE COMBINING FORMS PROVIDED.

The combining form cardi/o refers to the heart. Use it to write a term that means

1. pain in the heart _____
2. disease of the heart muscle _____
3. enlargement of the heart _____
4. abnormally fast heart rate _____
5. abnormally slow heart rate _____
6. inflammation of the heart _____

The combining form phleb/o refers to the vein. Use it to write a term that means

7. inflammation of a vein _____

C. ADD A PREFIX TO THE COMBINING FORM CARDI/O TO FORM THE TERM FOR

1. inflammation of the inner lining of the heart _____
2. inflammation of the outer layer of the heart _____
3. inflammation of the muscle of the heart _____

D. PROVIDE THE PRONUNCIATION FOR THE FOLLOWING WORDS.

1. atrial fibrillation _____
2. cardiopulmonary resuscitation _____
3. aneurysm _____
4. phlebitis _____

E. DEFINE EACH COMBINING FORM AND PROVIDE AN EXAMPLE OF ITS USE.

	Definition	Example
1. cardi/o		
2. vas/o		
3. steth/o		
4. arteri/o		
5. phleb/o		
6. angi/o		
7. ventricul/o		
8. thromb/o		

F. WRITE MEDICAL TERMS FOR THE FOLLOWING DEFINITIONS.

1. pertaining to a vein _____
2. fast heart beat _____
3. specialist in treating the heart _____
4. recording electrical activity of heart _____
5. high blood pressure _____
6. low blood pressure _____
7. inflammation of inner lining of heart _____
8. bluish coloring to skin _____
9. destruction of (dissolving) a clot _____

G. WRITE THE SUFFIX FOR EACH EXPRESSION AND PROVIDE AN EXAMPLE OF ITS USE.

	Suffix	Example
1. instrument for recording		
2. abnormal narrowing		
3. instrument to measure pressure		
4. enlargement		
5. record		

H. IDENTIFY THE FOLLOWING ABBREVIATIONS.

1. BP _____
2. CHF _____
3. MI _____
4. CCU _____
5. PVC _____
6. CPR _____
7. CAD _____

I. WRITE THE ABBREVIATIONS FOR THE FOLLOWING TERMS.

1. mitral valve prolapse _____
2. ventricular septal defect _____
3. percutaneous transluminal coronary angioplasty _____
4. jugular venous pulse _____
5. coronary intensive care _____
6. congestive heart failure _____

J. MATCH THE TERMS IN COLUMN A WITH THE DEFINITIONS IN COLUMN B.

	A		B
1. ____	arrhythmia	a.	swollen, distended veins
2. ____	thrombus	b.	inflammation of vein
3. ____	bradycardia	c.	abnormal connection
4. ____	bruit	d.	slow heart rate
5. ____	phlebitis	e.	insert thin tubing
6. ____	commissurotomy	f.	irregular heartbeat
7. ____	varicose	g.	murmur

K. USE THE FOLLOWING TERMS IN THE SENTENCES THAT FOLLOW.

angioma	angina	echocardiogram	MI
angiography	ischemia	aortic stenosis	Pro time
defibrillator	Holter monitor	hypertension	CCU
murmur	CHF	pacemaker	

1. Tiffany was born with a congenital condition that results in an abnormal heart sound. This is called a(n) _____

2. Porter's physician has placed him on medication that causes the blood to become thinner. His doctor wishes to measure the clotting time of his blood. He is ordering a(n) _____

3. Joseph suffered an arrhythmia while hospitalized that resulted in a cardiac arrest. The emergency physician and team used an instrument to give electric shocks to the heart in an attempt to create a normal heart

COMPANION WEBPAGE

Objectives

Step-by-step goals for each chapter of the text.

Check Your Progress

Ten multiple-choice questions offer a "mini-quiz" of basic material for each chapter.

End-of-Chapter Challenge

Ten additional multiple-choice questions for each chapter help students gauge their grasp of more difficult material.

Audio Glossary

Clear pronunciations orally reinforce key terms from the text.

Visit *www.prenhall.com/fremgen* for useful online study aids and research tools:

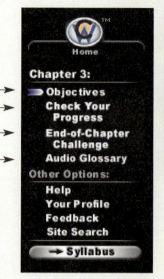

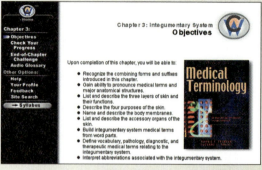

Audio Glossary

Students can hear the correct pronunciation for nearly 3,000 terms while also viewing the term's definition, for powerful visual and auditory reinforcement.

Word Building

Students view a definition, then drag prefixes, roots, and suffixes as needed to build the correct term.

Spelling Bee

Users hear a word, then type the correct spelling.

Flashcards

Allows students to easily create custom study aids for additional practice.

Practice Tests

Includes a mix of multiple-choice and true/false for each chapter, plus helpful "coaching comments" and immediate feedback.

Labeling Exercises

Users simply click and drag terms to label the appropriate section of an image.

COMPANION CD-ROM

Free with every copy of the text, this cross-platform CD-ROM offers a host of interactive study aids:

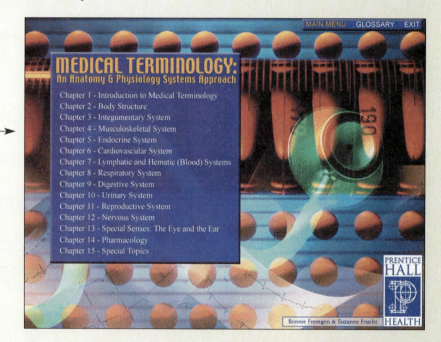

ONLINE COURSE

Available for **Blackboard**, **WebCT**, and **CourseCompass** platforms, the Online Course features many of the study aids noted above, as well as matching and web destination exercises, case studies, comprehensive exam, and an **eBook**.

BRIEF CONTENTS

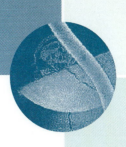

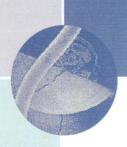

CONTENTS

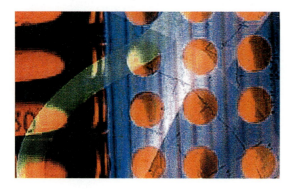

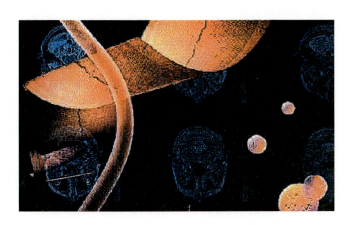

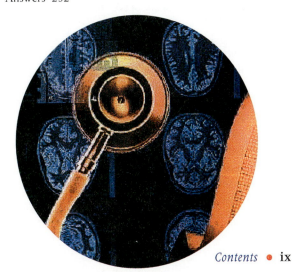

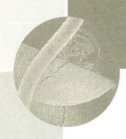

PREFACE

TO THE STUDENT

Welcome to the fascinating study of medical language—a vital part of your preparation for a career as a health professional. Throughout your career, in a variety of settings, you will use your understanding of medical terminology to communicate with other health professionals and patients. Employing a carefully constructed learning system, **Medical Terminology: An Anatomy and Physiology Systems Approach** is designed to guide you toward gaining a successful grasp of medical language, while giving you a real-world glimpse of its application in several professions.

The book will introduce you to the basic rules for using word parts to form medical terms. The use of phonetic pronunciation throughout the book will help you to easily say a word by spelling out the word part according to the way it sounds. You will find the integrated approach will help you learn by applying medical terminology to anatomy and physiology content by body system. Throughout the text there are many features, as well as real-life photographs and illustrations to enhance your comprehension of the material. A variety of end-of-chapter exercises allow you to review and master the content as you go along. An interactive CD-ROM and online study guide come free with the text and provide additional reinforcement of what you have learned in each chapter.

CHAPTER ORGANIZATION

INTRODUCTORY CHAPTERS

Chapters 1 and 2 contain the information necessary for an understanding of how medical terms are formed. In Chapter 1, you will learn about word parts, combining forms, prefixes, and suffixes, and general rules for building medical terms. You will also learn about terminology for medical records, managed care, and the different health care settings. Before the end-of-chapter activities begin, you will encounter the first of many new features in the text. "Professional Profile" boxes highlight different health professions and are intended to increase your knowledge of careers in the health care field. In Chapter 2, you will learn about terminology relating to the body structure, including organs and body systems. Here you will see another new feature, "Word Building" tables, which list medical terms and their respective word parts. Throughout each chapter are several "Med Term Tips" which are intended to stimulate your interest by describing quick facts about medical terms.

ANATOMY AND PHYSIOLOGY CHAPTERS

Chapters 3–13 are organized by body system. Each chapter begins with an overview of the organs in the system and is followed by lists of combining forms, prefixes, and/or suffixes with their meanings. Chapters are divided into the various components of the system, and each subsection begins with a list of key medical terms. Key terms are **boldfaced** and pronounced the first time they appear in the narrative. Following the anatomy and physiology section is a word building table, as well as medical terms with pronunciations. For ease of learning, the medical terms are divided into four separate sections: vocabulary, pathology, diagnostic procedures, and treatment procedures. Abbreviations and a list of key terms follow in the end-of-chapter material. For easy reference, there is a combination glossary and index at the end of the text with pronunciations and definitions of all of the terms in the text.

PHARMACOLOGY CHAPTER

Chapter 14 is a new chapter devoted to pharmacology. You will learn how different drugs are classified and how to administer drugs safely and effectively.

SPECIAL TOPICS CHAPTER

Chapter 15 contains timely information and appropriate medical terms relevant to the following medical specialties: emergency medicine, gerontology, radiology, oncology, rehabilitation services, surgery, mental health, and pediatrics. Knowledge of these topics is necessary for the well-rounded health care worker.

APPENDICES

The appendices contain helpful reference lists of word parts and definitions. This information is intended for quick access. Appendix A is an abbreviation listing; Appendix B contains prefixes; Appendix C contains suffixes, and Appendix D contains combining forms.

TEACHING AND LEARNING PACKAGE

An Interactive Student CD-ROM is packaged in the back of the book and contains a host of interactive study aids, including an audio glossary, practice tests, labeling exercises, word building exercises, a spelling bee game, and flashcards.

The Companion Website (www.prenhall.com/fremgen) is a free online study aid, tied chapter-by-chapter to the text, that provides interactive student activities and practice quizzes—complete with instant scoring and immediate user feedback—to enhance your learning.

A 90-minute audiocassette is available that provides students with the flexibility to practice and learn pronunciation in the classroom, at home, or while traveling to and from school.

TO THE INSTRUCTOR

The second edition of **Medical Terminology: An Anatomy and Physiology Systems Approach** uses an integrated approach for teaching the medical terminology to the health care student. It assists students in mastering terminology and incorporating this knowledge through an understanding of anatomy and physiology. In this way, beginning students learn the purpose and use of the medical terms they are learning.

FEATURES OF THE NEW EDITION

This edition contains many new features that facilitate student mastery, while maintaining the best features of the first edition. Each chapter is arranged in a similar format and the content has been reorganized with an emphasis on maintaining consistency and accuracy. More than one hundred new terms have been added. *Professional Profile* boxes highlight different career options to help students become more familiar with the health care field. *Word Building* tables within each chapter put much needed emphasis on building words rather than rote memorization. Learning objectives are listed at the beginning of each chapter. *Med Term Tips* help maintain student interest by presenting quick facts about medical terminology. A new chapter on Pharmacology has been added, and the special topics chapter covers medical terminology that is specific to a variety of health care fields, including emergency medicine, gerontology, nuclear medicine, oncology, rehabilitation services, surgery, mental health, and pediatrics. Four-color realistic photographs and illustrations of body systems, organs, and pathological conditions bring medical terminology to life and make learning more fun and effective. An at-a-glance summary chart of medical terms is presented in each chapter. Abbreviations used in the medical field are integrated in each chapter and are also listed for handy reference in an appendix. Pronunciations are based on Dorland's *Illustrated Medical Dictionary,* 29th edition.

We are pleased to welcome Sue Frucht from Northwest Missouri State University as a co-author on the second edition. Her knowledge and expertise have contributed enormously to the quality of the new edition.

END-OF-CHAPTER ACTIVITIES

The end-of-chapter activities have been significantly expanded in this edition and answers at the end of each chapter provide immediate feedback.

CHART NOTE TRANSCRIPTION

A patient scenario is presented and the student is asked to replace phrases used to describe maladies, procedures, tests, and conditions with the accurate medical terms.

CASE STUDIES WITH CRITICAL THINKING QUESTIONS

Students see practical applications of medical terminology for each body system.

EXERCISES

These problems allow students to test their knowledge of chapter material.

"GETTING CONNECTED" MULTIMEDIA EXTENSION EXERCISES

Students are directed to the activities on the student CD-ROM or the Companion Website at www.prenhall.com/fremgen.

ADDITIONAL LEARNING AND TEACHING RESOURCES

An **interactive student CD-ROM** is *free* with every text and offers a host of study aids including an audio glossary that allows students to practice and hear correct pronunciation; practice tests that include multiple-choice and true/false questions; labeling exercises which allow students to click and drag word parts to build terms; a spelling bee in which users hear a word, then type the correct spelling; and flashcards that allow students to easily create custom study aids for additional practice.

A **companion website** (www.prenhall.com/fremgen) with online learning tools including learning objectives for each chapter; an audio glossary with pronunciations of key terms; *Check Your Progress* sections consisting of ten multiple-choice questions relating to basic material in each chapter; and an *End-of-Chapter Challenge* with ten additional multiple-choice questions relating to more difficult material in each chapter. The website instantly tabulates student results and allows those results to be sent to instructors via e-mail. Educators can also post a syllabus online at this site using a template that is provided.

An **online course** is available for *Blackboard, WebCT,* and *CourseCompass* platforms. The online course features enhanced study aids such as matching and web destination exercises, case studies, and a comprehensive exam. The online course is accessible via a special access code that can be purchased separately from Prentice Hall or packaged with the book. For more information about Prentice Hall's online course offerings visit www.prenhall.com/demo.

A **test bank** for IBM PC and MAC formats with 375 multiple-choice, true/false, and fill-in questions.

An **instructor's guide** providing educators with additional labeling activities, handout quizzes, and teaching hints.

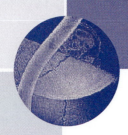

ACKNOWLEDGMENTS

Karen R. Hardney, M.S., Ed.
Recruitment Director
College of Health Sciences
Chicago State University
Chicago, Illinois

Andrew La Marca, EMT-P
EMT and Paramedic Instructor/Coordinator
Mobile Life Support Services
Middletown, New York

Kimberley Hontz , RN
Antonelli Medical and Professional Institute
Pottstown, Pennsylvania

Jamie Erskine, Ph.D., R.D.
Associate Professor
Department of Community Health and
Nutrition
University of Northern Colorado
Greeley, Colorado

Pamela S. Huber, M.S., MT(ASCP)
Assistant Professor
Medical Laboratory Technology Department
Erie Community College
Williamsville, New York

Joan Walker Brittingham
Program Coordinator
Adult Education and Training
Sussex Tech Adult Division
Georgetown, Delaware

Deborah J. Bedford, CMA, AAS
Program Coordinator
Medical Assisting Program
North Seattle Community College
Seattle, Washington

Linda Reigel
Assistant Professor
Department of Business
Glenville State College
Glenville, West Virginia

Sister M. Marguerite Polcyn, Ph.D.
Professor
Health Education
Lourdes College
Sylvania, Ohio

Toni Cade, MBA, RHIA, CCS
Assistant Professor
University of Louisiana at Lafayette
Lafayette, Louisiana

Pam Besser, Ph.D.
Professor of Rhetoric
Jefferson Community College
Louisville, Kentucky

Janet Stehling, RHIA
McLennan Community College
Waco, Texas

Sara J. Wellman, RHIT
Clinical Coordinator
Health Information Technology Program
Indiana University Northwest
Gary, Indiana

Ann Queen Giles, MHS, CMA
Program Director
Medical Assisting Program
Western Piedmont Community College
Morganton, North Carolina

Kathryn Gruber
Applied Sciences
Globe College
Oakdale, Minnesota

Lola McGourty, MSN, RN
Bossier Parish Community College
Bossier City, Louisiana

About the Authors

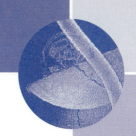

Bonnie F. Fremgen, Ph.D., is a former associate dean of the Allied Health Program at Robert Morris College. She has taught medical law and ethics courses as well as clinical and administrative topics. In addition, she has served as an advisor for students' career planning. She has broad interests and experiences in the health care field, including hospitals, nursing homes, and physicians' offices.

Dr. Fremgen holds a nursing degree as well as a master's in health care administration. She received her Ph.D. from the College of Education at the University of Illinois. She has performed postdoctoral studies in Medical Law at Loyola University Law School in Chicago.

Dr. Fremgen is currently co-director of the Center for Business Ethics at the University of Notre Dame in South Bend, Indiana.

Suzanne S. Frucht is an Assistant Professor of Physiology at Northwest Missouri State University. She received a BA in Biological Sciences in 1975 and a BS in Physical Therapy in 1977, both from Indiana University. She worked full-time as a physical therapist in various health care settings, including acute care hospitals, extended care facilities, and home health from 1977 to 1991.

Dr. Frucht received a MS degree in Biological Sciences from NWMSU in 1987. Based on her health care experience and graduate degree, she was invited to teach Medical Terminology part-time in 1988. Discovering a love for the challenge of teaching at the college level she joined the NWMSU biology faculty full-time in 1991. While continuing to work full-time on the faculty she obtained a Ph.D. from the University of Missouri-Kansas City in Molecular Biology and Biochemistry in 1999.

Today, she teaches a varied course load including Medical Terminology, Basic Physiology and Anatomy, Human Physiology, Comparative Anatomy, and Histology. To remain up-to-date in health care she continues to work as a PT on an occasional basis and takes continuing education courses to maintain her physical therapy license.

Chapter 1

Introduction to Medical Terminology

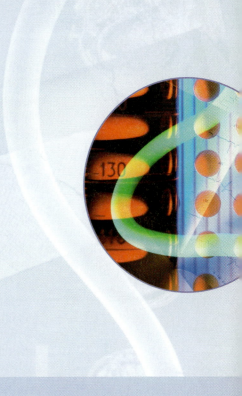

Learning Objectives

Upon completion of this chapter, you will be able to:

- Discuss the four parts to medical terms.

- State the importance of correct spelling of medical terms.

- Recognize word roots and the combining forms.

- Identify the most common prefixes and suffixes.

- State the rules for determining singular and plural endings.

- Define word building.

- Discuss the importance of using caution with abbreviations.

- Recognize the documents found in a medical record.

- Define the terms associated with managed care, health care settings, and billing codes.

- Understand the importance of confidentiality.

Overview

Learning medical terminology can seem at first like studying a strange new language. But once you understand some of the basic rules as to how medical terms are formed using word building, it will become much like piecing together a puzzle. The general guidelines for forming words, an understanding of word roots, combining forms, prefixes and suffixes pronunciation, and spelling are discussed in this chapter. Each chapter about a specific system contains examples of words containing word roots, combining vowels, prefixes, and suffixes, and exercises to help you gain experience with the word-building concept. In addition, "Med Term Tips" are sprinkled throughout the text to assist in clarifying some of the material. New medical terms discussed in each section are listed separately at the beginning of the section. You can use them as an additional study tool for previewing and reviewing terms.

Understanding medical terms requires you to be able to put words together or build words from their parts. It is impossible to memorize thousands of medical terms; however, once you understand the basic word roots, you can distinguish the meaning of medical terms by analyzing their prefixes, suffixes, and word roots. Remember that there will always be some exceptions to every rule, and medical terminology is no different. We will try to point out those exceptions. Most medical terms, however, do follow the general rule that there is a word root or fundamental meaning for the word, a combining vowel to make the pronunciation easier, and in many cases, a prefix and/or suffix.

MED TERM TIP

The general rule for forming medical terms is that most medical terms will consist of four parts:

Word Building Part	Example
1. Word root	cardi (heart)
2. Prefix	peri- (around)
3. Combining form	cardi/o (heart)
4. Suffix	-itis (inflammation)

When these four components are put together, the word **pericarditis** (per ih car **DYE** tis) is formed, meaning inflammation of the pericardium of the heart.

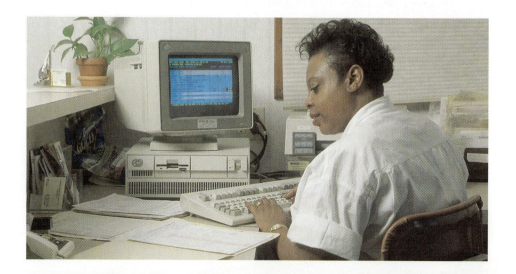

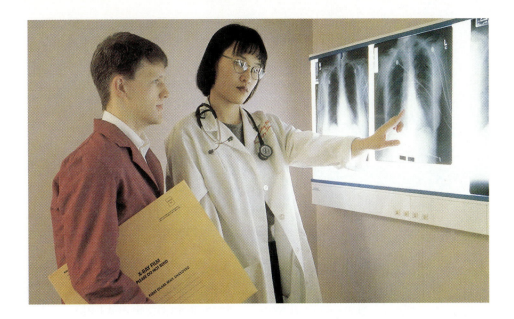

You will be amazed at the seemingly difficult words you are able to build and understand when you follow the simple steps in word building.

PRONUNCIATION

You will hear different pronunciations for the same terms depending on where people were born or educated. As long as it is clear which term people are discussing, differing pronunciations are acceptable. Some people are difficult to understand over the telephone or on a transcription tape. If you have any doubt about a term being discussed, ask for the term to be spelled.

Each new term in the book is introduced in boldface type, with the phonetic or "sounds like" pronunciation in parentheses immediately following. The part of the word that should receive the greatest emphasis during pronunciation appears in capital letters: for example, **pericarditis** (per ih car **DYE** tis). Pronounce the word to yourself or out loud.

Some words have the same pronunciation but very different meanings.

Ileum (**ILL** ee um), which means a part of the small intestine, is pronounced the same as the word **ilium,** which is a part of the hipbone. Ile/o with an e is the combining form for small intestine. Ili/o with an i is the combining form meaning hipbone.

SPELLING

Although you will hear differing pronunciations of the same term, there will be only one correct spelling. If you have any doubt about the spelling of a term or of its meaning, always look it up in a medical dictionary. If only one letter of the word is changed, it could make a critical difference for the patient. For example, imagine the problem that could arise if you note for insurance purposes that a portion of a patient's ileum, or small intestine, was removed when in reality he had surgery for removal of a piece of his ilium, or hipbone.

There are also words that have the same beginning sounds but are spelled differently. Some examples follow.

Sounds like *si*

psy	**psychiatry** (sigh **KIGH** ah tree)
cy	**cystitis** (siss **TYE** tis)
sy	**symptom** (**SIM** tom)
si	**silicosis** (sill ih **KOH** sis)

Sounds like *dis*

dys	**dyspnea** (disp **NEE** ah)
des	**desmoid** (**DEZ** moyd)
dis	**disease** (dih **ZEEZ**)

SINGULAR AND PLURAL ENDINGS

Many medical terms originate from Greek and Latin words. The rules for setting up the singular and plural forms of some words follow the rules of these languages. Other words, such as virus and viruses, are changed from singular to plural by following English rules. Each medical term needs to be considered individually when changing from the singular to the plural form. Following are some general rules in setting up plural forms.

Rule	Example: Singular to Plural
1. A word ending in -a will keep the -a and add -e for the plural.	*vertebra* to *vertebrae*
2. A word ending in -ax will drop the -ax and add -aces for the plural form.	*thorax* to *thoraces*
3. A word ending in -ex or -ix will drop these letters and add -ices for the plural form.	*appendix* to *appendices*
4. A word ending in -ma will keep the -ma and add -ta for the plural form.	*sarcoma* to *sarcomata*
5. A word ending in -is will drop the -is and add -es for the plural form	*metastasis* to *metastases*
6. A word ending in -on will drop the -on and add -a for the plural form.	*ganglion* to *ganglia*
7. A word ending in -us will drop the -us and add -i for the plural form.	*nucleus* to *nuclei*
8. A word ending in -um will drop the -um and add -a for the plural form.	*ovum* to *ova*
9. A word ending in -y will drop the -y and add -ies for the plural form.	*biopsy* to *biopsies*
10. A word ending in -nx will change the x to g and add -es.	*phalanx* to *phalanges*

WORD ROOTS

The main part of the word, or word root, is the foundation of the word. This provides us with the general meaning of the word. The word root will tell us the body system or part of the body that is being discussed, such as *cardi* for *heart*. The word root represents the fundamental meaning of the word: for example, cardi = heart.

A word may have more than one word root. For example, **osteoarthritis** (oss tee oh ar **THRY** tis) combines the word root *oste* meaning bone and *arthr* meaning the joints. When the suffix -itis, meaning inflammation, is added, we have the entire word, meaning an inflammation involving bone at the joints.

COMBINING VOWEL/FORM

To make it possible to pronounce long medical terms with ease and to combine several word roots, a combining vowel is used. This is usually the vowel *o*. When this vowel is combined with a word root in this book, it will be shown as root/o: for example, cardi/o.

A combining form for a word will consist of a word root and a vowel, usually *o*, such as cardi/o. A word root can be joined with another word root and/or with a suffix. If the suffix begins with a vowel (a,e,i,o,u), such as -itis, a combining vowel is usually not used. For example, **carditis** (car-**DYE**-tis) is correct rather than cardi*o*itis.

The combining vowel should be kept between two word roots: for example, **nephrolithectomy** (neh froh lith **ECK** toh mee), not nephrlithectomy. As you can tell from pronouncing these two terms, the combining vowel, *o*, lessens the difficulty of pronunciation. Following are some common word roots with their combining forms.

Combining Form	Meaning	Example (Definition)
abdomin/o	abdomen	abdominal (pertaining to the abdomen)
acu/o	needle, sharp	acupuncture (placing sharp needles into the body)
aden/o	gland	adenopathy (gland disease)
amni/o	amnion	amnionic (pertaining to the amnion)
andr/o	male	androgenic (pertaining to male generating)
angi/o	vessel	angioplasty (surgical repair of a vessel)
arter/o	artery	arterial (pertaining to an artery)
arthr/o	joint	arthritis (inflammation of a joint)
axill/o	armpit	axillary (pertaining to the armpit area)
blephar/o	eyelid	blepharoptosis (drooping eyelid)
bronch/o	bronchus	bronchial (pertaining to the bronchus)
carcin/o	cancer	carcinoma (cancerous tumor)
cardi/o	heart	cardiac (pertaining to the heart)
carp/o	wrist	carpal (pertaining to the wrist)
cephal/o	head	cephalic (pertaining to the head)
cerebr/o	cerebrum	cerebral (pertaining to the cerebrum)
chem/o	chemical	chemotherapy (treatment with chemicals)
cholecyst/o	gall bladder	cholecystitis (gall bladder inflammation)
chondr/o	cartilage	chondromalacia (softening of the cartilage)
chron/o	time	chronic (occurring over a long period of time)
cis/o	to cut	incision (process of cutting into)
col/o	colon	colonoscope (instrument for viewing the colon)
cost/o	rib	costal (pertaining to the ribs)
cutane/o	skin	cutaneous (pertaining to the skin)
cyst/o	bladder	cystic (pertaining to the bladder)

Combining Form	Meaning	Example (Definition)
cyt/o	cell	leukocyte (white blood cell)
dactyl/o	fingers, toes	dactylus (digits, fingers, toes)
derm/o	skin	dermal (pertaining to the skin)
dermat/o	skin	dermatology (study of the skin)
duct/o	duct	ductus (a duct)
encephal/o	brain	encephalic (pertaining to the brain)
enter/o	small intestines	enteric (pertaining to the small intestines)
erythr/o	red	erythrocyte (red blood cell)
esophag/o	esophagus	esophageal (pertaining to the esophagus)
flex/o	to bend	flexion (process of bending)
gastr/o	stomach	gastric (pertaining to the stomach)
gloss/o	tongue	glossal (pertaining to the tongue)
glyc/o	sugar	glycogenic (pertaining to producing sugar)
gynec/o	female	gynecology (study of female)
hem/o	blood	hemolysis (destruction of blood cells)
hemat/o	blood	hematic (pertaining to the blood)
hepat/o	liver	hepatic (pertaining to the liver)
hydr/o	water	hydrocele (protrusion of water [in the scrotum])
hyster/o	uterus	hysterectomy (surgical removal of the uterus)
ile/o	ileum	ileal (pertaining to the ileum)
immun/o	immune	immunology (study of immunity)
inguin/o	groin	inguinal (pertaining to the groin region)
lapar/o	abdomen	laparoscope (instrument for viewing the abdomen)
laryng/o	voice box	laryngeal (pertaining to the voice box)
leuk/o	white	leukorrhea (white discharge)
lingu/o	tongue	lingual (pertaining to the tongue)
lymph/o	lymph	lymphatic (pertaining to the lymph)
mamm/o	breast	mammary (pertaining to the breast)
mast/o	breast	mastoplasty (surgical repair of the breast)
morph/o	shape	morphology (study of shape)
muc/o	mucus	mucous (pertaining to mucus)
my/o	muscle	myoblast (immature muscle cell)
myel/o	spinal cord, bone marrow	myelopathy (spinal cord disease)
nat/o	birth	prenatal (before birth)
necr/o	death	necrosis (abnormal condition of being dead)
nephr/o	kidney	nephromegaly (enlarged kidney)
neur/o	nerve	neural (pertaining to a nerve)
norm/o	rule, order	abnormal (not the normal order)
onc/o	tumor	oncogen (producing a tumor)
ophthalm/o	eye	ophthalmic (pertaining to the eye)
oste/o	bone	osteocyte (bone cell)

Combining Form	Meaning	Example (Definition)
ot/o	ear	otic (pertaining to the ear)
ox/o	oxygen	hypoxemia (low level of oxygen in the blood)
path/o	disease	pathology (study of disease)
ped/o	child	pediatrics (branch of medicine relating to children)
peritone/o	peritoneum	peritoneal (pertaining to the peritoneum)
phag/o	eat	dysphagia (pertaining to difficulty eating)
pharyng/o	throat	pharyngeal (pertaining to the throat)
pleur/o	pleura	pleural (pertaining to the pleura)
pneumon/o	lung	pneumonic (pertaining to the lungs)
pulmon/o	lung	pulmonary (pertaining to the lungs)
rect/o	rectum	rectal (pertaining to the rectum)
ren/o	kidney	renal (pertaining to the kidney)
rhin/o	nose	rhinorrhea (discharge from the nose)
sarc/o	flesh	sarcoma (flesh tumor)
seps/o	infection	sepsis (condition of being infected)
somno/o	sleep	somnolence (sleepiness; unnatural drowsiness)
son/o	sound	sonography (procedure of recording sound waves)
splen/o	spleen	splenic (pertaining to the spleen)
staphyl/o	grape-like clusters	staphylococcus (round bacteria in grape-like clusters)
thel/o	nipple	theleplasty (surgical repair of the nipple)
thorac/o	chest	thoracic (pertaining to the chest)
thromb/o	clot	thrombosis (abnormal condition of being clotted)
tonsill/o	tonsils	tonsillitis (inflamed tonsils)
tox/o	toxin	toxic (pertaining to toxins)
trache/o	trachea	tracheal (pertaining to the trachea)
ur/o	urine, urinary tract	urology (study of the urinary tract)
ven/o	vein	venous (pertaining to veins)

PREFIXES

A new medical term is formed when a prefix is added in front of the word root. It will frequently give information about the location of the organ, the number of parts, or the time (frequency). For example, the prefix bi- stands for two of something, such as **bilateral** (bye **LAH** ter al), which means having two sides.

Remember to break down every word into its components (prefix, word root/combining form, and suffix) when you are learning medical terminology. Do not try to memorize every medical term. Instead, figure out how the word is formed from its components. In a short time you will be able to do this automatically when you see a term.

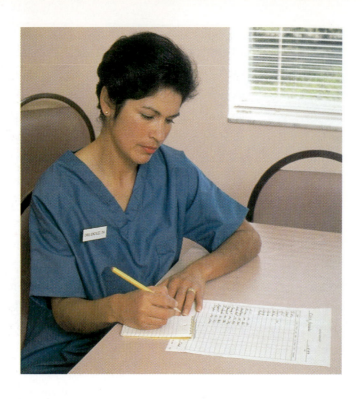

COMMON PREFIXES

Following are some of the more common prefixes, their meanings, and examples of their use.

Prefix	Meaning	Example (Definition)
a-	without, away from	aphasia (without speech)
ab-	away from	abduction (away from the midline)
ad-	toward	adduction (toward the midline)
ambi-	both, both sides	ambidextrous (able to use both hands well)
an-	without	anoxia (without oxygen)
ante-	before, in front of	antepartum (before birth)
antero-	before, in front of	anterior (the front side)
anti-	against	antibiotic (against life)
auto-	self	autograft (a graft from one's own body)
brady-	slow	bradycardia (slow heart beat)
circum-	around	circumoral (around the mouth)
con-	with, together	congenital (born with)
contra-	against	contraindicated (against what is indicated)
de-	down	descend (to come down)
dextro-	to the right of	dextrocardia (heart shifted in the chest to the right)
dia-	through, across	diagnosis (knowledge through testing)
dorso-	back	dorsal (the back side)
dys-	painful, difficult	dyspnea (painful breathing)
ec-	out, out from	ectopic (outside of its normal location)

Prefix	Meaning	Example (Definition)
endo-	within, inner	endoscope (instrument to view within)
epi-	upon, over	epigastric (upon or over the stomach)
eu-	normal, good	eupnea (normal breathing)
ex-	out from	exhale (breath out)
exo-	out	exophthalmia (eyeballs bulge outward)
hetero-	different	heterograft (a graft from another person's body)
homo-	same	homozygous (having two identical genes)
hydro-	water	hydrotherapy (water therapy)
hyper-	over, above	hypertrophy (over development)
hypo-	under, below	hypoglossal (under the tongue)
im-	not	impotent (not able to achieve a penile erection)
in-	not, into	incompetent (not able)
infra-	under, beneath, below	infraorbital (below, under the eye socket)
inter-	among, between	intervertebral (between the vertebrae)
intra-	within, inside	intravenous (inside, within a vein)
latero-	side	lateral (to the side)
mal-	bad, ill	malignant (tendency to become worse)
medi-	middle	medial (towards the middle of a structure)
meso-	middle	mesoderm (the middle embryonic cell layer)
meta-	change, beyond	metamorphosis (change shape)
mid-	middle	midline (line dividing body into left and right halves)
neo-	new	neonate (newborn)
pachy-	thick	pachyderma (thick skin)
pan-	all	pancarditis (inflammation of the entire heart)
para-	beside, beyond, near	paranasal (near or alongside the nose)
per-	through	percutaneous (through the skin)
peri-	around	pericardial (around the heart)
post-	after	postpartum (after birth)
postero-	after, behind	posterior (the back side)
pre-	before, in front of	prefrontal (in front of the frontal bone)
pro-	before, in front of	prodrome (very earliest symptoms of a disease)
pseudo-	false	pseudocyesis (false pregnancy)
re-	again, back	recurrent (to occur again)
retro-	backward, behind	retrograde (movement in a backwards direction)
sinistro-	left	sinistrotorsion (twisted to the left)
sub-	below, under	subcutaneous (under, below the skin)
super-	above, excess	supernumerary (above the normal number)
supra-	above	suprapubic (above the pubic bone)
sym-	together	symphysis (to grow together)
syn-	together	syndactyly (born with fused fingers)
tachy-	rapid, fast	tachycardia (fast heart beat)
trans-	through, across	transurethral (across the urethra)
ultra-	beyond, excess	ultrasound (high frequency sound waves)

Following are some common prefixes pertaining to the number of items or measurement, their meanings, and examples of their use.

Prefix	Meaning	Example (Definition)
bi-	two	bilateral (two sides)
di-	two	diplegic (paralysis of two extremities)
diplo-	double	diplopia (double vision)
hemi-	half	hemiplegia (paralysis of one side, or half, of the body)
macro-	large	macrocephalic (having a large head)
micro-	small	microcephalic (having a small head)
mono-	one	monoplegia (paralysis of one extremity)
multi-	many	multigravida (woman pregnant more than once)
nulli-	none	nulligravida (woman with no pregnancies)
poly-	many	polyuria (large amounts of urine)
quad-	four	quadriplegia (paralysis of all four extremities)
semi-	partial	semiconscious (partially conscious)
tri-	three	triceps (muscle with three heads)
uni-	one	unilateral (one side)

TERMINOLOGY RELATING TO COLOR

Following are some common prefixes and combining forms that pertain to color, their meanings, and examples of their use.

Prefix	Combining Form	Meaning	Example (Definition)
alb-		white	albino (person without any skin pigment)
chlor-	chlor/o	green	chloroma (greenish cancerous tumor)
cyan-	cyan/o	blue	cyanosis (abnormal condition of being blue)
	eosin/o	rosy	eosinophil (granular leukocyte)
erythr-	erythr/o	red	erythrocyte (red blood cell)
leuk-	leuk/o	white	leukocyte (white blood cell)
melan-	melan/o	black	melanocyte (skin cell with black pigment)
	purpur/o	purple	purpura (purplish skin bruises)
	rose/o	rose, pink	roseola (rose-colored rash)
rube-		red	rubella (viral infection with red skin rash [measles])
xanth-	xanth/o	yellow	xanthoderma (yellow skin)

SUFFIXES

A suffix is a word attached to the end of a word to add meaning, such as a condition, disease, or procedure. Not all words have a suffix, but when a word does, it is added at the end of the combining form of the word. For example, the suffix -itis, which means *inflammation of,* when added to pericardi- forms the new word pericarditis, which means inflammation of the membrane surrounding the heart.

MED TERM *TIP*

If a suffix begins with a vowel, the combining vowel (usually *o*) is dropped: for example, **mastitis** (mas **TYE** tis) rather than mastoitis. A new medical term is formed when a suffix is added.

COMMON SUFFIXES

Following are some common suffixes, their meanings, and examples of their use.

Suffix	Meaning	Example (Definition)
-a	converts a word root to a noun	gravida (pregnant)
-algia	pain	gastralgia (stomach pain)
-blast	immature, embryonic	osteoblast (immature bone cell)
-cele	hernia, protrusion	cystocele (protrusion of the bladder)
-cide	kill	bactericide (to kill bacteria)
-cise	cut	incision (to cut into)
-cle	small	vesicle (a small bladder or blister)
-coccus	berry-shaped	streptococcus (berry-shaped bacteria in twisted chains)
-cyte	cell	leukocyte (white blood cell)
-dynia	pain	cardiodynia (heart pain)
-ectasis	dilatation	bronchiectasis (dilated bronchi)
-ectopia	displacement	corectopia (pupil of the eye not centered)
-emia	condition of the blood	oxemia (oxygen in the blood)
-er	one who	radiographer (one who processes X-rays)
-gen	that which produces	mutagen (that which produces mutations)
-genesis	produces, generates	osteogenesis (produces bone)
-genic	producing	carcinogenic (producing cancer)
-ia	state, condition	hemiplegia (condition of being half paralyzed)
-iasis	abnormal condition	lithiasis (abnormal condition of stones)
-iatric	medicine, physician	psychiatric (medical field relating to the mind)
-ion	process	incision (process of cutting into)
-ism	state of	hypothyroidism (state of low thyroid)
-ist	one who specializes in	pharmacist (specialist in dispensing drugs)
-itis	inflammation	cellulitis (inflammation of cells)

Suffix	Meaning	Example (Definition)
-ium	converts word root into a noun	cranium (skull)
-ize	to make, to use, take away	anesthetize (to take away feeling)
-lapse	to slide, sag	relapse (to slide backwards)
-lith	stone	cystolith (bladder stone)
-logist	one who studies	cardiologist (one who studies the heart)
-logy	study of	cardiology (study of the heart)
-lysis	destruction	osteolysis (bone destruction)
-malacia	abnormal softening	chondromalacia (abnormal cartilage softening)
-megaly	enlargement, large	cardiomegaly (enlarged heart)
-ole	small	arteriole (small artery)
-oma	tumor, mass	carcinoma (cancerous tumor)
-osis	abnormal condition	cyanosis (abnormal condition of being blue)
-paresis	weakness	paraparesis (weak lower extremities)
-parous	bearing, give birth	nulliparous (given birth to no viable children)
-partum	birth, labor	postpartum (after birth)
-pathy	disease	myopathy (muscle disease)
-penia	few	cytopenia (too few cells)
-phasia	speech	aphasia (lack of speech)
-phobia	abnormal fear	photophobia (abnormal fear of light)
-phoria	feeling, mental state	euphoria (normal, good mental state)
-physis	to grow	symphysis (to grow together)
-plasia	development, growth	dysplasia (abnormal development)
-plasm	formation, development	neoplasm (new formation)
-plegia	paralysis	paraplegia (paralysis of both lower extremities)
-pnea	breathing	dyspnea (difficult, labored breathing)
-ptosis	drooping	proctoptosis (drooping rectum)
-rrhage	excessive, abnormal flow	hemorrhage (excessive bleeding)
-rrhea	discharge, flow	rhinorrhea (discharge from the nose)
-rrhexis	rupture	hysterorrhexis (ruptured uterus)
-sclerosis	hardening	arteriosclerosis (hardening of an artery)
-sis	condition	enuresis (condition of involuntary urination)
-spasm	involuntary muscle contraction	bronchospasm (involuntary contraction of bronchi muscles)
-stalsis	constriction, contraction	peristalsis (wavelike movement that propels food along the esophagus and other gastrointestinal tubes)
-stasis	stopping	hemostasis (stopping blood flow)
-stenosis	narrowing	angiostenosis (narrowing of a vessel)
-therapy	treatment	chemotherapy (treatment with chemicals)
-trophy	nourishment, development	hypertrophy (excessive nourishment)
-ule	small	venule (small vein)
-um	converts word root into a noun	duodenum (section of small intestine)
-uria	condition of the urine	hematuria (blood in the urine)
-us	converts word root into a noun	dactylus (digits, fingers, toes)

ADJECTIVE SUFFIXES

Following are suffixes that are used to convert a word root into an adjective. These suffixes usually are translated as *pertaining to* or *resembling*.

Suffix	Meaning	Example (Definition)
-ac	pertaining to	cardiac (pertaining to the heart)
-al	pertaining to	duodenal (pertaining to the duodenum)
-an	pertaining to	ovarian (pertaining to the ovary)
-ar	pertaining to	ventricular (pertaining to a ventricle)
-ary	pertaining to	pulmonary (pertaining to the lungs)
-eal	pertaining to	esophageal (pertaining to the esophagus)
-iac	pertaining to	iliac (pertaining to the ilium)
-ic	pertaining to	gastric (pertaining to the stomach)
-ical	pertaining to	neurological (pertaining to the study of the nerves)
-ile	pertaining to	penile (pertaining to the penis)
-ior	pertaining to	superior (pertaining to above)
-oid	resembling	lipoid (resembling fat)
-ory	pertaining to	auditory (pertaining to hearing)
-ose	pertaining to	adipose (pertaining to fat)
-ous	pertaining to	intravenous (pertaining to within a vein)
-tic	pertaining to	hepatic (pertaining to the liver)

SURGICAL SUFFIXES

Following are suffixes that are used to indicate surgical procedures, their meanings, and examples of their use.

Suffix	Meaning	Example (Definition)
-centesis	puncture to withdraw fluid	arthrocentesis (puncture to withdraw fluid from a joint)
-ectomy	surgical removal	gastrectomy (surgically remove the stomach)
-ostomy	surgically create an opening	colostomy (surgically create an opening for the colon through the abdominal wall)
-otomy	cutting into	thoracotomy (cutting into the chest)
-pexy	surgical fixation	nephropexy (surgical fixation of a kidney)
-plasty	surgical repair	dermatoplasty (surgical repair of the skin)
-rrhaphy	suture	myorrhaphy (suture together muscle)

Following are suffixes that indicate procedural processes or instruments, their meanings, and examples of their use.

Suffix	Meaning	Example (Definition)
-gram	record or picture	electrocardiogram (record of heart's electricity)
-graph	instrument for recording	electrocardiograph (instrument for recording the heart's electrical activity)
-graphy	process of recording	electrocardiography (process of recording the heart's electrical activity)
-meter	instrument for measuring	audiometer (instrument to measure hearing)
-metry	process of measuring	audiometry (process of measuring hearing)
-scope	instrument for viewing	gastroscope (instrument to view stomach)
-scopy	process of visually examining	gastroscopy (process of visually examining the stomach)

GENERAL RULES FOR MEDICAL TERMINOLOGY

General rules relating to the study of medical terminology are listed below. Once you understand this process you should be able to break any term into its parts to discover its meaning.

Rule	Example
1. The word root is the base of the word.	cardi = heart
2. A prefix is the beginning of the word.	*peri*carditis = around the heart
3. A suffix is the ending of the word.	card*itis* = inflammation of the heart
4. The combining vowel is a vowel (usually *o*) that links the word root to another word root or a suffix.	cardi*o*myopathy = disease of the heart muscle
5. A combining form is created by the word root, the combining vowel, and another word root or suffix.	cardiomyopathy

MED TERM TIP

To gain a quick understanding of a term, read the term from the end of the word (or the suffix) back to the beginning (the prefix) and then pick up the word root. For example, **pericarditis** reads inflammation of (-itis) the membrane surrounding (peri) the heart (cardi).

WORD BUILDING

Word building consists of putting together several parts of a word to form a variety of terms. The combining form of a word may be added to another combining form along with a suffix to create a new descriptive term. For example, adding hyster/o (meaning uterus) to salping/o (meaning fallopian tubes) along with the suffix-ectomy (meaning surgical removal of) forms **hysterosalpingectomy** (hiss ter oh sal pin **JEK** toh mee), the removal of both the uterus and the fallopian tubes. You will note that the combining vowel *o* is dropped when adding the suffix -ectomy since two vowels are not necessary.

ABBREVIATIONS

Abbreviations are commonly used in the medical profession as a way of saving time. However, some abbreviations can be confusing, such as *SM* for simple mastectomy and *sm* for small. Using the incorrect abbreviation can result in problems for a patient, as well as with insurance records and processing. If you have any concern that you will confuse someone by using an abbreviation, spell out the word instead. It is never a good idea to use one's own abbreviations. Throughout the book abbreviations are included, when possible, immediately following terms. In addition, a list of abbreviations for each body system is included at the end of each chapter (see appendix for a complete list of abbreviations).

THE MEDICAL RECORD

The medical record or chart documents the details of a patient's hospital stay. Each health care professional who has contact with the patient in any capacity completes the appropriate report of that contact and adds it to the medical chart. This results in a permanent physical record of the patient's day-to-day condition, when and what services he or she receives, and the response to treatment. Each institution adopts a specific format for each document and its location within the chart. This is necessary because each health care professional needs to be able to locate quickly and efficiently the information they need in order to provide proper care for the patient. The medical record is also a legal document. Therefore, it is essential that all chart components are completely filled out and signed. Each page must contain the proper patient identification information: the patient's name, age, gender, physician, admission date, and identification number.

While the patient is still in the hospital, the unit clerk is responsible for placing documents in the proper place. After discharge, the medical records department ensures that all documents are present, complete, signed, and in the correct order. If a person is readmitted, especially for the same diagnosis, parts of this previous chart can be pulled and added to the current chart for reference. Physicians' offices and other outpatient care providers such as clinics and therapists also maintain a medical record detailing each patient's visit to their facility.

The following is a list of the most common elements of a hospital chart with a brief description of each.

History and Physical—Written or dictated by the admitting physician; details the patient's history, results of the physician's examination, initial diagnoses, and physician's plan of treatment

Physician's Orders—A complete list of the care, medications, tests, and treatments the physician orders for the patient

Nurse's Notes—Record of the patient's care throughout the day; includes vital signs, treatment specifics, patient's response to treatment, and patient's condition

Physician's Progress Notes—The physician's daily record of the patient's condition, results of the physician's examinations, summary of test results, updated assessment and diagnoses, and further plans for the patient's care

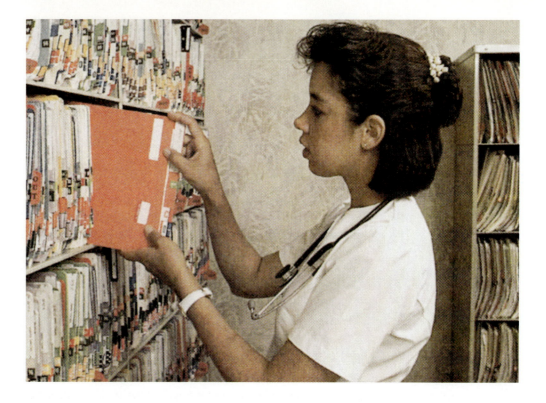

Consultation Reports—The report given by a specialist whom the physician has asked to evaluate the patient

Ancillary Reports—Reports from various treatments and therapies the patient has received, such as rehabilitation, social services, respiratory therapy, or the dietician

Diagnostic Reports—Results of all diagnostic tests performed on the patient, principally from the lab and medical imaging (for example:X-rays and ultrasound)

Informed Consent—A document voluntarily signed by the patient or a responsible party that clearly describes the purpose, methods, procedures, benefits, and risks of a diagnostic or treatment procedure

Operative Report—Report from the surgeon detailing an operation; includes a pre- and post-operative diagnosis, specific details of the surgical procedure itself, and how the patient tolerated the procedure

Anesthesiologist's Report—Relates the details regarding the drugs given to a patient, the patient's response to anesthesia, and vital signs during surgery

Pathologist's Report—The report given by a pathologist who studies tissue removed from the patient (for example: bone marrow, blood, or tissue biopsy)

Discharge Summary—A comprehensive outline of the patient's entire hospital stay; includes condition at time of admission, admitting diagnosis, test results, treatments and patient's response, final diagnosis, and follow-up plans

MANAGED CARE

Managed care is a systematic approach to delivering high quality, comprehensive health care while controlling costs. In this approach a third-party player, such as an insurance company, the federal government, or a corporation, oversees or manages a medical practice. This level of control results in cost containment by the elimination of duplicate and unwarranted facilities and services. There are several different managed care plans, with **health maintenance organizations (HMO)** and **preferred provider organizations (PPO)** being the most common.

An HMO is an organization that contracts with a group of physicians and other health care workers to provide care exclusively for its members. The HMO pays the health care workers a fixed amount per member, whether that member requires medical attention or not. Then members provide a co-payment for actual services received. If care beyond the primary care level is required, the member must seek prior authorization.

A PPO enters into contracts with individual medical professionals who agree to provide services to the PPO members at a reduced rate. The PPO pays most of the reduced fee and the patient pays the remainder (co-payment). Additionally, the patient may choose to use a nonpreferred provider and pay all the fees that are higher than the PPO has agreed to pay.

One method of controlling cost is to classify medical care into levels. Patients receive the level of care necessary for their problem. **Preventive care** emphasizes immunizations, check-ups, and patient education to prevent disease. **Primary care** providers, such as family practice physicians or nurse practitioners, treat routine medical problems and make referrals to specialists when indicated. **Specialty care providers,** such as orthopedists or surgeons, see patients who have been referred by the primary care provider for problems known to require the services of a specialist. **Urgent care** is for patients who need immediate attention, but whose condition is not life threatening or does not require hospitalization. A small child with an ear infection or a teenager with a simple fracture is a good example of this level of care. On the other hand, **emergency care** is reserved for life-threatening illnesses that probably require hospitalization, such as a heart attack. Outpatient care is encouraged; therefore, **hospitalization** requires pre-admission authorization to prevent unnecessary hospital stays.

PROCEDURAL AND DIAGNOSTIC BILLING CODES

Different agencies have established procedural and diagnostic codes for billing purposes. These numerical codes improve communication between providers and payers because they are universally accepted.

Diagnosis Related Groups (DRG)—This method of classification, which places patients into groups based on their primary and secondary diagnoses, was developed for Medicare. Each diagnostic group is assigned a dollar figure based on an estimate of the cost of caring for patients with this diagnosis. Providers receive this reimbursement regardless of the actual expenses incurred. This is referred to as a **prospective payment system.**

International Classification of Diseases, 9th Revision Clinical Modification (ICD-9-CM)—This official list of diseases was developed by the World Health Organization. The ICD-9-CM number consists of 3–5 digits that conveys general and specific information regarding a diagnosis.

Current Procedural Terminology (CPT)—The CPT was developed by the American Medical Association. Providers use this coding system to report the procedures it provides to a patient.

HEALTH CARE SETTINGS

The use of medical terminology is widespread. It provides health care professionals with a precise and efficient method of communicating very specific patient information to one

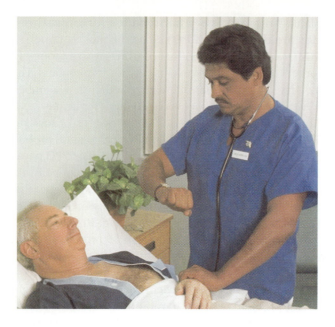

another, whether they are in the same type of facility or not. Following is a description of the different types of settings where medical terminology is used.

Acute Care or General Hospitals—These hospitals typically provide services to diagnose (laboratory, diagnostic imaging) and treat (surgery, medications, therapy) diseases for a short period of time. In addition, they usually provide emergency and obstetrical care.

Specialty Care Hospitals—These hospitals provide care for very specific types of diseases. A good example is a psychiatric hospital.

Nursing Homes or Long-term Care Facilities—These facilities provide long-term care for patients who need extra time to recover from an illness or injury before they return home, or for persons who can no longer care for themselves.

Ambulatory Care/Surgical Centers or Outpatient Clinics—These facilities provide services that do not require overnight hospitalization. The services range from simple surgeries to diagnostic testing or therapy.

Physicians' Offices—Individual or groups of physicians providing diagnostic and treatment services in a private office setting.

Health Maintenance Organizations—A group of primary-care physicians, specialists, and other health care professionals who provide a wide range of services in a prepaid system.

Home Health Care—Agencies that provide nursing, therapy, personal care, or housekeeping services in the patient's own home.

Rehabilitation Centers—These facilities provide intensive physical and occupational therapy. They include inpatient and outpatient treatment.

Hospices—An organized group of health care workers that provides supportive treatment to dying patients and their families.

CONFIDENTIALITY

Anyone who works with medical terminology and is involved in the medical profession must have a firm understanding of confidentiality. Any information or record relating to a patient must be considered privileged. This means that you have a moral and legal responsibility to keep all information about the patient confidential. If you are asked to supply documentation relating to a patient, the proper authorization form must be signed by the patient. Give only the specific information that the patient has authorized.

FINAL WORD

If you have any doubt about the meaning or spelling of a word, *look it up* in your medical dictionary. Medical personnel who have been practicing in their profession for many years still need to look up a few words. The student who is just learning medical terminology needs to look up words even more frequently.

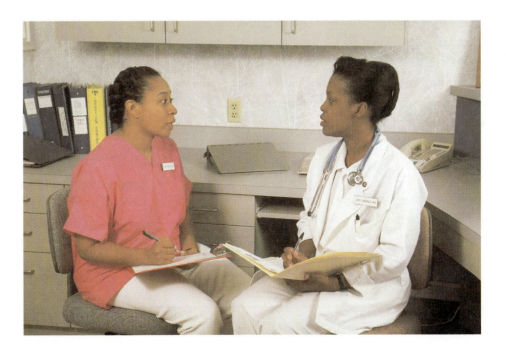

Medical Records

Medical records workers are responsible for keeping accurate, orderly, and permanent records of patients' condition and treatment. Medical records are often important in guiding patient care, and they have several other critical functions. Insurance companies use medical records to determine if a patient's care is to be covered by insurance. Medical records can also be introduced as evidence in a court of law in a lawsuit or criminal proceeding to document the severity of an injury or illness. Medical records workers play an important role in acute and long-term care facilities, health maintenance organizations, clinics, physician's offices, public health departments, and insurance companies. One possible career path for those interested in medical records is medical transcription. Medical transcriptionists are responsible for transcribing dictated medical notes. They must have an excellent grasp of medical terminology, pharmacology, anatomy, and physiology. To become a medical transcriptionist, students must either complete a vocational education program or receive extensive on-the-job training. They may opt to take an examination to become a certified medical transcriptionist (CMT). Visit the American Association for Medical Transcription's web site at www.aamt.org for more information on becoming a medical transcriptionist.

Medical Records/Health Information Management

Medical records workers keep accurate, orderly, and permanent records of each patient's condition and treatment. They also prepare patient information for release to health personnel, insurance companies, researchers, lawyers, and the courts. They work in

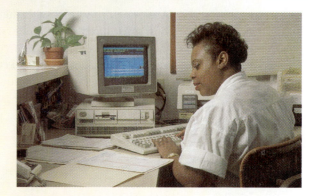

acute and long-term care facilities, health maintenance organizations, clinics, physicians' offices, public health departments, and insurance companies.

Registered Health Information Administrator (RHIA)

- **Graduates from an accredited four-year bachelor's degree program in Health Information Administration**
- **Passes national certification examination**

Registered Health Information Technician (RHIT)

- **Graduates from an accredited two-year degree program in Health Information Technology**
- **Passes national certification examination**

Medical Transcriptionist

- **Responsible for transcribing dictated medical notes**
- **Completes a vocational education program or receives on-the-job training**
- **May opt to take an examination to become a Certified Medical Transcriptionist (CMT)**

Practice Exercises

A. COMPLETE THE FOLLOWING STATEMENTS.

1. The combination of a word root and the combining vowel is called a(n) _____ .
2. The vowel that usually connects two word roots or a suffix with a word root is usually _____ .
3. A short word used at the end of a word root to change the meaning of the word is called a(n) _____ .
4. A(n) _____ is used at the beginning of a word to indicate number, location, or time.
5. Although the pronunciation of medical terms may differ slightly from one person to another, the _____ must never change.
6. The four components of a medical term are _____ , _____ , _____ , and _____ .

B. DEFINE THE FOLLOWING COMBINING FORMS.

1. arthr/o _____
2. enter/o _____
3. derm/o _____
4. hepat/o _____
5. cyst/o _____
6. ren/o _____
7. rect/o _____
8. cardi/o _____
9. cholecyst/o _____
10. esophag/o _____
11. onc/o _____
12. ot/o _____
13. neur/o _____
14. ur/o _____
15. path/o _____
16. rhin/o _____
17. ped/o _____
18. hemat/o _____
19. carcin/o _____
20. gynec/o _____
21. thromb/o _____
22. leuk/o _____
23. gastr/o _____
24. dermat/o _____
25. splen/o _____

C. DEFINE THE FOLLOWING SUFFIXES.

1. -plasty _____
2. -stenosis _____
3. -itis _____

4. -al _____

5. -algia _____

6. -otomy _____

7. -megaly _____

8. -ectomy _____

9. -rrhage _____

10. -centesis _____

11. -gram _____

12. -ac _____

13. -malacia _____

14. -ism _____

15. -rrhaphy _____

16. -ostomy _____

17. -pexy _____

18. -rrhea _____

19. -scopy _____

D. JOIN A COMBINING FORM AND A SUFFIX TO FORM WORDS WITH THE FOLLOWING MEANINGS.

1. pertaining to a nerve _____

2. pain relating to a nerve _____

3. excessive discharge from the nose _____

4. abnormal softening of a kidney _____

5. relating to the heart _____

6. cutting into the stomach _____

7. inflammation of the stomach _____

8. surgical removal of the spleen _____

9. inflammation of the joint _____

E. WRITE A PREFIX FOR EACH OF THE FOLLOWING EXPRESSIONS.

1. out from _____

2. large _____

3. before/in front of _____

4. around _____

5. toward _____

6. away from/absent _____

7. half _____

8. painful _____

9. above _____

10. excess/beyond _____

11. without _____

12. slow _____

13. self _____

14. across _____

F. CIRCLE THE PREFIX IN THE FOLLOWING TERMS AND DEFINE THE PREFIX.

1. acephalic _____

2. dysuria _____

3. hyperglycemia _____

4. intercostal _____

5. polycystic _____

6. postoperative _____

7. pericardium _____

8. suprapubic _____

G. MATCH THE PREFIX IN COLUMN A WITH THE DEFINITION IN COLUMN B.

A	B
1. _____ semi-	a. three
2. _____ hemi-	b. many
3. _____ micro-	c. two
4. _____ purpur/o-	d. partial
5. _____ erythr/o-	e. blue
6. _____ macro-	f. half
7. _____ mono-	g. yellow
8. _____ tri-	h. purple
9. _____ alb-	i. small
10. _____ bi-	j. white
11. _____ melan/o-	k. red
12. _____ cirrh/o-	l. four
13. _____ cyan/o-	m. black
14. _____ poly-	n. one
15. _____ quad-	o. large

H. CHANGE THE FOLLOWING SINGULAR TERMS TO PLURAL TERMS.

1. metastasis _____

2. ovum _____

3. diverticulum _____

4. lumen _____

5. diagnosis _____

6. vertebra _____

I. USING THE SUFFIX -OLOGY, MEANING THE STUDY OF, WRITE A TERM FOR EACH OF THE FOLLOWING MEDICAL SPECIALTIES.

1. heart _____

2. stomach _____

3. skin _____

4. eye _____

5. urinary tract _____

6. tumors _____

7. blood _____

8. pertaining to females _____

J. BUILD A MEDICAL TERM BY COMBINING THE WORD PARTS REQUESTED IN EACH QUESTION.

For example, use the combining form for spleen with the suffix meaning enlargement to form a word meaning enlargement of the spleen (answer: splenomegaly).

1. combining form for *heart* _____
   suffix meaning *abnormal softening* _____
   term meaning *a softening of the heart* _____

2. word root form for *stomach* _____
   suffix meaning *to surgically create an opening* _____
   term meaning *creating an opening into the stomach through the abdominal wall* _____

3. combining form for *nose* _____
   suffix meaning *discharge or flow* _____
   term meaning *runny nose* _____

4. combining form for *blood* _____
   suffix meaning *abnormal flow* _____
   term meaning *excessive bleeding* _____

5. word root meaning *disease* _____
   suffix meaning *the study of* _____
   term meaning *the study of disease* _____

6. prefix meaning *slow* _____
   word root for *heart* _____
   suffix meaning *pertaining to* _____
   term meaning *slow heart rate* _____

7. prefix meaning *under* _____
   word root for *stomach* _____
   suffix for *pertaining to* _____
   term meaning *under or below the stomach* _____

8. prefix meaning *around* _____
   combine with the term *oral* _____
   term meaning *around the mouth* _____

9. combining form meaning *tongue* _____
   word root meaning *pharynx* _____
   suffix meaning *pertaining to* _____
   term meaning *pertaining to the tongue and pharynx* _____

10. prefix meaning *before* _____
    combine with the word *cubital*, which means pertaining to the elbow _____
    term meaning *in front of the elbow* _____

11. prefix meaning *two* _____
    combine with the term *lateral* _____
    term meaning *pertaining to two sides* _____

12. prefix meaning *all* _____
    word root for *uterus* _____
    suffix meaning *surgical removal* _____
    term meaning *the removal of the entire uterus including the cervix* _____

13. combining form meaning *red* _____
    suffix meaning *cell* _____
    term meaning *red blood cell* _____

14. prefix meaning *without* _____

   word root for *brain* _____

   term meaning *without a brain* _____

15. prefix meaning *negative* _____

   combine with the word *normal* _____

   term meaning *not normal* _____

K. USE THE FOLLOWING TERMS IN THE SENTENCES THAT FOLLOW.

gastritis	urethritis	hemorrhage	polycystic
cholecystectomy	gastrotomy	dysuria	amniocentesis
prenatal	urethrostenosis		

1. Latonia is going to have her gallbladder removed due to gallstones. This surgery is called _____ .

2. Ralph's surgeon will cut an opening into his stomach to insert a feeding tube. This procedure is called

   _____ .

3. Amy is going to see her obstetrician for a pregnancy checkup. This type of visit is called a _____

   visit.

4. Amy is 40 years old and her doctor wishes to withdraw some amniotic fluid from her amniotic sac to test

   the baby's development. This procedure is called _____ .

5. Maria has developed many cysts in her breasts. The term that is used to describe this condition is

   _____ .

6. Shantel is having excessive bleeding from a nasal injury, which she cannot control. This is called _____ .

7. James has been admitted to the hospital with a stricture of the urethra. This condition is _____ .

8. Jerry is experiencing painful urination. This symptom is called _____ .

Getting Connected

Multimedia Extension Activities

CD-ROM

Use the CD-ROM enclosed with your textbook to gain additional reinforcement through interactive word building exercises, spelling games, labeling activities, and additional quizzes.

www.prenhall.com/fremgen

Use the above address to access the free, interactive Companion Website created for this textbook. Get hints, instant feedback, and textbook references to chapter-related multiple choice questions, and labeling and matching exercises. In addition, you will find an audio glossary, case studies, Internet exploration exercises, flashcards, and a comprehensive exam.

Answers

PRACTICE EXERCISES

A. 1. combining form   2. *o*   3. suffix   4. prefix   5. spelling   6. word root, combining form, prefix, suffix

B. 1. joint   2. intestine   3. skin   4. liver   5. bladder   6. kidney   7. rectum   8. heart   9. gallbladder
10. esophagus   11. tumor   12. ear   13. nerve   14. urinary tract   15. disease   16. nose   17. child   18. blood
19. cancer   20. female   21. clot   22. white   23. stomach   24. skin   25. spleen

C. 1. surgical repair   2. narrowing or stricture   3. inflammation of   4. pertaining to   5. pain   6. cutting into
7. enlargement   8. surgical removal of   9. excessive flow   10. surgical puncture to remove fluid   11. record of
12. pertaining to   13. abnormal softening   14. state of   15. to suture   16. surgical creation of opening
17. fixation   18. discharge or flow   19. to visualize with equipment

D. 1. neural   2. neuralgia   3. rhinorrhea   4. nephromalacia   5. cardiac   6. gastrotomy   7. gastritis
8. splenectomy   9. arthritis

E. 1. ex-   2. macro-   3. pro-/ante-   4. circum-   5. ad-   6. ab-   7. hemi-   8. dys-   9. supra-   10. ultra-
11. ar-   12. brady-   13. auto-   14. trans-

F. 1. a, without   2. dys, painful   3. hyper, over   4. inter, among   5. poly, many   6. post, after   7. peri, around
8. supra, above

G. 1. d   2. f   3. i   4. h   5. k   6. o   7. n   8. a   9. j   10. c   11. m   12. g   13. e   14. b   15. l

H. 1. metastases   2. ova   3. diverticula   4. lumina   5. diagnoses   6. vertebrae

I. 1. cardiology   2. gastrology   3. dermatology   4. ophthalmology   5. urology   6. oncology   7. hematology
8. gynecology

J. 1. cardiomalacia   2. gastrostomy   3. rhinorrhea   4. hemorrhage   5. pathology   6. bradycardia   7. hypogastric
8. circumoral   9. glossopharyngeal   10. antecubital   11. bilateral   12. panhysterectomy   13. erythrocyte
14. anencephalic   15. abnormal

K. 1. cholecystectomy   2. gastrostomy   3. prenatal   4. amniocentesis   5. polycystic   6. hemorrhage
7. urethrostenosis   8. dysuria

Chapter 2

BODY
STRUCTURE

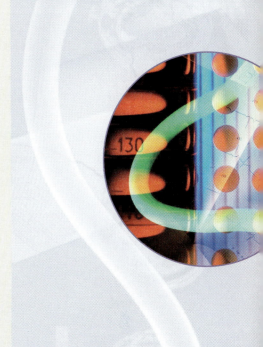

LEARNING OBJECTIVES

Upon completion of this chapter, you will be able to:

- Recognize the combining forms and prefixes introduced in this chapter.
- Gain the ability to pronounce medical terms.
- Discuss the organization of the body in terms of cells, tissues, organs, and systems.
- Define the four types of tissues.
- List the major organs found in the twelve organ systems.
- Describe the anatomical position.
- Define the body planes.
- Define directional and positional terms.
- Locate and describe the nine anatomical divisions of the abdomen.
- Locate and describe the four clinical divisions of the abdomen.
- List the body cavities and their contents.
- Identify the divisions of the back.
- Interpret abbreviations associated with body structure.

Overview

COMBINING FORMS RELATING TO BODY STRUCTURE

abdomin/o	abdomen	**medi/o**	middle
anter/o	front	**my/o**	muscle
caud/o	tail	**neur/o**	nerve
cephal/o	head	**pelv/o**	hip, pelvic
cervic/o	neck	**poster/o**	back
chondr/o	cartilage	**proxim/o**	near
coccyg/o	coccyx	**sacr/o**	sacrum
crani/o	skull	**somat/o**	body
cyt/o	cell	**spin/o**	spine, backbone
dist/o	away	**super/o**	above
dors/o	back of body	**system/o**	system
epitheli/o	epithelium	**thorac/o**	chest
hist/o	tissue	**umbilic/o**	navel
ili/o	ilium (pelvic bone)	**ventr/o**	belly
infer/o	below	**vertebr/o**	vertebra
later/o	side	**viscer/o**	internal organ
lumb/o	lower back		

MED TERM TIP — Remember that the prefixes and suffixes introduced in Chapter 1 will be used over and over again in your medical terminology course. There are a few that are frequently used in body structure terms. Examples of these prefixes follow:

PREFIXES RELATING TO BODY STRUCTURE

Prefix	Meaning	Example	Definition
epi-	above	epigastric	above the stomach
ex-	away from or out	external	on the outside
inter-	between	intermuscular	between the muscles
intra-	within	intramuscular	within the muscle
peri-	around or about	pericardium	around the heart
post-	behind or after	postnasal	behind the nose
retro-	behind or backward	retrosternal	behind the sternum
semi-	half	semicircular	half circle
sub-	under or below	substernal	below the sternum
supra-	above	suprasternal	above the sternum
trans-	through or across	transurethral	across the urethra
tri-	three	tricuspid	having three cusps or points

ORGANIZATION OF THE BODY

cell   systems

organism   tissues

organs

Before taking a look at the whole human body, we need to examine its parts. The human body consists of **cells (SELLS), tissues, organs,** and **systems** that come together to form the **organism.**

CELLS

The **cell** is the basic unit of all living things. In other words, it is the fundamental unit of life. All the tissues and organs in the body are composed of cells. Cells perform survival functions for either the cell or the body through reproduction, respiration, metabolism, and excretion.

Special cells are also able to carry on very specific functions, such as contraction by muscle cells and electrical impulse transmission by nerve cells. Figures 2.1 and 2.2 illustrate several types of cells.

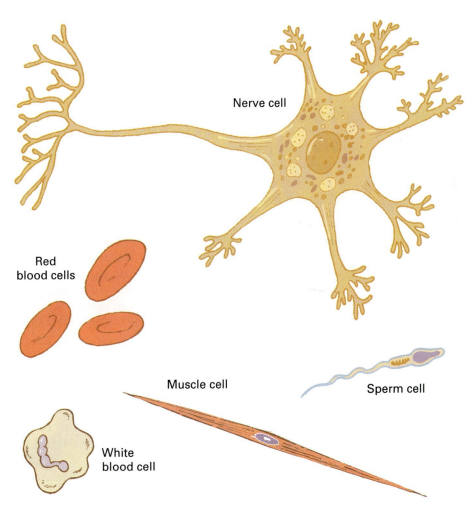

Nerve cell

Red
blood cells

Muscle cell

Sperm cell

White
blood cell

FIGURE 2.1   Nerve, muscle, and red blood cells.

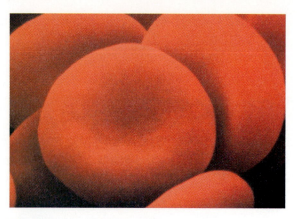

FIGURE 2.2 Red blood cells.

MED TERM TIP

Remember that the body's organization progresses from cells to tissues to organs to systems to the organism. Thus, the organism is the total of all its smaller parts.

TISSUES

adipose tissue	epithelial tissue	nervous tissue
bone	histology	neurons
cartilage	involuntary muscle tissue	voluntary muscle tissue
connective tissue	mucous membranes	

Histology (hiss **TALL** oh jee) is the study of tissue. Tissues are formed when cells are grouped together to perform one activity. For example, nerve cells, also called **neurons** (**NOO** rons), combine to form nerve fibers. Neurons have the ability to communicate between cells and conduct impulses throughout the body. The knee-jerk reaction that occurs when a physician taps the patellar tendon and the muscles in the leg extend the leg is an example of neurons responding to stimuli.

Following are the four tissue types:

1. **Muscle tissue,** which produces movement, is composed of both **voluntary** (**VOL** un ter ee) **tissue** and **involuntary tissue.** Voluntary muscle tissue is found in areas that we control, such as our arms and legs. Involuntary muscle tissue, over which we have little or no control, is found in the heart and digestive system. Muscle tissue allows for the contraction mechanism to operate within the body and its organs. For instance, the heart is mainly muscle tissue, which allows the heart to contract and pump the blood throughout the body (see Figure 2.3).

2. **Epithelial** (ep ih **THEE** lee al) **tissue** is found throughout the body as lining for internal organs as well as covering or skin tissue. The stomach is mainly epithelial and muscle tissue. The epithelial tissue secretes gastric juices that aid in digestion. The muscular tissue's movement allows food to come into contact with gastric juices, causing digestion to occur. **Mucous** (**MYOO** kus) **membranes** are a type of epithelial tissue that lines body surfaces and excretes a thick substance (see Figure 2.4).

3. **Connective tissue** is the supporting and protecting tissue in body structures. Fat or **adipose** (**ADD** ih pohs) **tissue, bone,** and **cartilage** (**CAR** tih lij) are examples of connective tissue (see Figure 2.5).

4. **Nervous tissue** allows for the conduction of impulses to and from the brain from throughout the body (see Figure 2.6).

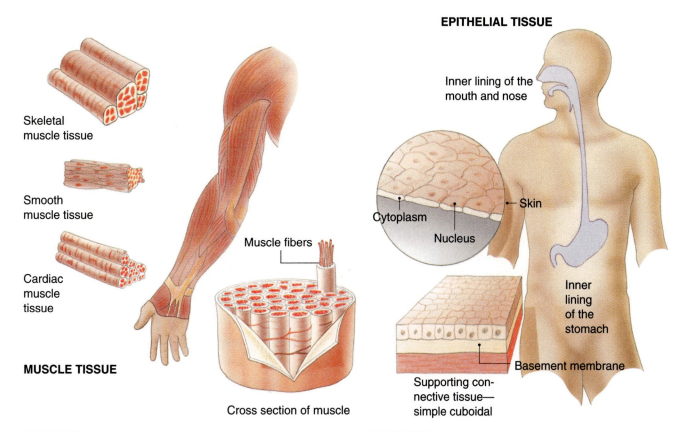

Skeletal muscle tissue

Smooth muscle tissue

Cardiac muscle tissue

MUSCLE TISSUE

Muscle fibers

Cross section of muscle

FIGURE 2.3   Muscle tissue makes all body movement possible.

EPITHELIAL TISSUE

Inner lining of the mouth and nose

Cytoplasm

Nucleus

Skin

Inner lining of the stomach

Supporting connective tissue— simple cuboidal

Basement membrane

FIGURE 2.4   Epithelial tissue forms the outer skin and lines internal organs of the body.

CONNECTIVE TISSUE

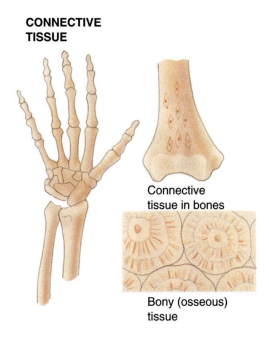

Connective tissue in bones

Bony (osseous) tissue

FIGURE 2.5   Connective tissue supports and protects body structures.

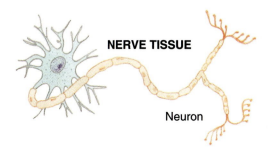

NERVE TISSUE

Neuron

FIGURE 2.6   Nervous tissue receives stimuli and responds to stimuli.

adrenal glands	nervous system
arteries	nose
blood	ovaries
blood vessels	pancreas
bones	parathyroid glands
brain	penis
bronchial tubes	pharynx
capillaries	pineal gland
cardiovascular (CV) system	pituitary gland
circulatory system	plasma
colon	prostate gland
digestive system	red blood cells
ears	reproductive system
endocrine system	respiratory system
esophagus	salivary glands
eyes	skin
fallopian tubes	small intestines
gallbladder (GB)	special sense organs
gastrointestinal (GI) system	spinal cord
hair	spleen
heart	stomach
hematic system	tendons
integumentary system	testes
joints	thymus gland
kidneys	thyroid gland
larynx	tongue
liver	trachea
lungs	ureters
lymph nodes	urethra
lymph vessels	urinary bladder
lymphatic system	urinary system
mammary glands	uterus
mouth	vagina
muscles	vas deferens
musculoskeletal (MS) system	veins
nails	white blood cells
nerves	

When groups of tissue come together to perform special functions they are called organs. Organs are composed of several different types of tissue that perform special functions. For example, the **heart** contains muscular fibers, nerve tissue, and blood vessels that allow the heart to contract and send along electrical impulses to regulate the heartbeat and pump blood throughout the body.

The skin is considered to be the largest organ of the body. In an adult it may weigh more than 20 pounds, which can also make it the heaviest organ in the human body.

A system is composed of several organs working in a compatible manner to perform a complex function or functions.

The **integumentary** (in teg you **MEN** tah ree) **system** includes the **skin, hair, sweat glands, sebaceous** or **oil glands,** and **nails** (see Figure 2.7).

The **musculoskeletal (MS) system** includes the **muscles, tendons, bones,** and **joints** and **cartilage** (see Figure 2.8).

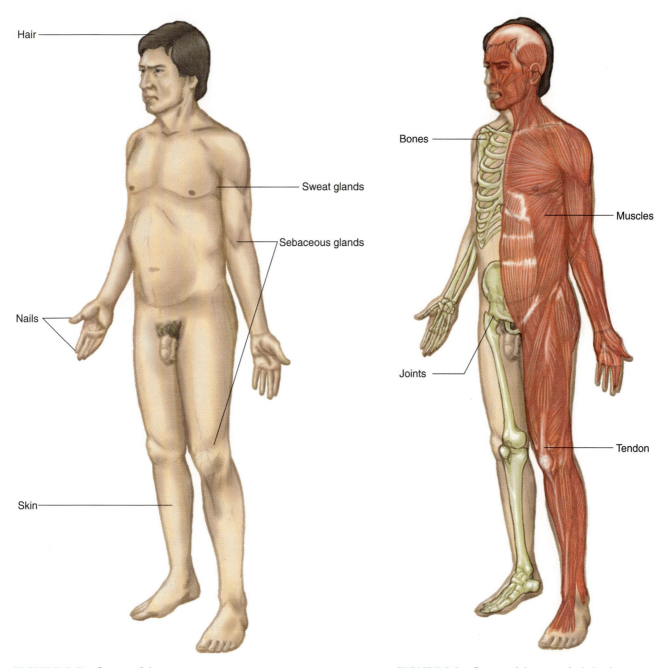

FIGURE 2.7   Organs of the integumentary system.

FIGURE 2.8   Organs of the musculoskeletal system.

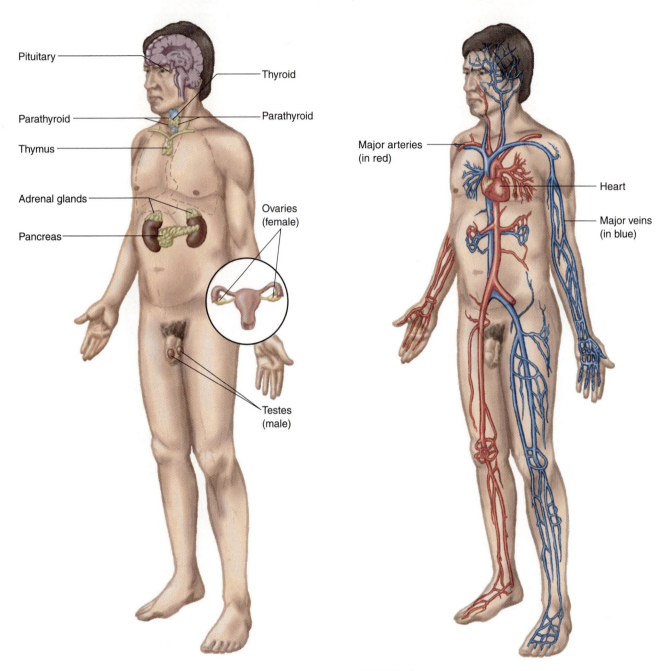

FIGURE 2.9   Organs of the endocrine system.

FIGURE 2.10   Organs of the cardiovascular system.

The **endocrine** (**EN** doh krin) **system** consists of the **thyroid** (**THIGH** royd) **gland** (located in the neck), **pituitary** (pih **TOO** ih tair ee) **gland** (located at the base of the brain), sex glands **testes** (**TESS** teez) and **ovaries** (**OH** vah reez), **adrenal** (ad **REE** nal) **glands** (located on top of the kidneys), **pancreas** (**PAN** kree ass), **parathyroid** (pair ah **THIGH** royd) **glands** (located behind the thyroid gland), and **thymus** (**THIGH** mus) **gland** (located in the chest cavity (see Figure 2.9).

The **cardiovascular** (car dee oh **VAS** kew lar) **(CV)** or **circulatory system** includes the **heart** and **blood vessels** (**arteries, veins,** and **capillaries**) (see Figure 2.10).

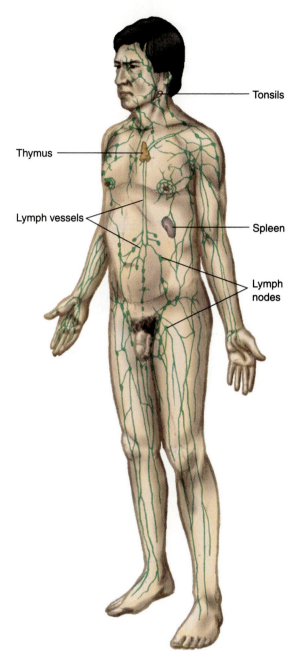

FIGURE 2.11 Organs of the lymphatic system.

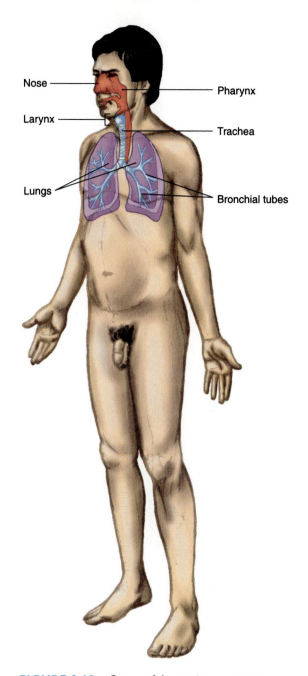

FIGURE 2.12 Organs of the respiratory system.

The **lymphatic** (lim **FAT** ik) **system** includes the **thymus gland, spleen, tonsils, lymph vessels,** and **lymph nodes** (see Figure 2.11).

The **hematic system** consists of the **blood** found within the blood vessels. Blood is composed of watery **plasma** (**PLAZ** mah), **red blood cells,** and **white blood cells.**

The **respiratory system** is composed of the **nose, pharynx** (**FAIR** inks) or *throat,* **larynx** (**LAR** inks) or *voice box,* **trachea** (**TRAY** kee ah) or *windpipe,* **bronchial** (**BRONG** kee al) **tubes,** and **lungs** (see Figure 2.12).

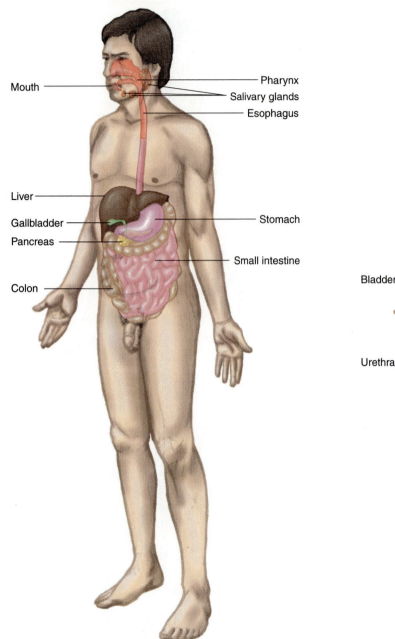

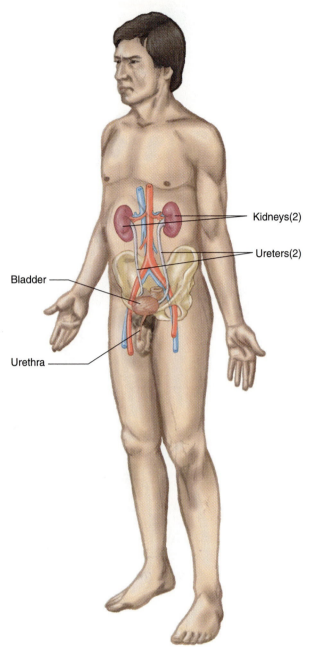

FIGURE 2.13 Organs of the gastrointestinal system.

FIGURE 2.14 Organs of the urinary system.

The **digestive** or **gastrointestinal** (gas troh in **TESS** tin al) **(GI) system** consists of the **mouth, salivary** (**SAL** ih vair ee) **glands, pharynx, esophagus, stomach, small intestines, large intestines** or **colon** (**COH** lon), **liver, gallbladder** (**GALL** blad er) **(GB),** and **pancreas** (see Figure 2.13).

The **urinary** (**YOO** rih nair ee) **system** includes the **kidneys, urinary** (**YOO** rih nair ee) **bladder, ureters** (yoo **REE** ters), and **urethra** (yoo **REE** thrah) (see Figure 2.14).

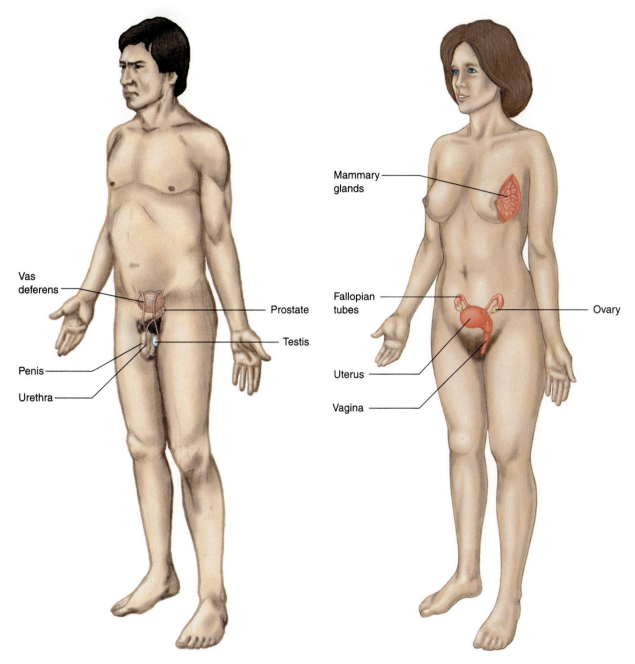

Vas deferens

Prostate

Testis

Penis

Urethra

Mammary glands

Fallopian tubes

Ovary

Uterus

Vagina

FIGURE 2.15 Organs of the female and male reproductive systems.

The female **reproductive system** contains the **ovaries, fallopian** (fah **LOH** pee an) **tubes, uterus** (**YOO** ter us) or *womb*, **vagina** (vah **JIGH** nah), and **mammary** (**MAM** ah ree) **glands;** the male system consists of the **testes, vas deferens** (vas **DEF** er enz), **urethra, prostate** (**PROS** tayt) **gland,** and **penis** (**PEE** nis) (see Figure 2.15). The **nervous system** consists of the **brain, spinal cord,** and **nerves** (see Figure 2.16).

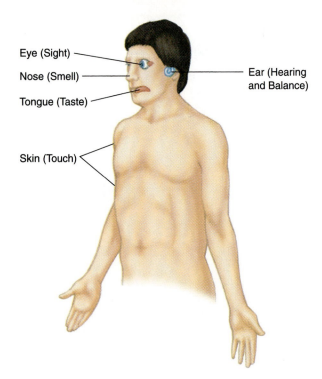

FIGURE 2.17   Organs of the special senses.

Eye (Sight)
Nose (Smell)
Tongue (Taste)
Ear (Hearing and Balance)
Skin (Touch)

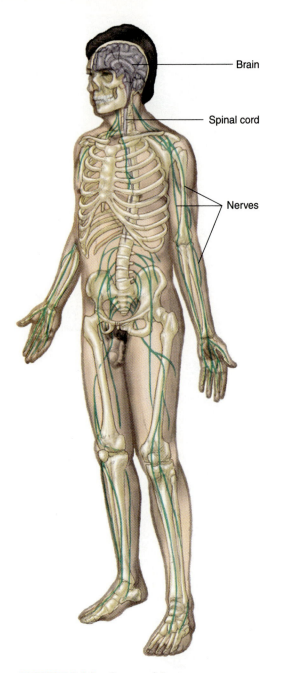

Brain
Spinal cord
Nerves

FIGURE 2.16   Organs of the nervous system.

The **special sense organs** are the **eyes** (sight), **ears** (hearing), **nose** (smell), **tongue** (taste), and **skin** (touch) (see Figure 2.17).

Table 2.1 lists the major organ systems and the medical specialty commonly found involved in the treatment of conditions relating to each organ system.

ANATOMICAL POSITION

The **anatomical position** is used when describing the positions and relationships of a structure in the human body. This term describes the position of the body in which the body is standing erect with the arms at the side of the body, the palms of the hands facing forward, and the eyes looking straight ahead. In this position the legs are parallel with the feet and the toes are pointing forward. For descriptive purposes the assumption is always

Table 2.1 — Organ Systems of the Human Body

Body System	Organs in the System	Combining Form	Medical Specialty
Integumentary	Skin	dermat/o	**dermatology** (der mah **TALL** oh jee)
	Hair	trich/o	
	Nails	onych/o	
	Sweat glands	sud/o	
	Sebaceous glands	seb/o	
Musculoskeletal	Muscles	my/o	**orthopedics** (or thoh **PEE** diks)
	Bones	oste/o	
	Joints	arthr/o	
Endocrine	Thyroid gland	thyr/o	**endocrinology** (en doh krin **ALL** oh jee)
	Pituitary gland	pituit/o	**internal** (in **TUR** nal) **medicine**
	Testes	test/o	
	Ovaries	ovari/o	**gynecology** (gigh neh **KOL** oh jee)
	Adrenal glands	adren/o	
	Pancreas	pancreat/o	
	Parathyroid glands	parathyroid/o	
	Pineal gland	pineal/o	
	Thymus gland	thym/o	
Cardiovascular	Heart	cardi/o	**cardiology** (car dee **ALL** oh jee)
	Blood	hemat/o	**hematology** (hee mah **TALL** oh jee)
	Arteries	arteri/o	**internal medicine**
	Veins	ven/o	
Lymphatic and Immune	Spleen	splen/o	**immunology** (im yoo **NALL** oh jee)
	Lymph	lymph/o	
	Thymus gland	thym/o	
Respiratory	Nose	nas/o	**otorhinolaryngology** (oh toh rye noh lair ing **GALL** oh jee)
	Pharynx	pharyng/o	**thoracic** (tho **RASS** ik) **surgery**
	Larynx	laryng/o	
	Trachea	trache/o	
	Lungs	pneum/o	**pulmonology** (pull mon **ALL** oh jee)
	Bronchial tubes	bronch/o	**internal medicine**
Gastrointestinal	Mouth	or/o	**gastroenterology** (gas troh en ter **ALL** oh jee)
	Pharynx	pharyng/o	**internal medicine**
	Salivary glands	sialaden/o	
	Esophagus	esophag/o	
	Stomach	gastr/o	
	Small intestine	enter/o	
	Colon	col/o	**proctology** (prok **TOL** oh jee)
	Liver	hepat/o	
	Gallbladder	cholecyst/o	
	Pancreas	pancreat/o	
Urinary	Kidneys	nephr/o	**nephrology** (neh **FROL** oh jee)
	Ureters	ureter/o	**urology** (yoo **RALL** oh jee)
	Bladder	cyst/o	
	Urethra	urethr/o	
Reproductive	Ovaries	hyster/o	**gynecology**
	Uterus	uter/o	**obstetrics** (ob **STET** riks)
	Fallopian tubes	salping/o	
	Vagina	vagin/o	
	Mammary glands	mamm/o	
	Testes	orchid/o	**urology**
	Prostate	prostat/o	
	Urethra	urethr/o	
	Vas deferens	vas/o	
Nervous	Brain	encephal/o	**neurology** (noo **RAL** oh jee)
	Spinal cord	myel/o	**neurosurgery** (noo roh **SIR** jer ee)
	Nerves	neur/o	
Special senses	Eye	ocul/o	**ophthalmology** (off thal **MALL** oh jee)
	Ear	ot/o	**otolaryngology** (oh toh lair ing **GALL** oh jee)

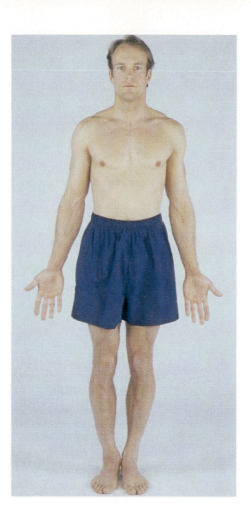

that the person is in the anatomical position even if the body or parts of the body are in any other position (see Figure 2.18).

BODY PLANES

coronal plane	horizontal plane	sagittal plane
frontal plane	midsagittal plane	transverse plane

The terminology for body planes is used to assist medical personnel in describing the body and its parts. To understand body planes, you must imagine cuts slicing through the body at various angles. This imaginary slicing would allow us to use more specific language when describing parts of the body. These body planes, illustrated in Figure 2.19, include the following:

1. **Sagittal** (**SAJ** ih tal) **plane:** This vertical plane is lengthwise and divides the body or any of its parts into right and left portions. The right and left sides do not have to be equal in a sagittal cut. If we were to divide the body or any of its parts into two *equal* parts, this would be called the **midsagittal** (mid **SAJ** ih tal) **plane.**

2. **Frontal plane:** The frontal or **coronal** (kor **RONE** al) plane divides the body into front and back portions. In other words, this is a vertical lengthwise plane running from side to side.

3. **Transverse** (trans **VERS**) **plane:** The transverse or **horizontal** plane is a crosswise plane that runs parallel to the ground. This imaginary cut would divide the body or its parts into upper and lower portions.

FIGURE 2.19   Planes of the body.

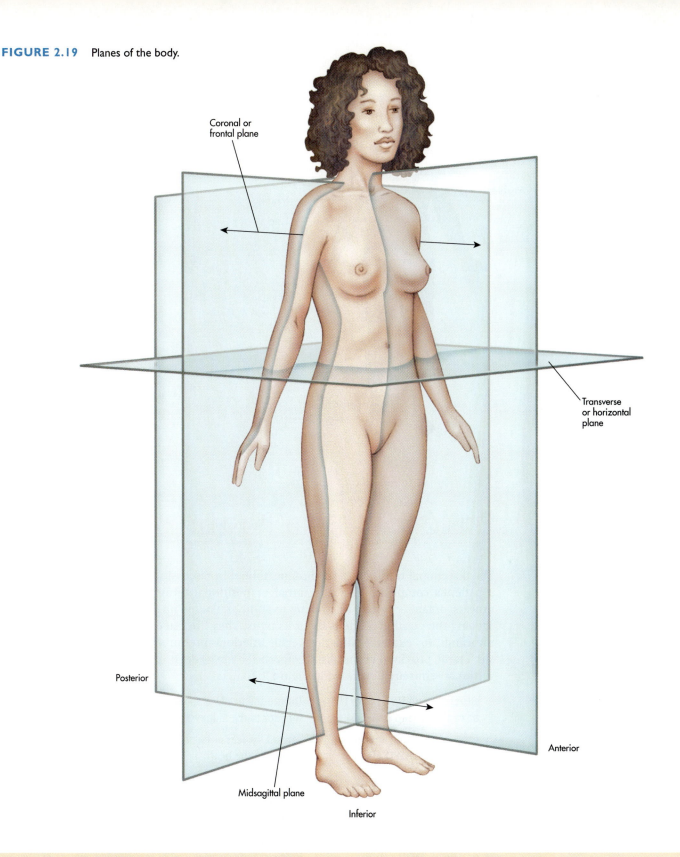

Coronal or
frontal plane

Transverse
or horizontal
plane

Posterior

Anterior

Midsagittal plane

Inferior

MED
TERM
TIP

Remember that when we use the body planes for descriptive purposes, the body we are
describing will be in the anatomical position—standing erect with arms at the sides and
palms facing forward.

Body Structure ● **41**

FIGURE 2.20
Directional terms.

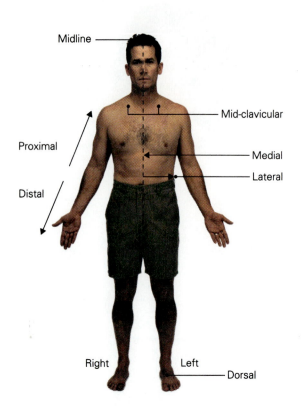

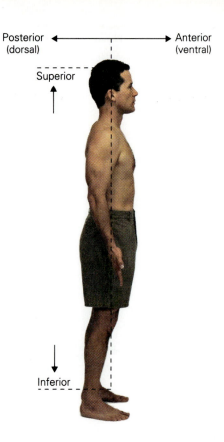

DIRECTIONAL AND POSITIONAL TERMS

The directional terms assist medical personnel in discussing the position or location of a patient's complaint. The directional or positional terms also help to describe one process, organ, or system as it relates to another. Following are the general terms for describing the position of the body or its parts. They are listed in pairs that have opposite meanings: for example, superior versus inferior, anterior versus posterior, medial versus lateral, proximal versus distal, superficial versus deep, and supine versus prone. Directional terms are illustrated in Figure 2.20.

superior (soo PEE ree or) or cephalic (seh FAL ik)	Toward the head, or above. *Example:* The adrenal glands are superior to the kidneys.
inferior (in FEE ree or) or caudal (KAWD al)	Toward the feet or tail, or below. *Example:* The intestine is inferior to the heart.
anterior (an TEE ree or) or ventral (VEN tral)	Near or on the front or belly-side of the body. *Example:* The umbilicus (um **BILL** ih kus), or navel, is located on the anterior surface of the body.
posterior (poss TEE ree or) or dorsal (DOR sal)	Near or on the back or spinal cord side of the body. *Example:* The posterior wall of the right kidney was excised.
medial (MEE dee al)	Refers to the middle or near the middle of the body or the structure. *Example:* The heart is medially located in the chest cavity.
lateral (lat) (LAT er al)	Refers to the side. *Example:* The lateral wall of the right lung was excised.

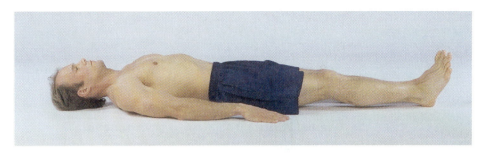

FIGURE 2.21　The supine position.

apex (AY peks)	Tip or summit. *Example:* We hear the apical pulse by listening with a stethoscope over the apex of the heart.
base	Bottom or lower part. *Example:* On the X-ray, a fracture was noted at the base of the skull.
abduction (ab DUCK shun)	To move away from the median or middle line of the body. *Example:* The arm is abducted from the body when it is placed over the head.
adduction (ad DUCK shun)	To move toward the median or middle line of the body. *Example:* The physical therapist adducted the lower extremities by moving the legs together.
proximal (PROK sim al)	Located closest to the point of attachment to the body. *Example:* In the anatomical position, the elbow is proximal to the hand.
distal (DISS tal)	Located farthest from the point of attachment to the body. *Example:* The ankle is distal to the knee.
superficial	Toward the surface of the body. *Example:* The cut was superficial.
deep	Away from the surface of the body. *Example:* An incision into an abdominal organ is a deep incision.
supine (soo PINE)	The body lying horizontally and facing upward (see Figure 2.21). *Example:* The patient is placed in the supine position for abdominal surgery.
prone (PROHN)	The body lying horizontally facing downward (see Figure 2.22). *Example:* The patient is placed in the prone position for spinal surgery.
inversion (in VER zhun)	A turning inward or inside out. *Example:* The patient has an inversion of both feet.
eversion (ee VER zhun)	A turning outward. *Example:* The lower leg brace prevented ankle eversion.

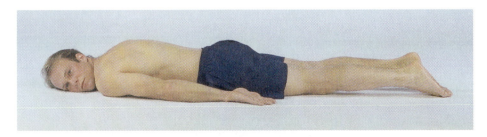

FIGURE 2.22　The prone position.

BODY CAVITIES

abdominal cavity	parietal peritoneum	thoracic cavity
abdominopelvic cavity	parietal pleura	viscera
aorta	pelvic cavity	visceral
cranial cavity	peritoneum	visceral peritoneum
diaphragm	pleura	visceral pleura
mediastinum	serous membrane	
parietal	spinal cavity	

The body is not a solid structure and has many open spaces or cavities. The cavities are part of the normal body structure and are illustrated in Figure 2.23. We can divide the body into four major cavities using the frontal or coronal plane to make two dorsal cavities and two ventral cavities.

FIGURE 2.23 Body cavities.

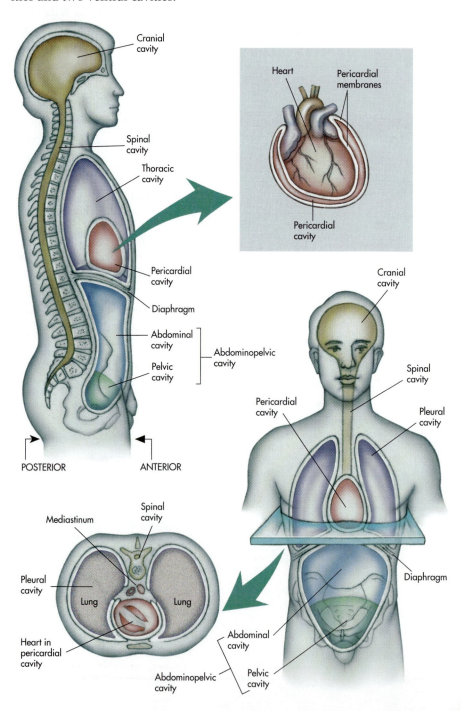

The dorsal cavities include the **cranial cavity** (KRAY nee al CAV ih tee), containing the brain; and the **spinal cavity,** containing the spinal cord.

The ventral cavities include the **thoracic cavity** (tho RASS ik CAV ih tee) and the **abdominopelvic cavity** (ab dom ih noh PELL vik CAV ih tee). The thoracic cavity contains the lungs on either side and a central region called the **mediastinum** (mee dee ass TYE num). The heart, **aorta,** esophagus, trachea, and thymus gland are located in the mediastinum. The abdominopelvic cavity is generally subdivided into a superior **abdominal cavity** (ab DOM ih nal CAV ih tee) and an inferior **pelvic cavity** (PELL vik CAV ih tee). The organs of the digestive, excretory, and reproductive systems are located in these cavities.

There is an actual physical wall between the thoracic cavity and the abdominopelvic cavity called the **diaphragm** (DYE ah fram). The diaphragm is a muscle used for respiration or breathing.

The organs within the ventral cavities are referred to as a group as the internal organs or **viscera** (VISS er ah). The cavities are lined by, and the viscera are encased in, a two-layer **serous** (SEER us) **membrane.** These membranes are called the **pleura** (PLOO rah) in the thoracic cavity and the **peritoneum** (pair ih toh NEE um) in the abdominopelvic cavity.

Additionally, within the thoracic cavity, the pleura is subdivided, forming the **pleural cavity** (PLOO ral CAV ih tee), containing the lungs, and the **pericardial cavity** (pair ih CAR dee al CAV ih tee), containing the heart. The outer layer that lines the cavities is called the **parietal** (pah RYE eh tal) layer (i.e., **parietal pleura** [pah RYE eh tal PLOO rah] and **parietal peritoneum** [pah RYE eh tal pair ih toh NEE um] and the inner layer that encases the viscera is called the **visceral** (VISS er al) layer (i.e., **visceral pleura** [VISS er al PLOO rah] and **visceral peritoneum** [VISS er al pair ih toh NEE um].

Table 2.2 describes the body cavities and their major organs.

ABDOMINOPELVIC REGION TERMINOLOGY

anatomical divisions	left inguinal	right inguinal
clinical divisions	left lower quadrant (LLQ)	right lower quadrant (RLQ)
epigastric	left lumbar	right lumbar
hypogastric	left upper quadrant (LUQ)	right upper quadrant (RUQ)
left hypochondriac	right hypochondriac	umbilical
left iliac	right iliac	

Table 2.2	*Body Cavities and Their Major Organs*
Cavity	**Major Organs**
Dorsal cavity	
Cranial cavity	Brain, pituitary gland
Spinal cavity	Spinal cord
Ventral cavity	
Thoracic cavity	Lungs *Mediastinum:* heart, esophagus, trachea, thymus gland, aorta
Abdominopelvic cavity	
Abdominal cavity	Stomach, spleen, liver, gallbladder, pancreas, and portions of the small intestines and colon
Pelvic cavity	Urinary bladder, ureters, urethra, and portions of the small intestines and colon *Female:* uterus, ovaries, fallopian tubes, vagina *Male:* prostate gland, seminal vesicles, portion of the vas deferens

FIGURE 2.24 Anatomical divisions of the abdomen.

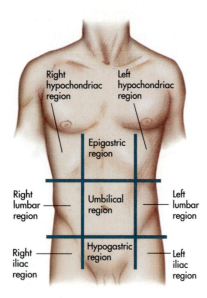

To be able to discuss and identify the positions of the abdominal organs, the abdomen has been divided into nine sections or regions, which are frequently referred to in operative reports. The nine regions, called the **anatomical divisions** of the abdomen, are as follows (see Figure 2.24):

1. **Right hypochondriac** (high poh **KON** dree ak): Right lateral region of upper row just beneath the ribs.
2. **Epigastric** (ep ih **GAS** trik): Middle area of upper row near the stomach.
3. **Left hypochondriac:** Left lateral region of the upper row just beneath the ribs.
4. **Right lumbar:** Right lateral region of the middle row near the waist.
5. **Umbilical** (um **BILL** ih kal): Central area near the navel.
6. **Left lumbar:** Left lateral region of the middle row near the waist.
7. **Right inguinal** (**ING** gwih nal) or **iliac** (**IL** eh ak): Right lateral region of the lower row near the groin.
8. **Hypogastric** (high poh **GAS** trik): Middle region of the lower row beneath the navel.
9. **Left inguinal** or **iliac:** Left lateral region of the lower row near the groin.

MED TERM TIP

To visualize the nine sections of the abdomen, imagine a tic-tac-toe diagram over this region.

The area referred to as the abdominopelvic region can also be divided into four equal areas or quadrants by visualizing two imaginary lines. One will run horizontally through the body and the other will run vertically, crossing at the navel. These four quadrants are referred to as the **clinical divisions** of the abdomen. These terms and their abbreviations (for example: right upper quadrant or RUQ) are useful when charting patient assessments and writing operative reports. These quadrants are as follows (see Figure 2.25):

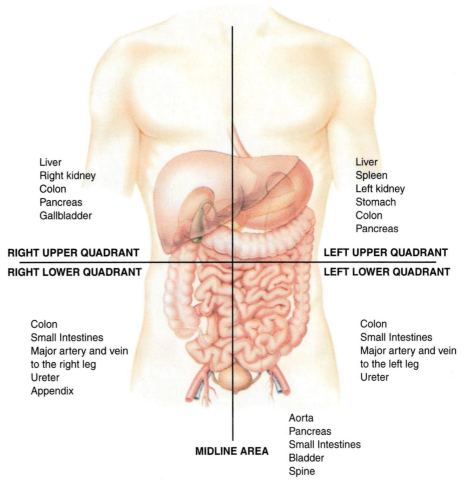

Liver
Right kidney
Colon
Pancreas
Gallbladder

Liver
Spleen
Left kidney
Stomach
Colon
Pancreas

RIGHT UPPER QUADRANT

LEFT UPPER QUADRANT

RIGHT LOWER QUADRANT

LEFT LOWER QUADRANT

Colon
Small Intestines
Major artery and vein
to the right leg
Ureter
Appendix

Colon
Small Intestines
Major artery and vein
to the left leg
Ureter

Aorta
Pancreas
Small Intestines
Bladder
Spine

MIDLINE AREA

FIGURE 2.25 Clinical divisions of the abdomen.

1. **Right upper quadrant (RUQ):** Contains right lobe of liver, gallbladder, portions of the pancreas, small intestines, and colon.

2. **Right lower quadrant (RLQ):** Contains portions of small intestines and colon, right ovary and fallopian tube, appendix, and right ureter.

3. **Left upper quadrant (LUQ):** Contains left lobe of liver, spleen, stomach, and portions of the pancreas, small intestines, and colon.

4. **Left lower quadrant (LLQ):** Contains portions of small intestines and colon, left ovary and fallopian tube, and left ureter.

THE BACK

cervical	**sacrum**	**vertebral column**
coccyx	**thoracic**	
lumbar	**vertebra**	

The back can be divided into five divisions that correspond to regions of the spinal column. Figure 2.26 illustrates the divisions of the back. The spinal column, also called

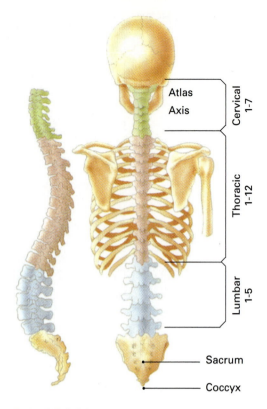

Atlas

Axis

Cervical 1-7

Thoracic 1-12

Lumbar 1-5

Sacrum

Coccyx

FIGURE 2.26 The spinal column.

the **vertebral** (**VER** teh bral) **column,** consists of the bones from the neck down to the tailbone. Each bone is called a **vertebra** (**VER** teh brah). The spinal column is composed of bones and encases the spinal cord, which contains nerve tissue. The divisions of the back are listed in Table 2.3.

Table 2.3	*Divisions of the Back*		
Term	**Area of the Back**	**Number of Bones**	**Abbreviation**
Cervical	Neck	7	C (C1–C7)
Thoracic (tho **RASS** ik)	Chest	12	T (T1–T12)
Lumbar	Loin	5	L (L1–L5)
Sacrum (**SAY** krum)	Lower back	5 fused parts	S (S1–S5)
Coccyx (**COCK** six)	Tailbone	4 fused parts	

Word Building Relating to Body Structure

When using medical terms to indicate different areas of the body or organs it is usually necessary to turn the combining form into an adjective. For example, gastr/o becomes gastric or ventr/o becomes ventral. This is done by adding a suffix to the combining form that translates as *pertaining to*. The following list contains examples of frequently used medical terms relating to body structure that are built directly from word parts. It is important to study this list because there are no rules about which of the several *pertaining to* suffixes to use.

Combining Form	Suffix	Medical Term	Definition
abdomin/o	-al	abdominal (ab **DOM** ih nal)	pertaining to the abdomen
anter/o	-ior	anterior (an **TEE** ree or)	pertaining to the front side
caud/o	-al	caudal (**KAWD** al)	pertaining to the tail
cephal/o	-ic	cephalic (she **FAL** ik)	pertaining to the head
cervic/o	-al	cervical (**SER** vih kal)	pertaining to the neck
coccyg/o	-eal	coccygeal (cock **SIJ** ee al)	pertaining to the tailbone
crani/o	-al	cranial (**KRAY** nee al)	pertaining to the skull
dist/o	-al	distal (**DISS** tal)	pertaining to away (from point of reference)
dors/o	-al	dorsal (**DOR** sal)	pertaining to the spinal cord side
epitheli/o	-al	epithelial (ep ih **THEE** lee al)	pertaining to the epithelium
infer/o	-ior	inferior (in **FEE** ree or)	pertaining to below
later/o	-al	lateral (**LAT** er al)	pertaining to the side
lumb/o	-ar	lumbar (**LUM** bar)	pertaining to the lower back
medi/o	-al	medial (**MEE** dee al)	pertaining to the middle
muscul/o	-ar	muscular (**MUSS** kew lar)	pertaining to muscles
neur/o	-al	neural (**NOO** ral)	pertaining to nerves
pelv/o	-ic	pelvic (**PELL** vik)	pertaining to the pelvis
poster/o	-ior	posterior (poss **TEE** ree or)	pertaining to the back side
proxim/o	-al	proximal (**PROK** sim al)	pertaining to near (to a point of reference)
sacr/o	-al	sacral (**SAY** cral)	pertaining to the sacrum
spin/o	-al	spinal	pertaining to the spine
super/o	-ior	superior (soo **PEE** ree or)	pertaining to above
system/o	-ic	systemic (sis **TEM** ik)	pertaining to systems
thorac/o	-ic	thoracic (tho **RASS** ik)	pertaining to the chest
ventr/o	-al	ventral (**VEN** tral)	pertaining to the belly side
vertebr/o	-al	vertebral (**VER** teh bral)	pertaining to vertebrae
viscer/o	-al	visceral (**VISS** er al)	pertaining to internal organs

Physicians and Assistants

Medical assistants have various duties in the physician's office. Some work in the front office managing the operation of the physician's office and are responsible for duties such as record keeping, billing, and preparing insurance forms. Others perform medical duties such as taking a client/patient's vital signs, taking patient history, and making sure that the examination rooms are clean and well stocked with supplies. Medical assistants can also work in clinics, schools, acute and long-term care facilities, and research. In order to become a medical assistant, students must graduate from an accredited medical assisting program and pass a certification exam given by the American Association of Medical Assistants. To learn more about a career in medical assisting, visit the American Association of Medical Assistants' web site at http://www.aama-ntl.org/.

Physicians oversee patients' care. They examine patients, diagnose diseases, order treatments, perform surgery, and educate patients on health issues. Physicians and their assistants work in acute and long-term care facilities, health maintenance organizations, private practices, clinics, schools, public health facilities, and research.

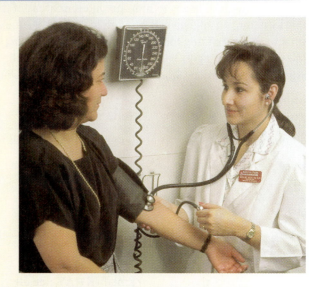

Doctor of Medicine (MD)

- **Graduates from an approved four-year medical school after attending at least three years of college**
- **Passes national board examinations**
- **Completes postgraduate internship and residency years**
- **Licensed by the state in which he or she practices medicine**

Doctor of Osteopathy (DO)

- **A branch of medicine that emphasizes the role of the musculoskeletal system in the health of the body**
- **Graduates from an approved four-year osteopathic school after attending at least three years of college**

- **Passes national board examinations**
- **Completes postgraduate internship and residency years**
- **Licensed by the state in which he or she practices osteopathic medicine**

Physician's Assistant (PA)

- **Trained in certain aspects of the medical practice in order to assist a physician**
- **Graduates from two-year physician's assistant program after attending four years of college**
- **Passes national certification examination**

Certified Medical Assistant (CMA)

- **Works under the supervision of a physician**
- **Graduates from an accredited clinical medical assistant program**
- **Passes a certification exam**

Nurse (RN)

- **Graduates from a two-year, three-year, or four-year program**
- **Provides hands-on patient care**
- **Works under direction of a physician**
- **Must pass a national licensing exam**

Abbreviations Relating to Body Structure

AP	anterioposterior		**LK&S**	liver, kidney, and spleen
C1, C2, etc.	first cervical vertebra, second cervical vertebra, etc.		**LLQ**	left lower quadrant
			LUQ	left upper quadrant
CNS	central nervous system		**MS**	musculoskeletal
CV	cardiovascular		**PNS**	peripheral nervous system
GB	gallbladder		**RLQ**	right lower quadrant
GI	gastrointestinal		**RUQ**	right upper quadrant
GU	genitourinary		**S1, S2, etc.**	first sacral vertebra, second sacral vertebra, etc.
KUB	kidney, ureter, bladder			
L1, L2, etc.	first lumbar vertebra, second lumbar vertebra, etc.		**T1, T2, etc.**	first thoracic vertebra, second thoracic vertebra, etc.
lat	lateral		**UGI**	upper gastrointestinal
LB	large bowel			

KEY TERMS

- abdominal (ab **DOM** ih nal)
- abdominal cavity (ab **DOM** ih nal **CAV** ih tee)
- abdominopelvic cavity (ab dom ih noh **PELL** vik **CAV** ih tee)
- abduction (ab **DUCK** shun)
- adduction (ad **DUCK** shun)
- adipose tissue (**ADD** ih pohs)
- adrenal glands (ad **REE** nal)
- anatomical divisions
- anatomical position
- anterior (an **TEE** ree or)
- aorta (ay **OR** ta)
- apex (**AY** peks)
- arteries (**AR** teh reez)
- base
- blood
- blood vessels
- bone
- brain
- bronchial tubes (**BRONG** kee al)
- capillaries (**CAP** ih lair eez)
- cardiology (car dee **ALL** oh jee)
- cardiovascular (CV) (car dee oh **VAS** kew lar)
- cartilage (**CAR** tih lij)
- caudal (**KAWD** al)
- cell (**SELL**)
- cephalic (seh **FAL** ik)
- cervical (**SER** vih kal)
- circulatory system
- clinical divisions
- coccygeal (cock **SIJ** ee al)
- coccyx (**COCK** siks)
- colon (**COH** lon)
- connective tissue
- coronal plane (kor **RONE** al)
- cranial (**KRAY** nee al)
- cranial cavity (**KRAY** nee al **CAV** ih tee)
- deep
- dermatology (der mah **TALL** oh jee)
- diaphragm (**DYE** ah fram)
- digestive system
- distal (**DISS** tal)
- dorsal (**DOR** sal)
- ears
- endocrine system (**EN** doh krin)
- endocrinology (en doh krin **ALL** oh jee)
- epigastric (ep ih **GAS** trik)
- epithelial (ep ih **THEE** lee al)
- epithelial tissue (ep ih **THEE** lee al)
- esophagus (es **SOF** ah gus)
- eversion (ee **VER** zhun)
- external
- eyes
- fallopian tubes (fah **LOH** pee an)
- frontal plane
- gallbladder (GB) (**GALL** blad er)
- gastroenterology (gas troh en ter **ALL** oh jee)
- gastrointestinal system (GI) (gas troh in **TESS** tin al)
- gynecology (gigh neh **KOL** oh jee)
- hair
- heart
- hematic system
- hematology (hee mah **TALL** oh jee)
- histology (hiss **TALL** oh jee)
- horizontal plane
- hypogastric (high poh **GAS** trik)
- immunology (im yoo **NALL** oh jee)
- inferior (in **FEE** ree or)
- integumentary system (in teg you **MEN** tah ree)
- intermuscular (in ter **MUSS** kyoo lar)
- internal medicine (in **TUR** nal)
- intramuscular (in trah **MUSS** kyoo lar)
- inversion (in **VER** zhun)
- involuntary muscle tissue
- joints
- kidneys

- larynx (**LAIR** inks)
- lateral (lat) (**LAT** er al)
- left hypochondriac (high poh **KON** dree ak)
- left iliac (**ILL** ee ak)
- left inguinal (**ING** gwih nal)
- left lower quadrant (LLQ)
- left lumbar (**LUM** bar)
- left upper quadrant (LUQ)
- liver
- lumbar (**LUM** bar)
- lungs
- lymph nodes (**LIMF**)
- lymph vessels (**LIMF**)
- lymphatic system (lim **FAT** ik)
- mammary glands (**MAM** ah ree)
- medial (**MEE** dee al)
- mediastinum (mee dee ass **TYE** num)
- midsagittal plane (mid **SAJ** ih tal)
- mouth
- mucous membranes (**MYOO** kus)
- muscle tissue
- muscles
- muscular (**MUSS** kyoo lar)
- musculoskeletal (MS) system
- nails
- nephrology (neh **FROL** oh jee)
- nerves
- nervous system
- nervous tissue
- neural (**NOO** ral)
- neurology (noo **RAL** oh jee)
- neurons (**NOO** rons)
- neurosurgery (noo roh **SIR** jer ee)
- nose
- obstetrics (ob **STET** riks)
- ophthalmology (off thal **MALL** oh jee)
- organism
- organs
- orthopedics (or tho **PEE** diks)
- otolaryngology (oh toh lair ing **GALL** oh jee)
- ovaries (**OH** vah reez)
- pancreas (**PAN** kree ass)
- parathyroid glands (pair ah **THIGH** royd)
- parietal (pah **RYE** eh tal)
- parietal peritoneum (pah **RYE** eh tal
  pair ih toh **NEE** um)
- parietal pleura (pah **RYE** eh tal **PLOO** rah)
- pelvic (**PELL** vik)
- pelvic cavity (**PELL** vik **CAV** ih tee)
- penis (**PEE** nis)
- pericardial cavity (pair ih **CAR** dee al **CAV** ih tee)
- pericardium (pair ih **CAR** dee um)
- peritoneum (pair ih toh **NEE** um)
- pharynx (**FAIR** inks)
- pineal gland (**PIN** ee al)
- pituitary gland (pih **TOO** ih tair ee)
- plasma (**PLAZ** mah)
- pleura (**PLOO** rah)
- pleural cavity (**PLOO** ral **CAV** ih tee)
- posterior (poss **TEE** ree or)
- postnasal
- proctology (prok **TALL** oh jee)
- prone (**PROHN**)
- prostate gland (**PROS** tayt)
- proximal (**PROK** sim al)

- pulmonology (pull mon **ALL** oh jee)
- red blood cells
- reproductive system
- respiratory system (**RES** pih rah tor ee)
- retrosternal
- right hypochondriac (high poh **KON** dree ak)
- right iliac (**ILL** ee ak)
- right inguinal (**ING** gwih nal)
- right lower quadrant (RLQ)
- right lumbar (**LUM** bar)
- right upper quadrant (RUQ)
- sacral (**SAY** kral)
- sacrum (**SAY** krum)
- sagittal plane (**SAJ** ih tal)
- salivary glands (**SAL** ih vair ee)
- semicircular
- serous membrane (**SEER** us)
- skin
- small intestine
- special sense organs
- spinal
- spinal cavity
- spinal cord
- spleen
- stomach (**STUM** ak)
- substernal
- superficial
- superior (soo **PEE** ree or)
- supine (soo **PINE**)
- suprasternal
- systemic (sis **TEM** ik)
- systems
- tendons
- testes (**TESS** teez)
- thoracic (tho **RASS** ik)
- thoracic cavity (tho **RASS** ik **CAV** ih tee))
- thoracic surgery (tho **RASS** ik)
- thymus gland (**THIGH** mus)
- thyroid gland (**THIGH** royd)
- tissues
- tongue
- trachea (**TRAY** kee ah)
- transurethral (trans yoo **REE** thral)
- transverse plane (trans **VERS**)
- tricuspid (try **CUSS** pid)
- umbilical (um **BILL** ih kal)
- ureters (yoo **REE** ters)
- urethra (yoo **REE** thrah)
- urinary bladder (**YOO** rih nair ee)
- urinary system (**YOO** rih nair ee)
- urology (yoo **RALL** oh jee)
- uterus (**YOO** ter us)
- vagina (vah **JIGH** nah)
- vas deferens (vas **DEF** er enz)
- veins
- ventral (**VEN** tral)
- vertebra (**VER** teh brah)
- vertebral column (**VER** teh bral)
- viscera (**VISS** er ah)
- visceral (**VISS** er al)
- visceral peritoneum (**VISS** er al pair ih toh **NEE** um)
- visceral pleura (**VISS** er al **PLOO** rah)
- voluntary muscle tissue (**VOL** un ter ee)
- white blood cells

Practice Exercises

A. COMPLETE THE FOLLOWING STATEMENTS.

1. The study of tissue is called _____ .
2. The tissue that lines internal organs and serves as a covering for the skin is _____ tissue.
3. The position that describes the body standing erect with arms at the sides and the palms of the hands facing forward is the _____ .
4. The _____ plane of the body is an imaginary line running lengthwise and dividing the body into right and left components.
5. The _____ quadrant of the abdomen contains the appendix.
6. The spinal column is also called the _____ column.
7. The dorsal cavity contains the _____ cavity and the _____ cavity.
8. There are _____ regional positions in the abdominal cavity.
9. The _____ region of the abdominal cavity is located in the right lower lateral region near the groin.
10. The upper left region located just beneath the ribs is called the _____ region.
11. The total of all the body systems is called the _____ .

B. MATCH THE PLANES OF THE BODY IN COLUMN A WITH THE DEFINITIONS IN COLUMN B.

A	B
1. _____ frontal plane	a. divides the body into right and left
2. _____ sagittal plane	b. divides the body into upper and lower
3. _____ transverse plane	c. divides the body into anterior and posterior

C. MATCH THE TERMS IN COLUMN A WITH THE DEFINITIONS IN COLUMN B.

A	B
1. _____ distal	a. away from the surface
2. _____ prone	b. toward the surface
3. _____ lateral	c. located closer to point of attachment to the body
4. _____ inferior	d. caudal
5. _____ deep	e. move toward middle line of the body
6. _____ adduction	f. lying face down
7. _____ abduction	g. cephalic
8. _____ posterior	h. ventral
9. _____ superficial	i. dorsal
10. _____ supine	j. lying face up
11. _____ anterior	k. to the side
12. _____ medial	l. middle
13. _____ proximal	m. move away from middle line of the body
14. _____ superior	n. located further away from point of attachment to the body

D. CIRCLE THE COMBINING FORM(S) IN THE FOLLOWING TERMS AND DEFINE.

1. epigastric _____
2. lumbosacral _____
3. umbilical _____
4. intervertebral _____
5. thoracotomy _____
6. histology _____
7. coccygeal _____
8. visceral _____

E. BUILD TERMS FOR THE FOLLOWING EXPRESSIONS USING THE CORRECT PREFIXES, SUFFIXES, AND COMBINING FORMS.

1. pertaining to the heart _____
2. pertaining to the chest _____
3. cell formation _____
4. below the sternum _____
5. above the sternum _____
6. between the muscles _____
7. specialist in urinary disorders _____
8. specialist in disorders of bones _____
9. surrounding the heart _____
10. pertaining to the muscles _____
11. study of cells _____
12. specialist in the nervous system _____
13. refers to the head _____
14. refers to the skull _____

F. WRITE THE ABBREVIATIONS FOR THE FOLLOWING TERMS.

1. central nervous system _____
2. lateral _____
3. right upper quadrant _____
4. cardiovascular _____
5. peripheral nervous system _____
6. fifth lumbar bone _____
7. first cervical bone _____
8. left lower quadrant _____

G. IDENTIFY THE FOLLOWING ABBREVIATIONS.

1. LUQ _____
2. UGI _____
3. MS _____
4. AP _____
5. GI _____
6. GU _____
7. RLQ _____
8. T11 _____
9. C5 _____
10. S2 _____
11. L4-S2 _____
12. C1-C7 _____
13. T11-L3 _____

H. DEFINE THE FOLLOWING COMBINING FORMS.

1. viscer/o _____
2. poster/o _____
3. abdomin/o _____
4. cervic/o _____
5. medi/o _____
6. ventr/o _____
7. anter/o _____
8. hist/o _____
9. coccyg/o _____
10. crani/o _____
11. lumb/o _____
12. my/o _____
13. cephal/o _____

I. USE THE FOLLOWING TERMS IN THE SENTENCES THAT FOLLOW.

internal medicine	endocrinology	gastroenterology	gynecology
ophthalmology	urology	orthopedics	immunology
otolaryngology	proctology	obstetrics	

1. John is a musician who plays an electric bass guitar and is experiencing difficulty in hearing soft voices. He would consult a physician in _____ .
2. Ruth is a stock trader with the Chicago Board of Trade. She has had persistent laryngitis since taking her new position. She would consult a physician specializing in _____ .
3. Mary Ann is experiencing excessive bleeding from fibroid tumors. She would consult a specialist in _____ .
4. Jose has persistent pain in his lower back. He would be seen for an examination by a physician in _____ .
5. A physician who performs eye exams is specializing in the field of _____ .

Getting Connected

Multimedia Extension Activities

CD-ROM

Use the CD-ROM enclosed with your textbook to gain additional reinforcement through interactive word building exercises, spelling games, labeling activities, and additional quizzes.

www.prenhall.com/fremgen

Use the above address to access the free, interactive Companion Website created for this textbook. Get hints, instant feedback, and textbook references to chapter-related multiple choice questions, and labeling and matching exercises. In addition, you will find an audio glossary, case studies, Internet exploration exercises, flashcards, and a comprehensive exam.

Answers

PRACTICE EXERCISES

A. 1. histology   2. epithelial   3. anatomical position   4. sagittal   5. right lower   6. vertebral   7. cranial, spinal   8. nine   9. right inguinal   10. left hypochondriac   11. organism

B. 1. c   2. a   3. b

C. 1. n   2. f   3. k   4. d   5. a   6. e   7. m   8. i   9. b   10. j   11. h   12. l   13. c   14. g

D. 1. gastr: area over the pit of the stomach   2. lumbo, sacr: lumbar vertebra and the sacrum area   3. umbilic: referring to the naval area   4. vertebr: between the vertebra   5. thorac: cutting into the chest   6. histo: study of tissues   7. coccyg: pertaining to coccyx area   8. viscer: pertaining to internal organs

E. 1. cardiac   2. thoracic   3. cytoplasm   4. substernal   5. suprasternal   6. intermuscular   7. urologist   8. orthopedist   9. pericardium   10. muscular   11. cytology   12. neurologist   13. cephalic   14. cranial

F. 1. CNS   2. lat   3. RUQ   4. CV   5. PNS   6. L5   7. C1   8. LLQ

G. 1. left upper quadrant   2. upper gastrointestinal   3. musculoskeletal   4. anteroposterior   5. gastrointestinal   6. genitourinary   7. right lower quadrant   8. eleventh thoracic vertebra   9. fifth cervical vertebra   10. second sacral vertebra   11. fourth lumbar vertebra to second sacral vertebra   12. first cervical vertebra to seventh cervical vertebra   13. eleventh thoracic vertebra to third lumbar vertebra

H. 1. internal organ   2. back   3. abdomen   4. neck   5. middle   6. belly   7. front   8. tissues   9. coccyx   10. skull   11. lower back   12. muscle   13. head

I. 1. otolaryngology   2. otolaryngology   3. gynecology   4. orthopedics   5. ophthalmology

Chapter 3

INTEGUMENTARY SYSTEM

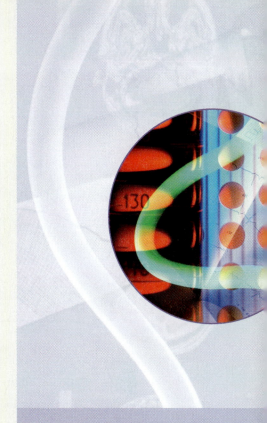

LEARNING OBJECTIVES

Upon completion of this chapter, you will be able to:

- Recognize the combining forms and suffixes introduced in this chapter.

- Gain the ability to pronounce medical terms and major anatomical structures.

- List and describe the three layers of skin and their functions.

- Describe the four purposes of the skin.

- Name and describe the body membranes.

- List and describe the accessory organs of the skin.

- Build integumentary system medical terms from word parts.

- Define vocabulary, pathology, diagnostic, and therapeutic medical terms relating to the integumentary system.

- Interpret abbreviations associated with the integumentary system.

Overview

ORGANS OF THE INTEGUMENTARY SYSTEM

skin
    dermis
    epidermis
    subcutaneous layer

accessory organs
    hair
    nails
    sebaceous (oil) glands (se BAY shus)
    sweat glands

COMBINING FORMS OF THE INTEGUMENTARY SYSTEM

adip/o	fat	**lip/o**	fat
albin/o	white	**macul/o**	stain, spot
caus/o	burn, burning	**melan/o**	black
chrom/o	color	**myc/o**	fungus
cry/o	cold	**onych/o**	nail
cutane/o	skin	**papul/o**	pimple
cyan/o	blue	**pil/o**	hair
derm/o	skin	**py/o**	pus
dermat/o	skin	**rhytid/o**	wrinkle
diaphor/o	profuse sweating	**scler/o**	hard
erythem/o	flush	**seb/o**	sebum, oil
erythemat/o	redness	**squam/o**	scale-like
hidr/o	sweat	**steat/o**	fat
hist/o	tissue	**trich/o**	hair
histi/o	tissue	**ungu/o**	nail
ichthy/o	scaly, dry	**vesic/o**	blister
kerat/o	hard, horny	**vit/o**	blemish
leuk/o	white	**xer/o**	dry

SUFFIXES RELATING TO THE INTEGUMENTARY SYSTEM

Suffix	Meaning	Example
-derma	skin	leukoderma
-tome	instrument used to cut	dermatome

ANATOMY AND PHYSIOLOGY OF THE INTEGUMENTARY SYSTEM

dermatology

erythema

hyperemia

pathogens

sebaceous glands

sebum

sensory receptors

sweat glands

The skin and its appendages—sweat glands, oil glands, hair, and nails—are known as the **integumentary** (in teg you **MEN** tah ree) **system.** *Integument* is another term for skin. Sense organs that allow us to respond to changes in temperature, pain, touch, and pressure are located in the skin.

The skin is the largest organ of the body; it can weigh more than 20 pounds in an adult and covers more than 16 percent of the body. **Dermatology** (der mah **TALL** oh jee) (**Derm**), the study of the skin, is a particularly important specialty in the care of the elderly.

The skin serves many purposes for the body: protecting, housing nerve receptors, secreting fluids, and regulating temperature. The primary purpose of the skin is protection. Under normal conditions, the skin stops all bacteria, harmful chemicals, and injury to the body's internal organs. Since the skin's secretions are slightly acidic, bacteria are less likely to invade the body. Critical body fluids are kept in and **pathogens** (**PATH** oh jenz), disease-bearing organisms, are kept out.

Nerve fibers that are located directly under the surface of the skin are **sensory receptors** (**SEN** soh ree ree **SEP** tors) for the sensations of temperature, pain, touch, and pressure. The messages for these sensations are conveyed to the brain and spinal cord from the nerve endings in the skin.

Fluids are produced in two types of glands: sweat and sebaceous. **Sweat glands** assist the body in maintaining its internal temperature by creating a cooling effect when sweat evaporates. The **sebaceous** (see **BAY** shus) **glands,** or *oil glands,* produce a substance called **sebum** (**SEE** bum). This oily substance lubricates the skin surface.

The complex structure of the skin and tissues aids in the regulation of body temperature through a variety of means. In addition to the cooling action inherent in the evaporation of sweat, changes occur in body temperature as a result of messages from the nerve fibers to the brain. These messages cause an increase or decrease in body temperature. When blood vessels dilate, more blood is brought to the surface of the skin, which results in heat. Sweat glands react to this change by producing a secretion, sweat, which helps to eliminate the heat.

Flushing of the skin is a normal response to an increase in temperature in the environment or to a fever. However, in some people, it is also a response to embarrassment and not easily controlled. **Erythema** (er ih **THEE** mah), which means redness, comes from the combining form *erythem/o.* This term is commonly used to denote any abnormal flushing or redness of the skin. **Hyperemia** (high per **EE** mee ah) is another term that refers to redness caused by increased blood flow to the skin.

BODY MEMBRANES

connective tissue

cutaneous membrane

epithelial

membranes

mucous membrane

serous membrane

synovial membrane

To understand the structure of the skin, it is helpful to have an understanding of the classifications of body membranes. The thin structures called **membranes** cover and protect the body surface, line body cavities, and line some of the internal organs, such as the digestive and respiratory passages. Membranes also secrete lubricating fluids to reduce friction during some processes, such as respiration, and serve to anchor organs and bones.

The two major types of membranes are **epithelial** (ep ih **THEE** lee al) and **connective tissue.** Epithelial membranes contain two layers of tissue: a superficial layer of epithelial tissue and an underlying layer of connective tissue. However, connective tissue membranes contain no epithelial cells.

There are three types of epithelial membranes:

1. **Cutaneous** (kew **TAY** nee us) **membrane** is another term for the skin. It contains both epithelial and connective tissue.

2. **Serous** (**SEER** us) **membrane** is found as a lining in body cavities. It secretes a thin, watery fluid that acts as a lubricant when organs rub against each other.

3. **Mucous** (**MYOO** kus) **membranes** line body passages that open directly to the exterior of the body, such as the mouth and reproductive tract.

The most common connective tissue membrane forms the lining in spaces between bones of a joint. It is called a **synovial** (sin **OH** vee al) **membrane.**

MED TERM TIP An understanding of the designations of membranes and skin layers is important for the health care worker because much of the terminology relating to types of injections and medical conditions, such as burns, is described using these designations.

THE SKIN

albino

basal layer

collagen

dermis (corium)

epidermis

horny cells

keratin

lipocytes

malignant melanoma

melanin

melanocytes

stratified squamous epithelium

subcutaneous layer

FIGURE 3.1 Epidermis.

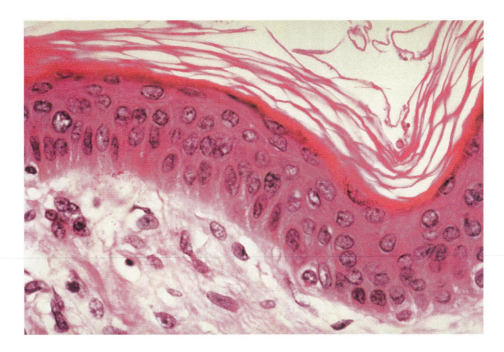

Moving from the outer surface of the skin inward, the three layers are as follows (see also Figure 3.4):

1. **Epidermis** (ep ih **DER** mis) is the thin, outer membrane layer (see Figure 3.1).
2. **Dermis** (**DER** mis) or **corium** (**KOH** ree um) is the middle, fibrous connective tissue layer.
3. **Subcutaneous** (sub kyoo **TAY** nee us) (**Subcu, Subq**) is the innermost layer, containing fatty tissue.

Epidermis

The epidermis is composed of squamous epithelium cells. These flat scale-like cells are arranged in layers or strata and are called **stratified squamous epithelium** (**STRAT** ih fyd **SKWAY** mus ep ih **THEE** lee um). The epidermis does not have a blood supply or any connective tissue, so it is dependent for nourishment on the deeper layers of skin.

The epidermis has many layers of cells, which allows the skin to repair itself as a barrier to infection. The deep layer within the epidermis is called the **basal** (**BAY** sal) **layer.** Cells in this layer continually grow and multiply. New cells that are forming push the old cells toward the outer layer of the epidermis. As the basal layer cells shrink and die, they become filled with a protein called **keratin** (**KAIR** ah tin). This hard protein material then forms **horny cells,** which, as they reach the surface of the skin, slough off as dead cells.

MED TERM *TIP*

We are constantly losing old dead cells, called horny cells, and replacing them with new young cells. In fact, because of this process, our skin is replaced entirely about every seven years.

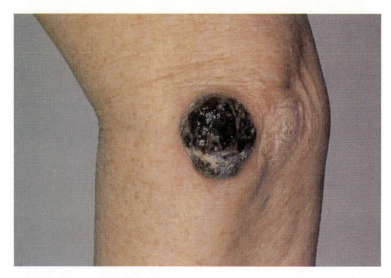

FIGURE 3.2 Malignant melanoma. (BioPhoto Associates/Science Source/Photo Researchers, Inc.)

The basal layer of cells is important because it contains special cells called **melanocytes** (mel **AN** oh sights), which form the black pigment **melanin** (**MEL** ah nin). This pigment gives skin its color and protects it against the ultraviolet rays of the sun. Melanin therefore protects against skin cancer, called **malignant melanoma** (mah **LIG** nant mel ah **NOH** mah) (see Figure 3.2).

A suntan can be thought of as a protective response to the rays of the sun. However, when the melanin in the skin is not able to absorb all the rays of the sun, the skin burns.

When people are exposed to the sun's rays over a long period of time, they have a tendency to form wrinkles and develop skin cancer. Dark-skinned people have more melanin and are generally less likely to have wrinkles and skin cancer.

The term **albino** (al **BYE** noh) refers to someone who is not able to produce melanin. A person with this characteristic has white hair and skin, and red pupils due to the lack of pigment.

Dermis

The dermis, also referred to as the corium, is located between the epidermis and the subcutaneous tissue. It is referred to as the *true skin.* Unlike the thinner epidermis, the dermis is living tissue. The dermis includes hair follicles, sweat glands and sebaceous glands, blood vessels, lymph vessels, nerve fibers, and muscle fibers. It also contains connective tissue and collagen fibers. **Collagen** (**KOL** ah jen), an insoluble fibrous protein present in connective tissue, forms a flexible *glue* that protects the skin and other parts of the body.

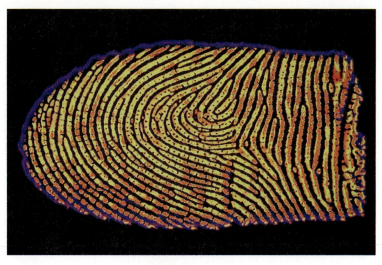

FIGURE 3.3　Enhanced color fingerprint. (Scott Camazine/Photo Researchers, Inc.)

The dermis also contains nerves and nerve endings that provide sensory information to the brain about pain, temperature, touch, and pressure.

MED TERM *TIP* Ridges formed in the dermal layer on our fingertips are what gives each of us unique fingerprints (see Figure 3.3). These do not change during a person's lifetime and are thus a positive means of identification.

Subcutaneous Layer

This third and much smaller layer of the skin is where fat is formed. This layer of fatty tissue with **lipocytes** (**LIP** oh sights) or *fat cells* protects the deeper tissues of the body, and acts as insulation for heat and cold.

ACCESSORY ORGANS

Hair

alopecia　　　　　　　　**systemic lupus erythematosus**
hair follicle

The fibers that make up our hair are composed of the protein keratin, the same hard protein material that fills the horny cells of the epidermis. The process of hair formation is much like the process of growth in the epidermal layer of the skin. The deeper cells in the hair root (see Figure 3.4) force horny cells to move upward through the **hair follicles** (**FALL** ikls). The hair follicles are tiny sacs or cavities that hold individual hair fibers. These sacs are formed from cells in the epidermal layer growing down into the dermal layer of the skin. Color-producing cells, melanocytes, are at the root of the hair follicle and contain the pigment for the hair fibers.

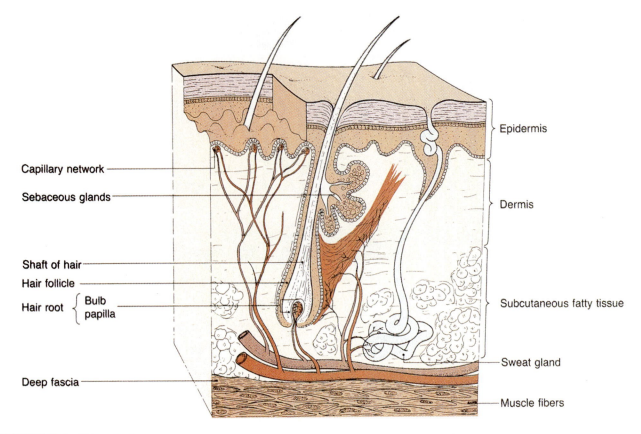

Capillary network

Sebaceous glands

Shaft of hair

Hair follicle

Hair root { Bulb
             papilla

Deep fascia

Epidermis

Dermis

Subcutaneous fatty tissue

Sweat gland

Muscle fibers

FIGURE 3.4   Skin structures.

**MED
TERM
*TIP***

Our hair turns gray when we no longer produce melanin. This is a normal part of the aging process. Hair loss or **alopecia** (al oh **PEE** she ah) is also a normal part of aging in some people (see Figure 3.5). However, a rapid hair loss in patches may indicate a disease such as **systemic lupus erythematosus** (sis **TEM** ik **LOO** pus air ih them ah **TOH** sis) (**SLE**).

FIGURE 3.5   Alopecia.
(BioPhoto Associates/Photo
Researchers, Inc.)

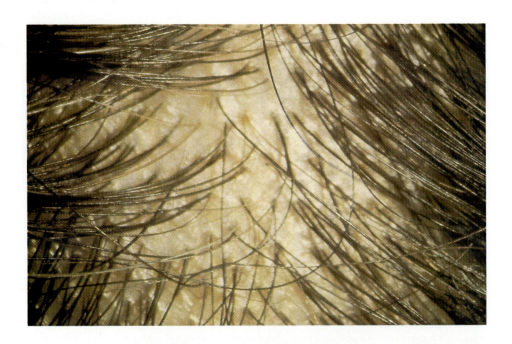

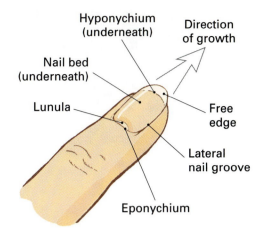

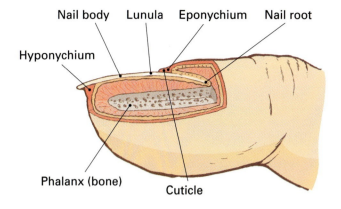

FIGURE 3.6 Nail bed and structure.

Nails

cuticle	keratin
cyanosis	lunula

Nails are also formed from the hard protein **keratin,** by cells in the epidermis. They are formed over the ends of fingers and toes and will continue to grow unless trimmed. The nail consists of the nail edge, nail body, **lunula** (**LOO** nyoo lah) or *half-moon* **cuticle** (**KEW** tikl) at the base of the nail, and nail root (see Figure 3.6).

MED TERM TIP

There is a rich blood supply to the nailbed, and if blood oxygen levels drop, the nailbed will show a distinctive **cyanosis** (sigh ah **NOH** sis) or bluish tinge. When testing for a patient's circulation, press down on the fingernail edge until the nail body takes on a whitish cast. If there is proper circulation, the nail body will immediately return to its normal color when the pressure is released.

Glands

Sebaceous Glands

acne rosacea	comedo	papules
acne vulgaris	hypertrophy	pustules

Sebaceous glands, found in the dermis (corium) layer of the skin, secrete the oil sebum. These oil ducts open into hair follicles and lubricate the hair and skin, thereby helping to prevent drying of the skin (see also Figure 3.4). Secretion from the sebaceous glands increases during adolescence and begins to diminish as age increases. A loss of sebum in old age can account for wrinkles and dry skin.

When sebum accumulates, it can cause congestion in the sebaceous glands, and whiteheads or pimples may form. When the sebum becomes dark it is referred to as a **comedo** (**KOM** ee do) or *blackhead*.

Acne rosacea (**ACK** nee roh **ZAY** she ah) refers to **hypertrophy** (high **PER** troh fee) of sebaceous glands, which causes thickened skin, generally on the nose, forehead, and cheeks.

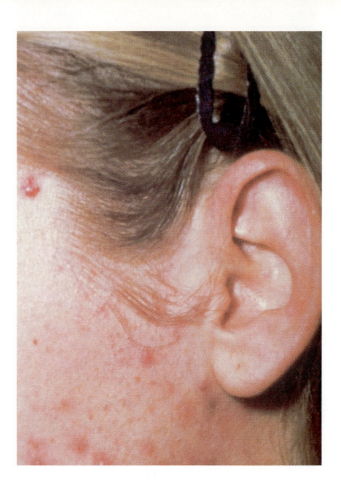

FIGURE 3.7 Case of acne vulgaris (severe acne) on face. (BioPhoto Associates/Science Source/Photo Researchers, Inc.)

Acne vulgaris (**ACK** nee vul **GAY** ris) is a common form of acne occurring during adolescence from an oversecretion of the oil glands (see Figure 3.7). It is characterized by **papules** (**PAP** yools), **pustules** (**PUS** tyools), blackheads, and whiteheads. Papules are small, elevated inflammations on the surface of the skin as a result of inflammation in the oil glands. Pustules, which can rupture and cause a secondary infection, occur when pimples become pus-filled.

Sweat Glands

apocrine glands	**pore**
diaphoresis	

Sweat glands are found throughout the body. There are about two million of these small glands, which originate in the dermis layer and reach into the epidermis of the skin. The surface opening of a sweat gland is called a **pore** (see also Figure 3.4).

Sweat glands have the function of cooling the body as sweat evaporates. Excessive sweating is called **diaphoresis** (dye ah for **REE** sis). Sweat or perspiration is normally colorless and odorless. However, there are sweat glands called **apocrine** (**APP** oh krin) **glands** that open into hair follicles located in the pubic, anal, and mammary areas. These glands secrete a milky substance that can produce an odor when it comes into contact with bacteria on the skin. This is what we recognize as body odor.

Word Building Relating to the Integumentary System

The following list contains examples of medical terms built directly from word parts. The definition for these terms can be determined by a straightforward translation of the word parts.

Combining Form	Combined With	Medical Term	Definition
cutane/o	sub- -ous	subcutaneous (sub kyoo **TAY** nee us)	pertaining to under the skin
derm/o	epi- -al	epidermal (ep ih **DER** mal)	pertaining to upon the skin
	erythro- -a	erythroderma (eh rith roh **DER** mah)	red skin
	hypo- -ic	hypodermic (high poh **DER** mik)	pertaining to under the skin
	intra- -al	intradermal (in trah **DER** mal)	pertaining to within the skin
	leuko- -a	leukoderma (loo koh **DER** mah)	white skin
	pachy- -a	pachyderma (pak ee **DER** mah)	thick skin
	scler/o -a	scleroderma (sklair ah **DER** mah)	hard skin
	xantho- -a	xanthoderma (zan thoh **DER** mah)	yellow skin
	xero- -a	xeroderma (zee roh **DER** mah)	dry skin
dermat/o	-fibr/o -oma	dermatofibroma (der mah toh figh **BROH** ma)	fibrous skin tumor
	-itis	dermatitis (der mah **TYE** tis)	inflammation of the skin
	-logist	dermatologist (der mah **TALL** oh jist)	specialist in skin (diseases)
	-logy	dermatology (der mah **TALL** oh jee)	study of the skin
	-pathy	dermatopathy (der mah **TOP** ah thee)	skin disease
	-plasty	dermatoplasty (**DER** mah toh plas tee)	surgical repair of the skin
	-tome	dermatome (**DER** mah tohm)	instrument to cut this skin
lip/o	-ectomy	lipectomy (lih **PECK** toh mee)	excision of fat
	-oma	lipoma (lip **OH** mah)	fatty growth
melan/o	-oma	melanoma (mel ah **NOH** mah)	black tumor
necr/o	-osis	necrosis (neh **KROH** sis)	abnormal condition of death
onych/o	-ectomy	onychectomy (on ee **KECK** toh mee)	excision of a nail
	-malacia	onychomalacia (on ih koh mah **LAY** she ah)	softening of nails
	myc/o -osis	onychomycosis (on ih koh my **KOH** sis)	abnormal condition of nail fungus
	par- -ia	paronychia (pair oh **NICK** ee ah)	(diseased) condition around the nail
	-phagia	onychophagia (on ih koh **FAY** jee ah)	nail eating (nail biting)
py/o	-genic	pyogenic (pye oh **JEN** ik)	pus forming
rhytid/o	-ectomy	rhytidectomy (rit ih **DECK** toh mee)	excision of wrinkles
	-plasty	rhytidoplasty (**RIT** ih doh plas tee)	surgical repair of wrinkles
seb/o	-rrhea	seborrhea (seb or **EE** ah)	oily discharge
trich/o	myc/o -osis	trichomycosis (trick oh my **KOH** sis)	abnormal condition of hair fungus
ungu/o	-al	ungual (**UNG** gwal)	pertaining to the nails

Vocabulary Relating to the Integumentary System

alopecia **(al oh PEE she ah)**	Absence or loss of hair, especially of the head (see Figure 3.8).
cicatrix (SICK ah trix)	A scar.
depigmentation **(dee pig men TAY shun)**	Loss of normal skin color or pigment.
dermatographia **(der mah toh GRAF ee ah)**	Skin writing. Wheals develop on the skin of some people as a result of tracing on the skin with an instrument or fingernail. This type of skin is susceptible to infection.
dermatologist **(der mah TALL oh jist)**	Physician who specializes in the treatment of the integumentary system.
dermatology **(der mah TALL oh jee)(derm)**	Study of diseases and conditions of the integumentary system.
diaphoresis **(dye ah for REE sis)**	Profuse sweating.
ecchymosis (ek ih MOH sis)	Skin discoloration or bruise caused by blood collecting under the skin.
erythema (er ih THEE mah)	Redness or flushing of the skin.
frostbite	Freezing or the effect of freezing a part of the body. Exposed areas such as ears, nose, cheeks, fingers, and toes are generally affected (see Figure 3.9).
hirsutism (HER soot izm)	Excessive hair growth over the body.
hyperpigmentation **(high per pig men TAY shun)**	Abnormal amount of pigmentation in the skin seen in diseases such as acromegaly and adrenal insufficiency.
necrosis (neh KROH sis)	Tissue death.
onychophagia **(on ih koh FAY jee ah)**	Nail biting.
pediculosis **(peh dik you LOH sis)**	Infestation with lice.
petechiae (peh TEE kee eye)	Flat, pinpoint, purplish spots from bleeding under the skin.
photosensitivity **(foh toh sen sih TIH vih tee)**	Condition in which the skin reacts abnormally when exposed to light, such as the ultraviolet rays of the sun.
pruritus (proo RIGH tus)	Severe itching.
purpura (PER pew rah)	Hemorrhages into the skin and mucous membranes.
ulcer (ULL sir)	Open sore or lesion in skin or mucous membrane.
vitiligo (vit ill EYE go)	Disappearance of pigment from the skin in patches, causing a milk-white appearance. Also called *leukoderma*.
xeroderma (zee roh DER ma)	Dry skin.

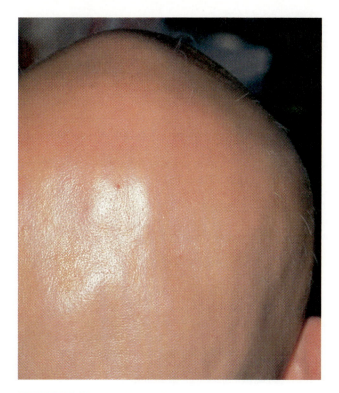

FIGURE 3.8 Complete baldness.

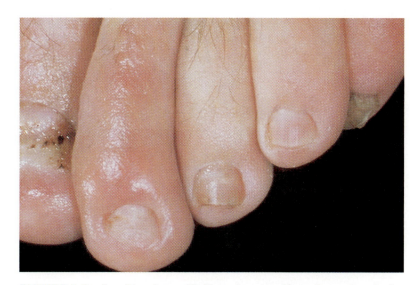

FIGURE 3.9 Frostbite of toes. (BioPhoto Associates/Photo Researchers, Inc.)

Pathology of the Integumentary System

acne (ACK nee)	Inflammatory disease of the sebaceous glands and hair follicles that results in papules and pustules.
dermatitis (der mah TYE tis)	Inflammation of the skin.
gangrene (GANG green)	Necrosis (death of tissue) usually due to deficient blood supply.
leukoderma (loo koh DER mah)	Disappearance of pigment from the skin in patches, causing a milk-white appearance. Also called *vitiligo*.
onychia (oh NICK ee ah)	Infected nailbed.
pachyderma (pak ee DER mah)	Thickening of the skin.
paronychia (pair oh NICK ee ah)	Infection around a nail.
pemphigus vulgaris (PEM fi gus vul GAY ris)	Blisters forming in the skin and mucous membranes.
sebaceous cyst (see BAY shus SIST)	Sac under the skin filled with sebum or oil from a sebaceous gland. This can grow to a large size and may need to be excised (see Figure 3.10).
seborrhea (seb or EE ah)	Excessive discharge of sebum.
shingles (SHING lz)	Eruption of vesicles along a nerve, causing a rash and pain. Caused by the same virus as chickenpox.
systemic lupus erythematosus (sis TEM ik LOO pus air ih them ah TOH sis) (SLE)	Chronic disease of the connective tissue that injures the skin, joints, kidneys, nervous system, and mucous membranes. May produce a characteristic butterfly rash across the cheeks and nose.

MED TERM TIP When trying to remember the meaning of the term *pachyderma,* remember that the elephant and hippopotamus are animals, called pachyderms, with thick skins.

FIGURE 3.10 Sebaceous cyst. (Charles Stewart and Associates)

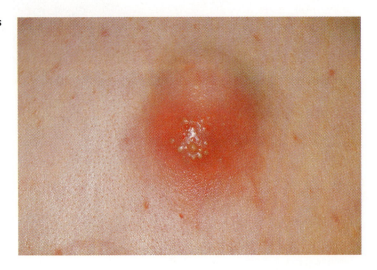

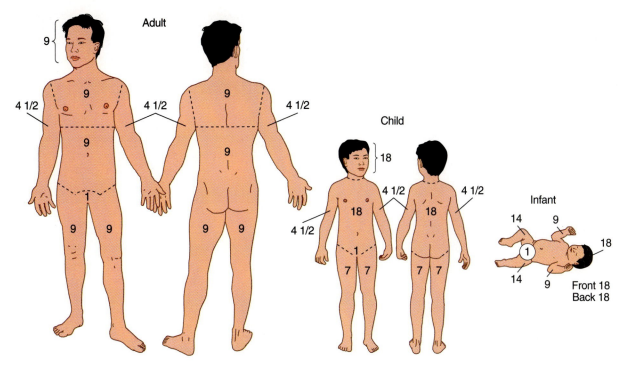

FIGURE 3.11   Rule of Nines for burns (all numbers are % of body surface). (Dr. P. Marazzi/Science Photo Library/Photo Researchers, Inc.)

BURNS

hyperemia

vesicles

Burns are one of the most serious medical problems that affect the integumentary system. A burn can result from exposure to open fire, electricity, ultraviolet light from the sun, or caustic chemicals. The seriousness of a burn depends on the amount of body surface involved and the depth or severity of the actual burn. Health care workers use a common terminology to determine the extent of a burn called the *rule of nines.* Figure 3.11 illustrates this rule, in which the body is divided into 11 areas, each containing 9 percent of body surface. The genital area accounts for the remaining 1 percent of body surface.

The actual classification of a burn depends on the number of layers of skin involved. A mild burn will cause some discomfort and a reddening of skin. However, a serious burn will destroy all skin layers, subcutaneous tissue, and underlying tissues. Burns are classified as follows:

1. *First-degree:* **Hyperemia** (redness caused by increased blood flow to the skin) involving a superficial layer of skin or outer layer of epidermis. Generally, there is no scarring (see Figure 3.12).

2. *Second-degree:* Burn damage that extends through the epidermis and into the dermis, causing small fluid-filled raised spots called **vesicles** (**VESS** iklz) to form. Scarring may occur (see Figure 3.13).

3. *Third-degree:* Burn damage to full thickness of skin (epidermis and dermis) and into underlying tissues. Infection is a major concern with third-degree burns, and fluid loss can be life threatening. Scarring will occur.

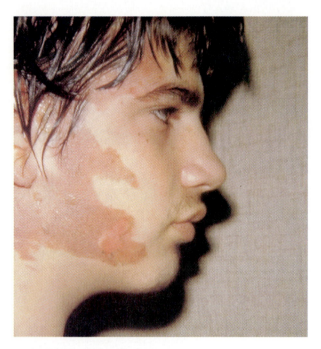

FIGURE 3.12   First degree burns on face.

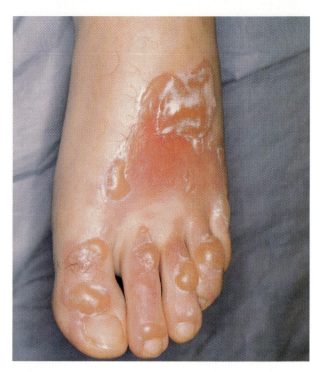

FIGURE 3.13   Second degree burns on feet. (Moynahan Medical Center)

SKIN LESIONS

Skin lesions are considered to be a disorder of the skin. However, they are not always a sign of disease and may simply be a variation from the normal surface of the skin. Most skin conditions and diseases are diagnosed, in part, by observing the lesions. There is generally some discoloration or change in coloration with a skin lesion. The most common lesions are described below and illustrated in Figure 3.14.

cyst (SIST)	Fluid-filled sac under the skin.
fissure (FISH er)	Crack-like lesion or groove on the skin.
macule (MACK yool)	Flat, discolored area that is flush with the skin surface. An example would be a freckle or a birthmark.
nodule (NOD yool)	Solid, raised group of cells.
papule (PAP yool)	Small, solid, circular raised spot on the surface of the skin.
polyp (POLL ip)	Small tumor with a pedicle or stem attachment. They are commonly found in vascular organs such as the nose, uterus, and rectum.
pustule (PUS tyool)	Raised spot on the skin containing pus.
vesicle (VESS ikl)	Small, fluid-filled raised spot on the skin.
wheal (WEEL)	Small, round, raised area on the skin that may be accompanied by itching.

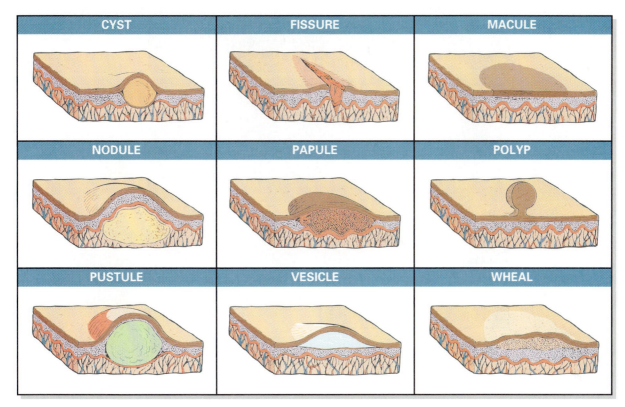

A

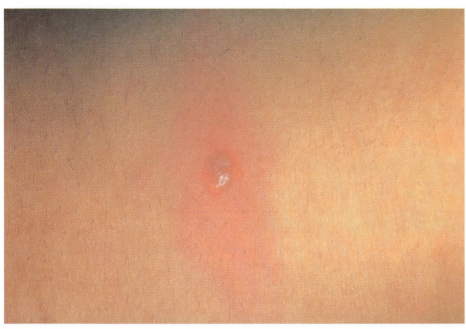

B

FIGURE 3.14   (A) Skin lesions; (B) vesicle associated with chicken pox. (Charles Stewart and Associates)

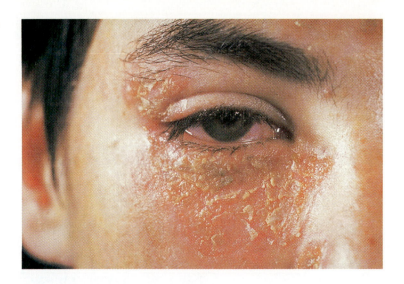

FIGURE 3.15 Impetigo. (Charles Stewart and Associates)

SKIN INFECTIONS

Bacteria, viruses, fungi, and parasites can all invade the skin if its protective barrier is broken down. Some of the more common skin infections are listed below.

boil	Acute inflammation of subcutaneous layer of skin, gland, or hair follicle. Also called a *furuncle*.
carbuncle (CAR bung kl)	Inflammation and infection of the skin and hair follicle that may result from several untreated boils. Most commonly found on neck, upper back, or head.
furuncle (FOO rung kl)	Staphylococcal skin abscess with redness, pain, and swelling. Also called a *boil*.
impetigo (im peh TYE goh)	Inflammatory skin disease with pustules that become crusted and rupture (see Figure 3.15).
scabies (SKAY bees)	Contagious skin disease caused by an egg-laying mite that causes intense itching; often seen in children.
tinea (TIN ee ah)	Fungal skin disease resulting in itching, scaling lesions.
verruca (ver ROO kah)	Warts; a benign neoplasm (tumor) caused by a virus. Has a rough surface that is removed by chemicals and/or laser therapy.

INFLAMMATORY SKIN DISORDERS

cellulitis (sell you LYE tis)	Inflammation of the cellular or connective tissues (see Figure 3.16).
decubitus (dee KYOO bih tus) ulcers	Bedsores or pressure sores caused by pressure over bony prominences on the body are due to a lack of blood flow. These can appear in bedridden patients who lie in one position too long and can be difficult to heal.
eczema (EK zeh mah)	Superficial dermatitis accompanied by papules, vesicles, and crusting.
psoriasis (soh RYE ah sis)	Chronic inflammatory condition consisting of crusty papules forming patches with circular borders (see Figure 3.17).
scleroderma (sklair ah DER mah)	Disorder in which the skin becomes taut, thick, and leatherlike.
urticaria (er tih KAY ree ah)	Hives, a skin eruption of pale reddish wheals (circular elevations of the skin) with severe itching. Usually associated with food allergy, stress, or drug reactions (see Figure 3.18).

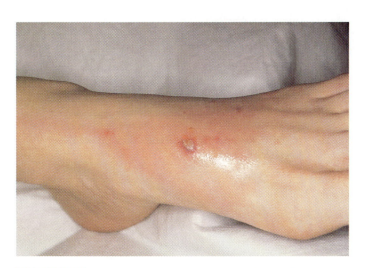

FIGURE 3.16 Cellulitus on foot. (Barts Medical Library/Phototake NYC)

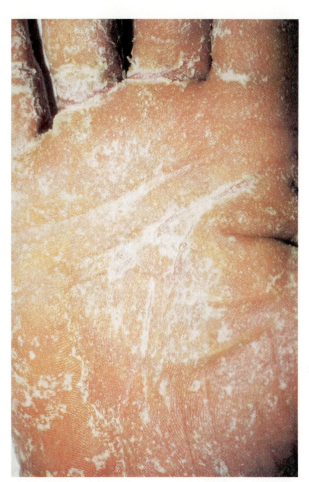

FIGURE 3.17 Psoriasis on hand. (Charles Stewart and Associates)

SKIN NEOPLASMS

Neoplasms (**NEE** oh plazms) or **tumors** (**TOO** mors) can be either **benign** (bee **NINE**), which means they are noncancerous, or **malignant** (mah **LIG** nant), which means they are cancerous. Skin neoplasms are described below.

Benign (Noncancerous) Neoplasms

dermatofibroma (der mah toh figh BROH mah)	Fibrous tumor of the skin. It is painless, round, firm, red, and generally found on the extremities.
hemangioma (hee man jee OH ma)	Benign tumor of dilated blood vessels (see Figure 3.19).
keloid (KEE loyd)	Formation of a scar after an injury or surgery, which results in a raised, thickened red area (see Figure 3.20).
keratosis (KAIR ah TOH sis)	Overgrowth and thickening of the epithelium.
leukoplakia (loo koh PLAY kee ah)	Change in mucous membrane that results in thick, white patches on the mucous membrane of the tongue and cheek. Considered precancerous, it is associated with smoking.
lipoma (lip OH mah)	Fatty tumor that generally does not metastasize.
nevus (NEV us)	Pigmented (colored) congenital skin blemish, birthmark, or mole. Usually benign but may become cancerous.

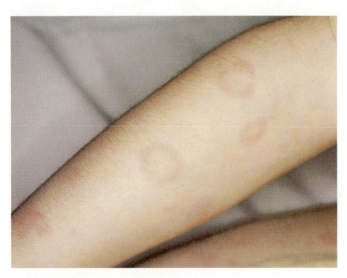

FIGURE 3.18 Severe itching can be caused by a rash such as found in urticaria. (CNRI/Phototake NYC)

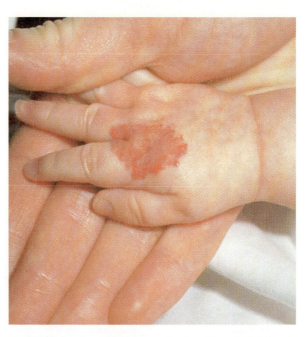

FIGURE 3.19 Hemangioma (birthmark) on baby's hand. (Dr. H. C. Robinson/Science Photo Library/Photo Researchers, Inc.)

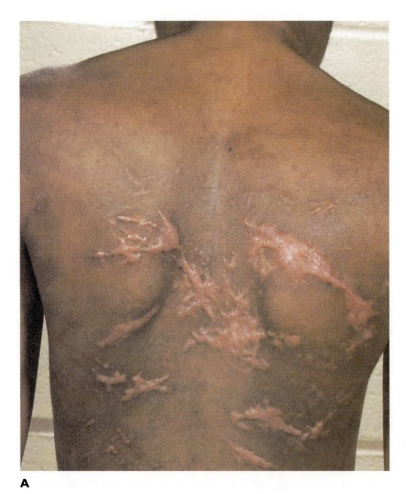

A

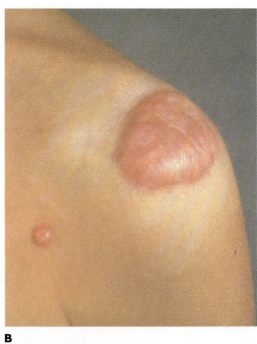

B

FIGURE 3.20 (A) Keloids on back (Martin Rotker/Phototake NYC); (B) Keloids on shoulder. (BioPhoto Associates/Photo Researchers, Inc.)

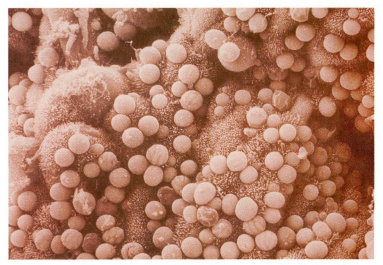

A

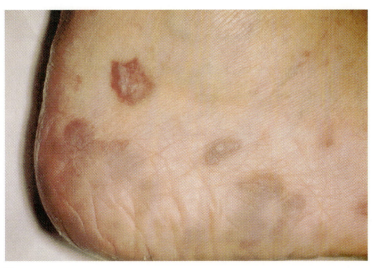

B

FIGURE 3.21 (A) Cells of Kaposi's sarcoma (Ralph Eagle, MD/Photo Researchers, Inc.); (B) Kaposi's sarcoma of heel and foot. (CDC/Phototake NYC)

Malignant (Cancerous) Neoplasms

basal cell carcinoma
(BAY sal sell kar sin NOH ma)

Epithelial tumor of the basal cell layer of the epidermis. A frequent type of skin cancer that rarely metastasizes or spreads. Usually found between the hairline and the upper lip. These cancers can arise on sun-exposed skin.

Kaposi's sarcoma
(KAP oh seez sar KOH mah)

Form of skin cancer frequently seen in acquired immunodeficiency syndrome (AIDS) patients. Consists of brownish-purple papules that spread from the skin and metastasize to internal organs (see Figure 3.21). Named for Moritz Kaposi, an Austrian dermatologist.

malignant melanoma
(mah LIG nant mel a NOH ma)

Dangerous form of skin cancer caused by an overgrowth of melanin. May metastasize or spread.

squamous cell carcinoma
(SKWAY mus sell kar sih NOH mah)

Epidermal cancer that may go into deeper tissue but does not generally metastasize.

Diagnostic Procedures Relating to the Integumentary System

biopsy (BYE op see) (BX, bx)	A piece of tissue is removed by syringe and needle, knife, punch, or brush to examine under a microscope. Used to aid in diagnosis.
culture and sensitivity (C&S)	A laboratory test that grows a colony of pathogens removed from an infected area in order to identify the pathogen and then determine its sensitivity to a variety of antibiotics.
exfoliative cytology (ex FOH lee ah tiv sigh TALL oh jee)	Scraping cells from tissue and then examining them under a microscope.
frozen section (FS)	A thin piece of tissue is cut from a frozen specimen for rapid examination under a microscope.
fungal (FUN gal) scrapings	Scrapings, taken with a curette or scraper, of tissue from lesions are placed on a growth medium and examined under a microscope to identify fungal growth.
needle biopsy	Using a sterile needle to remove tissue for examination under a microscope.
skin tests (ST)	Test to determine the patient's reaction to a suspected allergen by injecting a small amount under the skin (intradermal) with a needle. The reaction of the patient to this material is then read to indicate any allergy. Examples of such tests are the tuberculin (TB) test, Mantoux (PPD) test, patch test, and Schick test.
sweat test	Test performed on sweat to determine the level of chloride. There is an increase in skin chloride in the disease cystic fibrosis.

Abbreviations Relating to the Integumentary System

BX, bx	biopsy	**SLE**	systemic lupus erythematosus
C&S	culture and sensitivity	**ST**	skin test
Derm	dermatology	**STD**	skin test done; sexually transmitted disease
FS	frozen section		
H	hypodermic	**STSG**	split-thickness skin graft
I&D	incision and drainage	**Subcu**	subcutaneous
ID	intradermal	**Subq**	subcutaneous
LE	lupus erythematosus	**ung**	ointment
SCLE	subacute cutaneous lupus erythematosus	**UV**	ultraviolet
SG	skin graft		

Treatment Procedures Relating to the Integumentary System

abrasion (ah BRAY zhun)	Scraping away a portion of the surface of the skin. Performed to remove acne scars, tattoos, and scar tissue.
adipectomy (add ih PECK toh mee)	Surgical removal of fat.
cauterization (kaw ter ih ZAY shun)	Destruction of tissue with a caustic chemical, electric current, freezing, or hot iron.
chemobrasion (kee moh BRAY zhun)	Abrasion using chemicals. Also called a *chemical peel*.
cryosurgery (cry oh SER jer ee)	Using extreme cold to freeze and destroy tissue.
curettage (koo REH tahz)	Removal of superficial skin lesions with a curette (surgical instrument shaped like a spoon) or scraper.
debridement (day breed MON)	Removal of foreign material and dead or damaged tissue from a wound.
dermabrasion (DERM ah bray shun)	Abrasion or rubbing using wire brushes or sandpaper.
dermatome (DER mah tohm)	Instrument for cutting the skin or thin transplants of skin.
dermatoplasty (DER mah toh plas tee)	Skin grafting; transplantation of skin. May be used to treat large birthmarks (hemangiomas).
electrocautery (ee leck troh KAW teh ree)	To destroy tissue with an electric current.
incision and drainage (I&D)	Making an incision to create an opening for the drainage of material such as pus.
laser therapy	Removal of skin lesions and birthmarks using a laser beam that emits intense heat and power at a close range. The laser converts frequencies of light into one small, powerful beam.
lipectomy (lih PECK toh mee)	Surgical removal of fat.
liposuction (LIP oh suck shun)	Removal of fat beneath the skin by means of suction.
marsupialization (mahr soo pee al ih ZAY shun)	Creating a pouch to promote drainage by surgically opening a closed area such as a cyst.
plication (plye KAY shun)	Taking tucks surgically in a structure to shorten it.
rhytidectomy (rit ih DECK toh mee)	Surgical removal of excess skin to eliminate wrinkles. Commonly referred to as a *face-lift*.
skin graft	The transfer of skin from a normal area to cover another site. Used to treat burn victims and after some surgical procedures.

Emergency Medical Technician

Emergency Medical Technicians (EMTs) provide basic and advanced pre-hospital emergency care for traumatic or medical emergencies. They are often the first to arrive on the scene. They evaluate the patient's condition, relay the information to an emergency physician, initiate the medical care ordered by the physician and stabilize and transport the patient to the hospital. Often EMTs are volunteers who hold down full-time jobs in other fields; others are employed as EMTs on a full-time basis. They work in a variety of challenging and fast-paced environments such as police and fire departments, hospital emergency rooms, and private ambulance services. An Emergency Medical Technician completes an approved EMT-paramedic training program and six months of field experience, and must pass a national certification examination. For more information regarding a career as an Emergency Medical Technician, visit the National Association of Emergency Medical Technicians at http://naemt.org/.

Nursing Service

Nursing Service workers assess patients, plan and carry out patient treatments, and evaluate the patient's response to treatment. Skilled nursing care includes intravenous therapy, administering medication and anesthesia, wound care, and patient education. Nursing Service personnel are found in acute and long-term care facilities, clinics, physician's offices, health maintenance organizations, home health agencies, public health agencies, and schools.

Nurse Practitioner (NP)

- **Receives advanced training in a specialized area of nursing such as nurse midwife, nurse anesthetist, or nurse clinician**
- **Meets all the requirements for becoming a registered nurse**

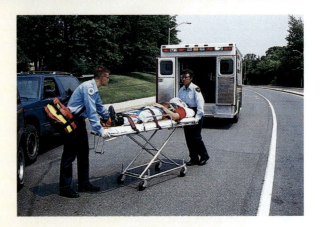

- **Completes advanced training and clinical experience in an accredited nurse practitioner program**
- **Licensed by the state of employment**

Registered Nurse (RN, BSN, MSN)

- **Graduates from an accredited two-year associate, four-year bachelor's, or five-year master's degree nursing program**
- **Passes national licensing examination**
- **Licensed by the state of employment**

Licensed Practical/Vocational Nurse (LPN or LVN)

- **Trained in basic nursing techniques**
- **Works under the supervision of a physician or registered nurse**
- **Graduates from a recognized one-year vocational education practical nursing program**
- **Licensed by the state of employment**

Certified Nurse Aide (CNA)

- **Trained in basic patient care such as bathing and feeding**
- **Works under supervision of RN or LPN**
- **Completes approved on-the-job certification program**

- abrasion (ah **BRAY** zhun)
- acne (**ACK** knee)
- acne rosacea (**ACK** knee roh **ZAY** she ah)
- acne vulgaris (**ACK** nee vul **GAY** ris)
- adipectomy (add ih **PECK** toh mee)
- albino (al **BYE** noh)
- alopecia (al oh **PEE** she ah)
- apocrine glands (**APP** oh krin)
- basal cell carcinoma
  (**BAY** sal sell kar sin **NOH** mah)
- basal layer (**BAY** sal)
- benign (bee **NINE**)
- biopsy (**BYE** op see)
- boil
- carbuncle (**CAR** bung kl)
- cauterization (kaw ter ih **ZAY** shun)
- cellulitis (sell you **LYE** tis)
- chemobrasion (kee moh **BRAY** zhun)
- cicatrix (**SIK** ah trix)
- collagen (**KOL** ah jen)
- comedo (**KOM** ee doh)
- connective tissue
- corium (**KOH** ree um)
- cryosurgery (cry oh **SER** jer ee)
- culture and sensitivity
- curettage (koo **REH** tazh)
- cutaneous membrane (kew **TAY** nee us)
- cuticle (**KEW** tikl)
- cyanosis (sigh ah **NOH** sis)
- cyst (**SIST**)
- debridement (day breed **MON**)
- decubitus ulcers (dee **KYOO** bih tus **ULL** sers)
- depigmentation (dee pig men **TAY** shun)
- dermabrasion (**DERM** ah bray shun)
- dermatitis (der mah **TYE** tis)
- dermatofibroma (der mah toh figh **BROH** mah)
- dermatographia (der mah toh **GRAF** ee ah)
- dermatologist (der mah **TALL** oh jist)
- dermatology (der mah **TALL** oh jee)
- dermatome (**DER** mah tohm)
- dermatopathy (der mah **TOP** ah thee)

- dermatoplasty (**DER** mah toh plas tee)
- dermis (**DER** mis)
- diaphoresis (dye ah for **REE** sis)
- ecchymosis (ek ih **MOH** sis)
- eczema (**EK** zeh mah)
- electrocautery (ee leck troh **KAW** teh ree)
- epidermal (ep ih **DER** mal)
- epidermis (ep ih **DER** mis)
- epithelial (ep ih **THEE** lee al)
- erythema (er ih **THEE** mah)
- erythroderma (eh rith roh **DER** ma)
- exfoliative cytology (ex **FOH** lee ah tiv
  sigh **TALL** oh jee)
- fissure (**FISH** er)
- frostbite
- frozen section
- fungal scrapings (**FUN** gal)
- furuncle (**FOO** rung kl)
- gangrene (**GANG** green)
- hair follicles (**FALL** ikls)
- hemangioma (hee man jee **OH** mah)
- hirsutism (**HER** soot izm)
- horny cells
- hyperemia (high per **EE** mee ah)
- hyperpigmentation (high per pig men **TAY** shun)
- hypertrophy (high **PER** troh fee)
- hypodermic (high poh **DERM** ik)
- impetigo (im peh **TYE** goh)
- incision and drainage
- integumentary system (in teg you **MEN** tah ree)
- intradermal (in trah **DER** mal)
- Kaposi's sarcoma (**KAP** oh seez sar **KOH** mah)
- keloid (**KEE** loyd)
- keratin (**KAIR** ah tin)
- keratosis (kair ah **TOH** sis)
- laser therapy
- leukoderma (loo koh **DER** mah)
- leukoplakia (loo koh **PLAY** kee ah)
- lipectomy (lih **PECK** toh mee)
- lipocytes (**LIP** oh sights)
- lipoma (lip **OH** mah)

- liposuction (**LIP** oh suck shun)
- lunula (**LOO** nyoo lah)
- macule (**MACK** yool)
- malignant (mah **LIG** nant)
- malignant melanoma (mah **LIG** nant mel ah **NOH** mah)
- marsupialization (mahr soo pee al ih **ZAY** shun)
- melanin (**MEL** an in)
- melanocytes (mel **AN** oh sights)
- melanoma (mel ah **NOH** ma)
- membranes
- mucous membrane (**MYOO** kus)
- necrosis (neh **KROH** sis)
- needle biopsy
- neoplasms (**NEE** oh plazms)
- nevus (**NEV** us)
- nodule (**NOD** yool)
- onychectomy (on ee **KECK** toh me)
- onychia (oh **NICK** ee ah)
- onychomalacia (on ih koh mah **LAY** she ah)
- onychomycosis (on ih koh my **KOH** sis)
- onychophagia (on ih koh **FAY** jee ah)
- pachyderma (pak ee **DER** mah)
- papule (**PAP** yool)
- paronychia (pair oh **NICK** ee ah)
- pathogens (**PATH** oh jenz)
- pediculosis (peh dik you **LOH** sis)
- pemphigus vulgaris (**PEM** fih gus vul **GAY** ris)
- petechiae (peh **TEE** kee eye)
- photosensitivity (foh toh sen sih **TIH** vih tee)
- plication (plye **KAY** shun)
- polyp (**POLL** ip)
- pore
- pruritus (proo **RIGH** tus)
- psoriasis (soh **RYE** ah sis)
- purpura (**PER** pew rah)
- pustule (**PUS** tyool)
- pyogenic (pye oh **JEN** ik)
- rhytidectomy (rit ih **DECK** toh mee)
- rhytidoplasty (**RIT** ih doh plas tee)
- scabies (**SKAY** bees)
- scleroderma (sklair ah **DER** mah)
- sebaceous cyst (see **BAY** shus **SIST**)
- sebaceous gland (see **BAY** shus)
- seborrhea (seb or **EE** ah)
- sebum (**SEE** bum)
- sensory receptors (**SEN** soh ree)
- serous membrane (**SEER** us)
- shingles (**SHING** lz)
- skin graft
- skin tests
- squamous cell carcinoma (**SKWAY** mus sell kar sih **NOH** mah)
- stratified squamous epithelium (**STRAT** ih fyde **SKWAY** mus ep ih **THEE** lee um)
- subcutaneous (sub kyoo **TAY** nee us)
- subcutaneous layer (sub kyoo **TAY** nee us)
- sweat glands
- sweat test
- synovial membrane (sin **OH** vee al)
- systemic lupus erythematosus (sis **TEM** ik **LOO** pus air ih them ah **TOH** sis)
- tinea (**TIN** ee ah)
- trichomycosis (trik oh mye **KOH** sis)
- tumors (**TOO** mors)
- ulcer (**ULL** ser)
- ungual (**UNG** gwal)
- urticaria (er tih **KAY** ree ah)
- verruca (ver **ROO** kah)
- vesicle (**VESS** ikl)
- vitiligo (vit ill **EYE** go)
- wheal (**WEEL**)
- xanthoderma (zan thoh **DER** mah)
- xeroderma (zee roh **DER** ma)

Case Study

DERMATOLOGY CONSULTATION REPORT

Reason for Consultation: Evaluate patient for excision of recurrent basal cell carcinoma, left cheek.

History of Present Illness: Patient is a 74-year-old male first seen by his regular physician 5 years ago for persistent facial lesions. Biopsies revealed basal cell carcinoma in two lesions, one on the nasal tip and the other on the left cheek. These were excised and healed with a normal cicatrix. The patient noted that the left cheek lesion returned approximately one year ago. Patient admits to not following his physician's advice to use sunscreen and a hat. The patient reports pruritis and states the lesion is growing larger. Patient has been referred for dermatology evaluation regarding deep excision of the lesion and dermatoplasty.

Past Medical History: Patient's activity level is severely restricted due to congestive heart failure (CHF) with dyspnea, lower extremity edema, and cyanosis. He takes several cardiac medications daily and occasionally requires oxygen by nasal canula. History is negative for other types of cancer.

Results of Physical Exam: Examination revealed a 10 x 14 mm lesion on left cheek 20 mm anterior to the ear. The lesion displays marked erythema and poorly defined borders. The area immediately around the lesion shows de-pigmentation with vesicles. There is a well-healed cicatrix on the nasal tip with no evidence of the neoplasm returning.

Assessment: Even without a biopsy, this is most likely a recurrence of this patient's basal cell carcinoma.

Recommendations: Due to the lesion's size, shape, and reoccurrence, recommend deep excision of the neoplasm through the epidermis and dermis layers. The patient will then require dermatoplasty. The most likely donor site will be the proximal-medial thigh. This patient is at high risk for basal cell carcinoma and should never go outside without sunscreen and a hat. I have discussed the surgical procedure with the patient and he fully understands the procedure, risks, and alternate treatment choices. In light of his cardiac status, if he decides to proceed with the surgery, he will need a thorough workup by his cardiologist.

CRITICAL THINKING QUESTIONS

1. Which of the following symptoms was reported by the patient?

   a. easy bruising

   b. excessive scarring

   c. intense itching

   d. yellow skin

2. In your own words, describe the lesion on the patient's face.

3. What advice did this patient fail to follow? What happened, in part, because he did not follow instructions?

4. This patient has a serious health condition other than his facial lesion. Name that condition and describe it in your own words. What is the abbreviation for this condition? This patient has three symptoms of this condition. List the three symptoms and describe each in your own words. This condition and its symptoms use terminology that has not been introduced yet. You will need to use your text as a reference to answer this question.

   The condition is _____

   The abbreviation for this condition is _____

   The three symptoms are _____

5. What procedure was performed on the original lesion that confirmed the diagnosis? Explain, in your own words, what this procedure involves.

6. Briefly describe, in your own words, the two stages of the surgical procedure the physician recommends.

Chart Note Transcription

Chart Note

The chart note below contains ten phrases that can be reworded with a medical term that you learned in this chapter. Each phrase is identified with an underline. Determine the medical term and write your answers in the space provided.

Current Complaint: A 64-year-old female with an open sore[1] on her right leg is seen by the specialist in treating diseases of the skin.[2]

Past History: Patient states she first noticed an area of pain, severe itching,[3] and redness of the skin[4] just below her right knee about 6 weeks ago. One week later raised spots containing pus[5] appeared. Patient states the raised spots containing pus ruptured and the open sore appeared.

Signs and Symptoms: Patient has a deep open sore 5 × 3 cm. It is 4 cm distal to the knee on the lateral aspect of the right leg. It appears to extend into the middle skin layer,[6] and the edges show signs of tissue death.[7] The open sore has a small amount of drainage but there is no odor. A sample of the drainage that was grown in the lab to identify the microorganism and determine the best antibiotic[8] of the drainage revealed *Staphylococcus* bacteria in the open sore.

Diagnosis: Inflammation of skin cells and tissues.[9]

Treatment: Removal of damaged tissue[10] of the open sore followed by application of an antibiotic cream. Patient was instructed to return to the specialist in treating diseases of the skin's office in two weeks, or sooner if the open sore does not heal, or if it begins draining pus.

1 _____

2 _____

3 _____

4 _____

5 _____

6 _____

7 _____

8 _____

9 _____

10 _____

Practice Exercises

A. STATE THE TERMS DESCRIBED USING THE COMBINING FORMS PROVIDED.

The combining form dermat/o refers to the skin. Use it to write a term that means

1. inflammation of the skin _____
2. any abnormal skin condition _____
3. an instrument for cutting the skin _____
4. white skin _____
5. surgical repair of the skin _____
6. study of the skin _____
7. pertaining to within the skin _____
8. pertaining to under the skin _____
9. pertaining to upon the skin _____

The combining form melan/o means black. Use it to write a term that means

10. a cancerous tumor with black pigmentation _____
11. a black cell _____

The combining form leuk/o means white. Use it to write a term that means

12. white spots on mucous membranes _____
13. white skin _____

The combining form trich/o refers to the hair. Use it to write a term that means

14. a disease of the hair caused by a fungus _____

The combining form onych/o refers to the nail. Use it to write a term that means

15. softening of the nails _____
16. infection around the nail _____
17. nail eating (biting) _____
18. inflammation of the nailbed _____

B. DEFINE THE FOLLOWING COMBINING FORMS.

1. cry/o _____
2. cutane/o _____
3. hist/o _____
4. py/o _____
5. papul/o _____
6. onych/o _____
7. lip/o _____
8. kerat/o _____

C. DEFINE THE FOLLOWING TERMS.

1. integumentary _____
2. melanin _____
3. sebum _____
4. cutaneous membrane _____

5. epidermis _____

6. keratin _____

7. lipoma _____

8. hair follicle _____

D. DESCRIBE THE FOLLOWING TYPES OF BURNS.

1. first degree _____

2. second degree _____

3. third degree _____

E. MATCH THE TERMS IN COLUMN A WITH THE DEFINITIONS IN COLUMN B.

A	B
1. _____ eczema	a. decubitus ulcer
2. _____ nevus	b. lack of skin pigment
3. _____ lipoma	c. hypertrophy of oil glands
4. _____ urticaria	d. thick, leatherlike skin
5. _____ bedsore	e. papules, vesicles, crusts
6. _____ acne rosacea	f. white patches
7. _____ acne vulgaris	g. birthmark
8. _____ leukoplakia	h. excessive hair growth
9. _____ hirsutism	i. death of tissue
10. _____ alopecia	j. fatty tumor
11. _____ gangrene	k. hives
12. _____ scleroderma	l. baldness
13. _____ albinism	m. acne of adolescence

F. MATCH THE TERMS IN COLUMN A WITH THE PROCEDURES IN COLUMN B.

A	B
1. _____ debridement	a. surgical removal of wrinkled skin
2. _____ cauterization	b. instrument to cut thin slices of skin
3. _____ lipectomy	c. removal of fat with suction
4. _____ dermatoplasty	d. surgical removal of fat
5. _____ liposuction	e. skin grafting
6. _____ rhytidectomy	f. removal of lesions with scraper
7. _____ curettage	g. remove skin with brushes
8. _____ dermabrasion	h. remove damaged skin
9. _____ dermatome	i. destruction of tissue with electric current

G. WRITE THE ABBREVIATIONS FOR THE FOLLOWING TERMS.

1. frozen section _____

2. incision and drainage _____

3. intradermal _____

4. subcutaneous _____

5. ultraviolet _____

6. ointment _____

7. biopsy _____

H. USE THE FOLLOWING TERMS IN THE SENTENCES THAT FOLLOW.

cyst	impetigo	malignant melanoma	pustule
fissure	furuncle	petechiae	vesicle
macule	carbuncle	dermis	keloid
nodule	scabies	epidermis	Kaposi's sarcoma
papule	tinea	paronychia	xeroderma
polyp	verruca	pachyderma	shingles

1. The middle layer of the skin is called the _____ .
2. Meyer has a painful eruption of vesicles along a nerve. This condition is called _____ .
3. The winter climates can cause dry skin. The medical term for this is _____ .
4. Kim has experienced small pinpoint purplish spots caused by bleeding under the skin. This is called

   _____ .
5. Janet has a fungal skin disease. This is called _____ .
6. A contagious skin disease caused by a mite is _____ .
7. An infection around the entire nail is called _____ .
8. A form of skin cancer affecting AIDS patients is called _____ .
9. An especially dangerous type of skin cancer caused by an overproduction of melanin is called _____ .
10. Latrivia has an inflammatory skin disease that results in pustules crusting and rupturing. It is called

    _____ .
11. A pus-containing raised spot on the skin is called a _____ .
12. A small, flat, discolored area, such as a freckle, is called a _____ .
13. A small tumor with a pedicle or stem is called a _____ .
14. A solid raised group of cells is called a _____ .
15. A crack or groove in the skin is referred to as a _____ .

I. USE THE FLLOWING PREFIXES TO WRITE A WORD THAT MEANS

epi-	on, upon, over	sub-	under
intra-	within	hypo-	under, below

1. under the skin   _____ or _____
2. within the skin   _____
3. on the surface of the skin _____

Getting Connected

Multimedia Extension Activities

CD-ROM

Use the CD-ROM enclosed with your textbook to gain additional reinforcement through interactive word building exercises, spelling games, labeling activities, and additional quizzes.

www.prenhall.com/fremgen

Use the above address to access the free, interactive Companion Website created for this textbook. Get hints, instant feedback, and textbook references to chapter-related multiple choice questions, and labeling and matching exercises. In addition, you will find an audio glossary, case studies, Internet exploration exercises, flashcards, and a comprehensive exam.

Answers

Case Study (Critical Thinking Questions)

1. c—intense itching (urticaria)   2. translated into student's own words: size of 10 × 14 mm; left cheek 20 mm anterior to the ear; erythema; poorly define borders, depigmentation, vesicles   3. wear sunscreen and a hat
4. congestive heart failure; CHF; dyspnea, lower extremity edema, cyanosis   5. biopsy   6. excision; dermatoplasty

Chart Note

1. ulcer—open sore   2. dermatologist's—specialist in treating diseases of the skin   3. pruritis—severe itching
4. erythema—redness of the skin   5. pustules—raised spots containing pus   6. dermis—middle skin layer
7. necrosis—tissue death   8. culture and sensitivity—sample was grown in the lab to identify the microorganism and determine the best antibiotic   9. cellulitis—inflammation of skin cells and tissue   10. debridement—removal of damaged tissue

Practice Exercises

A. 1. dermatitis   2. dermatosis   3. dermatome   4. leukoderma   5. dermatoplasty   6. dermatology   7. intradermal
8. hypodermal   9. epidermal   10. melanoma   11. melanocyte   12. leukoplakia   13. leukoderma   14. trichomycosis
15. onychomalachia   16. paronychia   17. onychophagia   18. onchitis
B. 1. cold   2. skin   3. tissue   4. pus   5. pimple   6. nail   7. fat   8. horny/hard
C. 1. skin   2. black   3. oil   4. skin   5. outer layer of skin   6. protein, hard   7. fatty tumor   8. hair chamber
D. 1. Redness involving superficial layer of skin.   2. Burn damage through epidermis and into dermis causing vesicles.
3. Burn damage to full thickness of epidermis and dermis.
E. 1. e   2. g   3. j   4. k   5. a   6. c   7. m   8. f   9. h   10. l   11. i   12. d   13. b
F. 1. h   2. i   3. d   4. e   5. c   6. a   7. f   8. g   9. b
G. 1. FS   2. I&D   3. ID   4. subq   5. UV   6. ung   7. BX
H. 1. dermis   2. shingles   3. xeroderma   4. petechiae   5. tinea   6. scabies   7. paronychia   8. Kaposi's sarcoma
9. malignant melanoma   10. impetigo   11. pustule   12. macule   13. polyp   14. nodule   15. fissure
I. 1. hypodermic, or subcutaneous   2. intradermal   3. epidermal

Chapter 4

MUSCULOSKELETAL SYSTEM

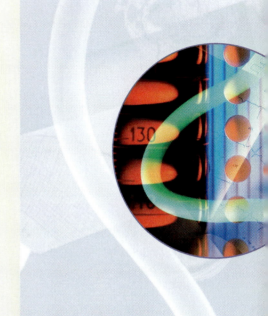

LEARNING OBJECTIVES

Upon completion of this chapter, you will be able to:

- Recognize the combining forms and suffixes introduced in this chapter.

- Gain the ability to pronounce medical terms and major anatomical structures.

- List the major organs of the musculoskeletal system and describe their functions.

- Correctly place bones in either the axial or the appendicular skeleton.

- Recognize the components of a long bone.

- Identify bony projections and depressions.

- Identify the parts of a synovial joint.

- Describe the characteristics of the three types of muscle tissue.

- Distinguish the major muscles of the body.

- Use movement terminology correctly.

- Build musculoskeletal system medical terms from word parts.

- Define vocabulary, pathology, diagnostic, and therapeutic medical terms relating to the musculoskeletal system.

- Interpret abbreviations associated with the musculoskeletal system.

Overview

ORGANS OF THE MUSCULOSKELETAL SYSTEM

bones   muscles

joints

COMBINING FORMS RELATING TO THE MUSCULOSKELETAL SYSTEM

acetabul/o	acetabulum	**maxill/o**	maxilla, upper jawbone
ankyl/o	stiff joint	**metacarp/o**	metacarpus, hand bones
arthr/o	joint	**metatars/o**	metatarsals, foot bones
brachi/o	arm	**muscul/o**	muscle
burs/o	sac	**my/o**	muscle
calc/o	calcium	**myel/o**	bone marrow
calcane/o	calcaneus, heel bone	**olecran/o**	olecranon, bony projection in elbow
carp/o	wrist		
caud/o	tail	**orth/o**	straight
cephal/o	head	**oste/o**	bone
cervic/o	neck	**patell/o**	patella, kneecap
chondr/o	cartilage	**ped/o**	foot
clavicul/o	clavicle, collarbone	**pelv/o**	pelvis
cleid/o	clavicle, collarbone	**phalang/o**	phalanges, bones of fingers and toes
condyl/o	condyle, bony projection		
cost/o	rib	**pub/o**	pubis, part of hipbone
crani/o	head, skull	**radi/o**	radius, lower arm bone
dactyl/o	digit, one finger or toe	**scapul/o**	scapula, shoulder blade
femor/o	femur, thigh bone	**scoli/o**	vertebra, backbone
fibul/o	fibula, smaller outer bone of lower leg	**spondyl/o**	vertebrae, backbone
		stern/o	sternum, breastbone
humer/o	humerus, upper arm bone	**tars/o**	ankle
ili/o	ilium, part of hipbone	**ten/o**	tendon
ischi/o	ischium, part of hipbone	**tend/o**	tendon
kyph/o	hump	**tendin/o**	tendon
lamin/o	lamina, part of vertebra	**tens/o**	stretch
lord/o	swayback, curve	**thorac/o**	chest
lumb/o	loin, lower back	**tibi/o**	tibia, inner bone of lower leg
malleol/o	malleolus, ankle process	**uln/o**	ulna, lower arm
mandibul/o	mandible, jawbone	**vertebr/o**	vertebra, backbone

SUFFIXES RELATING TO THE MUSCULOSKELETAL SYSTEM

Suffix	Meaning	Example
-blast	immature, embryonic	osteoblast
-clasia	to surgically break	osteoclasia
-desis	stabilize, fuse	arthrodesis
-kinesia	movement	bradykinesia
-malacia	softening	osteomalacia
-physis	to grow	epiphysis
-plasty	surgical repair	arthroplasty
-porosis	porous	osteoporosis
-scopy	procedure to visually examine	arthroscopy

ANATOMY AND PHYSIOLOGY OF THE MUSCULOSKELETAL SYSTEM

BONES

appendicular skeleton

axial skeleton

The human body contains 206 bones (see Figure 4.1). Each bone is a unique organ that carries its own blood supply, nerves, and lymphatic system.

All the bones form the skeleton, which serves as the body's frame, protects vital organs, and works together with muscles to produce movement. In fact, the bone must have muscles attached to it for movement to take place. The human skeleton has two divisions: the **axial** (**AK** see al) **skeleton** and the **appendicular** (app en **DIK** yoo lar) **skeleton.** Figures 4.2 and 4.3 illustrate the axial and appendicular skeleton. See Table 4.1 for a listing of the main divisions of the skeleton.

Axial Skeleton

cervical vertebrae	lacrimal	palatine	temporal
coccyx	lumbar vertebrae	parietal	thoracic vertebrae
cranium	mandible	rib cage	vertebral column
ethmoid	maxilla	sacrum	vomer
frontal	nasal	sphenoid	zygomatic
hyoid	occipital	sternum	

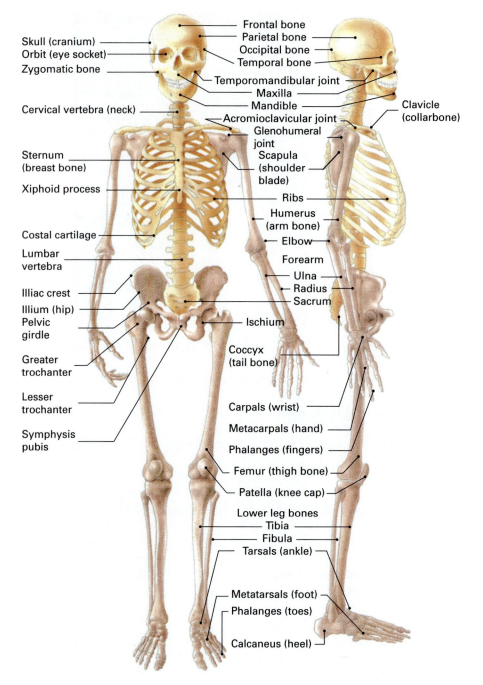

FIGURE 4.1 The human skeleton.

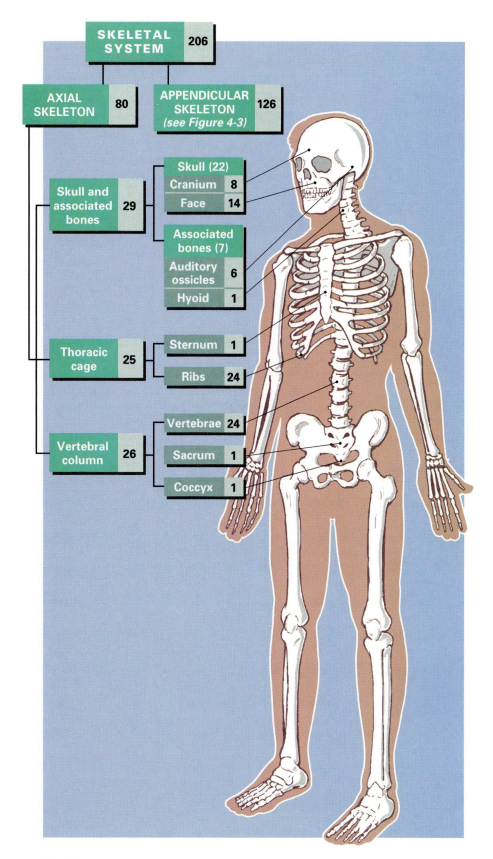

FIGURE 4.2 The axial skeleton.

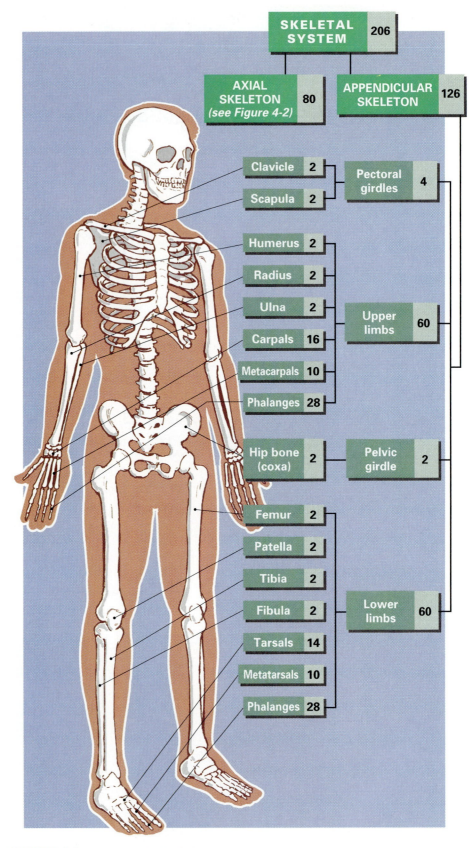

FIGURE 4.3 The appendicular skeleton.

Table 4.1	Division of the Skeleton (total 206 bones)	
Axial skeleton (total 80 bones)		
Skull	Cranium	
	Ear bones	
	Facial bones	
Spinal column	Vertebra	
Thorax	Ribs	
	Sternum	
Appendicular skeleton (total 126 bones)		
Lower extremities (LE)	Hip girdle	
	Legs	
	Ankles	
	Feet	
Upper extremities (UE)	Shoulder girdle	
	Arms	
	Wrists	
	Hands	

The axial skeleton includes the bones in the head, spine, chest, and trunk of the body. The head or skull is divided into two parts consisting of the cranium and facial bones. The cranial bones consist of the **frontal, parietal** (pah **RYE** eh tal), **temporal** (**TEM** por al), **ethmoid** (**ETH** moyd), **sphenoid** (**SFEE** noyd), and **occipital** (ock **SIP** eh tal) bones. The facial bones are the **mandible** (**MAN** dih bl), **maxilla** (mack **SIH** lah), **zygomatic** (zeye go **MAT** ik), **vomer** (**VOH** mer), **palatine** (**PAL** ah tine), **hyoid** (**HIGH** oyd), and small **nasal** (**NAY** sl) and **lacrimal** (**LACK** rim al) bones. The cranial and facial bones are illustrated in Figure 4.4 and described in Tables 4.2 and 4.3.

FIGURE 4.4 The cranial and facial bones.

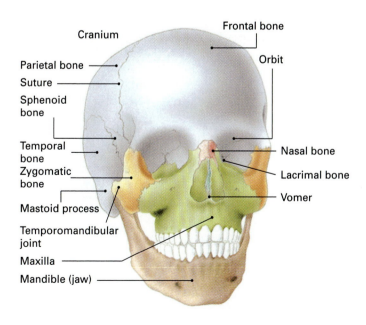

Table 4.2	Cranial Bones	
Name	**Number**	**Description**
Frontal	1	Forehead
Parietal	2	Upper sides of cranium and roof of skull
Occipital	1	Back and base of skull
Temporal	2	Sides and base of cranium
Sphenoid	1	Bat-shaped bone that forms part of the base of the skull, floor, and sides of eye orbit
Ethmoid	1	Forms part of eye orbit, nose, and floor of cranium

Table 4.3	Facial Bones	
Name	**Number**	**Description**
Lacrimal	2	Inner corner of each eye
Nasal	2	Form part of nasal septum and support bridge of nose
Maxilla	2	Upper jaw
Mandible	1	Lower jawbone; only movable bone of the skull
Zygomatic	2	Cheekbones
Vomer	1	Base of nasal septum
Palatine	1	Hard palate (PAH lat) of mouth and floor of the nose
Hyoid	1	Separate from skull between mandible and larynx

The **cranium (KRAY** nee um) is the protective portion of the skull that covers the brain. The cranial and facial bones protect the brain and special sense organs from injury. Muscles for chewing and head movements are attached to the cranial bones. The cranial bones come together at joints called sutures. The actual cranial joint mark resembles a suture or stitch line.

The hyoid bone is a single U-shaped bone suspended in the neck between the mandible and larynx. It is a point of attachment for swallowing and speech muscles.

The trunk of the body consists of the **vertebral (VER** teh bral) **column, sternum (STER** num), and **rib cage.** The vertebral or spinal column can be divided into five sections: **cervical vertebrae (SER** vih kal **VER** teh bray), **thoracic vertebrae** (tho **RASS** ik **VER** teh bray), **lumbar vertebrae (LUM** bar **VER** teh bray), **sacrum (SAY**

Table 4.4	*Bones of the Vertebral/Spinal Column*	
Name	**Number**	**Description**
Cervical vertebra	7	First bones in the neck region
Thoracic vertebra	12	Next bones with ribs attached
Lumbar vertebra	5	Next bones after thoracic; located in the small of the back
Sacrum	1	Five separate bones in the child that become fused into one in the adult
Coccyx	1	Three to five bones in the child that become fused into one in the adult

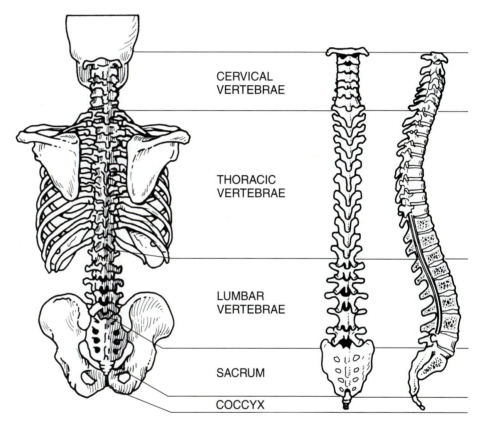

CERVICAL
VERTEBRAE

THORACIC
VERTEBRAE

LUMBAR
VERTEBRAE

SACRUM

COCCYX

FIGURE 4.5 The spinal column.

crum), and **coccyx** (**COCK** six) (see Table 4.4 and Figure 4.5). The rib cage has 12 pairs of ribs attached at the back to the vertebral or spinal column. Ten of the pairs are also attached to the breastbone or sternum in the front (see Figure 4.6). The remaining two pairs are called floating ribs and are attached only to the vertebral column. The rib cage serves to provide support for other organs, such as the heart and lungs.

FIGURE 4.6   The rib cage.

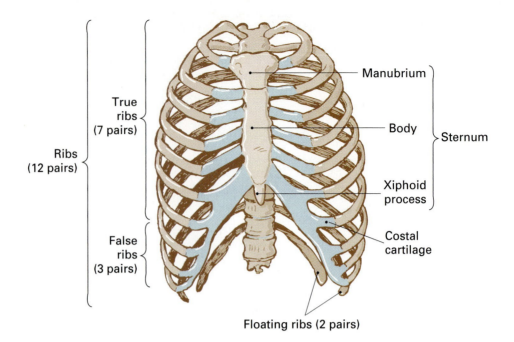

True ribs (7 pairs)

Ribs (12 pairs)

False ribs (3 pairs)

Manubrium

Body

Xiphoid process

Costal cartilage

Sternum

Floating ribs (2 pairs)

Table 4.5	Bones in the Upper Extremities	
Name	**Number**	**Description**
Clavicle	2	Collar bone
Scapula	2	Shoulder blade
Humerus	2	Upper arm bone
Radius	2	Bone on thumb side of lower arm
Ulna	2	Bone on little finger side of lower arm
Carpal	16	Bones of wrist
Metacarpals	10	Bones in palm of hand
Phalanges	28	Finger bones; three in each finger and two in each thumb

Appendicular Skeleton

acetabulum	**ilium**	**os coxae**	**tarsals**
carpals	**innominate bone**	**patella**	**tibia**
clavicle	**ischium**	**phalanges**	**ulna**
femur	**metacarpals**	**pubis**	
fibula	**metatarsals**	**radius**	
humerus	**olecranon process**	**scapula**	

The appendicular skeleton consists of the upper and lower extremities, shoulder, and pelvis (see Figure 4.3). The upper extremities include the **clavicle** (**CLAV** ih kl), **scapula** (**SKAP** yoo lah), **humerus** (**HYOO** mer us), **ulna** (**UHL** nah), **radius** (**RAY** dee us), **carpals** (**CAR** pals), **metacarpals** (met ah **CAR** pals), and **phalanges** (fah **LAN** jeez). The bones are listed in Table 4.5 and illustrated in Figure 4.7.

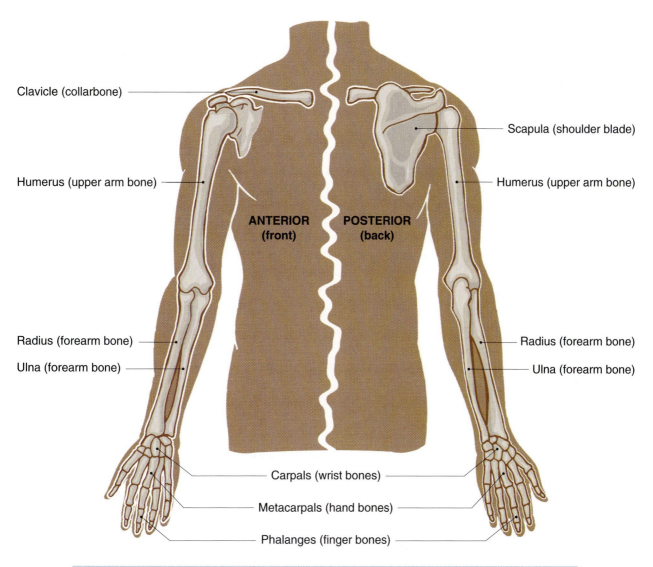

Clavicle (collarbone)

Scapula (shoulder blade)

Humerus (upper arm bone)

Humerus (upper arm bone)

ANTERIOR (front)

POSTERIOR (back)

Radius (forearm bone)

Radius (forearm bone)

Ulna (forearm bone)

Ulna (forearm bone)

Carpals (wrist bones)

Metacarpals (hand bones)

Phalanges (finger bones)

THE UPPER EXTREMITIES

COMMON NAME	ANATOMICAL NAME
Shoulder girdle	Pectoral girdle: clavicle, scapula, and head of humerus
Collarbone (1/side)	Clavicle
Shoulder blade (1/side)	Scapula
Arm bone (1/limb, from shoulder to elbow)	Humerus
Forearm bones (2/limb, from elbow to wrist: 1/medial, 1/lateral)	Ulna – medial Radius – lateral
Wrist bones (8/wrist)	Carpals
Hand bones (5/palm, palm bones)	Metacarpals
Finger bones (14/hand)	Phalanges

FIGURE 4.7 Bones of the upper extremities.

The elbow is commonly referred to as the *funny bone*. It is actually a projection of the ulna bone called the **olecranon** (oh **LEK** ran on) **process.**

The lower extremities include the **os coxae (OSS KOK** sigh), **femur (FEE** mer), **patella** (pah **TELL** ah), **tibia (TIB** ee ah), **fibula (FIB** yoo lah), **tarsals (TAHR** sals), **metatarsals** (met ah **TAR** sals), and **phalanges** (fah **LAN** jeez). They are illustrated in Figure 4.8.

The os coxae is also known as the **innominate** (ih **NOM** ih nayt) **bone** or hipbone. It contains the **ilium (ILL** ee um), **ischium (ISS** kee um), and **pubis (PYOO** bis). It unites with the sacrum and coccyx to form the pelvis. The os coxae is illustrated in Figure 4.9.

The term girdle, meaning something that encircles or confines, refers to the entire bony structure of the shoulder and the pelvis. Therefore, if just one bone from these two areas is being discussed, such as the ilium of the pelvis, it would be named. If the entire pelvis is being discussed, it would be called the pelvic girdle.

The **femur** is the strongest bone in the body. The head of the femur fits into the **acetabulum** (ass eh **TAB** yoo lum), which is the large cup-shaped cavity formed by the juncture of the ilium, ischium, and pubis. This is the site where hip fractures are common or damage from osteoporosis takes place. **Total hip replacements** (THRs) have become quite common and successful.

The bones in the lower extremities are listed in Table 4.6.

It is easier to remember the extremity bones when you note that the bones in the arms and legs are almost identical in number and placement. Although it is easier to see the similarity between the fingers and toes, even the ankle and wrist bones have common functions of movement and support.

Bone Structure

cancellous bone	epiphysis	ossification	short bones
cartilaginous tissue	flat bones	osteoblasts	spongy bone
compact bone	irregular bones	osteocytes	yellow bone marrow
cortical bone	long bones	periosteum	
diaphysis	osseous tissue	red bone marrow	

Bone, called **osseous (OSS** ee us) **tissue,** is actually one of the hardest materials in the body. Bones are formed from a gradual process beginning before birth called **ossification** (oss ih fih **KAY** shun). The fetal skeleton is formed from **cartilaginous** (car tih **LAJ** ih nus) **tissue.** This flexible tissue is gradually replaced by **osteoblasts** (**OSS** tee oh blasts), immature bone cells. In adult bone, the osteoblasts have matured into **osteocytes (OSS** tee oh sights). The formation of strong bones is greatly dependent on an adequate supply of minerals.

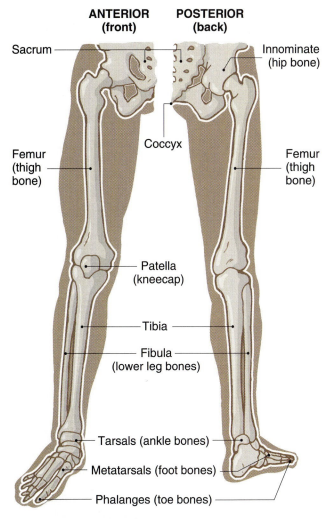

ANTERIOR (front) — POSTERIOR (back)

Sacrum

Innominate (hip bone)

Coccyx

Femur (thigh bone)

Femur (thigh bone)

Patella (kneecap)

Tibia

Fibula (lower leg bones)

Tarsals (ankle bones)

Metatarsals (foot bones)

Phalanges (toe bones)

THE LOWER EXTREMITIES

COMMON NAME	ANATOMICAL NAME
Pelvic girdle (pelvis or hips)	Innominate on each side made up of the fused ilium, ischium, and pubis bones, as well as sacrum and coccyx posteriorly
Thigh bone (1/limb)	Femur
Kneecap (1/limb)	Patella
Leg bones (shin bones, 2/leg, 1 medial, 1 lateral)	Tibia – medial Fibula – lateral
Ankle bones (7/foot)	Tarsals
Foot bones (5/foot)	Metatarsals
Toe bones (14/foot. Some people have two bones in their little toe, others may have three.)	Phalanges

FIGURE 4.8 Bones of the lower extremities.

FIGURE 4.9 The pelvis: (A) anterior view of os coxae; (B) posterior view of os coxae.

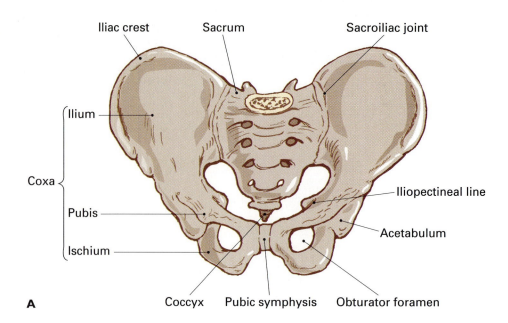

Iliac crest   Sacrum   Sacroiliac joint

Ilium

Coxa

Pubis

Ischium

Iliopectineal line

Acetabulum

A

Coccyx   Pubic symphysis   Obturator foramen

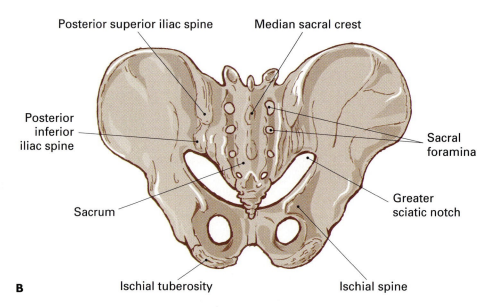

Posterior superior iliac spine   Median sacral crest

Posterior inferior iliac spine

Sacral foramina

Sacrum

Greater sciatic notch

B

Ischial tuberosity   Ischial spine

Table 4.6	Bones in the Lower Extremities	
Name	**Number**	**Description**
Os coxae	2	Hipbone (ilium, ischium, pubis)
Femur	2	Upper leg bone; thigh bone
Patella	2	Knee cap
Tibia	2	Shin bone; thicker lower leg bone
Fibula	2	Thinner, long bone in lateral side of lower leg
Tarsals	14	Ankle and heel bones
Metatarsals	10	Foot bones
Phalanges	28	Toe bones: three in each toe and two in each great toe

FIGURE 4.10
Composition of bone.

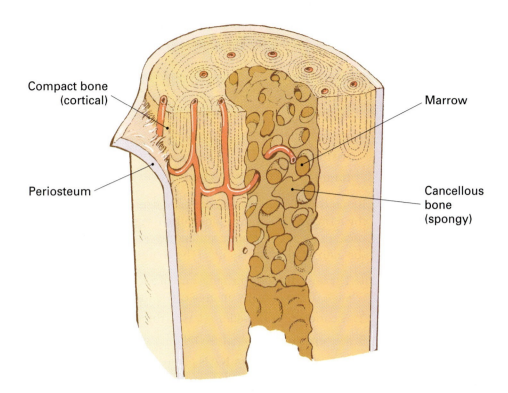

The major components of bone are the **diaphysis** (dye **AFF** ih sis) or middle shaft of a long bone, and the **epiphysis** (eh **PIFF** ih sis) or wide end of a long bone. Most bones are covered with a membrane called **periosteum** (pair ee **AH** stee um), which contains numerous nerves and lymphatic vessels. The hard exterior surface of bone is called **cortical** (**KOR** ti kal) or **compact bone. Cancellous** (**CAN** sell us) or **spongy bone** is found inside the bone. The spaces within cancellous bone contain both red and yellow bone marrow. **Red bone marrow** manufactures most of the blood cells and is found in some parts of all bones. The **yellow bone marrow** is located mainly in the center of the long bones and contains mainly fat cells. Figure 4.10 contains an illustration of bone composition.

There are several different types of bones found throughout the body. They basically fall into four categories: **long bones, short bones, flat bones,** and **irregular bones** (see Figure 4.11). Long bones are the thigh, lower leg bones, and arm bones. Short and

FIGURE 4.11
Classification of bones.

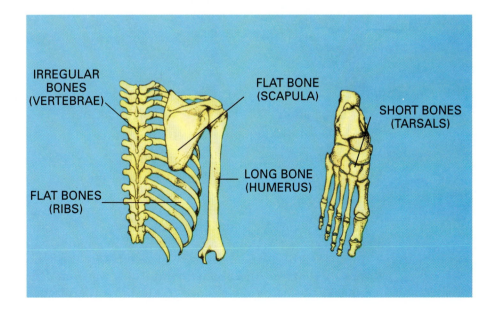

irregular bones are found in the wrist, ankle, and vertebra. Flat bones cover the soft body parts and include the ribs, shoulder bones, and pelvic bones.

Bone Projections and Depressions

condyle	fossa	trochanter
epicondyle	head	tubercle
fissure	process	tuberosity
foramen	sinus	

Bones contain many projections and depressions that allow muscles to attach. Generally, the term **process** is used when discussing bony projections. These terms are commonly used on operative reports and in physicians' records for clear identification of areas on the individual bones. Some of the common bony processes include the following:

1. The bone **head** is the large end of a long bone. It may be separated from the body or shaft of the bone by an area called the neck.
2. A **condyle** (**KON** dile) refers to the rounded portion at the end of a bone.
3. The **epicondyle** (ep ih **KON** dile) is a projection located above or on a condyle.
4. The **trochanter** (tro **KAN** ter) refers to the large blunt process on the femur for the attachment of a muscle.
5. A **tubercle** (**TOO** ber kl) is a small, rounded process that provides the attachment for tendons and muscles.
6. The **tuberosity** (too ber **OSS** ih tee) is the large, rounded process that provides the attachment of tendons and muscles.

See Figure 4.12 for an illustration of the processes on the femur.

In addition, there are hollow regions or depressions in bones that allow one bone to join another for the transport of nerves and blood vessels. The most common depressions are as follows:

1. A **sinus** (**SIGH** nus), which is a hollow cavity within a bone.
2. A **foramen** (for **AY** men), which is a smooth passage or opening for nerves and blood vessels.
3. A **fossa** (**FOSS** ah), which consists of a shallow cavity or depression within or on a bone.
4. A **fissure** (**FISH** er), which is a deep groove or slit-type opening.

JOINTS

articulation	**cartilaginous joints**	**sutures**
ball-and-socket joint	**fibrous joints**	**synovial fluid**
bursa	**ligaments**	**synovial joint**
bursitis	**prepatellar bursitis**	**synovial membrane**
cartilage	**pubic symphysis**	

Joints are formed when two or more bones meet. This is also referred to as **articulation** (ar tik yoo **LAY** shun). Most joints are freely moving **synovial** (sin **OH** vee al) **joints** and have a lubricating fluid secreted by the **synovial membrane** (sin **OH** vee al **MEM** brayn) called **synovial fluid.** The ends of bones in a synovial joint are covered by a layer of **cartilage** (**CAR** tih lij). Cartilage is very tough, but still flexi-

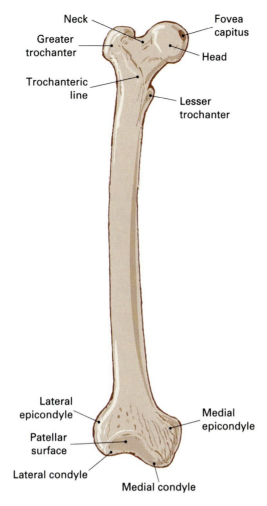

Neck
Fovea capitus
Greater trochanter
Head
Trochanteric line
Lesser trochanter

Lateral epicondyle
Medial epicondyle
Patellar surface
Lateral condyle
Medial condyle

FIGURE 4.12 Processes of the femur.

ble. It can withstand high levels of stress. It acts as a shock absorber for the joint and prevents bone from rubbing against bone. Cartilage is found in several other areas of the body, such as the nasal septum, external ear, eustachian tube, larynx, trachea, bronchi, and invertebral discs. One example of a synovial joint is the **ball-and-socket joint,** which is found at the shoulder and hip. The ball rotating in the socket allows for a wide range of motion. Bands of connective tissue called **ligaments** (**LIG** ah ments) bind bones together at the joint. Ligaments can also assist or limit motion.

Some joints contain a **bursa** (**BER** sah), which is a saclike cavity found in connecting tissue that protects moving parts from friction. It is also lined with synovial membrane. Some common bursal locations are the elbow, knee, and shoulder joints.

MED TERM *TIP*

Bursitis (bur **SIGH** tis) is an inflammation of the bursa located between bony prominences such as at the shoulder. Housemaid's knee is a form of bursitis and carries the medical name **prepatellar bursitis** (pre pah **TELL** er bur **SIGH** tis). The term is thought to have originated from the damage to the knees that occurred when maids knelt to scrub floors.

Not all joints are freely moving. **Fibrous (FYE** bruss) **joints** allow almost no movement since they do not contain synovial fluid and because the ends of the bones are joined together by thick fibrous tissue. The **sutures (SOO** chers) of the skull are an example of a fibrous joint. **Cartilaginous** (car tih **LAJ** ih nus) **joints** allow for slight movement but hold bones firmly in place by a solid piece of cartilage. An example of this type of joint is the **pubic symphysis (PYOO** bik **SIM** fih sis), the point at which the left and right pelvic bones meet in the front of the lower abdomen.

MUSCLES

adductor longus	gluteus maximus	skeletal muscle
biceps	myocardium	smooth muscle
cardiac muscle	rectus abdominis	tendon
fascia		

Muscles are bundles of parallel muscle tissue fibers. As these fibers contract (shorten in length) they pull whatever they are attached to together. This may move two bones closer together or make an opening narrower. A muscle contraction occurs when a message is transmitted from the brain through the nervous system to the muscles.

Three basic types of muscle tissue are **skeletal (SKELL** eh tal), **smooth,** and **cardiac (CAR** dee ak) (see Figure 4.13). These muscle tissues are either voluntary or

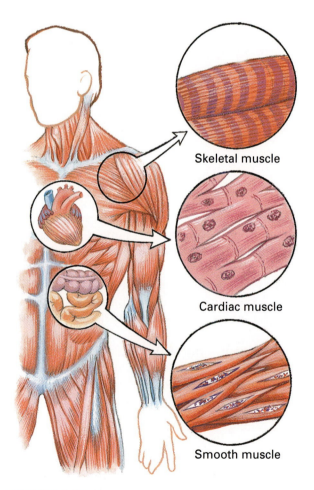

Skeletal muscle

Cardiac muscle

Smooth muscle

FIGURE 4.13   Types of muscles.

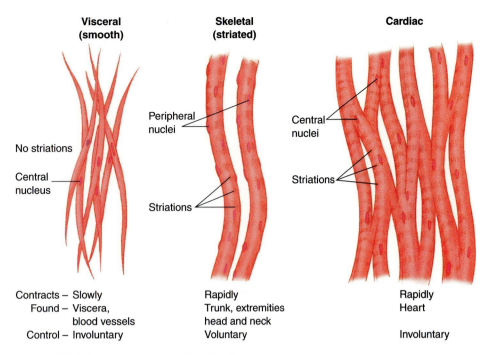

Visceral (smooth)	Skeletal (striated)	Cardiac

No striations

Central nucleus

Peripheral nuclei

Striations

Central nuclei

Striations

Contracts – Slowly	Rapidly	Rapidly
Found – Viscera, blood vessels	Trunk, extremities head and neck	Heart
Control – Involuntary	Voluntary	Involuntary

FIGURE 4.14 Characteristics of muscle tissue.

involuntary. Voluntary muscle tissue allows the person to dictate the function. **Skeletal muscle** is an example of this type of muscle. Involuntary muscles generally act without any direction from the person. Smooth and cardiac muscles are examples of involuntary muscle tissue (see Figure 4.14).

Skeletal muscle is attached to the skeletal bones and allows for voluntary movement that the person can command. These muscles are wrapped in layers of connective tissue called **fascia** (**FASH** ee ah). The fascia covering tapers at each end of a skeletal muscle to form a very strong **tendon** (**TEN** dun). The tendon then inserts into the periosteum covering a bone to attach the muscle to the bone. The skeletal muscles are stimulated by motor neurons of the nervous system.

The human body has more than 400 skeletal muscles, which accounts for almost 50 percent of the body weight.

Smooth muscle tissue is found in the walls of the hollow organs, such as the stomach, and the walls of ducts and blood vessels. It is responsible for the involuntary muscle action associated with digestion and respiration.

Cardiac muscle, or **myocardium** (my oh **CAR** dee um), occurs in the walls of the heart and allows for the involuntary action of the heart's pumping action. See Figure 4.15 for an illustration of the most commonly discussed muscles.

FIGURE 4.15   Muscles: anterior view.

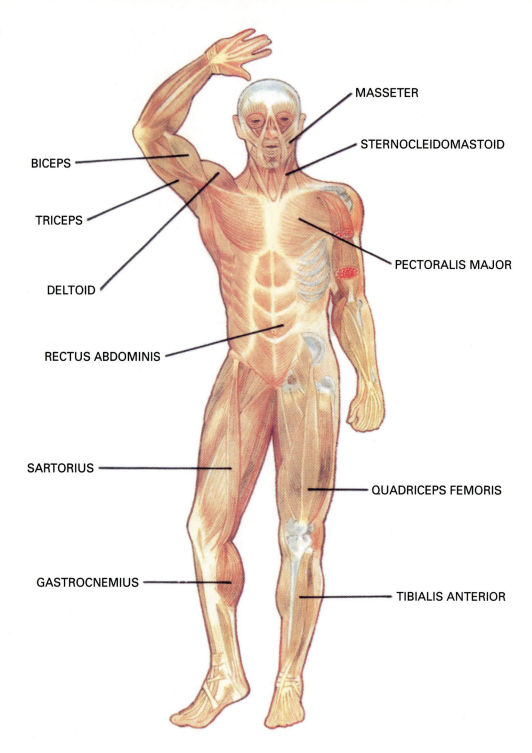

MASSETER

STERNOCLEIDOMASTOID

BICEPS

TRICEPS

PECTORALIS MAJOR

DELTOID

RECTUS ABDOMINIS

SARTORIUS

QUADRICEPS FEMORIS

GASTROCNEMIUS

TIBIALIS ANTERIOR

Terminology for Movement Produced by Muscles

Some common terminology for movement produced by muscles is as follows:

abduction (ab DUCK shun)	Movement away from midline of the body (see Figure 4.16).
adduction (ah DUCK shun)	Movement toward midline of the body (see Figure 4.17).
circumduction (sir kum DUCK shun)	Movement in a circular direction from a central point.
dorsiflexion (dor see FLEK shun)	Backward bending, as of hand or foot. (see Figure 4.18).

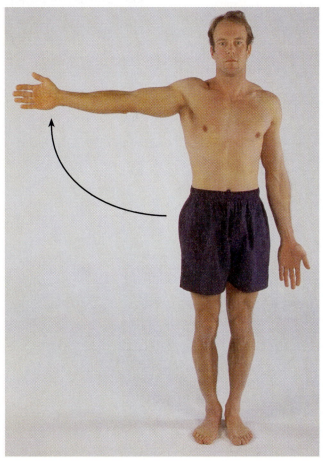

FIGURE 4.16   Abduction.

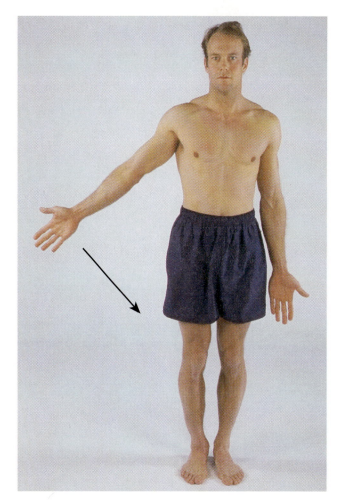

FIGURE 4.17   Adduction.

FIGURE 4.18   Dorsiflexion of toes.

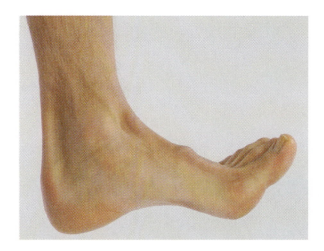

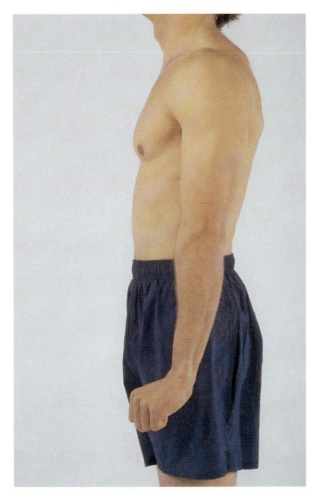

FIGURE 4.19   Extension of left arm.

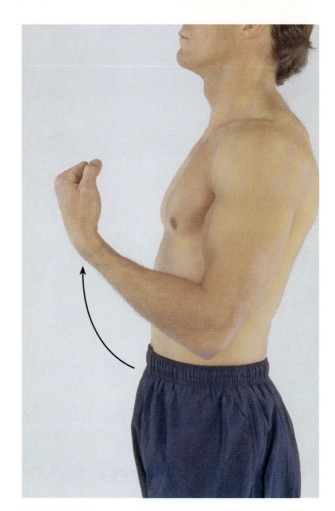

FIGURE 4.20   Flexion of left forearm.

eversion (ee VER zhun)	Turning outward.
extension (eks TEN shun)	Movement that brings limb into or toward a straight condition (see Figure 4.19).
flexion	Act of bending or being bent (see Figure 4.20).
inversion (in VER zhun)	Turning inward.
opposition	Moving thumb away from palm; the ability to move the thumb into contact with the other fingers.
plantar flexion (PLAN tar FLEK shun)	Bending sole of foot; pointing toes downward (see Figure 4.21).

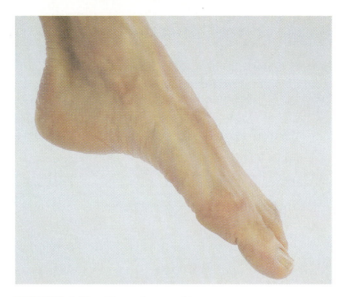

FIGURE 4.21 Plantar flexion of foot.

pronation (proh NAY shun)	To turn downward or backward as with the hand or foot.
rotation (roh TAY shun)	Moving around a central axis.
supination (soo pin NAY shun)	Turning the palm or foot upward.

MED TERM TIP

Muscles are generally named by their location, size, direction of fibers, or number of attachment points, as the following examples illustrate.

- Location: The term **rectus abdominis** (**REK** tus ab **DOM** ih nus) means straight (rectus) abdominal muscle.
- Size: When gluteus, meaning rump area, is combined with maximus, meaning large, we have the term **gluteus maximus** (**GLOO** tee us **MACKS** ih mus). This large muscle on the buttock area is the site generally used for the administration of intramuscular (IM) injections.
- Direction of fibers: The **adductor** (ad **DUCK** tor) **longus** is the long thigh muscle responsible for adduction.
- Number of attachment points: The term bi, meaning two, can form the medical term **biceps** (**BYE** seps), which stands for the muscle in the upper arm that has two heads or connecting points.

Word Building Relating to the Musculoskeletal System

The following list contains examples of medical terms built directly from word parts. The definition for these terms can be determined by a straightforward translation of the word parts.

Combining Form	Combined With	Medical Term	Definition
ankyl/o	-osis	ankylosis (ang kih **LOH** sis)	abnormal condition of stiffness
arthr/o	-algia	arthralgia (ar **THRAL** jee ah)	joint pain
	-centesis	arthrocentesis (ar thro sen **TEE** sis)	puncture to withdraw fluid from a joint
	-clasia	arthroclasia (ar throh **KLAY** see ah)	surgically breaking a joint
	-desis	arthrodesis (ar throh **DEE** sis)	fusion of a joint
	-itis	arthritis (ar **THRY** tis)	joint inflammation
	-otomy	arthrotomy (ar **THROT** oh mee)	incision into a joint
	-plasty	arthroplasty (**AR** throh plas tee)	surgical repair of a joint
	-scopy	arthroscopy (ar **THROS** koh pee)	visual examination of inside a joint
burs/o	-ectomy	bursectomy (ber **SEK** toh mee)	excision of a bursa
	-itis	bursitis (ber **SIGH** tis)	inflammation of a bursa
	-lith	bursolith (**BER** soh lith)	stone in a bursa
chondr/o	-ectomy	chondrectomy (kon **DREK** toh mee)	excision of cartilage
	-malacia	chondromalacia (kon droh mah **LAY** she ah)	cartilage softening
	-plasty	chondroplasty (**KON** droh plas tee)	surgical repair of cartilage
crani/o	intra- -al	intracranial (in trah **KRAY** nee al)	pertaining to inside the skull
	-otomy	craniotomy (kray nee **OTT** oh mee)	incision into the skull
	-plasty	cranioplasty (**KRAY** nee oh plas tee)	surgical repair of the skull
kyph/o	-osis	kyphosis (ki **FOH** sis)	abnormal condition of hump
lord/o	-osis	lordosis (lor **DOH** sis)	abnormal condition of swayback
my/o	electr/o -gram	electromyogram (ee lek troh **MY** oh gram) (EMG)	record of muscle electricity
	-pathy	myopathy (my **OPP** ah thee)	muscle disease

	-plasty	myoplasty (**MY** oh plas tee)	surgical repair of muscle
	poly- -itis	polymyositis (pol ee my oh **SIGH** tis)	inflammation of many muscles
	-rrhaphy	myorrhaphy (**MY** or ah fee)	suture a muscle
myel/o	-oma	myeloma (my ah **LOH** mah)	bone marrow tumor
oste/o	-blast	osteoblast (**OSS** tee oh blast)	embryonic bone cell
	carcin/o -oma	osteocarcinoma (oss tee oh kar sin **OH** mah)	cancerous bone tumor
	-clasia	osteoclasia (oss tee oh **KLAY** see ah)	to surgically break a bone
	-malacia	osteomalacia (oss tee oh mah **LAY** she ah)	bone softening
	myel/o -itis	osteomyelitis (oss tee oh mi ell **EYE** tis)	inflammation of bone and bone marrow
	-otomy	osteotomy (oss tee **OTT** ah me)	incision into a bone
	-pathy	osteopathy (oss tee **OPP** ah thee)	bone disease
	-porosis	osteoporosis (oss tee oh por **ROH** sis)	abnormal condition of porous bones
	-tome	osteotome (**OSS** tee oh tohm)	instrument to cut bone
scapul/o	sub- -ar	subscapular (sub **SCAP** yoo lar)	pertaining to under the shoulder blade
ten/o	-dynia	tenodynia (ten oh **DIN** ee ah)	tendon pain
	-rrhaphy	tenorrhaphy (tah **NOR** ah fee)	suture a tendon
vertebr/o	inter- -al	intervertebral (in ter **VER** teh bral)	pertaining to between vertebrae

Suffix	Combined With Prefix	Medical Term	Definition
-kinesia	brady-	bradykinesia (brad ee kih **NEE** see ah)	slow movement
	dys-	dyskinesia (dis kih **NEE** see ah)	difficult or painful movement
	hyper-	hyperkinesia (high per kih **NEE** see ah)	excessive movement
-trophy	a-	atrophy (**AT** rah fee)	lack of development
	dys-	dystrophy (**DIS** troh fee)	difficult (poor) development
	hyper-	hypertrophy (high **PER** troh fee)	excessive development

Vocabulary Relating to the Musculoskeletal System

chiropodist (kye ROPP ah dist)	Specialist in treating disorders of the feet. More modern term is podiatrist.
chiropractic (kye roh PRAK tik)	Practice of treating patients using manipulation of the vertebral column.
myopathy (my OPP ah thee)	Any disease of muscles.
orthopedics (or thoh PEE diks)	Branch of medicine specializing in the diagnosis and treatment of conditions of the musculoskeletal system.
orthopedist (or thoh PEE dist)	Physician who specializes in treatment of conditions of the musculoskeletal system.
orthotics (or THOT iks)	Fitting of orthopedic appliances used to prevent or correct deformities.
orthotist (or THOT ist)	Person skilled in orthotics.
ossification (oss sih fih KAY shun)	Bone formation.
osteopath (OSS tee oh path)	Physician who specializes in osteopathy. This physician would use the initials D.O.
osteopathy (oss tee OPP ah thee)	Form of medicine that places great emphasis on the musculoskeletal system and the body system as a whole. Manipulation is also used as part of the treatment.
physiatrist (fiz ee AT rist)	Physician specializing in rehabilitation or physical medicine.
podiatrist (po DYE ah trist)	Specialist in treating disorders of the feet.
prosthesis (pross THEE sis)	Artificial device that is used as a substitute for a body part that is either congenitally missing or is absent as a result of accident or disease (for instance, an artificial leg or hip).
prosthetist (PROSS thah tist)	Person who fabricates and fits prostheses.
rigor mortis (RIG ur MOR tis)	Stiffness of skeletal muscles that is seen in death.

Pathology of the Musculoskeletal System

arthritis (ar THRY tis)	Inflammation of the bone joints (see Figure 4.22).
bunion (BUN yun)	Inflammation of the bursa of the great toe.
bursitis (ber SIGH tis)	Inflammation of the bursa.
carpal tunnel syndrome (CTS) (CAR pal TUN el SIN drohm)	Pain caused by compression of the nerve as it passes between the bones and tendons of the wrist.
gout (GOWT)	Inflammation of the joints caused by excessive uric acid.
kyphosis (ki FOH sis)	Abnormal increase in the outward curvature of the thoracic spine. Also known as *hunchback* or *humpback*. See Figure 4.23 for an illustration of abnormal spine curvatures.
lordosis (lor DOH sis)	Abnormal increase in the forward curvature of the lumbar spine. Also known as *swayback*. See Figure 4.23 for an illustration of abnormal spine curvatures.
muscular dystrophy (MUSS kew ler DIS troh fee)	Inherited disease causing a progressive muscle weakness and atrophy.

myasthenia gravis (my ass THEE nee ah GRAV is)	Disorder causing loss of muscle strength and paralysis. This is an autoimmune disease.
osteoarthritis (oss tee oh ar THRY tis)	Noninflammatory type of arthritis resulting in degeneration of the bones and joints, especially those bearing weight.
osteomalacia (oss tee oh mah LAY she ah)	Softening of the bones caused by a deficiency of phosphorus or calcium. It is thought that in children the cause is insufficient sunlight and vitamin D.
osteomyelitis (oss tee oh my ell EYE tis)	Inflammation of the bone and bone marrow due to infection; can be difficult to treat.
osteoporosis (oss tee oh por ROH sis)	Decrease in bone mass that results in a thinning and weakening of the bone with resulting fractures. The bone becomes more porous, especially in the spine and pelvis.
Paget's (PAH jets) disease	A fairly common metabolic disease of the bone from unknown causes. It usually attacks middle-aged and elderly people and is characterized by bone destruction and deformity. Named for Sir James Paget, a British surgeon.
polymyositis (pol ee my oh SIGH tis)	Disease causing muscle inflammation and weakness from an unknown cause.
rheumatoid arthritis (ROO mah toyd ar THRY tis) (RA)	Chronic form of arthritis with inflammation of the joints, swelling, stiffness, pain, and changes in the cartilage that can result in crippling deformities (see Figure 4.24).
rickets (RIK ets)	Deficiency in calcium and vitamin D found in early childhood that results in bone deformities, especially bowed legs.
ruptured intervertebral (in ter VER tee bral) **disk**	Herniation or outpouching of a disk between two vertebrae—also called *herniated disk*. May require surgery.
scoliosis (skoh lee OH sis)	Abnormal lateral curvature of the spine. See Figure 4.23 for an illustration of abnormal spine curvatures.
spinal stenosis (ste NOH sis)	Narrowing of the spinal canal causing pressure on the cord and nerves.
supernumerary bone (soo per NOO mer ar ee)	Extra bone, generally a finger or toe, found in newborns.
systemic lupus erythematosus (sis TEM ik LOOP us air ih them ah TOH sis) (SLE)	Chronic inflammatory disease of connective tissue that causes injury to the joints, skin, kidneys, heart, lungs, and nervous system. A characteristic butterfly rash or erythema may be present.
talipes (TAL ih peez)	Congenital deformity of the foot. Also referred to as a *clubfoot*. The variations are:
equinus (eh KWI nus)	Only the front of the foot touches the ground, causing the person to walk on their toes.
planus (PLAY nus)	The arch is broken, causing the entire foot to be flat on the ground.
valgus (VAL gus)	The foot is everted, with the inner side of the foot resting on the ground.
varus (VAIR us)	The foot is inverted, and the outer side of the foot touches the ground.
torsion (TOR shun)	Twisting.
whiplash	Injury to the bones in the cervical spine as a result of a sudden movement forward and backward of the head and neck. Can occur as a result of a rear-end auto collision.

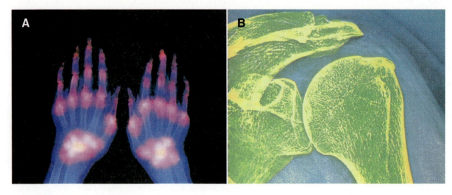

FIGURE 4.22 (A) Enhanced color X-ray of arthritis in hands and wrists (Science Photo Library/Photo Researchers, Inc.); (B) enhanced color X-ray of arthritic shoulder. (CNRI/Science Photo Library/Photo Researchers, Inc.)

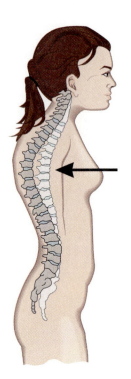

Excessive kyphosis
(slouch)

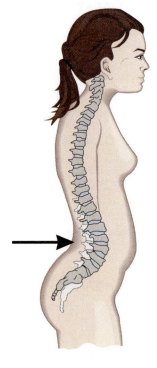

Excessive lordosis
(swayback)

FIGURE 4.23 Abnormal spinal curvature.

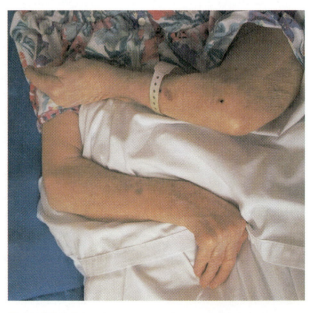

FIGURE 4.24 Contractures of rheumatoid arthritis.

FRACTURES

A **fracture** (**FX, Fx**) is an injury to a bone that causes a break. Fractures are named to describe the type of damage to the bone. The most common types are listed below.

Closed or Simple	Fracture with no open skin or wound (see Figure 4.25).
Colles' (COL eez)	Wrist fracture (see Figure 4.26).
Comminuted (kom ih NYOOT ed)	Fracture in which the bone is shattered, splintered, or rushed into many small pieces or fragments. The fracture is completely through the bone.

FIGURE 4.25 (A) Closed and (B) open fractures.

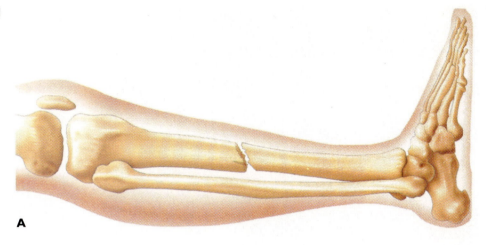

A

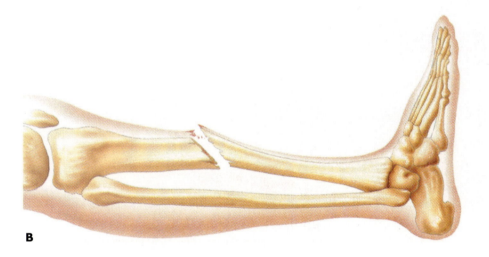

B

FIGURE 4.26 Colles' fracture. (Charles Stewart and Associates)

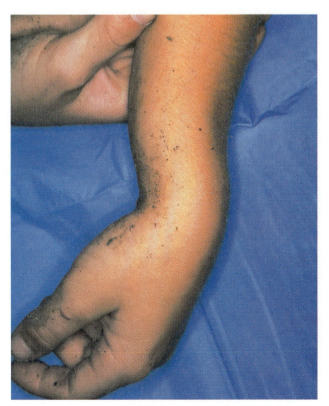

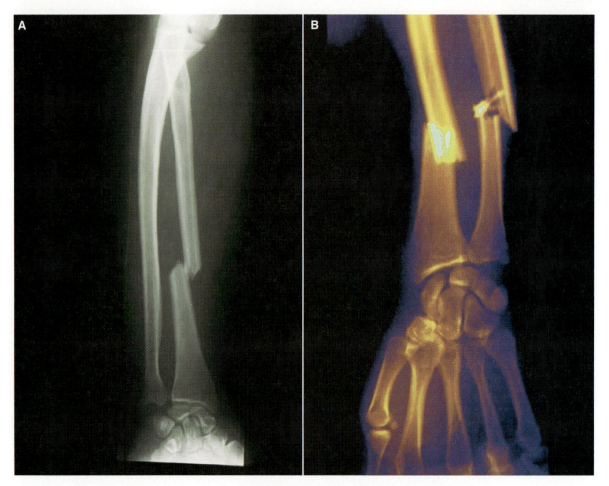

FIGURE 4.27 (A) X-ray of complete fracture of radius (James Stevenson/Science Photo Library/Photo Researchers, Inc.); (B) enhanced color X-ray of forearm fractures. (Scott Camazine/Photo Researchers, Inc.)

Complete	Bone is completely broken with neither fragment connected to the other (see Figure 4.27).
Compound or Open	Fracture in which the skin has been broken through to the fracture. (see also Figure 4.25)
Fissured (FISH erd)	Incomplete longitudinal fracture.
Greenstick	Fracture in which there is an incomplete break; one side of bone is broken and the other side is bent. This type of fracture is commonly found in children due to their softer and more pliable bone structure.
Impacted	Fracture in which bone fragments are pushed into each other.
Incomplete	Fracture in which the line of fracture does not include the entire bone.
Oblique (oh BLEEK)	Fracture at an angle to the bone (see Figure 4.28).
Pathologic (path a LOJ ik)	Fracture caused by diseased or weakened bone.
Spiral	Fracture in an *S* shape (spiral). Can be caused by a twisting injury.
Transverse (trans VERS)	Complete fracture that is straight across the bone at right angles to the long axis of the bone.

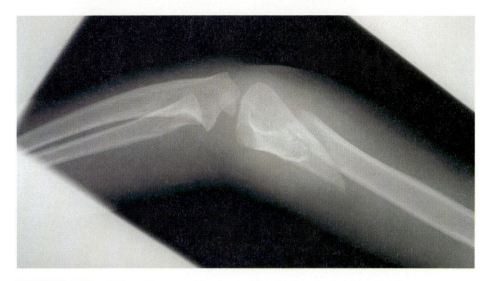

FIGURE 4.28 Oblique fracture of the femur. (Charles Stewart and Associates)

BONE TUMORS OR NEOPLASMS

MED TERM *TIP*

Remember that the words **tumor** (**TOO** mor) and **neoplasm** (**NEE** oh plazm) both mean *new growth*. A tumor can be either **benign** (bee **NINE**), meaning noncancerous, or **malignant** (mah **LIG** nant), which indicates a cancerous growth of tissue. However, many of your patients will equate the word tumor with cancer even though they may have only a benign growth. Be careful when you discuss these terms in front of patients.

Benign Tumors

epidermoid (ep ih DER moyd) cyst	Cyst in the skull and phalanges of the fingers.
ganglion (GANG lee on)	Cyst at the end of long bones.
giant cell tumor	Benign tumor that appears at the epiphysis but does not interfere with joint movement. May become malignant or return after removal.
hemangioma (hee man jee OH mah)	Common benign, vascular tumor usually located on the skull or vertebral body.
osteoblastoma (oss tee oh blas TOH mah)	Benign lesion or tumor generally found on the spine, where it may result in paralysis.
osteochondroma (oss tee oh kon DROH mah)	Tumor composed of both cartilage and bony substance.
osteoid osteoma (OSS tee oyd oss tee OH mah)	Painful tumor usually found in the lower extremities.

Malignant Tumors

Ewing's sarcoma **(YOO wings sar KOH mah)**	Malignant growth found in the shaft of long bones that spreads through the periosteum. Removal is treatment of choice, as this tumor will metastasize or spread to other organs. Named for James Ewing, an American pathologist.
fibrosarcoma **(figh broh sar KOH ma)** **of the bone**	Tumor containing connective tissue that occurs in bone marrow. It is found most frequently in the femur, humerus, and jaw bone.
myeloma (my ah LOH mah)	Malignant neoplasm originating in plasma cells in the bone.

Diagnostic Procedures Relating to the Musculoskeletal System

arthrocentesis **(ar throh sen TEE sis)**	Removal of synovial fluid with a needle from a joint space, such as in the knee, for examination.
arthrography **(ar THROG rah fee)**	Visualization of a joint by radiographic study after injection of a contrast medium into the joint space.
arthroscopy **(ar THROS koh pee)**	Examination of the interior of a joint by entering the joint with an arthroscope. Torn ligaments can be repaired while the patient is undergoing arthroscopy. The arthroscope contains a small television camera that allows the physician to view the interior of the joint on a monitor during the procedure.
bone scan	Patient is given a radioactive dye and then scanning equipment is used to visualize bones. It is especially useful in observing progress of treatment for osteomyelitis and cancer metastases to the bone.
computerized axial tomography **(toh MOG rah fee)**	Computer-assisted X-ray used to detect tumors and fractures. Also referred to as a *CAT* or *CT scan.*
electromyography **(ee lek troh my OG rah fee)**	Study and record of the strength of muscle contractions as a result of electrical stimulation.
magnetic resonance imaging **(mag NEH tik REHZ oh nance)** **(MRI)**	Medical imaging that uses radio-frequency radiation as its source of energy. It does not require the injection of contrast medium or exposure to ionizing radiation. The technique is useful for visualizing large blood vessels, the heart, the brain, and soft tissues.
muscle biopsy (BYE op see)	Removal of muscle tissue for pathological examination.
myelography **(my eh LOG rah fee)**	Study of the spinal column after injecting opaque contrast material.
photon absorptiometry **(FOH ton** **ab sorp she AHM eh tree)**	Measurement of bone density using an instrument for the purpose of detecting osteoporosis.

Treatment Procedures Relating to the Musculoskeletal System

amputation (am pew TAY shun)	Partial or complete removal of a limb for a variety of reasons, including tumors, gangrene, intractable pain, crushing injury, or uncontrollable infection.
anterior cruciate (an TEE ree or KROO she ate) ligament (ACL) reconstruction	Replacing a torn ACL with a graft by means of arthroscopy.
arthrodesis (ar throh DEE sis)	Fusion or stiffening of a joint to provide stability. This is sometimes done to relieve the pain of arthritis.
arthroplasty (AR throh plas tee)	Surgical reconstruction of a joint.
arthroscopic (ar throh SKOP ic) surgery	Use of an arthroscope to facilitate performing surgery on a joint (see Figure 4.29).
arthrotomy (ar THROT oh mee)	Surgically cutting into a joint.
bone graft	Piece of bone taken from the patient that is used to take the place of a removed bone or a bony defect at another site.
bunionectomy (bun yun ECK toh mee)	Removal of the bursa at the joint of the great toe.
carpal tunnel release (CAR pal TUN el)	Surgical cutting of the ligament in the wrist to relieve nerve pressure caused by carpal tunnel disease, which can result from repetitive motion such as typing.
cast	Application of a solid material to immobilize an extremity or portion of the body as a result of a fracture, dislocation, or severe injury. It is most often made of plaster of Paris (see Figure 4.30).
fasciectomy (fas ee EK tah mee)	Surgical removal of the fascia, which is the fibrous membrane that covers and supports muscles.
laminectomy (lam ih NEK toh mee)	Removal of the vertebral posterior arch to correct severe back problems and pain caused by compression of the lamina.
meniscectomy (men ih SEK toh mee)	Removal of the knee cartilage (meniscus).
osteoclasia (oss tee oh KLAY see ah)	Intentional breaking of a bone to correct a deformity.
reduction	Correcting a fracture by realigning the bone fragments. *Closed reduction* is doing this manipulation without entering the body. *Open reduction* is the surgical incision at the site of the fracture to do the reduction. This is commonly necessary where there are bony fragments to remove.
spinal fusion	Surgical immobilization of adjacent vertebrae. This may be done for several reasons, including correction for a herniated disk.
total hip replacement (THR)	Surgical reconstruction of a hip by implanting a prosthetic or artificial hip joint (see Figure 4.31).

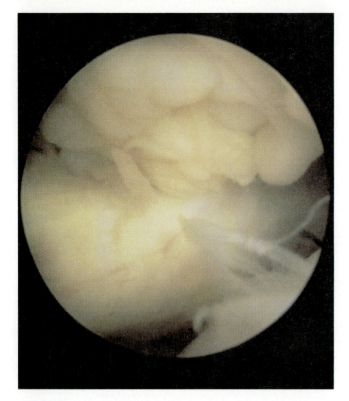

FIGURE 4.29 Arthroscopy of the knee. (Southern Illinois University/Photo Researchers, Inc.)

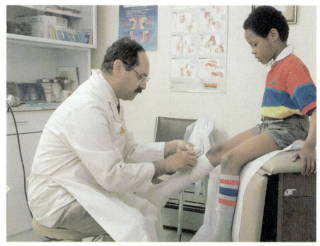

FIGURE 4.30 Physician applying cast to right leg.

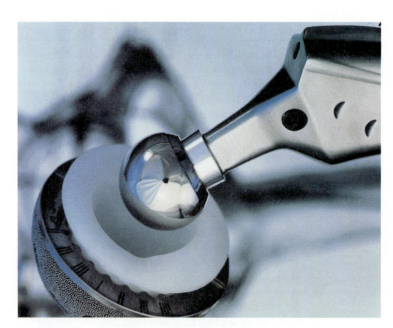

FIGURE 4.31 Prosthetic hip joint. (Lawrence Livermore National Library/Science Photo Library/Photo Researchers, Inc.)

Rehabilitation Services

Rehabilitation services consist of physical therapy and occupational therapy. These allied health personnel plan and carry out treatment programs to develop, restore, or maintain function. Occupational therapy specializes in programs for activities of daily living (ADLs); personal care; and work and leisure-time activities for persons with physical, mental, emotional, or developmental disabilities. Physical therapy specializes in programs for movement dysfunction and physical disabilities resulting from muscle, bone, joint, and nerve injuries or diseases. Rehabilitation services are found in acute and long-term facilities, rehabilitation centers, health maintenance organizations, schools, home health agencies, private practices, clinics, and mental health facilities.

Physical Therapist

Physical therapists specialize in programs for movement dysfunction and physical disabilities resulting from muscle, bone, joint, and nerve injuries or disease. They work with patients/clients to help them overcome these barriers to mobility. Physical therapists work in a variety of settings including acute and long-term facilities, rehabilitation centers, and private practice. To become a physical therapist, students must graduate from an accredited master's degree physical therapy program, complete a four month clinical internship, and pass a national licensing exam. For more information about a career in physical therapy, visit the American Physical Therapy Association's web site at www.apta.org.

Physical Therapist (PT)

- **Provides physical therapy as ordered by a physician**

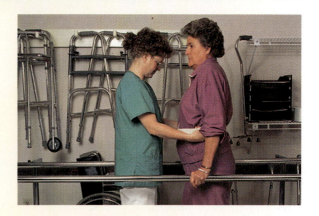

- **Graduates from an accredited four-year bachelor's or five-year master's degree physical therapy program**
- **Completes a four-month clinical internship**
- **Passes a national licensing examination**

Certified Occupational Therapy Assistant (COTA)

- **Works under the supervision of an occupational therapist**
- **Graduates from a two-year approved occupational therapy assistant program**
- **Completes supervised clinical fieldwork**
- **Passes a national certification examination**

Physical Therapy Assistant (PTA)

- **Works under the supervision of a physical therapist**
- **Graduates from an accredited two-year associate degree physical therapy assistant program**
- **Passes a national licensing examination**

Abbreviations Relating to the Musculoskeletal System

ACL	anterior cruciate ligament		**LIF**	left iliac fossa
ADLs	activities of daily living		**LLE**	left lower extremity
AP	anterioposterior		**LOM**	limitation of motion
C1, C2, etc.	first cervical vertebra, second cervical vertebra, etc.		**LUE**	left upper extremity
			ortho	orthopedics
CA	cancer		**RA**	rheumatoid arthritis
Ca	calcium, cancer		**RIF**	right iliac fossa
CDH	congenital dislocation of the hip		**RLE**	right lower extremity
CTS	carpal tunnel syndrome		**ROM**	range of motion
DTR	deep tendon reflex		**RUE**	right upper extremity
EMG	electromyogram		**SLE**	systemic lupus erythematosus
FX, Fx	fracture		**T1, T2, etc.**	first thoracic vertebra, second thoracic vertebra, etc.
Ga	gallium			
IM	intramuscular		**THR**	total hip replacement
KB	knee bearing		**TKA**	total knee arthroplasty
L1, L2, etc.	first lumbar vertebra, second lumbar vertebra, etc.		**TKR**	total knee replacement
			TX, Tx	traction, treatment
LAT, lat	lateral		**UE**	upper extremity
LE	lower extremity			

KEY TERMS

- abduction (ab **DUCK** shun)
- acetabulum (ass eh **TAB** yoo lum)
- adduction (ad **DUCK** shun)
- adductor longus (ad **DUCK** tor)
- amputation (am pew **TAY** shun)
- ankylosis (ang kih **LOH** sis)
- anterior cruciate ligament reconstruction (an **TEE** ree or **KROO** she ate)
- appendicular skeleton (app en **DIK** yoo lar)
- arthralgia (ar **THRAL** jee ah)
- arthritis (ar **THRY** tis)
- arthrocentesis (ar throh sen **TEE** sis)
- arthroclasia (ar throh **KLAY** see ah)
- arthrodesis (ar throh **DEE** sis)
- arthrography (ar **THROG** rah fee)
- arthroplasty (**AR** throh plas tee)
- arthroscopic surgery (ar throh **SKOP** ik)
- arthroscopy (ar **THROS** koh pee)
- arthrotomy (ar **THROT** oh mee)

- articulation (ar tik yoo **LAY** shun)
- atrophy (**AT** rah fee)
- axial skeleton (**AK** see al)
- ball-and-socket joint
- benign (bee **NINE**)
- biceps (**BYE** seps)
- bone graft
- bone scan
- bones
- bradykinesia (brad ee kih **NEE** see ah)
- bunion (**BUN** yun)
- bunionectomy (bun yun **ECK** toh mee)
- bursa (**BER** sah)
- bursectomy (ber **SEK** toh mee)
- bursitis (ber **SIGH** tis)
- bursolith (**BER** soh lith)
- cancellous bone (**CAN** sell us)
- cardiac muscle (**CAR** dee ak)
- carpal tunnel release (**CAR** pal **TUN** el)

- carpal tunnel syndrome (**CAR** pal **TUN** el **SIN** drohm)
- carpals (**CAR** pals)
- cartilage (**CAR** tih lij)
- cartilaginous joints (car tih **LAJ** ih nus)
- cartilaginous tissue (car tih **LAJ** ih nus)
- cast
- cervical vertebrae (**SER** vih kal **VER** teh bray)
- chiropodist (kye **ROPP** ah dist)
- chiropractic (kye ro **PRAK** tik)
- chondrectomy (kon **DREK** toh mee)
- chondromalacia (kon droh mah **LAY** she ah)
- chondroplasty (**KON** droh plas tee)
- circumduction (sir kum **DUCK** shun)
- clavicle (**CLAV** ih kl)
- closed fracture
- coccyx (**COCK** six)
- Colles' (**COL** eez)
- comminuted fracture (kom ih **NYOOT** ed)
- compact bone
- complete fracture
- compound fracture
- computerized axial tomography (**AK** see al toh **MOG** rah fee)
- condyle (**CON** dile)
- cortical bone (**KOR** tih kal)
- cranioplasty (**KRAY** nee oh plas tee)
- craniotomy (kray nee **OTT** oh mee)
- cranium (**KRAY** nee um)
- diaphysis (dye **AFF** ih sis)
- dorsiflexion (dor see **FLEK** shun)
- dyskinesia (dis kih **NEE** see ah)
- dystrophy (**DIS** troh fee)
- electromyogram (ee lek troh **MY** oh gram) (EMG)
- electromyography (ee lek troh my **OG** rah fee)
- epicondyle (ep ih **KON** dile)
- epidermoid cyst (ep ih **DER** moyd **SIST**)
- epiphysis (eh **PIFF** ih sis)
- ethmoid (**ETH** moyd)
- eversion (ee **VER** zhun)
- Ewing's sarcoma (**YOO** wings sar **KOH** ma)
- extension (eks **TEN** shun)
- fascia (**FASH** ee ah)
- fasciectomy (fas ee **EK** tah mee)
- femur (**FEE** mer)
- fibrosarcoma (figh broh sar **KOH** mah)
- fibrous joints (**FYE** bruss)
- fibula (**FIB** yoo lah)
- fissure (**FISH** er)
- fissured fracture
- flat bones
- flexion (**FLEK** shun)
- foramen (for **AY** men)
- fossa (**FOSS** ah)
- fracture
- frontal
- ganglion (**GANG** lee on)
- giant cell tumor
- gluteus maximus (**GLOO** tee us **MACKS** ih mus)
- gout (**GOWT**)
- greenstick fracture
- head
- hemangioma (hee man jee **OH** mah)
- humerus (**HYOO** mer us)
- hyoid bone (**HIGH** oyd)
- hyperkinesia (high per kih **NEE** see ah)
- hypertrophy (high **PER** troh fee)
- ilium (**ILL** ee um)
- impacted fracture
- incomplete fracture
- innominate bone (ih **NOM** ih nayt)
- intervertebral (in ter **VER** teh bral)
- intracranial (in trah **KRAY** nee al)
- inversion (in **VER** zhun)
- irregular bones
- ischium (**ISS** kee um)
- joints
- kyphosis (ki **FOH** sis)
- lacrimal (**LACK** rim al)
- laminectomy (lam ih **NEK** toh mee)
- ligaments (**LIG** ah ments)
- long bones
- lordosis (lor **DOH** sis)
- lumbar vertebrae (**LUM** bar **VER** teh bray)
- magnetic resonance imaging (mag **NEH** tik **REHZ** oh nance) (MRI)
- malignant (mah **LIG** nant)
- mandible (**MAN** dih bl)
- maxilla (mack **SIH** lah)
- meniscectomy (men eh **SEK** toh mee)
- metacarpals (met ah **CAR** pals)
- metatarsals (met ah **TAR** sals)
- muscle biopsy (**BYE** op see)
- muscles
- muscular dystrophy (**MUSS** kew ler **DIS** troh fee)
- myasthenia gravis (my ass **THEE** nee ah **GRAV** is)
- myelography (my eh **LOG** rah fee)
- myeloma (my ah **LOH** mah)
- myocardium (my oh **CAR** dee um)
- myopathy (my **OPP** ah thee)
- myoplasty (**MY** oh plas tee)
- myorrhaphy (my **OR** ah fee)
- nasal (**NAY** zl)
- neoplasm (**NEE** oh plazm)
- oblique fracture (oh **BLEEK**)
- occipital (ock **SIP** eh tal)
- olecranon process (oh **LEK** ran on)
- open fracture
- opposition
- orthopedics (or thoh **PEE** diks)

- orthopedist (or thoh **PEE** dist)
- orthotics (or **THOT** iks)
- orthotist (or **THOT** ist)
- os coxae (**OSS KOK** sigh)
- osseous tissue (**OSS** ee us)
- ossification (oss sih fih **KAY** shun)
- osteoarthritis (oss tee oh ar **THRY** tis)
- osteoblast (**OSS** tee oh blast)
- osteoblastoma (oss tee oh blas **TOH** mah)
- osteocarcinoma (oss tee oh kar sin **OH** ma)
- osteochondroma (oss tee oh kon **DROH** mah)
- osteoclasia (oss tee oh **KLAY** see ah)
- osteocytes (**OSS** tee oh sights)
- osteoid osteoma (**OSS** tee oyd oss tee **OH** mah)
- osteomalacia (oss tee oh mah **LAY** she ah)
- osteomyelitis (oss tee oh my ell **EYE** tis)
- osteopath (**OSS** tee oh path)
- osteopathy (oss tee **OP** ah thee)
- osteoporosis (oss tee oh por **ROH** sis)
- osteotome (**OSS** tee oh tohm)
- osteotomy (oss tee **OTT** ah mee)
- Paget's disease (**PAH** jets)
- palatine (**PAL** ah tine)
- parietal (pah **RYE** eh tal)
- patella (pah **TELL** ah)
- pathologic fracture (path ah **LOJ** ik)
- periosteum (pair ee **AH** stee um)
- phalanges (fah **LAN** jeez)
- photon absorptiometry
  (**FOH** ton ab sorp she **AHM** eh tree)
- physiatrist (fiz ee **AT** rist)
- plantar flexion (**PLAN** tar **FLEK** shun)
- podiatrist (po **DYE** ah trist)
- polymyositis (pol ee my oh **SIGH** tis)
- prepatellar bursitis (pre pah **TELL** er ber **SIGH** tis)
- process
- pronation (proh **NAY** shun)
- prosthesis (pross **THEE** sis)
- prosthetist (**PROSS** thah tist)
- pubic symphysis (**PYOO** bik **SIM** fih sis)
- pubis (**PYOO** bis)
- radius (**RAY** dee us)
- rectus abdominus (**REK** tus ab **DOM** ih nus)
- red bone marrow
- reduction
- rheumatoid arthritis (**ROO** mah toyd ar **THRY** tis)
  (RA)
- rib cage
- rickets (**RIK** ets)
- rigor mortis (**RIG** ur **MOR** tis)
- rotation (roh **TAY** shun)

- ruptured intervertebral disk (in ter **VER** tee bral)
- sacrum (**SAY** crum)
- scapula (**SKAP** yoo lah)
- scoliosis (skoh lee **OH** sis)
- short bones
- simple fracture
- sinus (**SIGH** nus)
- skeletal muscle (**SKELL** eh tal)
- smooth muscle
- sphenoid (**SFEE** noyd)
- spinal fusion
- spinal stenosis (ste **NOH** sis)
- spiral fracture
- spongy bone
- sternum (**STER** num)
- subscapular (sub **SCAP** yoo lar)
- supernumerary bone (soo per **NOO** mer ar ee)
- supination (soo pin **NAY** shun)
- sutures (**SOO** chers)
- synovial fluid (sin **OH** veeal)
- synovial joint
- synovial membrane (sin **OH** vee al **MEM** brayn)
- systemic lupus erythematosus (sis **TEM** ik **LOO** pus air ih them ah **TOH** sis)
- talipes (**TAL** ih peez)
- talipes equinus (eh **KWI** nus)
- talipes planus (**PLAY** nus)
- talipes valgus (**VAL** gus)
- talipes varus (**VAIR** us)
- tarsals (**TAHR** sals)
- temporal (**TEM** por al)
- tendon (**TEN** dun)
- tenodynia (ten oh **DIN** ee ah)
- tenorrhaphy (tah **NOR** ah fee)
- thoracic vertebrae (tho **RASS** ik **VER** teh bray)
- tibia (**TIB** ee ah)
- torsion (**TOR** shun)
- total hip replacement (THR)
- transurethral (trans yoo **REE** thral)
- transverse fracture (trans **VERS**)
- trochanter (tro **KAN** ter)
- tubercle (**TOO** ber kl)
- tuberosity (too ber **OSS** ih tee)
- tumor (**TOO** mor)
- ulna (**UHL** nah)
- vertebral column (**VER** teh bral)
- vomer (**VOH** mer)
- whiplash
- yellow bone marrow
- zygomatic (zeye go **MAT** ik)

Case Study

DISCHARGE SUMMARY

Admitting Diagnosis: Osteoarthritis bilateral knees

Final Diagnosis: Osteoarthritis bilateral knees with prosthetic right knee replacement

History of Present Illness: Patient is a 68-year-old male. He reports he has experienced occasional knee pain and swelling since he injured his knees playing football in high school. These symptoms became worse while he was in his 50s and working on a concrete surface. The right knee has always been more painful than the left. Arthroscopy 12 years ago revealed a torn lateral meniscus and chondromalacia of the patella on the right. He had an arthroscopic meniscectomy with a 50% improvement in symptoms at that time. He returned to his orthopedic surgeon 6 months ago because of constant knee pain and swelling severe enough to interfere with sleep and all activities. He required a cane to walk. CT-scan indicated severe bilateral osteoarthritis, with complete loss of the joint space on the right. He was referred to a physiatrist who prescribed Motrin; physical therapy for ROM; strengthening exercises; and a low-fat, low-calorie weight loss diet for moderate obesity that greatly added to the strain on his knees. Over the course of the next two months, the left knee improved, but the right knee did not. Due to the failure of conservative treatment, he is admitted to the hospital at this time for prosthetic replacement of the right knee. Patient's other medical history is significant for hypertension and coronary artery disease that is controlled with medication. He has lost weight through diet, which has improved his hypertension, if not his knee pain.

Summary of Hospital Course: Patient tolerated the surgical procedure well. He began intensive physical therapy for lower extremity ROM and strengthening exercises and gait training with a walker. He received occupational therapy instruction in ADLs, especially dressing and personal care. He was able to transfer himself out of bed by the 3rd post-op day and was able to ambulate 150 ft with a walker and dress himself on the 5th post-op day. His right knee flexion was 90° and he lacked 5° of full extension.

Discharge Plans: Patient was discharged home with his wife one week post-op. He will continue rehabilitation as an outpatient. Return to office for post-op checkup in one week.

CRITICAL THINKING QUESTIONS

1. What is the specialty of a physiatrist? Describe in your own words what the physiatrist ordered for this patient.

2. What surgical procedure did the patient have 12 years ago? What two pathologies were revealed by that procedure? What surgical procedure was performed to correct his problems at that time?

3. The following medical terms are not defined in your text. Based on your reading of this discharge summary, what do you think each term means in general — not the specifics of this patient.

   a. conservative treatment

   b. outpatient

4. What two types of post-op therapy did this patient receive? Describe the treatment each type of therapy provided for this patient.

5. Describe how much the patient could move his right knee when he was discharged from the hospital.

6. The following medical terms are introduced in a later chapter. Use your text as a dictionary to describe, in your own words, what each term means.

   a. coronary artery disease

   b. hypertension

Chart Note Transcription

Chart Note

The chart note below contains eleven phrases that can be reworded with a medical term that you learned in this chapter. Each phrase is identified with an underline. Determine the medical term and write your answers in the space provided.

Current Complaint: An 82-year-old female was transported to the Emergency Room via ambulance with severe left hip pain following a fall on the ice.

Past History: Patient suffered a wrist broken bone[1] two years earlier that required immobilization by solid material.[2] Following this broken bone,[3] her physician who specializes in treatment of bone conditions[4] diagnosed her with moderate porous bones[5] on the basis of a computer-assisted X-ray.[6]

Signs and Symptoms: Patient reported severe left hip pain, rating it as 8 on a scale of 1 to 10. She held her hip in a bent position[7] and could not tolerate movement toward a straight position.[8] X-rays of the left hip and leg were taken.

Diagnosis: Shattered broken bone[9] in the neck of the left thigh bone.[10]

Treatment: Implantation of an artificial hip joint[11] on the left.

1 _____

2 _____

3 _____

4 _____

5 _____

6 _____

7 _____

8 _____

9 _____

10 _____

11 _____

Practice Exercises

A. COMPLETE THE FOLLOWING STATEMENTS.

1. The two divisions of the human skeleton are the _____ and _____ .

2. The five regions of the spinal column are the _____ , _____ , _____ , _____ , and _____ .

3. The three functions of the skeletal system are to _____ , _____ , and _____ .

4. The strongest bone in the body is the _____ .

5. The medical term for kneecap is _____ .

6. The covering over bones is called the _____ .

7. A Colles' fracture occurs in the _____ .

8. There are _____ skeletal muscles.

9. There are _____ bones in the human body.

10. The three types of muscle are _____ , _____ , and _____ .

11. A physician specializing in diseases and injuries of the bones and muscles is a(n) _____ .

12. A physician specializing in rehabilitation is a(n) _____ .

B. STATE THE TERMS DESCRIBED USING THE COMBINING FORMS PROVIDED.

The combining form oste/o refers to bone. Use it to write a term that means

1. bone cell _____

2. developing bone cell _____

3. death of the bone tissue _____

4. surgical repair of the bone _____

5. incision of the bone _____

6. excision of the bone _____

7. inflammation of the bone and bone marrow _____

8. softening of the bones _____

9. tumor composed of both bone and cartilage _____

The combining form femor/o refers to the femur. Use it to write a term that means

10. pertaining to the femur _____

11. pertaining to the ilium and the femur _____

12. pertaining to the pubis and the femur _____

The combining form scapul/o refers to the scapula. Use it to write a term that means

13. pertaining to above the scapula _____

14. pertaining to below the scapula _____

The combining form vertebr/o refers to the vertebrae. Use it to write a term that means

15. pertaining to the vertebrae and the ribs _____

16. between the vertebrae _____

The combining form arthr/o refers to the joints. Use it to write a term that means

17. surgical fixation of a joint _____

18. surgical repair of a joint _____

19. incision into a joint _____

20. inflammation of a joint _____

21. inflammation of joint and cartilage _____

22. pain in the joints _____

The combining form crani/o refers to the head or skull. Use it to write a term that means

23. surgical incision into the skull _____

24. surgical repair of the skull _____

25. surgical removal of part of the skull _____

C. WRITE THE SUFFIX FOR EACH EXPRESSION AND PROVIDE AN EXAMPLE OF ITS USE.

Suffix   *Example*

1. the study of _____

2. surgical fixation _____

3. abnormal narrowing _____

4. incision into _____

D. DEFINE THE FOLLOWING SUFFIXES.

1. −ectomy _____

2. −itis _____

3. −blast _____

4. −al _____

5. −ar _____

6. −ic _____

7. −malacia _____

8. −oid _____

9. −gram _____

10. −algia _____

11. −pathy _____

12. −porosis _____

13. −scopy _____

14. −megaly _____

15. −oma _____

16. −clasia _____

E. DEFINE THE FOLLOWING WORD ROOTS/COMBINING FORMS.

1. lamin/o _____

2. humer/o _____

3. cleid/o _____

4. spondyl/o _____

5. my/o _____

6. dactyl/o _____

7. brachi/o _____

8. tend/o _____

9. ili/o _____

10. caud/o _____

F. DEFINE THE FOLLOWING TERMS.

1. chrondroplasty _____

2. periostitis (or periosteitis) _____

3. osteopathy _____

4. lordosis _____

5. kyphosis _____

6. metacarpals _____

7. phalanges _____

8. coccyx _____

9. occipital _____

10. laminectomy _____

G. NAME THE FIVE REGIONS OF THE SPINAL COLUMN AND INDICATE THE NUMBER OF BONES IN EACH AREA.

Name	Number of Bones
1. _____	_____
2. _____	_____
3. _____	_____
4. _____	_____
5. _____	_____

H. CIRCLE THE PREFIX AND SUFFIX AND PLACE A *P* FOR PREFIX OR AN *S* FOR SUFFIX OVER THESE WORD PARTS. IN THE SPACE PROVIDED, DEFINE THE TERM.

1. arthroscopy _____

2. quadriplegic _____

3. arthrocentesis _____

4. diskectomy _____

5. osteorrhaphy _____

6. submandibular _____

I. MATCH THE TERMS IN COLUMN A WITH THE DEFINITIONS IN COLUMN B.

A	B
1. _____ abduction	a. backward bending of hand or foot
2. _____ rotation	b. bending the foot toward the ground
3. _____ plantar flexion	c. straightening or stretching
4. _____ extension	d. motion around a central axis
5. _____ dorsiflexion	e. motion away from the body
6. _____ flexion	f. moving the thumb away from the palm
7. _____ adduction	g. motion toward the body
8. _____ opposition	h. bending motion

J. MATCH TYPES OF FRACTURES IN COLUMN A WITH THE DEFINITIONS IN COLUMN B.

A

1. _____ comminuted
2. _____ greenstick
3. _____ compound
4. _____ simple
5. _____ impacted
6. _____ transverse
7. _____ oblique
8. _____ spiral

B

a. break at an angle
b. *S*-shaped break
c. bone splintered or crushed
d. bone pressed into itself
e. broken straight across bone
f. skin has been broken
g. no open wound
h. bone only partially broken

K. DEFINE THE FOLLOWING MEDICAL SPECIALITIES AND SPECIALISTS.

1. orthopedics _____
2. osteopathy _____
3. chiropodist _____
4. podiatrist _____
5. orthotics _____
6. prosthetics _____

L. IDENTIFY THE FOLLOWING ABBREVIATIONS.

1. AP _____
2. EMG _____
3. CI _____
4. T6 _____
5. IM _____
6. ROM _____
7. RA _____
8. LLE _____

M. WRITE THE ABBREVIATIONS FOR THE FOLLOWING TERMS.

1. congenital dislocation of hip _____
2. total knee replacement _____
3. orthopedics _____
4. knee bearing _____
5. upper extremity _____
6. fifth cervical vertebra _____
7. carpal tunnel syndrome _____
8. cancer _____

N. USE THE FOLLOWING TERMS IN THE SENTENCES THAT FOLLOW.

talipes planus	myasthenia gravis	erythematosus	laminectomy
supernumerary bone	systemic lupus	scoliosis	
osteoporosis	muscular dystrophy	rickets	
whiplash	ganglion cyst	Ewing's sarcoma	

1. Mrs. Lewis, age 84, is being treated for a broken hip. Her physician will be running tests for what potential ailment? _____

2. Jamie, age 6 months, is being given orange juice and vitamin supplements to avoid what condition? _____

3. Baby Kesha was born with an extra digit at the side of her left hand. The doctor assures her mother that this can easily be removed. What is this condition called? _____

4. Marshall was involved in a rear-end collision. He is complaining of severe headaches and neck stiffness. What condition may he have suffered? _____

5. Mr. Jefferson's physician has discovered a tumor on his femur. He has been admitted to the hospital for a biopsy to rule out what type of bone cancer? _____

6. The school nurse has asked Janelle to bend over so that she may examine her back. What is the nurse looking for? _____

7. Gerald has experienced a gradual loss of muscle strength, especially in the face and throat, during the past five years. He is concerned that he may eventually have to face paralysis due to his chronic disease. What is that disease? _____

8. Roberta has suddenly developed arthritis in her hands and knees, an aversion to the sun, and a butterfly rash across her nose and cheeks. What is one of the diseases that her physician will wish to rule out? _____

Getting Connected

Multimedia Extension Activities

CD-ROM

Use the CD-ROM enclosed with your textbook to gain additional reinforcement through interactive word building exercises, spelling games, labeling activities, and additional quizzes.

www.prenhall.com/fremgen

Use the above address to access the free, interactive Companion Website created for this textbook. Get hints, instant feedback, and textbook references to chapter-related multiple choice questions, and labeling and matching exercises. In addition, you will find an audio glossary, case studies, Internet exploration exercises, flashcards, and a comprehensive exam.

Answers

CASE STUDY (CRITICAL THINKING QUESTIONS)

1. rehabilitation specialist; Motrin (a non-steroidal anti-inflammatory medication), physical therapy for range of motion and strengthening exercises, and low-fat, low-calorie diet   2. arthroscopy; torn lateral meniscus and chondromalacia; arthroscopic meniscectomy   3. (a) non-surgical treatments, such as medicine and therapy; (b) a patient who has not been admitted to the hospital   4. physical therapy for lower extremity ROM and strengthening exercises, and gait training with a walker; occupational therapy for ADL instruction, especially dressing and personal care   5. patient was able to bend knee to 90° but lacked 5° of being able to straighten it back out

CHART NOTE

1. Colles' fracture (fx) — wrist broken bone   2. cast — immobilization by solid material   3. fracture — broken bone   4. orthopedist — physician who specializes in treating bone conditions   5. osteoporosis — porous bones   6. computerized axial tomography (CT or CAT scan) — computer-assisted X-ray   7. flexion — a bent position   8. extension — movement toward a straight position   9. comminuted fracture (fx) — shattered broken bone   10. femur — thigh bone   11. total hip replacement (THR) — implantation of an artificial hip joint

PRACTICE EXERCISES

A. 1. axial, appendicular   2. cervical, thoracic, lumbar, sacrum, coccyx   3. frame, protect vital organs, work with muscles for movement   4. femur   5. patella   6. periosteum   7. wrist   8. 400   9. 206   10. skeletal, smooth, cardiac   11. orthopedist   12. physiatrist

B. 1. osteocyte   2. osteoblast   3. osteonecrosis   4. osteoplasty   5. osteotomy   6. ostectomy   7. osteomyelitis   8. osteomalacia   9. osteochondroma   10. femoral   11. iliofemoral   12. pubofemoral   13. suprascapular   14. subscapular   15. vertebrocostal   16. intervertebral   17. arthrodesis   18. arthroplasty   19. arthrotomy   20. arthritis   21. arthrochondritis   22. arthralgia   23. craniotomy   24. cranioplasty   25. craniectomy

C. 1. -ology   2. -pexy   3. -stenosis   4. -otomy

D. 1. surgical removal   2. inflammation of   3. germ cell   4. pertaining to   5. pertaining to   6. pertaining to   7. softening   8. like or resembling   9. record   10. pain   11. disease   12. cavity/pore   13. visual examination   14. large   15. tumor   16. to surgically break

E. 1. lamina   2. humerus   3. clavicle   4. vertebrae   5. muscle   6. digit   7. arm   8. tendon   9. ilium   10. tail

F. 1. surgical repair of cartilage   2. inflammation of periosteum   3. any bone disease   4. swayback   5. humpback   6. hand bones   7. finger bones, toe bones   8. tailbone   9. posterior wall of cranium   10. removal of spinal lamina

G. 1. cervical, 7   2. thoracic, 12   3. lumbar, 5   4. sacrum, 1   5. coccyx, 1

H. 1. scopy 5 S; examination of joint using an instrument   2. quad 5 P; ic 5 S; paralysis in arms and legs   3. centesis 5 S; surgical puncture with a needle into a joint   4. ectomy 5 S; surgical removal of disk   5. orrhaphy 5 S; suturing or wiring together of bones   6. sub 5 P; ar 5 S; under the mandible

I. 1. e   2. d   3. b   4. c   5. a   6. h   7. g   8. f

J. 1. c   2. h   3. f   4. g   5. d   6. e   7. a   8. b

K. 1. study of bones and muscles   2. study of musculoskeletal system; also uses manipulation of vertebral column   3. specialist in treating disorders of feet   4. foot specialist   5. fitting of orthopedic appliances   6. specialty of using artificial devices

L. 1. anteroposterior   2. electromyography   3. first cervical vertebra   4. sixth thoracic vertebra   5. intramuscular   6. range of motion   7. rheumatoid arthritis   8. left lower extremity

M. 1. CDH   2. TKR   3. Ortho   4. KB   5. UE   6. C5   7. CTS   8. Ca

N. 1. osteoporosis   2. rickets   3. supernumerary bone   4. whiplash   5. Ewing's sarcoma   6. scoliosis   7. myasthenia gravis   8. systemic lupus erythematosus

Chapter 5

ENDOCRINE SYSTEM

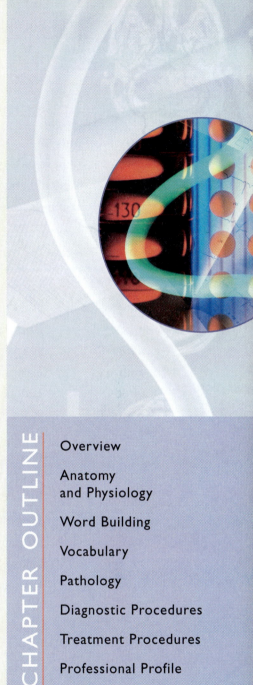

LEARNING OBJECTIVES

Upon completion of this chapter, you will be able to:

- Recognize the combining forms and suffixes introduced in this chapter.

- Gain the ability to pronounce medical terms and major anatomical structures.

- List the major glands of the endocrine system.

- List the major hormones secreted by each endocrine gland and discuss their functions.

- Build endocrine system medical terms from word parts.

- Define vocabulary, pathology, diagnostic, and therapeutic medical terms relating to the endocrine system.

- Interpret abbreviations associated with the endocrine system.

Overview

ORGANS OF THE ENDOCRINE SYSTEM

adrenal glands (2)   pituitary gland

ovaries (two in female)   testes (two in male)

pancreas (islets of Langerhans)   thymus gland

parathyroid glands (four)   thyroid gland

COMBINING FORMS RELATING TO THE ENDOCRINE SYSTEM

acr/o	extremities	kal/i	potassium
aden/o	gland	myx/o	mucus
adren/o	adrenal glands	natr/o	sodium
adrenal/o	adrenal glands	ophthalm/o	eye
andr/o	male	pancreat/o	pancreas
calc/i	calcium	parathyroid/o	parathyroid gland
cortic/o	cortex, outer layer	phys/o	growing
crin/o	secrete	pituitar/o	pituitary gland
dips/o	thirst	somat/o	body
estr/o	female	ster/o	steroid, solid
gluc/o	sugar	thym/o	thymus
glyc/o	sugar	thyr/o	thyroid gland
gonad/o	sex glands	thyroid/o	thyroid gland
home/o	sameness	toc/o	childbirth
hormon/o	hormone	toxic/o	toxic, poison
insulin/o	insulin		

SUFFIXES RELATING TO THE ENDOCRINE SYSTEM

Suffix	Meaning	Example
-crine	to secrete	endocrine
-dipsia	thirst	polydipsia
-emia	blood condition	hyperkalemia
-ine	a substance	thyroxine
-toxic	poison	thyrotoxicosis
-tropic	stimulate	adrenocorticotropic
-uria	urine condition	polyuria

ANATOMY AND PHYSIOLOGY OF THE ENDOCRINE SYSTEM

adrenal glands	endocrine system	ovaries	testes
endocrine glands	exocrine glands	pancreas	thymus gland
endocrinologists	glands	parathyroid glands	thyroid gland
endocrinology	hormones	pituitary gland	

The **endocrine** (**EN** doh krin) **system** is a glandular system that secretes **hormones** (**HOR** mohnz) directly into the bloodstream. Physicians who specialize in the medical practice of **endocrinology** (en doh krin **ALL** oh jee) are called **endocrinologists** (en doh krin **ALL** oh jists)

The organs of the endocrine system are called **glands** (see Figure 5.1). There are actually two distinct types of glands in the body: **exocrine** (**EKS** oh krin) and **endocrine** (**EN** doh krin). Exocrine glands release their secretions into a duct or another organ. Sweat glands that release sweat into a sweat duct are an example. Endocrine glands, on the other hand, release their secretions, called hormones, directly into the bloodstream. Since they have no ducts, they are referred to as *ductless glands*. The endocrine glands include two **adrenal** (ad **REE** nal) **glands,** two **ovaries** (**OH** vah reez) in the female, four **parathyroid** (pair ah **THIGH** royd) **glands,** the **pancreas** (**PAN** kree ass) or *islets of Langerhans,* the **pituitary** (pih **TOO** ih tair ee) **gland,** two **testes** (**TESS** teez) in the male, the **thymus** (**THIGH** mus) **gland,** and the **thyroid** (**THIGH** royd) **gland.** The endocrine glands as a whole affect the functions of the entire body. See Table 5.1 for a description of the glands and their hormones.

ADRENAL GLANDS (TWO)

adrenaline	corticosteroids	glucocorticoid	progesterone
aldosterone	cortisol	medulla	steroid sex hormones
androgens	epinephrine	mineralocorticoid	
cortex	estrogen	norepinephrine	

The two adrenal glands are located above each of the kidneys (see Figure 5.2 for the size of the adrenal glands). Each gland is composed of two sections: **cortex** (**KOR** tex) and **medulla** (meh **DOOL** lah). The outer portion, or adrenal cortex, manufactures several different hormones that are referred to collectively as **corticosteroids** (kor tih koh **STAIR** oydz). The **mineralocorticoid** (min er al oh **KOR** tih koyd) **hormone aldosterone** (al **DOSS** ter ohn) regulates sodium and potassium levels in the body. The **glucocorticoid** (gloo koh **KOR** tih koyd) **hormone cortisol** (**KOR** tih sal) regulates carbohydrates in the body. The adrenal cortex of both men and women secretes **steroid** (**STAIR** oyd) **sex hormones: androgen** (**AN** druh jen), **estrogen** (**ESS** troh jen), and **progesterone** (proh **JESS** ter ohn). These hormones regulate secondary sexual characteristics.

The inner portion, or medulla, is responsible for the hormones **epinephrine** (ep ih **NEF** rin) and **norepinephrine** (nor ep ih **NEF** rin). Epinephrine is also called **adrenaline** (ah **DREN** ah lin). These hormones are critical during emergency situations because they increase blood pressure, heart rate, and respiration levels.

Table 5.1   *Endocrine Glands and Their Hormones*

Gland and Hormone	Function
Adrenal cortex	
Glucocorticoids	
Cortisol	Regulates carbohydrate levels in the body
Mineralcorticoids	
Aldosterone	Regulates electrolytes and fluid volume in body
Steroid sex hormones	
Androgen, estrogen, progesterone	Responsible for reproduction and secondary sexual characteristics
Adrenal medulla	
Epinephrine (adrenalin)	Intensifies response during stress
Norepinephrine	Chiefly a vasoconstrictor
Ovaries	
Estrogen	Stimulates development of secondary sex characteristics in females; regulates menstrual cycle
Progesterone	Prepares for conditions of pregnancy
Pancreas	
Glucagon	Stimulates liver to release glucose into the blood
Insulin	Regulates and promotes entry of glucose into cells
Parathyroid Glands	
Parathyroid hormone	Stimulates bone breakdown; regulates calcium level in the blood
Pituitary anterior lobe	
Adrenocorticotropic hormone (ACTH)	Regulates function of adrenal cortex
Follicle-stimulating hormone (FSH)	Stimulates growth of eggs in female and sperm in males
Growth hormone (GH)	Stimulates growth of the body
Luteinizing hormone (LH)	Regulates function of male and female gonads and plays a role in releasing ova in females
Melanocyte-stimulating hormone (MSH)	Stimulates pigment in skin
Prolactin	Stimulates milk production
Thyroid-stimulating hormone (TSH)	Regulates function of thyroid gland
Pituitary posterior lobe	
Antidiuretic hormone (ADH)	Stimulates reabsorption of water by the kidneys
Oxytocin	Stimulates uterine contractions and releases milk into ducts
Testes	
Testosterone	Promotes sperm production and development of secondary sex characteristics in males
Thymus	
Thymosin	Promotes development of cells in immune system
Thyroid Gland	
Calcitonin	Stimulates deposition of calcium into bone
Thyroxine (T_4)	Stimulates metabolism in cells
Triiodothyronine (T_3)	Stimulates metabolism in cells

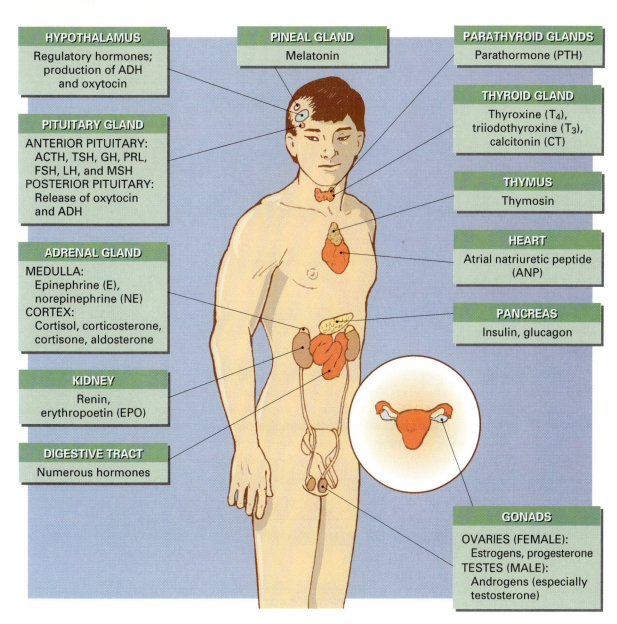

HYPOTHALAMUS
Regulatory hormones; production of ADH and oxytocin

PINEAL GLAND
Melatonin

PARATHYROID GLANDS
Parathormone (PTH)

PITUITARY GLAND
ANTERIOR PITUITARY: ACTH, TSH, GH, PRL, FSH, LH, and MSH
POSTERIOR PITUITARY: Release of oxytocin and ADH

THYROID GLAND
Thyroxine (T_4), triiodothyroxine (T_3), calcitonin (CT)

THYMUS
Thymosin

ADRENAL GLAND
MEDULLA:
  Epinephrine (E), norepinephrine (NE)
CORTEX:
  Cortisol, corticosterone, cortisone, aldosterone

HEART
Atrial natriuretic peptide (ANP)

PANCREAS
Insulin, glucagon

KIDNEY
Renin, erythropoetin (EPO)

DIGESTIVE TRACT
Numerous hormones

GONADS
OVARIES (FEMALE): Estrogens, progesterone
TESTES (MALE): Androgens (especially testosterone)

FIGURE 5.1 The endocrine system.

FIGURE 5.2 The adrenal glands. (Martin Rotker/ Phototake NYC)

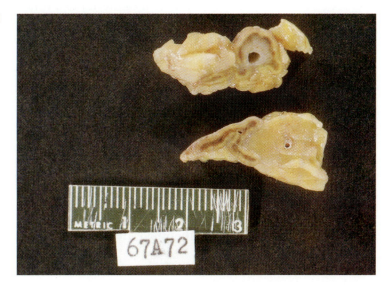

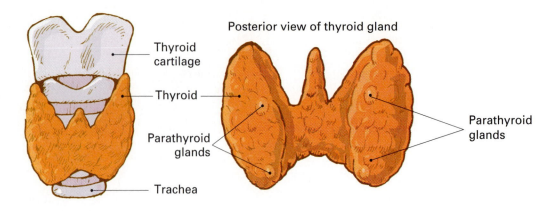

Thyroid cartilage

Thyroid

Parathyroid glands

Trachea

Posterior view of thyroid gland

Parathyroid glands

FIGURE 5.3 The parathyroid glands.

OVARIES (TWO)

estrogen	**ova**
gonads	**progesterone**

The two ovaries are located in the lower abdominopelvic region of the female. They are the female **gonads** (**GOH** nadz), which are responsible for the production of the female sex cells, **ova** (**OH** vah), each month. In addition, the ovaries produce the female sex hormones, **estrogen** and **progesterone.** Estrogen is responsible for the appearance of the female sexual characteristics and control of the menstrual cycle. Progesterone helps to maintain a suitable uterine environment for pregnancy.

PARATHYROID GLANDS (FOUR)

parathyroid hormone (PTH)

tetany

The four tiny parathyroid glands are located on the dorsal or back surface of the thyroid (see Figure 5.3). The **parathyroid hormone** (pair ah **THIGH** royd **HOR** mohn) **(PTH)** secreted by these glands assists in regulating the amount of calcium in the blood. If calcium levels in the blood fall too low, parathyroid hormone will stimulate bone breakdown to release more calcium into the blood.

A calcium deficiency in the system can result in a condition called **tetany** (**TET** ah nee) or muscle excitability and tremors. If the parathyroid glands are removed during thyroid surgery, calcium replacement in the body is often necessary.

PANCREAS (ISLETS OF LANGERHANS)

diabetes mellitus (DM)	**hypoglycemia**
glucagon	**insulin**
hyperglycemia	**islets of Langerhans**

The pancreas is located behind the stomach in front of the first and second lumbar vertebrae (see Figure 5.4). It is the only organ in the body that has both endocrine and exocrine functions. The exocrine portion of the pancreas releases digestive enzymes through a duct into the small intestines. The endocrine sections of the pan-

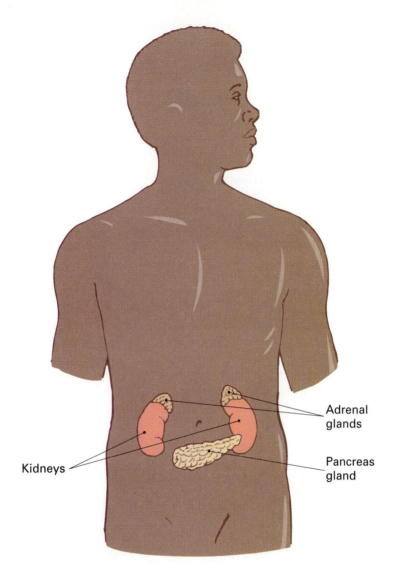

FIGURE 5.4 The pancreas.

creas, **islets of Langerhans** (**EYE** lets of **LAHNG** er hahnz), are named after Dr. Paul Langerhans, a German anatomist. The islets cells produce the hormone **insulin** (**IN** suh lin). Insulin stimulates the cells of the body to take in glucose from the blood stream. Destruction or impairment of the function of the islets results in **diabetes mellitus** (dye ah **BEE** teez **MELL** ih tus) **(DM)** and **hyperglycemia** (high per glye **SEE** mee ah), which is a high blood sugar level. On the other hand, overproduction of insulin will result in **hypoglycemia** (high poh glye **SEE** mee ah), or a low blood sugar level.

A person with Type 1 diabetes mellitus must take insulin injections to replace the insulin the pancreas is unable to produce. Persons with Type 2 diabetes mellitus are often able to take oral hypoglycemic agents—medication that stimulates the pancreas to secrete more insulin.

Another set of islet cells secrete a different hormone, **glucagon** (**GLOO** koh gon), in response to hypoglycemia. Glucagon stimulates the liver to release glucose, thereby raising the blood glucose level.

PITUITARY GLAND

adrenocorticotropic hormone (ACTH)	**luteinizing hormone (LH)**
anterior lobe	**melanocyte-stimulating hormone (MSH)**
antidiuretic hormone (ADH)	**oxytocin**
diabetes insipidus (DI)	**posterior lobe**
follicle-stimulating hormone (FSH)	**prolactin**
growth hormone (GH)	**thyroid-stimulating hormone (TSH)**
hypothalamus	

The pituitary gland is located behind the optic nerve in the brain (see Figure 5.5). It is often referred to as the *master gland* since many of its secretions regulate other endocrine glands. The small marble-shaped gland is divided into the **anterior lobe** and the **posterior lobe**. Both lobes are controlled by the **hypothalamus** (high poh **THAL** ah mus) in the brain.

The anterior pituitary secretes several different hormones (see Figure 5.6). **Growth hormone (GH)** promotes growth of the body by stimulating cells to rapidly increase in size and divide. **Thyroid-stimulating hormone** (**TSH**) regulates the function of the

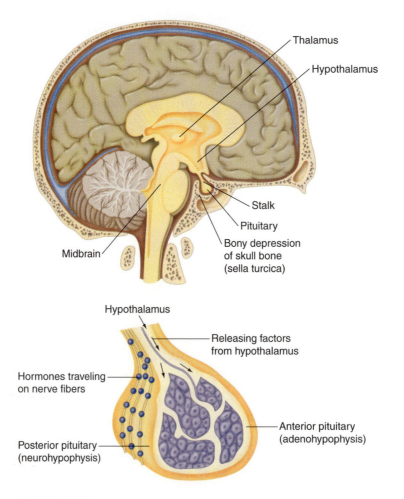

FIGURE 5.5 The pituitary gland and its relation to the brain.

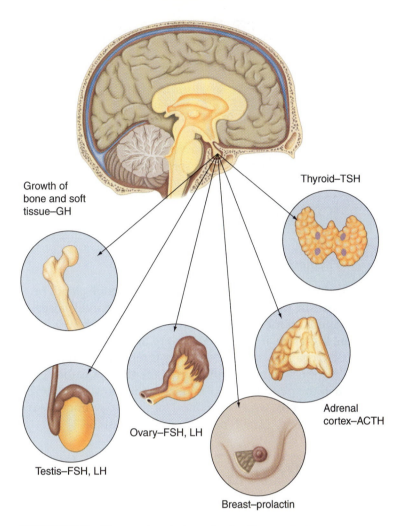

Growth of bone and soft tissue–GH

Thyroid–TSH

Testis–FSH, LH

Ovary–FSH, LH

Breast–prolactin

Adrenal cortex–ACTH

FIGURE 5.6 The anterior pituitary gland and its target organs.

thyroid gland. **Adrenocorticotropic hormone** (ah dree noh kor tih koh **TROH** pik **HOR** mohn) (**ACTH**) regulates the function of the adrenal cortex. **Prolactin** (proh **LAK** tin) stimulates milk production following pregnancy and birth. **Follicle-stimulating hormone** (**FOLL** ih kl **STIM** yoo lay ting **HOR** mohn) (**FSH**) and **luteinizing hormone** (**LOO** tee in eye zing **HOR** mohn) (**LH**) both exert their influence on the male and female gonads. FSH is responsible for the development of ova in ovaries and sperm in testes. It also stimulates the ovary to secrete estrogen. LH stimulates secretion of sex hormones in both males and females and plays a role in releasing ova in females. **Melanocyte-stimulating hormone** (**MSH**) stimulates melanocytes to produce more melanin, thereby darkening the skin.

The posterior pituitary secretes two hormones, **antidiuretic** (an tye dye yoo **RET** ik) **hormone** (**ADH**) and **oxytocin** (ok see **TOH** sin). ADH promotes water reabsorption by the kidney tubules. Oxytocin stimulates uterine contractions during labor and delivery, and after birth the release of milk from the mammary glands.

MED TERM *TIP*

The term *diabetes* usually refers to diabetes mellitus (DM), a disorder of the pancreas. Another type of diabetes, called **diabetes insipidus** (in **SIP** ih dus) **(DI),** is a result of the inadequate secretion of the **antidiuretic hormone (ADH)** from the pituitary gland.

TESTES (TWO)

gonads   **testosterone**

sperm

The testes are small, oval glands located in the scrotal sac of the male. They are the male **gonads,** which produce the male sex cells, **sperm,** and the male sex hormone, **testosterone** (tess **TOSS** ter own). Testosterone produces the male secondary sexual characteristics and regulates sperm production.

THYMUS

T cells

Thymosin

The thymus is considered one of the endocrine glands because it secretes the hormone **thymosin** (thigh **MOH** sin). The thymus gland is located in the mediastinal cavity in front of (anterior) and above the heart (see Figure 5.7). The thymus, a very small organ, is present at birth and grows to its largest size during puberty. After puberty it begins to change size and eventually is replaced with connective and adipose tissue.

The most important function of the thymus is the development of the immune system in the newborn. It is essential to the growth and development of thymic lymphoid cells or **T cells,** which are critical for the body's immune system. The complete function of the thymus gland is not very well understood.

THYROID GLAND

calcitonin   **T₃**   **triiodothyronine**

goiter   **T₄**

iodine   **thyroxine**

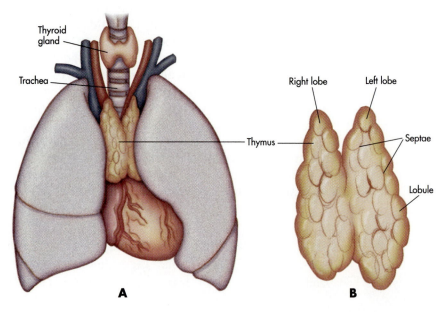

FIGURE 5.7   The thymus gland. (A) Appearance and position; (B) with anatomic structures.

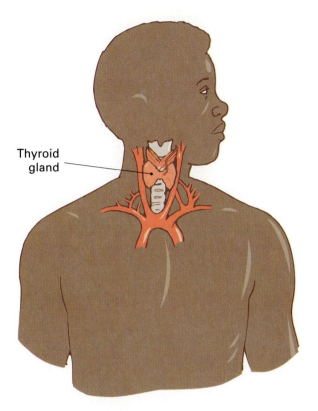

Thyroid gland

FIGURE 5.8 The thyroid gland.

The thyroid gland (see Figure 5.8), which resembles a butterfly in shape, has right and left lobes. It is located on either side of the trachea and larynx. Thyroid cartilage, or Adam's apple, is located just below the thyroid gland. This gland produces the hormones **thyroxine** (thigh **ROKS** in), which is also known as T_4, and **triiodothyronine** (try eye oh doh **THIGH** roh neen), which is called T_3. These hormones are produced in the thyroid gland from the mineral **iodine** (**EYE** oh dine). T_3 and T_4 help to regulate the production of energy and heat in the body to maintain normal metabolism.

The thyroid gland also secretes **calcitonin** (kal sih **TOH** nin) in response to hypercalcemia (too high blood calcium level). Its action is the opposite of parathyroid hormone and stimulates the increased deposition of calcium into bone, thereby lowering blood levels of calcium.

MED TERM TIP

Iodine is found in many foods, including vegetables and seafood. It is also present in iodized salt, which is one of the best sources of iodine for people living in the *Goiter belt*, composed of states located away from salt water. A lack of iodine in the diet can lead to thyroid disorders, including **goiter** (**GOY** ter).

Word Building Relating to the Endocrine System

The following list contains examples of medical terms built directly from word parts. The definitions of these terms can be determined by a straightforward translation of the word parts.

Combining Form	Combined With	Medical Term	Definition
acr/o	-megaly	acromegaly (ak roh **MEG** ah lee)	enlarged extremities
aden/o	-oma	adenoma (ad eh **NOH** mah)	gland tumor
adren/o	-megaly	adrenomegaly (ad ree noh **MEG** ah lee)	enlarged adrenal gland
	-pathy	adrenopathy (ad ren **OP** ah thee)	adrenal gland disease
adrenal/o	-ectomy	adrenalectomy (ad ree nal **EK** toh mee)	excision of adrenal glands
	-itis	adrenalitis (ad ree nal **EYE** tis)	inflammation of an adrenal gland
andr/o	-gen	androgen (**AN** druh jen)	male forming
calc/i	hyper- -emia	hypercalcemia (high per kal **SEE** mee ah)	excessive calcium in the blood
	hypo- -emia	hypocalcemia (high poh kal **SEE** mee ah)	low calcium in the blood
cortic/o	-al	cortical (**KOR** tih kal)	pertaining to the cortex
crin/o	endo- -ologist	endocrinologist (en doh krin **ALL** oh jist)	specialist in the endocrine system
	endo- -ology	endocrinology (en doh krin **ALL** oh jee)	study of the endocrine system
	endo- -pathy	endocrinopathy (en doh krin **OP** ah thee)	endocrine system disease
dips/o	poly- -ia	polydipsia (pall ee **DIP** see ah)	many (excessive) thirst
estr/o	-gen	estrogen (**ESS** troh jen)	female forming
glyc/o	hyper- -emia	hyperglycemia (high per glye **SEE** mee ah)	excessive sugar in the blood
	hypo- -emia	hypoglycemia (high poh glye **SEE** mee ah)	low sugar in the blood
glycos/o	-uria	glycosuria (glye kohs **YOO** ree ah)	sugar in the urine
kal/i	hyper- -emia	hyperkalemia (high per kal **EE** mee ah)	excessive potassium in the blood
natr/o	hypo- -emia	hyponatremia (high poh nah **TREE** mee ah)	low sodium in the blood
ophthalm/o	ex- -ic	exophthalmic (eks off **THAL** mik)	pertaining to outward eyes
pancreat/o	-ic	pancreatic (pan kree **AT** ik)	pertaining to the pancreas
parathyroid/o	-ectomy	parathyroidectomy (pair ah thigh royd **EK** toh mee)	excision of the parathyroid gland
	-oma	parathyroidoma (pair ah thigh royd **OH** ma)	parathyroid gland tumor
thyr/o	-megaly	thyromegaly (thigh roh **MEG** ah lee)	enlarged thyroid
	toxic/o -osis	thyrotoxicosis (thigh roh toks ih **KOH** sis)	abnormal condition of poisoning by the thyroid
thyroid/o	-ectomy	thyroidectomy (thigh royd **EK** toh mee)	excision of the thyroid
	eu-	euthyroid (yoo **THIGH** royd)	normal thyroid
	hyper- -ism	hyperthyroidism (hi per **THIGH** royd izm)	state of excessive thyroid
	hypo- -ism	hypothyroidism (high poh **THIGH** royd izm)	state of low thyroid
	-otomy	thyroidotomy (thigh royd **OTT** oh mee)	incision into thyroid gland
ur/o	poly- -ia	polyuria (pall ee **YOO** ree ah)	condition of (too) much urine

Vocabulary Relating to the Endocrine System

edema (eh DEE mah)	Condition in which the body tissues contain excessive amounts of fluid.
endocrinologist (en doh krin ALL oh jist)	Physician who specializes in the treatment of endocrine glands, including diabetes.
endocrinology (en doh krin ALL oh je)	Study of diseases and conditions of the endocrine glands.
exophthalmos (ex off THAL mohs)	Condition in which the eyeballs protrude, such as in Graves' disease. This is generally caused by an overproduction of thyroid hormone (see Figure 5.9).
glycosuria (glye kohs YOO ree ah)	Presence of an excess of sugar in the urine.
hirsutism (HER soot izm)	Condition of having an excessive amount of hair. Term generally used to describe females who have the adult male pattern of hair growth. Can be the result of a hormonal imbalance.
hypercalcemia (high per kal SEE mee ah)	Condition of having an excessive amount of calcium in the blood.
hyperglycemia (high per glye SEE mee ah)	Having an excessive amount of glucose (sugar) in the blood.
hyperkalemia (high per kal EE mee ah)	Condition of having an excessive amount of potassium in the blood.
metabolism (meh TAB oh lizm)	Sum of all chemical and physical changes that take place in the body.
obesity (oh BEE sih tee)	Having an abnormal amount of fat in the body.
oral hypoglycemic (high poh glye SEE mik) agent	Medication taken by mouth that causes a decrease in blood sugar. This is not used for insulin-dependent patients. There is no proof that this medication will prevent the long-term complications of diabetes mellitus.
polydipsia (pall ee DIP see ah)	Condition of having an excessive amount of thirst, such as in diabetes.
polyuria (pall ee YOO ree ah)	Condition of having excessive urine production. This can be a symptom of disease conditions such as diabetes.
syndrome (SIN drohm)	Group of symptoms and signs that, when combined, present a clinical picture of a disease or condition.

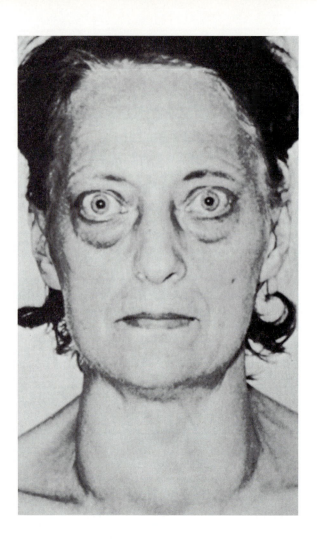

FIGURE 5.9 A patient with exophthalmos.

Pathology of the Endocrine System

acidosis (as ih DOH sis)	Excessive acidity of bodily fluids due to the accumulation of acids, as in diabetic acidosis.
acromegaly (ak roh MEG ah lee)	Chronic disease of adults that results in an elongation and enlargement of the bones of the head and extremities. There can also be mood changes.
Addison's disease (AD ih sons dih ZEEZ)	Disease named for Thomas Addison, a British physician, that results from a deficiency in adrenocortical hormones. There may be an increased pigmentation of the skin, generalized weakness, and weight loss.
adenoma (ad eh NOH mah)	Neoplasm or tumor of a gland.
cretinism (KREE tin izm)	Congenital condition in which a lack of thyroid may result in arrested physical and mental development.
Cushing's syndrome (CUSH ings SIN drohm)	Set of symptoms named after Harvey Cushing, an American neurosurgeon, that result from hypersecretion of the adrenal cortex. This may be the result of a tumor of the adrenal glands. The syndrome may present symptoms of weakness, edema, excess hair growth, skin discoloration, and osteoporosis (see Figures 5.10 and 5.11).

diabetes insipidus (DI) (dye ah BEE teez in SIP ih dus)	Disorder caused by the inadequate secretion of a hormone by the posterior lobe of the pituitary gland. There may be polyuria and polydipsia. This is more common in the young.
diabetes mellitus (DM) (dye ah BEE teez MELL ih tus)	Chronic disorder of carbohydrate metabolism that results in hyperglycemia and glycosuria. There are two distinct forms of diabetes mellitus: insulin-dependent diabetes mellitus (IDDM) or Type 1, and non–insulin-dependent diabetes mellitus (NDDM) or Type 2. See Figure 5.12 for examples of medication.
diabetic retinopathy (dye ah BET ik ret in OP ah thee)	Secondary complication of diabetes that affects the blood vessels of the retina, resulting in visual changes and even blindness.
dwarfism (DWARF izm)	Condition of being abnormally small. It may be the result of a hereditary condition or an endocrine dysfunction.
gigantism (JYE gan tizm)	Excessive development of the body due to the overproduction of the growth hormone by the pituitary gland. The opposite of dwarfism (see Figure 5.13).
goiter (GOY ter)	Enlargement of the thyroid gland (see Figure 5.14).
Graves' Disease	Condition named for Robert Graves, an Irish physician, that results in overactivity of the thyroid gland and can cause a crisis situation. Also called *hyperthyroidism*.
Hashimoto's disease (hash ee MOH tohz dih ZEEZ)	Chronic form of thyroiditis, named for a Japanese surgeon.
hyperthyroidism (hi per THIGH royd izm)	Condition that results from overactivity of the thyroid gland and can cause a crisis situation. Also called *Graves' disease*.
hypothyroidism (high poh THIGH royd izm)	Result of a deficiency in secretion by the thyroid gland. This results in a lowered basal metabolism rate with obesity, dry skin, slow pulse, low blood pressure, sluggishness, and goiter. Treatment is replacement with synthetic thyroid hormone.
insulin-dependent diabetes mellitus (dye ah BEE teez MELL ih tus)	Also called *Type 1 diabetes mellitus*. It develops early in life when the pancreas stops insulin production. Persons with IDDM must take daily insulin injections.
ketoacidosis (kee toh ass ih DOH sis)	Acidosis due to an excess of ketone bodies (waste products). A serious condition requiring immediate treatment that can result in death for the diabetic patient if not reversed.
myasthenia gravis (my ass THEE nee ah GRAV is)	Condition in which there is great muscular weakness and progressive fatigue. There may be difficulty in chewing and swallowing, and drooping eyelids. If a thymoma is causing the problem, it can be treated by removal of the thymus gland.
myxedema (miks eh DEE mah)	Condition resulting from a hypofunction of the thyroid gland. Symptoms can include anemia, slow speech, enlarged tongue and facial features, edematous skin, drowsiness, and mental apathy.
non-insulin-dependent diabetes mellitus (dye ah BEE teez MELL ih tus)	Also called *Type 2 diabetes mellitus*. It develops later in life when the pancreas produces insufficient insulin. Persons may take oral hypoglycemics to stimulate insulin secretion, or may eventually have to take insulin.
thyrotoxicosis (thigh roh toks ih KOH sis)	Condition that results from overproduction of the thyroid gland. Symptoms include a rapid heart action, tremors, enlarged thyroid gland, exophthalmos, and weight loss.
von Recklinghausen's disease (REK ling how zenz)	Excessive production of parathyroid hormone, which results in degeneration of the bones. Named for Friedrich von Recklinghausen, a German histologist.

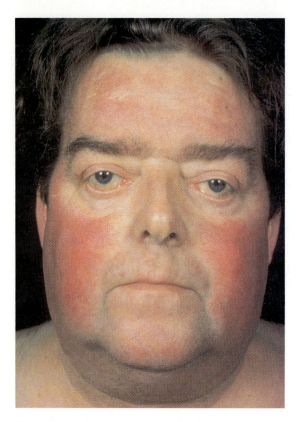

FIGURE 5.10 Cushing's disease. (BioPhoto Associates/Science Source/Photo Researchers, Inc.)

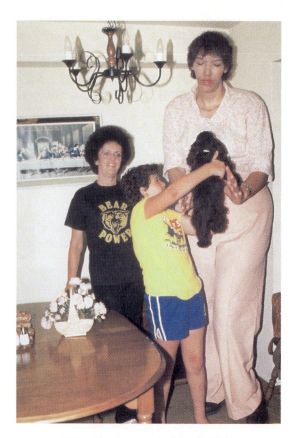

FIGURE 5.13 Gigantism of mother with normal son. (Bettina Cirrone/Photo Researchers, Inc.)

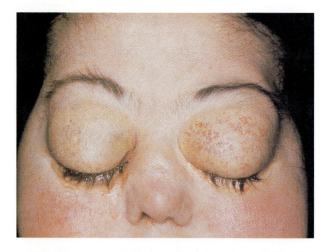

FIGURE 5.11 Facial features of Cushing's disease. (BioPhoto Associates/Science Source/Photo Researchers, Inc.)

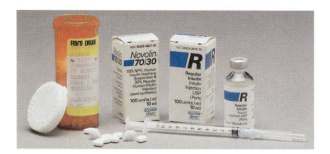

FIGURE 5.12 Insulin equipment for the diabetic patient.

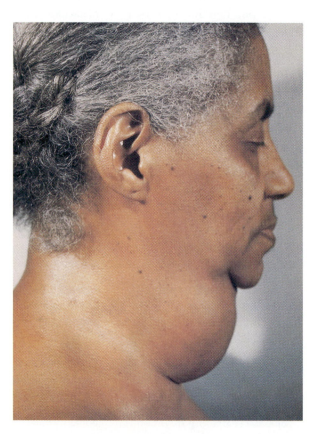

FIGURE 5.14 Goiter. (Martin Rotker/ Phototake NYC)

Diagnostic Procedures Relating to the Endocrine System

basal metabolic (BAY sal met ah BOLL ik) rate (BMR)	Somewhat outdated test to measure the energy used when the body is in a state of rest.
blood serum test	Blood test to measure the level of substances such as calcium, electrolytes, testosterone, insulin, and glucose. Used to assist in determining the function of various endocrine glands.
computerized tomography (toh MOG rah fee) (CT) scan	Radiographic scan of endocrine organs to assist in the diagnosis of pathology.
fasting blood sugar (FBS)	Blood test to measure the amount of sugar circulating throughout the body after a 12-hour fast.
glucose (GLOO kohs) tolerance test (GTT)	Test to determine the blood sugar level. A measured dose of glucose is given to a patient either orally or intravenously. Blood samples are then drawn at certain intervals to determine the ability of the patient to use glucose. Used for diabetic patients to determine their insulin response to glucose.
protein-bound iodine test (PBI)	Blood test to measure the concentration of thyroxine (T_4) circulating in the bloodstream. The iodine becomes bound to the protein in the blood and can be measured. Useful in establishing thyroid function.
radioactive iodine uptake test (RAIU)	Test in which radioactive iodine is taken orally (PO) or intravenously (IV). The amount that is eventually taken into the thyroid gland (the uptake) is measured to assist in determining thyroid function.
radioimmunoassay (RIA) (ray dee oh im yoo noh ASS ay)	Test used to measure the levels of hormones in the plasma of the blood.
serum glucose (SEE rum GLOO kohs) tests	Blood test performed to assist in determining insulin levels and useful for adjusting medication dosage. (See Figure 5.15 for illustration of a normal pancreas.)
thyroid echogram (THIGH royd EK oh gram)	Ultrasound examination of the thyroid that can assist in distinguishing a thyroid nodule from a cyst.
thyroid (THIGH royd) function tests (TFT)	Blood tests used to measure the levels of T_3, T_4, and TSH in the bloodstream to assist in determining thyroid function.
thyroid (THIGH royd) scan	Test in which a radioactive element is administered that localizes in the thyroid gland. The gland can then be visualized with a scanning device to detect pathology such as tumors.
total calcium	Blood test to measure the total amount of calcium to assist in detecting parathyroid and bone disorders.
two-hour postprandial (post PRAN dee al) glucose tolerance test	Blood test to assist in evaluating glucose metabolism. The patient eats a high-carbohydrate diet and fasts overnight before the test. A blood sample is then taken two hours after a meal.

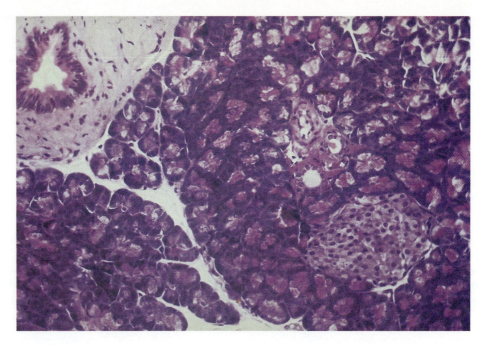

FIGURE 5.15 Enhanced color pancreas cells. (BioPhoto Associates/Photo Researchers, Inc.)

Treatment Procedures Relating to the Endocrine System

adrenalectomy **(ad ree nal EK toh mee)**	Excision of the adrenal gland.
parathyroidectomy **(pair ah thigh royd** **EK toh mee)**	Excision of one or more of the parathyroid glands. This is performed to halt the progress of hyperparathyroidism.
thymectomy **(thigh MEK toh mee)**	Removal of the thymus gland.
thyroidectomy **(thigh royd EK toh mee)**	Removal of the entire thyroid or a portion (partial thyroidectomy) to treat a variety of conditions, including nodes, cancer, and hyperthyroidism.
thyroparathyroidectomy **(thigh roh pair ah thigh** **royd EK toh mee)**	Surgical removal (excision) of the thyroid and parathyroid glands.

Endocrinologist

An endocrinologist diagnoses and treats patients with glandular disorders, which often interfere with the body's metabolism. Endocrinologists treat patients with diabetes, hyperthyroidism, and hypothyroidism by developing a course of treatment that will return the body to normal function. Endocrinologists must hold an M.D. or D.O. degree and may have their own medical practice or work in research or the pharmaceutical industry. For more information regarding a career as an endocrinologist, visit The American Association of Clinical Endocrinologist's web site at www.aace.com.

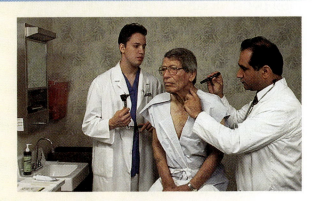

Abbreviations Relating to the Endocrine System

ACTH	adrenocorticotropic hormone	**NIDDM**	non-insulin-dependent diabetes mellitus
ADH	antidiuretic hormone	**NPH**	neutral protamine Hagedorn (insulin)
BMR	basal metabolic rate	**PBI**	protein-bound iodine
DI	diabetes insipidus	**PGH**	pituitary growth hormone
DM	diabetes mellitus	**PTH**	parathyroid hormone
FBS	fasting blood sugar	**RAI**	radioactive iodine
FSH	follicle-stimulating hormone	**RAIU**	radioactive iodine uptake
GH	growth hormone	**RIA**	radioimmunoassay
GTT	glucose tolerance test	**T$_3$**	triiodothyronine
HGH	human growth hormone	**T$_4$**	thyroxine
IDDM	insulin-dependent diabetes mellitus	**T$_7$**	free thyroxine index
K	potassium	**TFT**	thyroid function test
MSH	melanocyte-stimulating hormone	**TSH**	thyroid-stimulating hormone
Na	sodium		

KEY TERMS

- acidosis (ass ih **DOH** sis)
- acromegaly (ak roh **MEG** ah lee)
- Addison's disease (**AD** ih sons dih **ZEEZ**)
- adenoma (ad eh **NOH** mah)
- adrenal glands (ad **REE** nal)
- adrenalectomy (ad ree nal **EK** toh mee)
- adrenaline (ah **DREN** ah lin)
- adrenalitis (ad ree nal **EYE** tis)
- adrenocorticotropic hormone (ACTH) (ah dree noh kor tih koh **TROH** pik **HOR** mohn)
- adrenomegaly (ad ree noh **MEG** ah lee)

- adrenopathy (ad ren **OP** ah thee)
- aldosterone (al **DOSS** ter ohn)
- androgen (**AN** druh jen)
- anterior lobe
- antidiuretic hormone (ADH) (an tye dye yoo **RET** ik)
- basal metabolic rate (BMR) (**BAY** sal met ah **BOLL** ik)
- blood serum test
- calcitonin (kal sih **TOH** nin)
- computerized tomography (CT) scan (toh **MOG** rah fee)

- cortex (**KOR** tex)
- cortical (**KOR** tih kal)
- corticosteroids (kor tih koh **STAIR** oydz)
- cortisol (**KOR** tih sal)
- cretinism (**KREE** tin izm)
- Cushing's syndrome (**CUSH** ings **SIN** drohm)
- diabetes insipidus (DI)
  (dye ah **BEE** teez in **SIP** ih dus)
- diabetes mellitus (DM)
  (dye ah **BEE** teez **MELL** ih tus)
- diabetic retinopathy
  (dye ah **BET** ik ret in **OP** ah thee)
- dwarfism (**DWARF** izm)
- edema (eh **DEE** mah)
- endocrine glands (**EN** doh krin)
- endocrine system (**EN** doh krin)
- endocrinologist (en doh krin **ALL** oh jist)
- endocrinology (en doh krin **ALL** oh jee)
- endocrinopathy (en doh krin **OP** ah thee)
- epinephrine (ep ih **NEF** rin)
- estrogen (**ESS** troh jen)
- euthyroid (yoo **THIGH** royd)
- exocrine glands (**EKS** oh krin)
- exophthalmic (eks off **THAL** mik)
- exophthalmos (eks off **THAL** mohs)
- fasting blood sugar (FBS)
- follicle-stimulating hormone (FSH)
  (**FOLL** ih kl **STIM** yoo lay ting **HOR** mohn)
- gigantism (**JYE** gan tizm)
- glands
- glucagon (**GLOO** koh gon)
- glucocorticoid (gloo koh **KOR** tih koyd)
- glucose tolerance test (GTT) (**GLOO** kohs)
- glycosuria (glye kohs **YOO** ree ah)
- goiter (**GOY** ter)
- gonads (**GOH** nadz)
- Graves' disease
- growth hormone (GH)
- Hashimoto's disease (hash ee **MOH** tohz dih **ZEEZ**)
- hirsutism (**HER** soot izm)
- hormones (**HOR** mohnz)
- hypercalcemia (high per kal **SEE** mee ah)
- hyperglycemia (high per glye **SEE** mee ah)
- hyperkalemia (high per kal **EE** mee eah)
- hyperthyroidism (high per **THIGH** royd izm)
- hypocalcemia (high poh kal **SEE** mee ah)
- hypoglycemia (high poh glye **SEE** mee ah)
- hyponatremia (high poh nah **TREE** mee ah)
- hypothalamus (high poh **THAL** ah mus)
- hypothyroidism (high poh **THIGH** royd izm)
- insulin (**IN** soo lin)
- insulin-dependent diabetes mellitus
- iodine (**EYE** oh dine)
- islets of Langerhans (**EYE** lets of **LAHNG** er hahnz)
- ketoacidosis (kee toh ass ih **DOH** sis)
- luteinizing hormone
  (**LOO** tee in eye zing **HOR** mohn)
- medulla (meh **DULL** lah)
- melanocyte-stimulating hormone (MSH)
- metabolism (meh **TAB** oh lizm)

- mineralocorticoid (min er al oh **KOR** tih koyd)
- myasthenia gravis (my ass **THEE** nee ah **GRAV** is)
- myxedema (miks eh **DEE** mah)
- non-insulin dependent diabetes mellitus
- norepinephrine (nor ep ih **NEF** rin)
- obesity (oh **BEE** sih tee)
- oral hypoglycemic agent (high poh glye **SEE** mik)
- ova (**OH** vah)
- ovaries (**OH** vah reez)
- oxytocin (ok see **TOH** sin)
- pancreas (**PAN** kree ass)
- pancreatic (pan kree **AT** ik)
- parathyroid glands (pair ah **THIGH** royd)
- parathyroid hormone (PTH)
  (pair ah **THIGH** royd **HOR** mohn)
- parathyroidectomy (pair ah thigh royd **EK** toh mee)
- parathyroidoma (pair ah thigh royd **OH** mah)
- pituitary gland (pih **TOO** ih tair ee)
- polydipsia (pall ee **DIP** see ah)
- polyuria (pall ee **YOO** ree ah)
- posterior lobe
- progesterone (proh **JESS** ter ohn)
- prolactin (proh **LAK** tin)
- protein-bound iodine (PBI) test
- radioactive iodine uptake (RAIU) test
  (ray dee oh **AK** tiv **EYE** oh dine)
- radioimmunoassay (RIA)
  (ray dee oh im yoo noh **ASS** ay)
- serum glucose tests (**SEE** rum **GLOO** kohs)
- sperm
- steroid sex hormones (**STAIR** oyd)
- syndrome (**SIN** drohm)
- T_3
- T_4
- T cells
- testes (**TESS** teez)
- testosterone (tess **TOSS** ter own)
- tetany (**TET** ah nee)
- thymectomy (thigh **MEK** toh mee)
- thymosin (thigh **MOH** sin)
- thymus gland (**THIGH** mus)
- thyroid echogram (**THIGH** royd **EK** oh gram)
- thyroid function tests (TFT) (**THIGH** royd)
- thyroid gland (**THIGH** royd)
- thyroid scan (**THIGH** royd)
- thyroid-stimulating hormone (TSH)
- thyroidectomy (thigh royd **EK** toh mee)
- thyroidotomy (thigh royd **OTT** oh mee)
- thyromegaly (thigh roh **MEG** ah lee)
- thyroparathyroidectomy
  (thigh roh pair ah thigh royd **EK** toh mee)
- thyrotoxicosis (thigh roh toks ih **KOH** sis)
- thyroxine (T_4) (thigh **ROKS** in)
- total calcium
- triiodothyronine (T_3)
  (try eye oh doh **THIGH** roh neen)
- two-hour postprandial glucose tolerance test
  (post **PRAN** dee al)
- von Recklinghausen's disease
  (**REK** ling how zenz)

Case Study

DISCHARGE SUMMARY

Admitting Diagnosis: Hyperglycemia, ketoacidosis, glycosuria

Final Diagnosis: New-onset Type I diabetes mellitus

History of Present Illness: Patient presented to pediatrician's office with a two-month history of weight loss, fatigue, polyuria, and polydipsia. Her family history is significant for a grandfather, mother, and older brother with Type I diabetes mellitus. The pediatrician found hyperglycemia with a fasting blood sugar and glycosuria with a urine dipstick. Patient was also noted to be dehydrated and extremely lethargic. She is being admitted at this time for management of new-onset diabetes mellitus.

Summary of Hospital Course: At the time of admission, the FBS was 300 mg/100 ml and she was in ketoacidosis. She rapidly improved after receiving insulin; her serum glucose level normalized, and her lethargy disappeared. The next day a two-hour post-prandial glucose tolerance test confirmed the diagnosis of diabetes mellitus while an abdominal X-ray and a pancreas CT-scan were normal. There was no evidence of diabetic retinopathy. Attempts to control hyperglycemia with oral hypoglycemics were not successful and patient was started on insulin injections. She was discharged three days later on a protocol of b.i.d. insulin injections. The patient and her family were instructed in diet, exercise, symptoms of hypoglycemic coma, and long-term complications of diabetes mellitus.

Discharge Plans: Patient was discharged to home with her parents. She is on a 2,000-calorie ADA diet with three meals and two snacks. She may engage in any activity and may return to school next Monday. Her parents are to check her serum glucose levels b.i.d. (twice a day) and call the office for insulin dosage. She is to return to the office in two weeks.

CRITICAL THINKING QUESTIONS FOR THE ENDOCRINE SYSTEM

1. The patient's admitting diagnosis is three symptoms related to her final diagnosis. List the three symptoms and describe each in your own words.

   a.

   b.

   c.

2. This patient has Type I diabetes mellitus. Use your text to explain the difference between Type I and Type 2.

3. This discharge summary contains four medical terms that have not been introduced yet. Describe each of these terms in your own words. Use your text as a dictionary.

   a. retinopathy

   b. protocol

   c. coma

   d. b.i.d.

4. This patient had three different types of blood tests during her hospital stay. List the three blood tests and describe the differences among them in your own words.

   a.

   b.

   c.

5. This patient had two imaging procedures conducted by the radiology department while she was in the hospital. List them and describe the differences between the two.

   a.

   b.

6. Describe the patient's discharge instructions in your own words.

Chart Note Transcription

Chart Note

The chart note below contains ten phrases that can be reworded with a medical term that you learned in this chapter. Each phrase is identified with an underline. Determine the medical term and write your answers in the space provided.

Current Complaint: A 56-year-old female was referred to the specialist in the treatment of diseases of the endocrine glands[1] for evaluation of weakness, edema, an abnormal amount of fat in the body,[2] and an excessive amount of hair for a female.[3]

Past History: Patient reports she has been abnormally fat most of her life in spite of healthy diet and regular exercise. She was diagnosed with osteoporosis after incurring a pathological rib fracture following a coughing attack.

Signs and Symptoms: Patient has moderate edema in bilateral feet and lower legs as well as a puffy face and an upper lip moustache. She is 100 lbs. over normal body weight for her age and height. She moves slowly and appears generally lethargic. A test to measure the hormone levels in the blood plasma[4] reports increased steroid hormone that regulates carbohydrates in the body[5] levels in the blood. A computer-aided X-ray scan[6] demonstrates a mass in the right outer layer of the adrenal gland.[7]

Diagnosis: A group of symptoms associated with hypersecretion of the adrenal cortex[8] secondary to a gland tumor[9] in the right outer portion of the adrenal gland.

Treatment: Surgical removal of the right adrenal gland[10] to remove the gland tumor.

1 _____

2 _____

3 _____

4 _____

5 _____

6 _____

7 _____

8 _____

9 _____

10 _____

Practice Exercises

A. Complete the following statements.

1. The study of the endocrine system is called _____ .
2. The master endocrine gland is the _____ .
3. Another term for sexual organs is _____ .
4. The term for the hormones produced by the outer portion of the adrenal cortex is _____ .
5. The hormone produced by the testes is _____ .
6. The two hormones produced by the ovaries are _____ and _____ .
7. An inadequate supply of the hormone _____ causes diabetes insipidus.
8. Another term for thyroxine is _____ .
9. The term for a protrusion of the eyeballs in Graves' disease is _____ .
10. A general term for a neoplasm of a gland is _____ .

B. State the terms described using the combining forms provided.

The combining form thyr/o refers to the thyroid. Use it to write a term that means

1. excision of the thyroid gland _____
2. inflammation of the thyroid gland _____
3. toxic condition of the thyroid gland _____
4. enlargement of the thyroid gland _____

The combining form pancreat/o refers to the pancreas. Use it to write a term that means

5. inflammation of the pancreas _____
6. removal of the pancreas _____
7. incision into the pancreas _____

The combining form adren/o refers to the adrenal glands. Use it to write a term that means

8. excision of an adrenal gland _____
9. pertaining to the adrenal cortex _____
10. inflammation of the adrenal glands _____

The combining form thym/o refers to the thymus glands. Use it to write a term that means

11. removal of the thymus gland _____

C. Match the terms in column A with the definitions in column B.

A	B
1. _____ Cushing's disease	a. enlarged thyroid
2. _____ goiter	b. overactive adrenal cortex
3. _____ acidosis	c. hyperthyroidism
4. _____ gigantism	d. underactive adrenal cortex
5. _____ cretinism	e. a diabetic crisis
6. _____ myxedema	f. causes polyuria and polydipsia
7. _____ diabetes mellitus	g. thyroiditis
8. _____ diabetes insipidus	h. arrested growth
9. _____ Hashimoto's disease	i. poor carbohydrate metabolism
10. _____ Graves' disease	j. enlarged features and apathy
11. _____ Addison's disease	k. excessive growth hormone

D. IDENTIFY THE FOLLOWING ABBREVIATIONS.

1. PBI _____
2. K _____
3. T_4 _____
4. GTT _____
5. DM _____
6. BMR _____
7. Na _____
8. ADH _____

E. WRITE THE ABBREVIATIONS FOR THE FOLLOWING TERMS.

1. non-insulin-dependent diabetes mellitus _____
2. insulin-dependent diabetes mellitus _____
3. ACTH _____
4. parathyroid hormone _____
5. triiodothyronine _____

F. BUILD A TERM USING A WORD ROOT/COMBINING FORM FROM THE ENDOCRINE SYSTEM AND ONE OF THE FOLLOWING SUFFIXES.

-crine   -toxic   -uria   -in, -ine
-dipsia   -tropin   -trophy

1. the presence of sugar or glucose in the urine _____
2. the glandular system that secretes directly into the bloodstream _____
3. a toxic condition of the thyroid gland _____
4. a substance secreted by the adrenal medulla _____
5. excessive thirst, as in diabetes insipidus _____

G. DEFINE THE FOLLOWING TERMS.

1. corticosteroid _____
2. hirsutism _____
3. tetany _____
4. diabetic retinopathy _____
5. hyperglycemia _____
6. hypoglycemia _____
7. adrenaline _____
8. insulin _____
9. thyrotoxicosis _____
10. parathyroid glands _____

Getting Connected

Multimedia Extension Activities

CD-ROM

Use the CD-ROM enclosed with your textbook to gain additional reinforcement through interactive word building exercises, spelling games, labeling activities, and additional quizzes.

www.prenhall.com/fremgen

Use the above address to access the free, interactive Companion Website created for this textbook. Get hints, instant feedback, and textbook references to chapter-related multiple choice questions, and labeling and matching exercises. In addition, you will find an audio glossary, case studies, Internet exploration exercises, flashcards, and a comprehensive exam.

Answers

CASE STUDY (CRITICAL THINKING QUESTIONS)

1. hyperglycemia; ketoacidosis; glycosuria   2. student answers will vary   3. damage to the retina as a result of diabetes, a therapeutic plan, state of profound unconsciousness, twice a day   4. fasting blood sugar, serum glucose level, two-hour post-prandial glucose tolerance test   5. abdominal X-ray, pancreas CT-scan   6. 2,000-calorie ADA diet with 3 meals and 2 snacks, may engage in any activity, return to school next Monday, check serum glucose level b.i.d., and call office for insulin dosage

CHART NOTE

1. endocrinologist—specialist in the treatment of diseases of the endocrine glands   2. obesity—an abnormal amount of fat in the body   3. hirsutism—excessive amount of hair for a female   4. radioimmunoassay (RIA)—test to measure the hormone levels in blood plasma   5. cortisol—steroid hormone that regulates carbohydrates in the body   6. computerized tomography (CAT or CT scan)—computer-aided X-ray scan   7. adrenal cortex—outer layer of the adrenal gland   8. Cushing's syndrome—a group of symptoms associated with hypersecretion of the adrenal cortex   9. adenoma—gland tumor   10. adrenalectomy—surgical removal of the adrenal gland

PRACTICE EXERCISES

A. 1. endocrinology   2. pituitary   3. gonads   4. corticosteroids   5. testosterone   6. estrogen, progesterone
7. antidiuretic hormone (ADH)   8. T_4 9. exophthalmos   10. adenoma
B. 1. thyroidectomy   2. thyroiditis   3. thyrotoxicosis   4. thyromegaly   5. pancreatitis   6. pancreatectomy
7. pancreatotomy   8. adrenalectomy   9. adrenalcortical   10. adrenitis   11. thymectomy
C. 1. b   2. a   3. e   4. k   5. h   6. j   7. i   8. f   9. g   10. c   11. d
D. 1. protein-bound iodine   2. potassium   3. thyroxine   4. glucose tolerance test   5. diabetes mellitus   6. basal metabolic rate   7. sodium   8. antidiuretic hormone
E. 1. NIDDM   2. IDDM   3. ACTH   4. PTH   5. T_3
F. 1. glycosuria   2. endocrine   3. thyrotoxicosis   4. epinephrine   5. polydipsia
G. 1. Hormone obtained from cortex of adrenal gland.   2. Having excessive hair.   3. A nervous condition characterized with spasms of extremities. Can occur from imbalance of pH and calcium or disorder of parathyroid gland.   4. Disorder of the retina occurring with diabetes.   5. Increase of blood sugar in diabetes.   6. Decrease of blood sugar.   7. Another term for epinephrine. Produced by inner portion of adrenal gland.   8. Hormone produced by pancreas. Essential for metabolism of blood sugar.   9. Toxic condition due to hyperactivity of thyroid gland.
10. Four small glands located near thyroid. Assist in regulating amount of calcium in blood.

Chapter 6

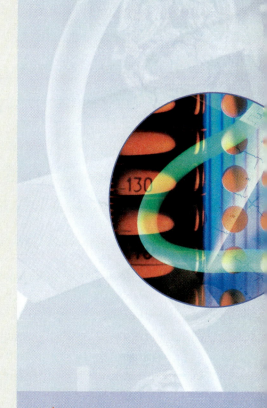

CARDIOVASCULAR SYSTEM

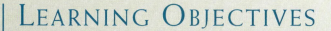

LEARNING OBJECTIVES

Upon completion of this chapter, you will be able to:

- Recognize the combining forms, prefixes, and suffixes introduced in this chapter.

- Gain the ability to pronounce medical terms and major anatomical structures.

- List the major organs of the cardiovascular system and their functions.

- Describe the flow of blood through the heart and the body.

- Explain how the electrical conduction system controls the heartbeat.

- Build cardiovascular system medical terms from word parts.

- Define vocabulary, pathology, diagnostic, and therapeutic medical terms relating to the cardiovascular system.

- Interpret abbreviations associated with the cardiovascular system.

Overview

ORGANS OF THE CARDIOVASCULAR SYSTEM

blood vessels
  arteries
  veins
  capillaries
heart

COMBINING FORMS RELATING TO THE CARDIOVASCULAR SYSTEM

angi/o	blood vessel	**pericardi/o**	pericardium
arteri/o	artery	**phleb/o**	vein
ather/o	fatty substance, plaque	**rrhythm/o**	rhythm
atri/o	atrium	**sphygm/o**	pulse
cardi/o	heart	**steth/o**	chest
coron/o	heart	**thromb/o**	clot
cyan/o	blue	**valv/o, valvul/o**	valve
embol/o	embolus	**vas/o**	vessel
hemangi/o	blood vessel	**ven/o**	vein
my/o	muscle	**ventricul/o**	ventricle
oxy/o, ox/i, ox/o	oxygen	**venul/o**	venule

PREFIXES RELATING TO THE CARDIOVASCULAR SYSTEM

Prefix	Meaning	Example
brady-	slow	bradycardia
endo-	inner	endocarditis
epi-	upon	epicardium
myo-	muscle	myocardial
peri-	around	pericarditis
sclero-	hard	arteriosclerosis
tachy-	fast	tachycardia

SUFFIXES RELATING TO THE CARDIOVASCULAR SYSTEM

Suffix	Meaning	Example
-gram	record	echocardiogram
-graphy	process of recording	angiography
-manometer	instrument to measure pressure	sphygmomanometer
-megaly	abnormally enlarged	cardiomegaly
-stenosis	narrowing	mitral stenosis
-tension	pressure	hypotension

Anatomy and Physiology of the Cardiovascular System

carbon dioxide	glucose	oxygen	pulmonary circulation
deoxygenated	metabolism	oxygenated	systemic circulation

The cardiovascular (CV) system is also called the circulatory system. This system, which maintains the distribution of blood throughout the body, is composed of the heart and blood vessels.

The actual circulatory system is composed of two parts: the **pulmonary circulation** (**PULL** mon air ee ser kew **LAY** shun) and the **systemic circulation** (sis **TEM** ik ser kew **LAY** shun). The pulmonary circulation, between the heart and lungs, transports **deoxygenated** (dee **OK** sih jen ay ted) blood to the lungs to get **oxygen,** and then back to the heart. The systemic circulation carries **oxygenated** (**OK** sih jen ay ted) blood away from the heart to the tissues and cells, and then back to the heart. In this way all the body cells receive blood and oxygen (see Figure 6.1).

In addition to distributing oxygen and other nutrients, such as **glucose** (**GLOO** kohs), the cardiovascular system collects the waste products from the cells. **Carbon dioxide** and other waste products from **metabolism** (meh **TAB** oh lizm) are transported to the lungs and kidneys by the cardiovascular system, where they are eliminated from the body.

HEART

apex	mediastinum
cardiac muscle	sternum
cardiopulmonary resuscitation (CPR)	

The heart is actually a muscular pump made up of **cardiac** (**CAR** dee ak) **muscle** fibers that could be called a muscle rather than an organ. It has four chambers or cavities and beats an average of 60 to 100 beats a minute (bpm) or about 100,000 times in one day. It is about the size of a fist and is shaped like an upside-down pear (see Figure 6.2). The tip of the heart at the lower edge is called the **apex** (**AY** peks).

The heart is located in the center of the chest cavity or **mediastinum** (mee dee ass **TYE** num). Most of the heart is actually to the left of the mediastinum. The **sternum** (**STER** num), or breastbone, is located directly in front of the heart.

MED TERM TIP

Locating the tip of the sternum is important when administering **cardiopulmonary resuscitation** (car dee oh **PULL** mon air ee ree suss ih **TAY** shun) (**CPR**). It is important to apply compressions over the center of the sternum and not over the tip (xiphoid process).

Heart Layers

endocarditis	myocardial infarction (MI)	pericarditis
endocardium	myocardium	pericardium
epicardium	parietal pericardium	visceral pericardium

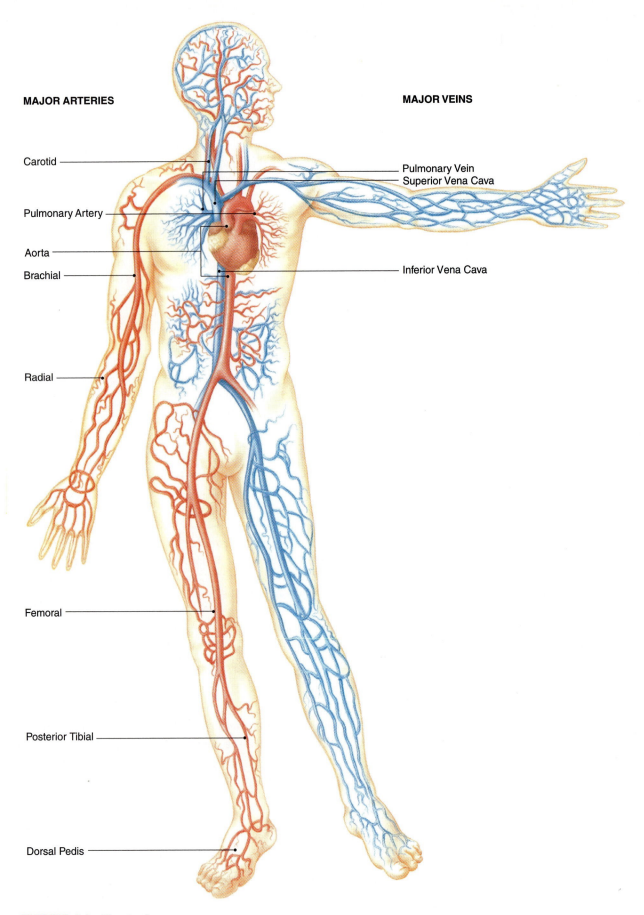

MAJOR ARTERIES

Carotid

Pulmonary Artery

Aorta

Brachial

Radial

Femoral

Posterior Tibial

Dorsal Pedis

MAJOR VEINS

Pulmonary Vein
Superior Vena Cava

Inferior Vena Cava

FIGURE 6.1 The circulatory system.

FIGURE 6.2 The heart: anterior view.

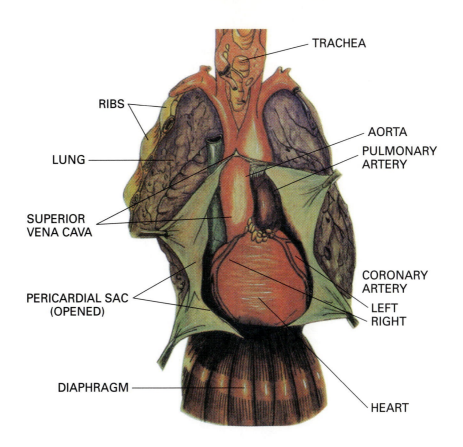

TRACHEA

RIBS

AORTA

PULMONARY ARTERY

LUNG

SUPERIOR VENA CAVA

CORONARY ARTERY

LEFT

RIGHT

PERICARDIAL SAC (OPENED)

DIAPHRAGM

HEART

FIGURE 6.3 Layers of the heart.

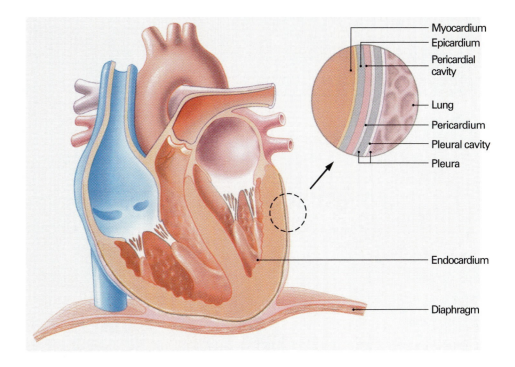

Myocardium
Epicardium
Pericardial cavity
Lung
Pericardium
Pleural cavity
Pleura

Endocardium

Diaphragm

The wall of the heart is composed of three layers (see Figure 6.3):

1. The **endocardium** (en doh **CAR** dee um) is the inner layer of the heart that lines the heart chambers.

2. The **myocardium** (my oh **CAR** dee um) is the muscular middle layer of the heart.

3. The **epicardium** (ep ih **CAR** dee um) is the outer layer of the heart. The heart is enclosed within the double-layer pleural sac, the **pericardium** (pair ih **CAR** dee um). The epicardium is the **visceral pericardium** (**VISS** er al pair ih **CAR** dee um), or inner layer of the sac. The outer layer of the sac is the **parietal pericardium** (pah **RYE** eh tal pair ih **CAR** dee um). Fluid between the two layers of the sac reduces friction as the heart beats.

MED TERM TIP

These layers become important when studying the disease conditions affecting the heart. For instance, when the prefix *endo-* is added to *carditis*, forming **endocarditis** (en doh car **DYE** tis), we know that the inflammation is within the inner layer of the heart. In discussing the muscular action of the heart the prefix **myo-,** meaning **muscle,** is added to *cardium* to form the word **myocardium.** The diagnosis **myocardial infarction** (my oh **CAR** dee al in **FARC** shun) **(MI),** or heart attack, means that the patient has an infarct or dead tissue in the muscle of the heart. The prefix *peri-*, meaning *around*, when added to the word *cardium*, refers to the sac surrounding the heart. Therefore, **pericarditis** (pair ih car **DYE** tis) is an inflammation of the outer sac of the heart.

Heart Chambers

atria	interventricular septum
interatrial septum	ventricles

The heart is divided into four chambers or cavities (see Figure 6.4). There are two **atria** (**AY** tree ah), or upper chambers, and two **ventricles** (**VEN** trik lz), or lower chambers. These are divided into right and left sides by walls called the **interatrial septum** (in ter **AY** tree al **SEP** tum) and the **interventricular septum** (in ter ven **TRIK** yoo lar **SEP** tum). The atria are the receiving chambers of the heart for all incoming blood vessels. The ventricles are the pumping chambers.

Heart Valves

aortic valve	cusps	semilunar valve
atrioventricular valve	mitral valve	tricuspid valve
bicuspid valve	pulmonary valve	

FIGURE 6.4 The heart: interior view of the heart chambers.

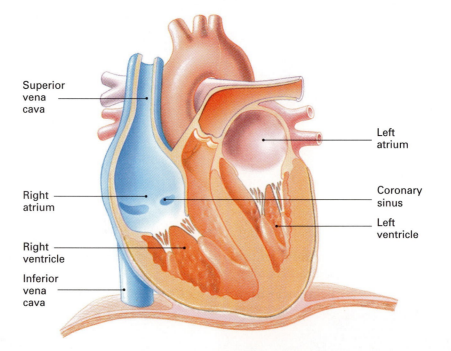

There are four valves that act as restraining gates to control the direction of blood flow. They are situated at the entrances and exits to the ventricles (see Figures 6.5 and 6.6). Properly functioning valves allow blood to flow only in the forward direction by blocking it from returning to the previous chamber. The valves are as follows:

1. **Tricuspid** (try **CUSS** pid) **valve:** This is an **atrioventricular** (ay tree oh ven **TRIK** yoo lar) **valve** (AV), meaning that it controls the opening between the right atrium and the right ventricle. It is a one-way valve, which means that once the blood enters the right ventricle it does not back up into the atrium again. The prefix *tri-*, meaning three, indicates that this valve has three leaflets or **cusps.**

2. **Pulmonary** (**PULL** mon air ee) **valve:** This is a **semilunar** (sem ih **LOO** nar) **valve.** The prefix *semi-*, meaning half, and the term *lunar*, meaning moon, indicate that this valve looks like a half-moon. Located between the right ventricle and the pulmonary artery, this important valve allows blood to flow from the right ventricle, through the pulmonary artery, and into the lungs.

3. **Mitral** (**MY** tral) **valve:** This is also called the **bicuspid** (bye **CUSS** pid) **valve,** indicating that it has two leaflets or cusps. Blood flows through this one-way atrioventricular valve to the left ventricle and does not back up into the left atrium.

4. **Aortic** (ay **OR** tik) **valve:** Blood leaves the left ventricle through this semilunar valve between the left ventricle and the aorta.

FIGURE 6.5 The valves of the heart.

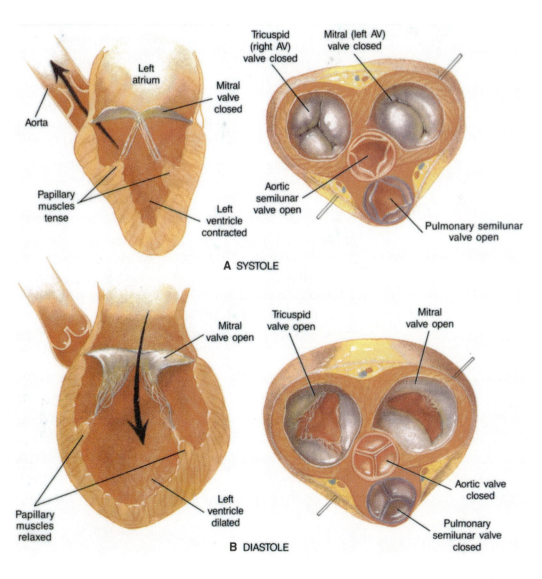

FIGURE 6.6 Heart valves. (Charles Stewart and Associates)

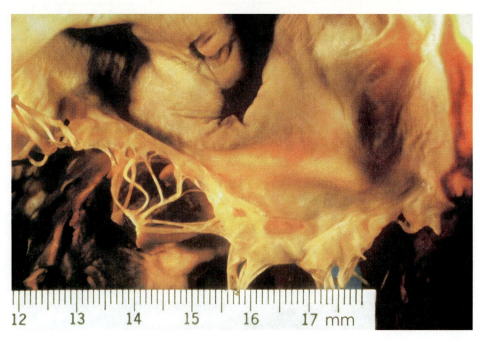

Blood Flow Through the Heart

aorta	pulmonary veins
diastolic pressure	systolic pressure
pulmonary artery	venae cavae

The flow of blood is quite orderly through the heart (see Figure 6.7). It progresses through the heart to the lungs, where it receives oxygen; back to the heart; and then out to the body tissues and parts. The normal blood flow is as follows:

1. Deoxygenated blood is received into the right atrium from all the tissues in the body, except lung tissue. It enters the right atrium through two large veins called the superior and inferior **venae cavae** (**VEE** nee **KAY** vee).

2. Blood flows from the right atrium by way of the tricuspid valve into the right ventricle.

3. The blood is pumped through the pulmonary valve by the ventricle. It moves into the **pulmonary** (**PULL** mon air ee) **artery,** where it can be carried to the lungs.

4. The left atrium receives blood that has been oxygenated by the lungs. This blood enters the left atrium from the four **pulmonary** (**PULL** mon air ee) **veins.**

5. The blood flows through the mitral valve into the left ventricle. From the left ventricle, the blood is pumped through the aortic valve and into the **aorta** (ay **OR** tah), the largest artery in the body. The aorta carries blood to all parts of the body except the lungs.

MED TERM *TIP*

A blood pressure reading is actually a measurement of two different sounds. The first sound, the *lubb* sound, is the **systolic** (sis **TOL** ik) **pressure.** This occurs when the ventricles contract and send blood through the body. It is the maximum pressure. The second, the *dubb* sound, occurs when the heart muscles relax before the cycle begins all over again. This is called the **diastolic** (dye ah **STOL** ik) **pressure** reading and is the lowest arterial pressure. In a reading of 120/90, the systolic pressure is 120 and the diastolic pressure is 90. The normal range for blood pressure in an adult is 90/60 to 140/90 (see Figure 6.8).

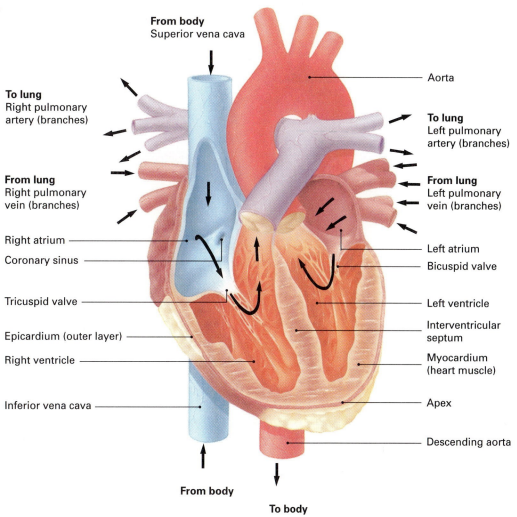

FIGURE 6.7 Circulation of the heart.

From body
Superior vena cava

Aorta

To lung
Right pulmonary artery (branches)

To lung
Left pulmonary artery (branches)

From lung
Right pulmonary vein (branches)

From lung
Left pulmonary vein (branches)

Right atrium

Coronary sinus

Left atrium

Bicuspid valve

Tricuspid valve

Left ventricle

Epicardium (outer layer)

Interventricular septum

Right ventricle

Myocardium (heart muscle)

Inferior vena cava

Apex

Descending aorta

From body

To body

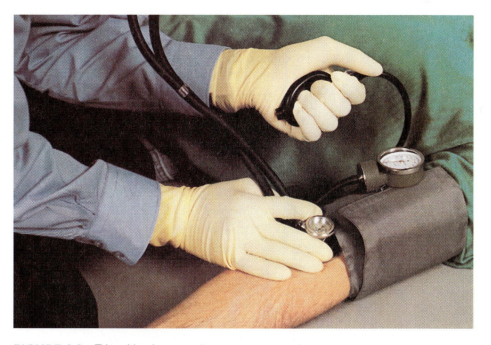

FIGURE 6.8 Taking blood pressure in an emergency setting.

171

FIGURE 6.9 The heart conduction system.

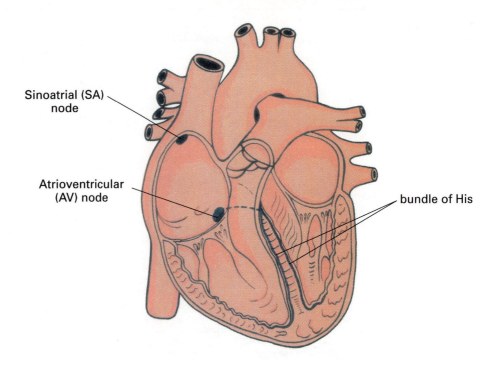

Sinoatrial (SA) node

Atrioventricular (AV) node

bundle of His

Heartbeat and Conduction System of the Heart

atrioventricular node	bundle of His	pacemaker
autonomic nervous system	electrocardiogram (ECG, EKG)	sinoatrial node

The **autonomic nervous system** (aw toh **NOM** ik **NER** vus **SIS** tem) controls the heartbeat; we have no direct control over the beating of our heart. Special tissue within the heart is responsible for the contraction impulses and the order in which they occur.

The order in which the impulses travel is as follows (see Figure 6.9):

1. The **sinoatrial** (sigh noh **AY** tree al) **node,** or **pacemaker,** is where the heartbeat begins.

2. The pacemaker causes a wave of impulse through the muscles of the atria, which causes them to contract.

3. Next, the **atrioventricular** (ay tree oh ven **TRIK** yoo lar) **node** is stimulated. The node sends a stimulation wave to the **bundle of His,** which carries the signal down the interventricular septum and out into the ventricular muscle.

4. The ventricles then contract almost simultaneously.

MED TERM TIP

The **electrocardiogram** (ee lek troh **CAR** dee oh gram), which is referred to as an EKG or ECG, is a measurement of the electrical activity of the heart (see Figure 6.10). This can give the physician information about the health of the heart.

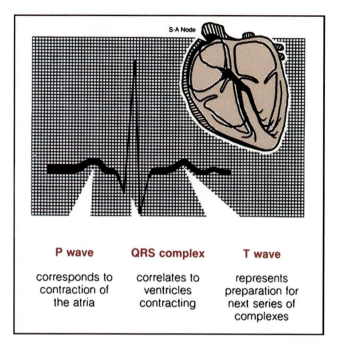

P wave	QRS complex	T wave
corresponds to contraction of the atria	correlates to ventricles contracting	represents preparation for next series of complexes

FIGURE 6.10 EKG tracing.

BLOOD VESSELS

aorta	capillaries	pulmonary artery	venules
arteries	coronary artery	superior vena cava	
arterioles	inferior vena cava	veins	

There are three types of blood vessels: arteries, veins, and capillaries. The **arteries** (**AR** teh reez) are the large thick-walled vessels that carry the blood away from the heart (see Figure 6.11). The **pulmonary artery** carries deoxygenated blood, or blood without oxygen, from the right ventricle to the lungs. The largest artery, the **aorta,** begins from the left ventricle of the heart and carries oxygenated blood, or blood with oxygen, to all the body systems. The **coronary artery** (**KOR** ah nair ee **AR** ter ee) then branches from the aorta and provides blood to the myocardium or heart muscle (see Figure 6.12). The small branches of the arteries are called **arterioles** (ar **TEE** ree ohlz). These branches carry blood to the **capillaries** (**CAP** ih lair eez).

The **veins** (**VAYNS**) carry blood back to the heart (see Figure 6.13). Blood leaving capillaries first enters small **venules** (**VEN** yools), which then turn into larger veins. Veins are smaller and much thinner than arteries, causing them to collapse easily. The veins also have valves that allow the blood to move only toward the heart. These valves prevent blood from backing away from the heart. The two large veins that enter the heart are the **superior vena cava** (soo **PEE** ree or **VEE** nah **KAY** vah), which carries blood from the upper body, and the **inferior vena cava** (in **FEE** ree or **VEE** nah **KAY** vah), which carries blood from the lower body. Blood pressure in the veins is much lower than it is in the arteries. Muscular action against the veins and skeletal muscle contractions help in the movement of blood.

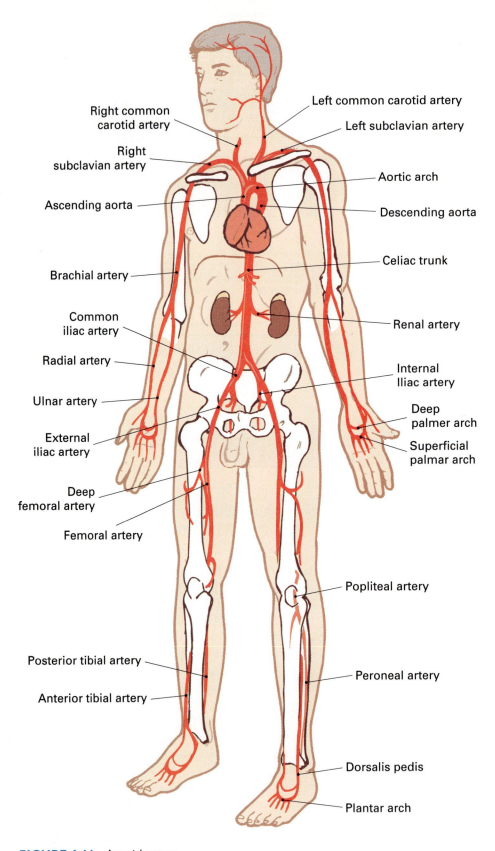

Right common
carotid artery

Left common carotid artery

Right
subclavian artery

Left subclavian artery

Ascending aorta

Aortic arch

Descending aorta

Brachial artery

Celiac trunk

Common
iliac artery

Renal artery

Radial artery

Internal
Iliac artery

Ulnar artery

Deep
palmer arch

External
iliac artery

Superficial
palmar arch

Deep
femoral artery

Femoral artery

Popliteal artery

Posterior tibial artery

Peroneal artery

Anterior tibial artery

Dorsalis pedis

Plantar arch

FIGURE 6.11   Arterial system.

FIGURE 6.12 Coronary arteries.

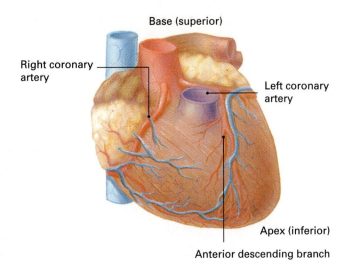

Base (superior)

Right coronary artery

Left coronary artery

Apex (inferior)

Anterior descending branch

FIGURE 6.13 Venous system.

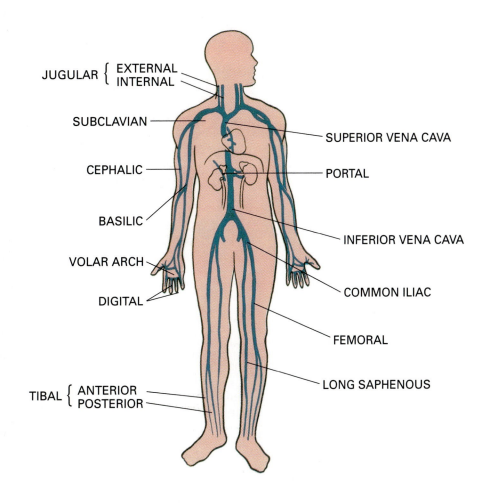

JUGULAR { EXTERNAL INTERNAL

SUBCLAVIAN

CEPHALIC

BASILIC

VOLAR ARCH

DIGITAL

TIBAL { ANTERIOR POSTERIOR

SUPERIOR VENA CAVA

PORTAL

INFERIOR VENA CAVA

COMMON ILIAC

FEMORAL

LONG SAPHENOUS

The tiny **capillaries** are actually the connecting units between the arteries and the veins. The capillaries are very thin and carry oxygen-rich blood from the arteries to the body cells. Since the capillaries are so small, the blood will not flow as quickly through them as it does through the arteries and veins. This means that the blood has time for an exchange of nutrients, oxygen, and waste material to take place between the surrounding cells and the tissue fluid.

See Figure 6.14 for an illustration of blood circulation through the cardiovascular system.

FIGURE 6.14 Circulation of blood through the cardiovascular system.

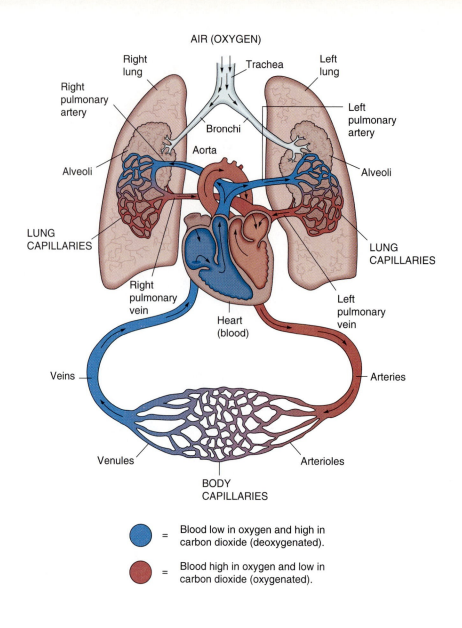

AIR (OXYGEN)

Right lung
Trachea
Left lung
Right pulmonary artery
Bronchi
Left pulmonary artery
Aorta
Alveoli
Alveoli
LUNG CAPILLARIES
LUNG CAPILLARIES
Right pulmonary vein
Heart (blood)
Left pulmonary vein
Veins
Arteries
Venules
Arterioles
BODY CAPILLARIES

🔵 = Blood low in oxygen and high in carbon dioxide (deoxygenated).

🔴 = Blood high in oxygen and low in carbon dioxide (oxygenated).

Word Building Relating to the Cardiovascular System

The following list contains examples of medical terms built directly from word parts. The definition for these terms can be determined by a straightforward translation of the word parts.

Combining Form	Combined With	Medical Term	Definition
angi/o	-graphy	angiography (an jee **OG** rah fee)	making a record of a vessel
	-plasty	angioplasty (**AN** jee oh plas tee)	surgical repair of a vessel
	-rrhaphy	angiorrhaphy (an jee **OR** rah fee)	suturing a vessel
	-scope	angioscope (**AN** jee oh scope)	instrument to view a vessel
	-scopy	angioscopy (an jee **OSS** koh pee)	viewing a vessel
	-spasm	angiospasm (**AN** jee oh spazm)	involuntary muscle contraction of a vessel
	-stenosis	angiostenosis (an jee oh sten **OH** sis)	narrowing of a vessel

aort/o	-gram	aortogram (ay **OR** toh gram)	record of the aorta
	-ic	aortic (ay **OR** tik)	pertaining to the aorta
arteri/o	-al	arterial (ar **TEE** ree al)	pertaining to the artery
	endo- -ectomy	endarterectomy (end ar teh **REK** toh mee)	excision of the inside of an artery
	poly- -itis	polyarteritis (pol ee ar ter **EYE** tis)	inflammation of many arteries
	-rrhexis	arteriorrhexis (ar tee ree oh **REK** sis)	ruptured artery
	-sclerosis	arteriosclerosis (ar tee ree oh skleh **ROH** sis)	hardening of an artery
ather/o	-ectomy	atherectomy (ath er **EK** toh mee)	excision of fatty substance
	-sclerosis	atherosclerosis (ath er oh skleh **ROH** sis)	hardening with fatty substance
atri/o	-al	atrial (**AY** tree al)	pertaining to the atrium
	inter- -al	interatrial (in ter **AY** tree al)	pertaining to between the atria
cardi/o	-ac	cardiac (**CAR** dee ak)	pertaining to the heart
	angi/o -itis	angiocarditis (an jee oh kar **DYE** tis)	inflammation of heart vessel
	brady- -ia	bradycardia (brad ee **CAR** dee ah)	state of slow heart
	-dynia	cardiodynia (car dee oh **DIN** ee ah)	heart pain
	electr/o -gram	electrocardiogram (ee lek tro **CAR** dee oh gram)	record of heart electricity
	electr/o -graphy	electrocardiography (ee lek tro car dee **OG** rah fee)	process of recording heart electricity
	endo- -itis	endocarditis (en doh car **DYE** tis)	inflammation of inner heart (layer)
	-megaly	cardiomegaly (car dee oh **MEG** ah le)	enlarged heart
	my/o -al	myocardial (my oh **CAR** de al)	pertaining to heart muscle
	my/o -itis	myocarditis (my oh car **DYE** tis)	inflammation of heart muscle
	my/o -pathy	cardiomyopathy (car dee oh my **OP** ah thee)	heart muscle disease
	-ologist	cardiologist (car dee **ALL** oh jist)	specialist in the cardiovascular system
	-ology	cardiology (car dee **ALL** oh jee)	study of the heart
	peri- itis	pericarditis (pair ih car **DYE** tis)	inflammation of outer heart (layer)
	-rrhaphy	cardiorrhaphy (car dee **OR** ah fee)	suture the heart
	tachy- -ia	tachycardia (tak ee **CAR** dee ah)	state of fast heart
coron/o	-ary	coronary (**KOR** ah nair ee)	pertaining to the heart
cyan/o	-osis	cyanosis (sigh ah **NOH** sis)	abnormal condition of (being) blue
phleb/o	-itis	phlebitis (fleh **BYE** tis)	inflammation of a vein
	-otomy	phlebotomy (fleh **BOT** oh me)	incision in a vein
rrhythm/o	a- -ia	arrhythmia (ah **RITH** mee ah)	state of no (heart) rhythm
steth/o	-scope	stethoscope (**STETH** oh scope)	chest instrument
thromb/o	-lysis	thrombolysis (throm **BOL** ih sis)	clot destruction
valvul/o	-itis	valvulitis (val vyoo **LYE** tis)	inflammation of a valve
ven/o	-ous	venous (**VEE** nus)	pertaining to a vein
ventricul/o	-ar	ventricular (ven **TRIK** yoo lar)	pertaining to a ventricle
	inter- -ar	interventricular (in ter ven **TRIK** yoo lar)	pertaining to between the ventricles

Vocabulary Relating to the Cardiovascular System

auscultation (oss kul TAY shun)	Process of listening to the sounds within the body by using a stethoscope (see Figure 6.15).
blood pressure (BP)	Measurement of the pressure that is exerted by blood against the walls of a blood vessel.
bruit (brew EE)	Term used interchangeably with the word *murmur*. A gentle, blowing sound that is heard during auscultation.
cardiologist (car dee ALL oh jist)	A physician specializing in treating diseases and conditions of the cardiovascular system.
cardiology (car dee ALL oh jee)	The branch of medicine relating to the cardiovascular system.
coronary (KOR ah nair ee)	Referring to the heart.
cyanosis (sigh ah NOH sis)	Slightly bluish color of the skin due to a deficiency of oxygen and an excess of carbon dioxide in the blood. It is caused by a variety of disorders, ranging from chronic lung disease to congenital and chronic heart problems.
defibrillator (dee fib rih LAY tor); **cardioverter** (CAR dee oh ver tor)	Instrument that uses electrodes placed externally over the heart to provide an electric shock for the purpose of converting an arrhythmia to normal sinus rhythm (see Figure 6.16).
embolus (EM boh lus)	Obstruction of a blood vessel by a blood clot that moves from another area.
infarct (IN farkt)	Area of tissue within an organ or part that undergoes necrosis (death) following the cessation of the blood supply.
ischemia (is KEYH mee ah)	Localized and temporary deficiency of blood supply due to an obstruction to the circulation.
lumen (LOO men)	The space, cavity, or channel within a tube or tubular organ or structure in the body.
murmur (MUR mur)	An abnormal heart sound such as a soft blowing sound or harsh click. They may be soft and heard only with a stethoscope, or so loud they can be heard several feet away.
pulse	Expansion and contraction produced by blood as it moves through an artery. The pulse can be taken at several pulse points throughout the body where an artery is close to the surface.
shunt	Abnormal connection between two cavities or organs. In a cardiovascular shunt there is an abnormal connection between the cavities of the heart.
sphygmomanometer (sfig moh mah NOM eh ter)	Instrument for measuring blood pressure. Also referred to as a *blood pressure cuff*.
stent	A stainless steel tube placed within a blood vessel or a duct to widen the lumen.
stethoscope (STETH oh scope)	Instrument for listening to body sounds, such as the chest, heart, or intestines.
thrombus (THROM bus)	Blood clot.

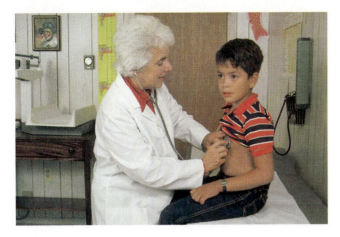

FIGURE 6.15 Auscultation.

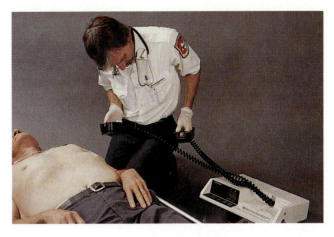

FIGURE 6.16 Defibrillator (cardioverter).

Pathology of the Cardiovascular System

aneurysm (AN yoo rizm)	Weakness in the wall of an artery that results in localized widening of the artery. Although an aneurysm may develop in any artery, common sites include the aorta in the abdomen and the cerebral arteries in the brain.
angina pectoris (an JYE nah PECK tor is)	Condition in which there is severe pain with a sensation of constriction around the heart. Caused by a deficiency of oxygen to the heart muscle.
angiocarditis (an je oh kar DYE tis)	Inflammation of blood vessels and the heart.
angioma (an jee OH ma)	Tumor, usually benign, consisting of blood vessels.
angiospasm (AN jee oh spazm)	Spasm or contraction of the blood vessels.
aortic (ay OR tik) insufficiency (AI)	Failure of the aortic valve to close completely, which causes leaking and inefficient heart action.
aortic stenosis (ay OR tik steh NOH sis)	Narrowing of the aorta.
arrhythmia (ah RITH mee ah)	Irregularity in the heartbeat or action.
arterial embolism (ar TEE ree al EM boh lizm)	Blood clot forming in an artery. Can be formed as a result of arteriosclerosis.
arteriosclerosis (ar tee ree oh skleh ROH sis)	Thickening, hardening, and loss of elasticity of the walls of the arteries.
arteriosclerotic (ar tee ree oh skleh ROT ik) heart disease (ASHD)	Chronic heart disorder caused by a hardening of the walls of the arteries.
atherosclerosis (ath er oh skleh ROH sis)	The most common form of arteriosclerosis. Caused by the formation of yellowish plaques of cholesterol on the inner walls of the arteries.

(continued)

Cardiovascular System • 179

atrioventricular (ay tree oh ven TRIK yoo lar) defect	Heart defect of the atrium and ventricle.
bradycardia (brad ee CAR dee ah)	Abnormally slow heart rate, below 60 bpm.
cardiomegaly (car dee oh MEG ah lee)	Abnormally enlarged heart.
cardiomyopathy (car dee oh my OP ah thee)	General term for a disease of the myocardium, or heart muscle. Can be caused by alcohol abuse, parasites, viral infection, and congestive heart failure.
coarctation (koh ark TAY shun) of the aorta	Severe congenital narrowing of the aorta.
congenital heart anomaly (ah NOM ah lee)	Heart defect that is present at birth.
congenital septal defect (CSD)	Defect, present at birth, in the wall separating two chambers of the heart. Results in a mixture of oxygenated and deoxygenated blood being carried to the surrounding tissues. There can be an atrial septal defect (ASD) and a ventricular septal defect (VSD).
congestive heart failure (CHF)	Pathological condition of the heart in which there is a reduced outflow of blood from the left side of the heart. Results in weakness, breathlessness, and edema.
coronary ischemia (KOR ah nair ee iss KEYH mee ah)	Insufficient blood supply to the heart muscle due to an obstruction.
coronary thrombosis (KOR ah nair ee throm BOH sis)	Blood clot in a coronary vessel of the heart causing the vessel to close completely or partially (see Figure 6.17).
endocarditis (en doh car DYE tis)	Inflammation of the lining membranes of the heart. May be due to microorganisms or to an abnormal immunological response.
fibrillation (fib ril AY shun)	Abnormal quivering or contractions of heart fibers. When this occurs within the fibers of the ventricle of the heart, arrest and death can occur. Emergency equipment to defibrillate, or convert the heart to a normal beat, is necessary.
heart valve prolapse	The cusps or flaps of the heart valve are too loose and fail to shut tightly, allowing blood to flow backwards through the valve when the heart chamber contracts. Most commonly occurs in the mitral valve, but may affect any of the heart valves.
heart valve stenosis	The cusps or flaps of the heart valve are too stiff. Therefore, they are unable to open fully, making it difficult for blood to flow through, or shut tightly, allowing blood to flow backwards. This condition may affect any of the heart valves.
hypertension (high per TEN shun)	Blood pressure above the normal range.
hypertensive (high per TEN siv) heart disease (dih ZEEZ)	Heart disease as a result of persistently high blood pressure, which damages the blood vessels and ultimately the heart.
hypotension (high poh TEN shun)	Decrease in blood pressure. Can occur in shock, infection, cancer, anemia, or as death approaches.
mitral stenosis (MY tral steh NOH sis) (MS)	Narrowing of the opening (orifice) of the mitral valve, which causes an obstruction in the flow of blood from the atrium to the ventricle.

mitral (MY tral) valve prolapse (PROH laps) (MVP)	Common and serious condition in which the cusp of the mitral valve drops down (prolapses) into the left atrium during systole.
myocardial infarction (my oh CAR dee al in FARC shun) (MI)	Condition caused by the partial or complete occlusion or closing of one or more of the coronary arteries (see Figure 6.18). Symptoms include a squeezing pain or heavy pressure in the middle of the chest. A delay in treatment could result in death. Also referred to as *MI or heart attack*.
patent ductus arteriosus (PAY tent DUCK tus ar tee ree OH sis)	Congenital heart anomaly in which the opening between the pulmonary artery and the aorta fails to close at birth. This condition requires surgery.
pericarditis (pair ih car DYE tis)	Inflammatory process or disease of the pericardium.
phlebitis (fleh BYE tiz)	Inflammation of a vein.
polyarteritis (pol ee ar ter EYE tis)	Inflammation of several arteries.
Raynaud's phenomenon (ray NOZ)	Periodic ischemic attacks affecting the extremities of the body, especially the fingers, toes, ears, and nose. The affected extremities become cyanotic and very painful. These attacks are brought on by arterial constriction due to extreme cold or emotional stress. Named after a French physician, Maurice Raynaud.
rheumatic (roo MAT ik) heart disease	Valvular heart disease as a result of having had rheumatic fever.
tachycardia (tak ee CAR dee ah)	Abnormally fast heart rate, over 100 bpm.
tetralogy of Fallot (teh TRALL oh jee of fal LOH)	Combination of four congenital anomalies: pulmonary stenosis, an interventricular septal defect, abnormal blood supply to the aorta, and hypertrophy of the right ventricle. Needs immediate surgery to correct. Named for Etienne-Louis Fallot, a French physician.
thrombophlebitis (throm boh fleh BYE tis)	Inflammation of a vein that results in the formation of blood clots within the vein.
varicose (VAIR ih kohs) veins	Swollen and distended veins, usually in the legs.

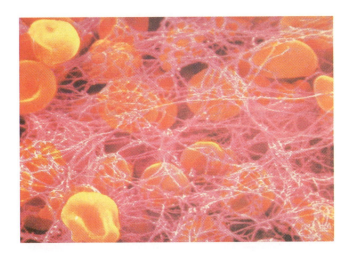

FIGURE 6.17 Enhanced color blood cell clot.

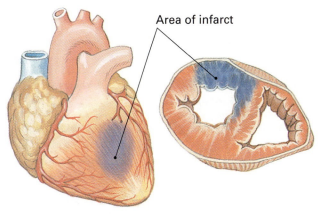

Area of infarct

FIGURE 6.18 Cross section of myocardial infarction.

Diagnostic Procedures Relating to the Cardiovascular System

angiocardiography (an jee oh kar dee OG rah fee)	Radiographic X-ray of the heart and large vessels after the injection of a radiopaque solution. X-rays are taken in rapid sequence as the material moves through the heart.
angiography (an jee OG rah fee)	X-rays taken after the injection of an opaque material into a blood vessel. Can be performed on the aorta as an aortic angiogram, on the heart as an angiocardiogram, and on the brain as a cerebral angiogram.
arterial (ar TEE ree al) blood gases (ABG)	Measurement of the amount of oxygen (O_2), carbon dioxide (CO_2), and nitrogen in the blood. Also gives a pH reading of the blood. Performed in emergency situations, it is valuable in evaluation of cardiac failure, hemorrhage, and kidney failure.
arteriography (ar tee ree OG rah fee)	X-ray of the arteries after a radiopaque dye has been inserted.
cardiac catheterization (CAR dee ak cath eh ter ih ZAY shun)	Passage of a thin tube (catheter) through an arm vein and the blood vessels leading into the heart. Done to detect abnormalities, to collect cardiac blood samples, and to determine the pressure within the cardiac area.
cardiac enzymes (CAR dee ak EN zyms)	Complex proteins that are capable of inducing chemical changes within the body. Cardiac enzymes are taken by blood sample to determine the amount of heart disease or damage.
cardiac magnetic resonance imaging (CAR dee ak mag NEH tik REHZ oh nance) (MRI)	Noninvasive procedure in which images of the heart and blood vessels are captured for examination to determine defects.
Doppler ultrasonography (DOP ler ul trah son OG rah fee)	Measurement of sound-wave echos as they bounce off tissues and organs to produce an image. Can assist in determining heart and blood vessel damage. Named for Christian Doppler, an Austrian physicist.
echocardiogram (ek oh CAR dee oh gram)	Noninvasive diagnostic method using ultrasound to visualize internal cardiac structures. Cardiac valves can be visualized using this method.
electrocardiogram (ee lek troh CAR dee oh gram) (ECG, EKG)	Record of the electrical activity of the heart. Useful in the diagnosis of abnormal cardiac rhythm and heart muscle (myocardium) damage.
Holter monitor	Portable ECG monitor worn by the patient for a period of a few hours to a few days to assess the heart and pulse activity as the person goes through the activities of daily living. Used to assess a patient who experiences chest pain and unusual heart activity during exercise and normal activities. Named for Norman Holter, an American biophysicist.
posteroanterior (PA) and lateral of the chest	Routine X-ray of the heart and lungs.
prothrombin (proh THROM bin) time (Pro time)	Measurement of the time it takes for a sample of blood to coagulate. Also called *Pro time*.
serum lipoprotein (SEE rum lip oh PROH teen) level	A laboratory test to measure the amount of cholesterol and triglycerides in the blood.
stress/exercise testing	Method for evaluating cardiovascular fitness. The patient is placed on a treadmill or a bicycle and then subjected to steadily increasing levels of work. An EKG and oxygen levels are taken while the patient exercises. The test is stopped if abnormalities occur on the EKG.
treadmill test	Also called a *stress test*.
venography (vee NOG rah fee)	X-ray of the veins by tracing the venous pulse. Also called *phlebography*.

Treatment Procedures Relating to the Cardiovascular System

aneurysmectomy (an yoo riz **MEK** toh mee)	Surgical removal of the sac of an aneurysm.
angioplasty (**AN** jee oh plas tee)	Surgical procedure of altering the structure of a vessel by dilating it using a balloon inside the vessel (see Figure 6.19).
artery graft	Piece of blood vessel that is transplanted from a part of the body to the aorta to repair a defect.
artificial pacemaker	Electrical device that substitutes for the natural pacemaker of the heart (see Figure 6.20). It controls the beating of the heart by a series of rhythmic electrical impulses. An external pacemaker has the electrodes on the outside of the body. An internal pacemaker has the electrodes surgically implanted within the chest wall (see Figure 6.21).
cardiolysis (car dee **OL** ih sis)	Surgical procedure to separate bands of scar tissue, called adhesions, that have formed between the pericardium and chest cavity wall. This procedure involves removing part of the sternum and ribs over the pericardium.
cardiorrhaphy (car dee **OR** ah fe)	Surgical suturing of the heart.
cardiotomy (car dee **OT** oh me)	Making an incision into the heart.
commissurotomy (com ih shur **OT** oh mee)	Surgical incision to change the size of an opening. For example, in mitral commissurotomy, a stenosis or narrowing is treated by cutting away at the adhesions around the mitral opening (orifice).
coronary (**KOR** ah nair ee) **artery** (**AR** ter ee) **bypass graft (CABG)**	Open-heart surgery in which a blood vessel is grafted to route blood around the point of constriction in a diseased vessel.
defibrillation (cardioversion) (dee fib rih **LAY** shun) (**CAR** dee oh ver shun)	A procedure that converts serious irregular heart beats, such as fibrillation, by giving electric shocks to the heart.
embolectomy (em boh **LEK** toh mee)	Removal of an embolus or clot from a blood vessel.
heart transplantation	Replacement of a diseased or malfunctioning heart with a donor's heart.
intracoronary artery stent (in trah **KOR** ah nair ee **AR** ter ee)	Placing a stent within a coronary artery to treat coronary ischemia due to atherosclerosis.
intravascular thrombolytic therapy (in trah **VAS** kew lar throm boh **LIT** ik **THAIR** ah pee)	Drugs, such as streptokinase or tissue-type plasminogen activator (tPA), are injected into a blood vessel to dissolve clots and restore blood flow.
open heart surgery	Surgery that involves incision of the heart, coronary arteries, or heart valves (see Figure 6.22).
percutaneous transluminal coronary angioplasty (per kyoo **TAY** nee us trans **LOO** mih nal **KOR** ah nair ee **AN** jee oh plas tee) **(PTCA)**	Method for treating localized coronary artery narrowing. A balloon catheter is inserted through the skin into the coronary artery and inflated to dilate the narrow blood vessel.

(continued)

pericardiectomy (pair ih car dee EK toh mee)	Surgical excision of part of the pericardium.
phleborrhaphy (fleh BOR ah fee)	Suturing of a vein.
phlebotomy (fleh BOT oh mee)	Creating an opening into a vein to withdraw blood.
thrombectomy (throm BEK toh mee)	Surgical removal of a thrombus or blood clot from a blood vessel.
valve replacement	Excision of a diseased heart valve and replacement with an artificial valve.
venipuncture (VEEN ih punk cher)	Puncture into a vein to withdraw fluids or insert medication and fluids.
venotomy (vee NOT oh mee)	Surgical incision into a vein.

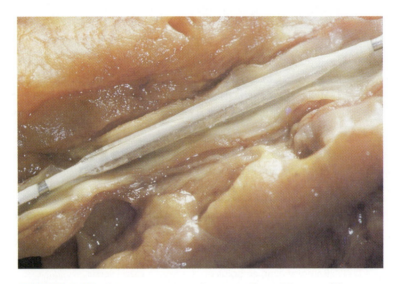

FIGURE 6.19 Balloon angioplasty. (Southern Illinois University/Photo Researchers, Inc.)

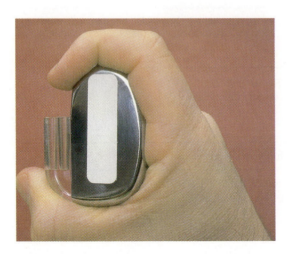

FIGURE 6.20 Heart pacemaker. (Science Photo Library/Photo Researchers, Inc.)

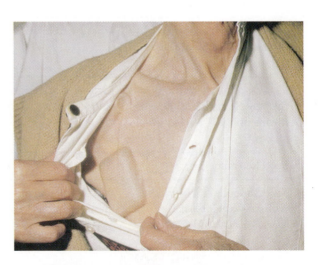

FIGURE 6.21 Pacemaker implanted into a patient's chest. (Yoav Levy/Phototake NYC)

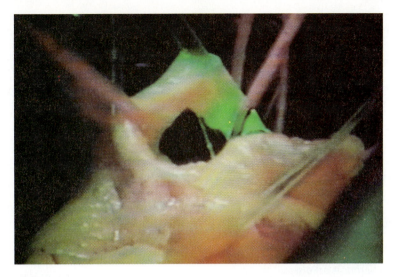

FIGURE 6.22 Enhanced color photo taken during open heart surgery as laser burns away blockage. (Daniel Choy/Phototake NYC)

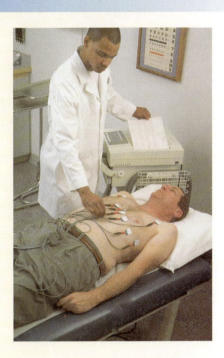

Abbreviations Relating to the Cardiovascular System

ABG	arterial blood gases
ADL	activities of daily living
AF	atrial fibrillation
AI	aortic insufficiency
AMI	acute myocardial infarction
APB	atrial premature beat
AS	aortic stenosis, arteriosclerosis
ASCVD	arteriosclerotic cardiovascular disease
ASD	atrial septal defect
ASHD	arteriosclerotic heart disease
AV, A-V	atrioventricular
BBB	bundle branch block (L for left; R for right)
BP	blood pressure
bpm	beats per minute
CABG	coronary artery bypass graft
CAD	coronary artery disease
cath	catheterization
CCU	coronary care unit
CHD	congestive heart disease
CHF	congestive heart failure
CIC	coronary intensive care
CP	chest pain
CPR	cardiopulmonary resuscitation
CSD	congenital septal defect
CV	cardiovascular
DVT	deep vein thrombosis
ECG, EKG	electrocardiogram
HDL	high-density lipoproteins
HTN	hypertension
IV	intravenous
IVCD	intraventricular conduction delay
JVP	jugular venous pulse
LDL	low-density lipoproteins
LVAD	left ventricular assist device
MI	myocardial infarction, mitral insufficiency
mmHg	millimeters of mercury
MR	mitral regurgitation
MRI	magnetic resonance imaging
MS	mitral stenosis
MVP	mitral valve prolapse
NSR	normal sinus rhythm
P	pulse
PA	posteroanterior
PAP	pulmonary arterial pressure
PAT	paroxysmal atrial tachycardia
Pro time	prothrombin time
PTCA	percutaneous transluminal coronary angioplasty
PVC	premature ventricular contraction
S1	first heart sound
S2	second heart sound
SA, S-A	sinoatrial
SBE	subacute bacterial endocarditis
SGOT	serum glutamic oxaloacetic transaminase
SK	streptokinase
SVT	supraventricular tachycardia
tPA	tissue-type plasminogen activator
VLDL	very low density lipoproteins
VPB	ventricular premature beat
VSD	ventricular septal defect
WPW	Wolff-Parkinson-White syndrome

- aneurysm (**AN** yoo rizm)
- aneurysmectomy (an yoo riz **MEK** toh mee)
- angina pectoris (an **JYE** nah **PECK** tor is)
- angiocardiography (an jee oh kar dee **OG** rah fee)
- angiocarditis (an jee oh kar **DYE** tis)
- angiography (an jee **OG** rah fee)
- angioma (an jee **OH** mah)
- angioplasty (**AN** jee oh plas tee)
- angiorrhaphy (an jee **OR** rah fee)
- angioscope (**AN** jee oh scope)
- angioscopy (an jee **OSS** koh pee)
- angiospasm (**AN** jee oh spazm)
- angiostenosis (an jee oh sten **OH** sis)
- aorta (ay **OR** tah)
- aortic (ay **OR** tik)
- aortic insufficiency (AI) (ay **OR** tik)
- aortic stenosis (AS) (ay **OR** tik steh **NOH** sis)
- aortic valve (ay **OR** tik)
- aortogram (ay **OR** toh gram)
- apex (**AY** peks)
- arrhythmia (ah **RITH** mee ah)
- arterial (ar **TEE** ree al)
- arterial blood gases (ABG) (ar **TEE** ree al)
- arterial embolism (ar **TEE** ree al **EM** boh lizm)
- arteries (**AR** teh reez)
- arteriography (ar tee ree **OG** rah fee)
- arterioles (ar **TEE** ree ohlz)
- arteriorrhexis (ar tee ree oh **REK** sis)
- arteriosclerosis (ar tee ree oh skleh **ROH** sis)
- arteriosclerotic heart disease (ASHD) (ar tee ree oh skleh **ROT** ik)
- artery graft
- artificial pacemaker
- atherectomy (ath er **EK** toh mee)
- atherosclerosis (ath er oh skleh **ROH** sis)
- atria (**AY** tree ah)
- atrial (**AY** tree al)
- atrioventricular defect (ay tree oh ven **TRIK** yoo lar)
- atrioventricular node (ay tree oh ven **TRIK** yoo lar)
- atrioventricular valve (AV) (ay tree oh ven **TRIK** yoo lar)
- auscultation (oss kul **TAY** shun)
- autonomic nervous system (aw toh **NOM** ik **NER** vus **SIS** tem)
- bicuspid valve (bye **CUSS** pid)
- blood pressure (BP)
- blood vessels
- bradycardia (brad ee **CAR** dee ah)
- bruit (brew **EE**)
- bundle of His (**HISS**)
- capillaries (**CAP** ih lair eez)
- carbon dioxide
- cardiac (**CAR** dee ak)
- cardiac catheterization (**CAR** dee ak cath eh ter ih **ZAY** shun)
- cardiac enzymes (**CAR** dee ak **EN** zyms)
- cardiac magnetic resonance imaging (**CAR** dee ak mag **NEH** tik **REHZ** oh nance)
- cardiac muscle (**CAR** dee ak)
- cardiodynia (car dee oh **DIN** ee ah)
- cardiologist (car dee **ALL** oh jist)
- cardiology (car dee **ALL** oh jee)
- cardiolysis (car dee **OL** ih sis)
- cardiomegaly (car dee oh **MEG** ah lee)
- cardiomyopathy (car dee oh my **OP** ah thee)
- cardiopulmonary resuscitation (CPR) (car dee oh **PULL** mon air ee ree suss ih **TAY** shun)
- cardiorrhaphy (car dee **OR** ah fee)
- cardiotomy (car dee **OT** oh mee)
- cardioversion (**CAR** dee oh ver shun)
- cardioverter (**CAR** dee oh ver ter)
- coarctation of the aorta (koh ark **TAY** shun)
- commissurotomy (com ih shur **OT** oh me)
- congenital heart anomaly (ah **NOM** ah lee)
- congenital septal defect (CSD)
- congestive heart failure (CHF) (kon **JESS** tiv)
- coronary (**KOR** ah nair ee)
- coronary artery (**KOR** ah nair ee **AR** ter ee)
- coronary artery bypass graft (CABG) (**KOR** ah nair ee **AR** ter ee)
- coronary ischemia (**KOR** ah nair ee iss **KEYH** mee ah)
- coronary thrombosis (**KOR** ah nair ee throm **BOH** sis)
- cusps
- cyanosis (sigh ah **NOH** sis)
- defibrillation (dee fib rih **LAY** shun)
- defibrillator (dee **FIB** rih lay tor)
- deoxygenated (dee **OK** sih jen ay ted)
- diastolic pressure (dye ah **STOL** ik)
- Doppler ultrasonography (**DOP** ler ul trah son **OG** rah fee)
- echocardiogram (ek oh **CAR** dee oh gram)
- electrocardiogram (ECG, EKG) (ee lek troh **CAR** dee oh gram)
- electrocardiography (ee lek troh car dee **OG** rah fee)
- electrolytes (ee **LEK** troh lites)
- embolectomy (em boh **LEK** toh mee)
- embolus (**EM** boh lus)
- endarterectomy (end ar teh **REK** toh mee)
- endocarditis (en doh car **DYE** tis)
- endocardium (en doh **CAR** dee um)
- epicardium (ep ih **CARD** ee um)
- fibrillation (fih brill **AY** shun)

- glucose (**GLOO** kohs)
- heart
- heart transplantation
- heart valve prolapse
- heart valve stenosis
- Holter monitor
- hypertension (high per **TEN** shun)
- hypertensive heart disease (high per **TEN** siv heart dih **ZEEZ**)
- hypotension (high poh **TEN** shun)
- infarct (**IN** farkt)
- inferior vena cava (in **FEE** ree or **VEE** nah **KAY** vah)
- interatrial (in ter **AY** tree al)
- interatrial septum (in ter **AY** tree al **SEP** tum)
- interventricular (in ter ven **TRIK** yoo lar)
- interventricular septum (in ter ven **TRIK** yoo lar **SEP** tum)
- intracoronary artery stent (in trah **KOR** ah nair ee **AR** ter ee)
- intravascular thrombolytic therapy (in trah **VAS** kew lar throm boh **LIT** ik **THAIR** ah pee)
- ischemia (iss **KEYH** mee ah)
- lumen (**LOO** men)
- mediastinum (mee dee ass **TYE** num)
- metabolism (meh **TAB** oh lizm)
- mitral stenosis (MS) (**MY** tral steh **NOH** sis)
- mitral valve (**MY** tral)
- mitral valve prolapse (MVP) (**MY** tral valve **PROH** laps)
- murmur
- myocardial (my oh **CAR** dee al)
- myocardial infarction (MI) (my oh **CAR** dee al in **FARC** shun)
- myocarditis (my oh car **DYE** tis)
- myocardium (my oh **CAR** dee um)
- open-heart surgery
- oxygen (**OK** sih jen)
- oxygenated (**OK** sih jen ay ted)
- pacemaker
- parietal pericardium (pah **RYE** eh tal pair ih **CAR** dee um)
- patent ductus arteriosus (**PAY** tent **DUCK** tus ar tee ree **OH** sis)
- percutaneous transluminal coronary angioplasty (PTCA) (per kyoo **TAY** nee us trans **LOO** mih nal **KOR** ah nair ree **AN** jee oh plas tee)
- pericardiectomy (pair ih car dee **EK** toh mee)
- pericarditis (pair ih car **DYE** tis)
- pericardium (pair ih **CAR** dee um)
- phlebitis (fleh **BYE** tis)

- phleborrhaphy (fleh **BOR** ah fee)
- phlebotomy (fleh **BOT** oh mee)
- polyarteritis (pol ee ar ter **EYE** tis)
- posteroanterior (PA) and lateral of the chest
- prothrombin time (proh **THROM** bin)
- pulmonary artery (**PULL** mon air ee)
- pulmonary circulation (**PULL** mon air ee ser kew **LAY** shun)
- pulmonary valve (**PULL** mon air ee)
- pulmonary vein (**PULL** mon air ee)
- pulse
- Raynaud's phenomenon (ray **NOZ**)
- rheumatic heart disease (roo **MAT** ik)
- semilunar valve (sem ih **LOO** nar)
- serum lipoprotein level (**SEE** rum lip oh **PROH** teen)
- shunt
- sinoatrial node (sigh noh **AY** tree al)
- sphygmomanometer (sfig moh mah **NOM** eh ter)
- stent
- sternum (**STER** num)
- stethoscope (**STETH** oh scope)
- stress/exercise testing
- superior venae cavae (soo **PEE** ree or **VEE** nee **KAY** vee)
- systemic circulation (sis **TEM** ik ser kew **LAY** shun)
- systolic pressure (sis **TOL** ik)
- tachycardia (tak ee **CAR** dee ah)
- tetralogy of Fallot (teh **TRALL** oh jee of fal **LOH**)
- thrombectomy (throm **BEK** toh mee)
- thrombolysis (throm **BOL** ih sis)
- thrombophlebitis (throm boh fleh **BYE** tis)
- thrombus (**THROM** bus)
- treadmill test
- tricuspid valve (try **CUSS** pid)
- valve replacement
- valvulitis (val vyoo **LYE** tis)
- varicose veins (**VAIR** ih kohs)
- veins (**VAYNS**)
- venae cavae (**VEE** nee **KAY** vee)
- venipuncture (**VEEN** ih punk cher)
- venography (vee **NOG** rah fee)
- venotomy (vee **NOT** oh mee)
- venous (**VEE** nus)
- ventricles (**VEN** trik lz)
- ventricular (ven **TRIK** yoo lar)
- venules (**VEN** yools)
- visceral pericardium (**VISS** er al pair ih **CAR** dee um)

Case Study

DISCHARGE SUMMARY

Admitting Diagnosis: Difficulty breathing, hypertension, tachycardia

Final Diagnosis: CHF secondary to mitral valve prolapse

History of Present Illness: Patient was brought to the Emergency Room by her family because of SOB, tachycardia (a racing heart rate), and anxiety. Patient reports that she has experienced these symptoms for the past six months, brought on by exertion. The current episode began while she was cleaning house and is more severe than any previous episode. Upon admission in the ER, HR was 120 beats per minute and blood pressure was 180/110. The patient was cyanotic around the lips and nail beds and had severe edema in feet and lower legs. The results of an EKG and cardiac enzyme blood tests were normal. Medication improved the symptoms but she was admitted for observation and a complete cardiac workup for tachycardia, hypertension.

Summary of Hospital Course: Patient underwent a full battery of cardiac diagnostic tests. A prolapsed mitral valve was observed on an echocardiogram. A treadmill test had to be stopped early due to onset of severe difficulty in breathing and cyanosis of the lips. Arterial blood gases showed low oxygen, and supplemental oxygen per nasal canula was required to resolve cyanosis. Angiocardiography failed to demonstrate significant coronary artery thrombosis. Blood pressure, tachycardia, anxiety, and pitting edema were controlled with medications. Patient took Lopressor to control blood pressure, Norpace to slow heart rate, Valium for the anxiety, and Lasix to reduce edema. At discharge, HR was 88 beats/minute, blood pressure was 165/98, and there was no evidence of edema unless she was on her feet too long.

Discharge Plans: There was no evidence of a myocardial infarction and with lack of significant coronary thrombosis, angioplasty is not indicated for this patient. Patient was placed on a low salt and low cholesterol diet. She received instructions on beginning a carefully graded exercise program. She is to continue Lasix, Norpace, Valium, and Lopressor. If symptoms are not controlled by these measures, a mitral valve replacement will be considered.

CRITICAL THINKING QUESTIONS

1. List the four medications this patient was given in the hospital and describe in your own words what condition each medication treats.

    a.

    b.

    c.

    d.

2. Two diagnostic tests conducted in the Emergency Room were normal. List them and describe each test in your own words. Because the results from these two tests were normal, a very serious heart condition could be ruled out. This is noted in the discharge plans. Identify the serious heart condition and describe it in your own words.

3. Explain in your own words why the treadmill test had to be stopped.

4. Which of the following is NOT one of the admitting diagnoses?

    a. high blood pressure

    b. dizziness

    c. difficulty breathing

    d. fast heart beat

5. The physician has two treatment options for this patient, medication and surgery. If the medication fails to control her condition, then describe what surgery will be considered.

6. Compare and contrast valve stenosis and valve prolapse.

Chart Note Transcription

Chart Note

The chart note below contains eleven phrases that can be reworded with a medical term that you learned in this chapter. Each phrase is identified with an underline. Determine the medical term and write your answers in the space provided.

Current Complaint: A 56-year-old male was admitted to the Cardiac Care Unit from the Emergency Room with left arm pain, severe pain around the heart,[1] an abnormally slow[2] heart beat, nausea, and vomiting.

Past History: Patient reports no heart problems prior to this episode. He has taken medication for high blood pressure[3] for the past five years. His family history is significant for a father and brother who both died in their 50s from death of heart muscle.[4]

Signs and Symptoms: Patient reports severe pain around the heart that radiates into his left jaw and arm. A record of the heart's electrical activity[5] and a blood test to determine the amount of heart damage[6] were abnormal.

Diagnosis: An acute death of heart muscle resulting from a blood clot in a coronary vessel.[7]

Treatment: First, provide supportive care during the acute phase. Second, evaluate heart damage by passing a thin tube through a blood vessel into the heart to detect abnormalities[8] and evaluate heart fitness by having patient exercise on a treadmill.[9] Finally, perform surgical intervention by either inflating a balloon catheter to dilate a narrow vessel[10] or by open heart surgery to create a shunt around a blocked vessel.[11]

1 _____

2 _____

3 _____

4 _____

5 _____

6 _____

7 _____

8 _____

9 _____

10 _____

11 _____

Practice Exercises

A. COMPLETE THE FOLLOWING STATEMENTS.

1. The study of the heart is called _____ .
2. The three layers of the heart are _____ , _____ , and
   _____ .
3. The impulse for the heartbeat (the pacemaker) originates in the _____ .
4. The artery that does not carry oxygenated blood is the _____ .
5. The four heart valves are _____ , _____ , _____ , and
   _____ .
6. Three procedures that are used to correct heart and cardiovascular problems are _____ ,
   _____ , and _____ .

B. STATE THE TERMS DESCRIBED USING THE COMBINING FORMS PROVIDED.

The combining form cardi/o refers to the heart. Use it to write a term that means

1. pain in the heart _____
2. disease of the heart muscle _____
3. enlargement of the heart _____
4. abnormally fast heart rate _____
5. abnormally slow heart rate _____
6. inflammation of the heart _____

The combining form phleb/o refers to the vein. Use it to write a term that means

7. inflammation of a vein _____
8. opening a vein (to withdraw blood) _____
9. clotting in a vein _____

The combining form arteri/o refers to the artery. Use it to write a term that means

10. pertaining to an artery _____
11. hardening of an artery _____

C. ADD A PREFIX TO THE COMBINING FORM CARDI/O TO FORM THE TERM FOR

1. inflammation of the inner lining of the heart   _____
2. inflammation of the outer layer of the heart   _____
3. inflammation of the muscle of the heart   _____

D. PROVIDE THE PRONUNCIATION FOR THE FOLLOWING WORDS.

1. atrial fibrillation   _____
2. cardiopulmonary resuscitation   _____
3. aneurysm   _____
4. phlebitis   _____
5. embolus   _____

E. Define each combining form and provide an example of its use.

Definition   Example

1. cardi/o _____
2. vas/o _____
3. steth/o _____
4. arteri/o _____
5. phleb/o _____
6. angi/o _____
7. ventricul/o _____
8. thromb/o _____
9. embol/o _____
10. oxy/o _____
11. sphygm/o _____

F. Write medical terms for the following definitions.

1. pertaining to a vein _____
2. fast heart beat _____
3. specialist in treating the heart _____
4. recording electrical activity of heart _____
5. high blood pressure _____
6. low blood pressure _____
7. inflammation of inner lining of heart _____
8. bluish coloring to skin _____
9. destruction of (dissolving) a clot _____
10. hardening of the arteries _____

G. Write the suffix for each expression and provide an example of its use.

Suffix   Example

1. instrument for recording _____
2. abnormal narrowing _____
3. instrument to measure pressure _____
4. enlargement _____
5. record _____

H. Identify the following abbreviations.

1. BP _____
2. CHF _____
3. MI _____
4. CCU _____
5. PVC _____
6. CPR _____
7. CAD _____

I. WRITE THE ABBREVIATIONS FOR THE FOLLOWING TERMS.

1. mitral valve prolapse   _____
2. ventricular septal defect   _____
3. percutaneous transluminal coronary angioplasty   _____
4. jugular venous pulse   _____
5. coronary intensive care   _____
6. congestive heart failure   _____

J. MATCH THE TERMS IN COLUMN A WITH THE DEFINITIONS IN COLUMN B.

A	B
1. _____ arrhythmia	a. swollen, distended veins
2. _____ thrombus	b. inflammation of vein
3. _____ bradycardia	c. abnormal connection
4. _____ bruit	d. slow heart rate
5. _____ phlebitis	e. insert thin tubing
6. _____ commissurotomy	f. irregular heartbeat
7. _____ varicose	g. murmur
8. _____ shunt	h. clot in blood vessel
9. _____ catheterization	i. to change the size of opening
10. _____ venography	j. X-ray of veins

K. USE THE FOLLOWING TERMS IN THE SENTENCES THAT FOLLOW.

angioma	angina	echocardiogram	MI
angiography	ischemia	aortic stenosis	Pro time
defibrillator	Holter monitor	hypertension	CCU
murmur	CHF	pacemaker	

1. Tiffany was born with a congenital condition that results in an abnormal heart sound. This is called a(n) _____ .

2. Porter's physician has placed him on medication that causes the blood to become thinner. His doctor wishes to measure the clotting time of his blood. He is ordering a(n) _____ .

3. Joseph suffered an arrhythmia while hospitalized that resulted in a cardiac arrest. The emergency physician and team used an instrument to give electric shocks to the heart in an attempt to create a normal heart rhythm. This is called a(n) _____ .

4. Marguerite has been placed on a low-sodium diet and medication to bring her blood pressure down to a normal range. She suffers from _____ .

5. Tony has had an artificial device called a(n) _____ inserted to control the beating of his heart by producing rhythmic electrical impulses.

6. Derrick has been admitted to the coronary care unit due to a heart condition occurring as a result of a circulatory obstruction causing a decreased blood supply. The term for this condition is _____ .

7. Laura has persistent chest pains that require medication. The term for the pain is _____ .

8. La Tonya is not receiving a sufficient blood supply due to a stricture in her aorta. This is called _____ .

9. La Tonya is going to have surgery to correct her heart condition. She will be admitted to what hospital unit after her surgery? _____

10. Stephen is going to have coronary bypass surgery to correct the constriction in his blood vessels. He recently suffered a heart attack as a result of this occlusion. His attack is called a(n) _____ .

11. Stephen's physician scheduled a test to determine the extent of his blood vessel damage. This test is called a(n) _____ .

12. In a patient who is not a good candidate for an invasive procedure such as a cardiac catheterization, what preliminary noninvasive test might be used? _____ .

13. Rolando has been diagnosed with a benign tumor of the blood vessels. This is a called a(n) _____ .

14. Eric must wear a device for 24 hours that will keep track of his heart activity as he performs his normal daily routine. This device is called a(n) _____ .

15. Lydia is 82 years old and is suffering from a heart condition that causes weakness, edema, and breathlessness. Her heart failure is the cause of her lung congestion. This condition is called _____ .

Getting Connected

Multimedia Extension Activities

CD-ROM

Use the CD-ROM enclosed with your textbook to gain additional reinforcement through interactive word building exercises, spelling games, labeling activities, and additional quizzes.

www.prenhall.com/fremgen

Use the above address to access the free, interactive Companion Website created for this textbook. Get hints, instant feedback, and textbook references to chapter-related multiple choice questions, and labeling and matching exercises. In addition, you will find an audio glossary, case studies, Internet exploration exercises, flashcards, and a comprehensive exam.

Answers

CASE STUDY (CRITICAL THINKING QUESTIONS)

1. Lopressor to control blood pressure, Norpace to slow down the heart rate, Valium to reduce anxiety, Lasix to reduce swelling   2. EKG, cardiac enzymes blood test; myocardial infarction   3. patient developed dyspnea and cyanosis   4. b — dizziness   5. mitral valve replacement   6. compare: both conditions allow blood to flow backwards   contrast: prolapse — too floppy, valve droops down   stenosis — too stiff, preventing it from opening all the way or closing all the way

CHART NOTE

1. angina pectoris — severe pain around the heart   2. bradycardia — abnormally slow heart beat   3. hypertension — high blood pressure   4. myocardial infarction (MI) — death of heart muscle   5. electrocardiogram (EKG, ECG) — record of the heart's electrical activity   6. cardiac enzymes — blood test to determine the amount of heart damage   7. coronary thrombosis — blood clot in a coronary vessel   8. cardiac catheterization — passing a thin tube through a blood vessel into the heart to detect abnormalities   9. stress test (treadmill test) — evaluate heart fitness by having patient exercise on a treadmill   10. percutaneous transluminal coronary angioplasty (PTCA)— inflating a balloon catheter to dilate a narrow vessel   11. coronary artery bypass graft (CABG) — open heart surgery to create a shunt around a blocked vessel

PRACTICE EXERCISES

A. 1. cardiology 2. endocardium myocardium epicardium 3. sinoatrial node 4. pulmonary artery 5. tricuspid pulmonary mitral aortic 6. name any three procedures

B. 1. cardiodynia 2. cardiomyopathy 3. cardiomegaly 4. tachycardia 5. bradycardia 6. carditis 7. phlebitis 8. phlebotomy 9. phlebothrombosis 10. arterial 11. arteriosclerosis

C. 1. endocarditis 2. epicarditis 3. myocarditis

D. 1. **AY** tree al fih brill **AY** shun 2. car dee oh **PULL** mon air ee ree suss ih **TAY** shun 3. **AN** yoo rizm 4. fleh **BYE** tis 5. **EM** boh lus

E. 1. heart 2. vessel 3. chest 4. artery 5. vein 6. blood vessel 7. ventricle 8. clot 9. embolus 10. oxygen 11. pulse

F. 1. venous 2. tachycardia 3. cardiologist 4. electrocardiogram 5. hypertension 6. hypotension 7. endocarditis 8. cyanosis 9. thrombolysis 10. arteriosclerosis

G. 1. -graph 2. -stenosis 3. -manometer 4. -megaly 5. -gram

H. 1. blood pressure 2. congestive heart failure 3. myocardial infarction 4. coronary care unit 5. premature ventricular contraction 6. cardiopulmonary resuscitation 7. coronary artery disease

I. 1. MVP 2. VSD 3. PTCA 4. JVP 5. CIC 6. CHF

J. 1. f 2. h 3. d 4. g 5. b 6. i 7. a 8. c 9. e 10. j

K. 1. murmur 2. Pro time 3. defibrillator 4. hypertension 5. pacemaker 6. ischemia 7. angina 8. aortic stenosis 9. CCU 10. MI 11. angiography 12. echocardiogram 13. angioma 14. Holter monitor 15. CHF

Chapter 7

LYMPHATIC AND HEMATIC (BLOOD) SYSTEMS

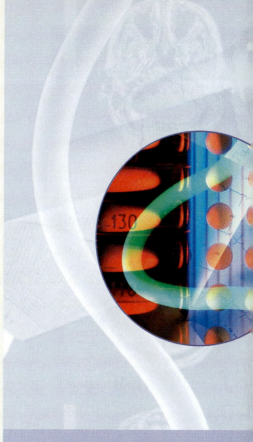

LEARNING OBJECTIVES

Upon completion of this chapter, you will be able to:

- Recognize the combining forms and suffixes introduced in this chapter.

- Gain the ability to pronounce medical terms and major anatomical structures.

- List the major organs of the lymphatic and hematic systems and their functions.

- Discuss the immune response.

- Describe the blood grouping systems.

- Build lymphatic and hematic system medical terms from word parts.

- Define vocabulary, pathology, diagnostic, and therapeutic medical terms relating to the lymphatic and hematic systems.

- Interpret abbreviations associated with the lymphatic and hematic systems.

Overview

PART I: *The Lymphatic System*

ORGANS OF THE LYMPHATIC SYSTEM

lymph nodes	spleen	tonsils
lymph vessels	thymus gland	

COMBINING FORMS RELATING TO THE LYMPHATIC SYSTEM

aden/o	gland	**lymphangi/o**	lymph vessel
fibrin/o	fibers, fibrous	**splen/o**	spleen
immun/o	protection	**thym/o**	thymus
lymph/o	lymph	**tonsill/o**	tonsils
lymphaden/o	lymph node	**tox/o**	poison

SUFFIXES RELATING TO THE LYMPHATIC SYSTEM

Suffix	Meaning	Example
-cyte	cell	lymphocyte
-cytosis	condition of cells	phagocytosis
-globulin	protein	immunoglobulin
-osis	abnormal condition	mononucleosis
-phage	eat, swallow	macrophage

ANATOMY AND PHYSIOLOGY OF THE LYMPHATIC SYSTEM

lymph	microorganisms
lymphocytes (lymphs)	

The lymphatic system is actually the body's immune or defense system against the invasion of foreign **microorganisms** (my kroh **OR** gan izmz). See Figure 7.1 for an illustration of its components. This system becomes a drainage system in conjunction with the circulatory system. The lymphatic system is actually a network of vessels and glands that assist in purifying the tissues. It is interfaced with the blood circulatory system at the point when blood and fluids mix outside the walls of blood vessels.

Fluid that has left the blood and come into contact with the tissues is called **lymph (LIMF).** Lymph fluid is composed of **lymphocytes** (**LIM** foh sights) (**lymphs**), water (H_2O), nutrients, hormones, salts, carbon dioxide (CO_2), oxygen (O_2), and urea.

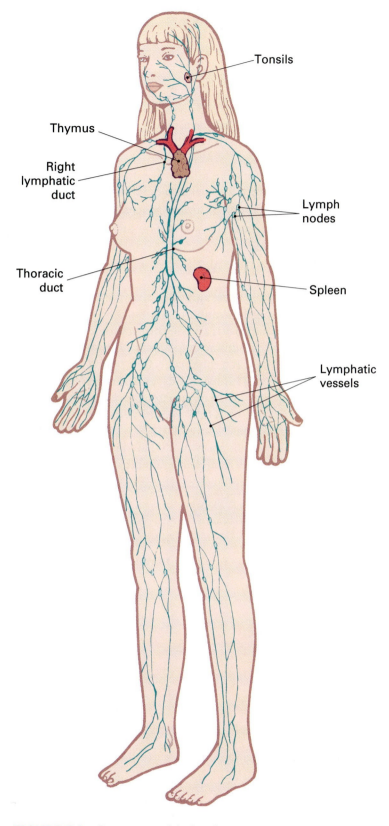

Tonsils

Thymus

Right
lymphatic
duct

Lymph
nodes

Thoracic
duct

Spleen

Lymphatic
vessels

FIGURE 7.1   Components of the lymphatic system.

LYMPH VESSELS

capillaries	lymph ducts	thoracic duct
cisterna chyli	lymphatic duct	valves
left subclavian vein	right subclavian vein	

Capillaries (**CAP** ih lair eez), which are the smallest lymphatic vessels, carry lymph fluid to the larger lymph vessels.

MED TERM *TIP* The term capillary is also used to describe the minute blood vessels within the circulatory system. This is one of several general medical terms, such as valves and cilia, or hair, that are used in several systems. The function is the same, but the structure may be somewhat different.

These large vessels have **valves** so that the fluid can only move in one direction (see Figure 7.2 for an illustration of a lymphatic valve). Lymph vessels drain into **lymph ducts.** The primary ducts are the **thoracic duct** (tho **RASS** ik) and the **lymphatic** (lim **FAT** ik) **duct.** The thoracic duct has the responsibility of draining most of the body (Figure 7.3). There is a large collection pouch at the beginning of the duct called the **cisterna chyli** (sis **TER** nah **KYE** lee). The cisterna chyli empties into the **left subclavian** (sub **KLAY** vee an) **vein** of the circulatory system. The lymphatic duct empties into the **right subclavian** (sub **KLAY** vee an) **vein.** It receives lymph fluid from the neck, head, thorax, and right upper extremity.

The lymphatic cells are actually blood cells from the hematic system including lymphocytes, monocytes, platelets, and erythrocytes.

LYMPH NODES

axillary	mediastinal
cervical	metastasized
inguinal	

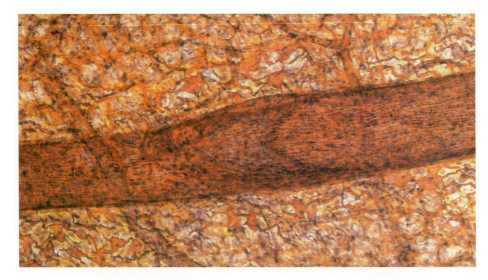

FIGURE 7.2 Enhanced color microscopic view of lymphatic vessel and valve. (Michael Abbey/Photo Researchers, Inc.)

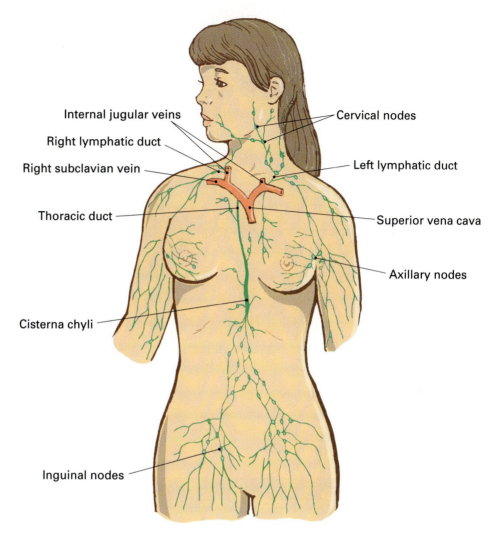

Internal jugular veins

Right lymphatic duct

Right subclavian vein

Thoracic duct

Cisterna chyli

Inguinal nodes

Cervical nodes

Left lymphatic duct

Superior vena cava

Axillary nodes

FIGURE 7.3 Vessels of the lymphatic system.

Lymph nodes are small knots of lymphatic tissue located along the route of the lymphatic vessels (see Figure 7.4). These specialized nodes have several functions, including the following:

1. Removing impurities from the body
2. Manufacturing lymphocytes
3. Producing antibodies to fight disease

Once lymph fluid is drained from the tissue, it is filtered in the node to remove impurities. Lymph nodes also serve to trap and contain cells from cancerous lesions.

MED TERM TIP

In surgical procedures to remove a malignancy from an organ, such as a breast, the adjacent lymph nodes are also tested for cancer. If cancerous cells are found in the tested lymph nodes, the disease is said to have **metastasized** (meh **TASS** tah sized). Tumor cells may then spread to other parts of the body by means of the lymphatic system.

FIGURE 7.4 Lymph node.

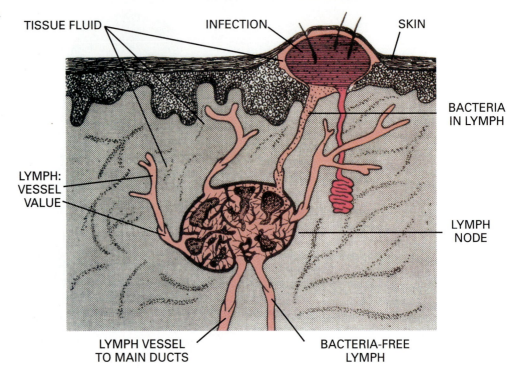

The nodes are numerous throughout the body and are usually found in groupings. These groups can range from one or two nodes to as many as one hundred. See Table 7.1 for a list of some of the most important sites for lymph nodes.

ACCESSORY LYMPH ORGANS

Tonsils

adenoids   palatine tonsils   pharynx

lingual tonsils   pharyngeal tonsils

The **tonsils** (**TON** sulls), composed of lymphatic tissue, are located on each side of the **pharynx** (**FAIR** inks). There are three sets of tonsils: **palatine** (**PAL** ah tyne) **tonsils;** **pharyngeal** (fair **IN** jee al) **tonsils,** commonly referred to as the **adenoids** (**ADD** eh noydz); and **lingual** (**LING** gwal) **tonsils.** All tonsils contain a large number of lymphocytes and act as filters to protect the body from the invasion of microorganisms

Table 7.1	Sites for Lymph Nodes	
Name	**Location**	**Function**
Axillary (**AK** sih lair ee)	Armpits	Become enlarged during infections of arms and breasts; cancer cells from breasts may be present
Cervical (**SER** vih kal)	Neck	Drains parts of head and neck; may be enlarged during upper respiratory infections
Inguinal (**ING** gwi nal)	Groin	Drains area of the legs and lower pelvis
Mediastinal (mee dee ass **TYE** nal)	Chest	Assists in draining infection from within the chest cavity

through the digestive or respiratory system. Tonsils are not required for life and can safely be removed if they become a continuous site of infection.

Spleen

lymphocytes (lymphs)	phagocytic cells
monocytes (monos)	phagocytosis
phagocytes	

The **spleen,** located in the upper left quadrant of the abdomen, consists of lymphatic tissue that is infiltrated with blood vessels. The spleen produces new red blood cells in the unborn baby. In adults it forms **lymphocytes (lymphs)** and **monocytes** (**MON** oh sights) **(monos);** filters out and destroys old red blood cells, recycling the iron; and stores some of the blood supply for the body. **Phagocytic** (fag oh **SIT** ik) **cells** lining the spleen actually remove bacteria, parasites, and other infectious materials.

MED TERM *Tip*

A **phagocyte (FAG** oh sight) is a cell that has the ability to ingest (eat) and destroy bacteria and other foreign particles. This function, **phagocytosis** (fag oh sigh **TOH** sis), is critical for the control of bacteria within the body.

The spleen is not an essential organ for life and can be removed due to injury or disease. However, without the spleen there may be an increased susceptibility to a bloodstream infection.

Thymus Gland

T cells	thymosin
T lymphocytes	

The **thymus** (**THIGH** mus) **gland,** located in the upper portion of the chest or mediastinum, has a function similar to that of lymph nodes. It assists the body with the immune function and the development of antibodies. This organ's hormone, **thymosin** (thigh **MOH** sin), changes lymphocytes to **T lymphocytes** (simply called **T cells**). These cells play an important role in the immune response. The thymus is active in the unborn child and throughout childhood until adolescence, when it begins to shrink in size.

IMMUNITY

active acquired immunity	immunizations	protozoans
aquired immunity	innate immunity	vaccinations
bacteria	macrophage	viruses
fungi	natural immunity	
immune response	passive acquired immunity	

Immunity is the body's ability to defend itself against pathogenic microorganisms and toxic substances, such as **bacteria** (bak **TEE** ree ah), **viruses, fungi** (**FUN** jee), **protozoa** (proh toh **ZOH** ah), toxins, and cancerous tumors. Immunity comes in two forms: **natural immunity** (im **YOO** nih tee) and **acquired immunity** (im **YOO** nih tee). Natural immunity, also called **innate immunity,** is not specific to a

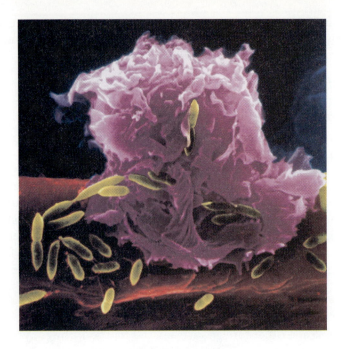

FIGURE 7.5 Enhanced color photo showing macrophage on lung blood cell wall attacking bacillus *Escherichia coli.*

particular disease and does not require prior exposure to the pathogenic agent. A good example of natural immunity is the **macrophage** (**MACK** roh fayj). These cells are present throughout all the tissues of the body, but are concentrated in areas of high exposure to invading bacteria, such as in the lungs and digestive system. They are very active phagocytic cells, ingesting and digesting bacteria that enters the body (see Figure 7.5).

Acquired immunity is the body's response to a specific pathogen. Acquired immunity may be established either passively or actively. **Passive acquired immunity** results when a person receives protective substances produced by another human or animal. This may take the form of maternal antibodies crossing the placenta to a baby, or an antitoxin or gamma globulin injection. **Active acquired immunity** develops following direct exposure to the pathogenic agent. The agent stimulates the **immune** (im **YOON**) **response,** a series of different mechanisms all geared to neutralize the agent. **Immunizations** (im yoo nih **ZAY** shuns) or **vaccinations** (vak sih **NAY** shuns) are special types of active acquired immunity. Instead of actually being exposed to the infectious agent and having the disease, a person is exposed to a modified or weakened pathogen that is still capable of stimulating the immune response.

Immune Response

acquired immunodeficiency syndrome (AIDS)

antibody

antibody-mediated immunity

antigen

B cells

B lymphocytes

cell-mediated immunity

cellular immunity

cytotoxic

human immunodeficiency virus (HIV)

humoral immunity

natural killer (NK) cells

T-helper cells

Disease-causing agents are recognized as being foreign because they have proteins that are different from the natural proteins in the body. Those foreign proteins, called **antigens** (**AN** tih jens), stimulate the immune response. The immune response results in two types of immunity: **humoral immunity** (**HYOO** mor al im **YOO** nih tee) (also called **antibody-mediated immunity**) and **cellular immunity** (also called **cell-mediated immunity**).

Humoral immunity refers to the production of **B lymphocytes** (called **B cells**). B cells respond to antigens by producing a protective protein, an **antibody** (**AN** tih bod ee). Antibodies combine with the antigen to form an antigen-antibody complex. This complex either marks the foreign substance for phagocytosis or prevents the infectious agent from damaging healthy cells.

Cellular immunity involves the production of T cells and **natural killer (NK) cells.** These defense cells are **cytotoxic** (sigh toh **TOK** sik). They physically attack and destroy pathogenic cells.

The immune response is better understood when we examine what happens to a person who has **acquired immunodeficiency syndrome (AIDS)** (acquired im yoo noh dee **FIH** shen see **SIN** drohm). In this disease, part of the body's immune system is destroyed. The **human immunodeficiency** (im yoo noh dee **FIH** shen see) **virus (HIV)** destroys one particular type of T cell, the **T-helper cell** (see Figure 7.6). This leaves the patient open to life threatening infections and cancers to which they would normally have immunity.

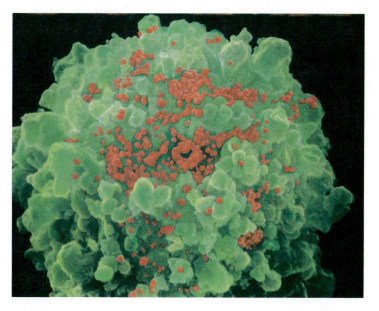

FIGURE 7.6   Enhanced color scanning electron micrograph of HIV virus infecting T-helper cells. (NIBSC/Science Photo Library/Photo Researchers, Inc.)

Word Building Relating to the Lymphatic System

The following list contains examples of medical terms built directly from word parts. The definition for these terms can be determined by a straightforward translation of the word parts.

Combining Form	Combined With	Medical Term	Definition
cyt/o	mono-	monocyte (**MON** oh sight)	single (nucleus) cell
	tox/o -ic	cytotoxic (sigh toh **TOK** sik)	pertaining to cell poisoning
immun/o	-globulin	immunoglobulin (im yoo noh **GLOB** yoo lin)	immunity protein
lymph/o	aden/o -ectomy	lymphadenectomy (lim fad eh **NEK** toh mee)	excision of lymph gland
	aden/o -graphy	lymphadenography (lim fad eh **NOG** rah fee)	recording of lymph glands
	aden/o -itis	lymphadenitis (lim fad en **EYE** tis)	inflammation of lymph glands
	aden/o -pathy	lymphadenopathy (lim fad eh **NOP** ah thee)	lymph gland disease
	angi/o -gram	lymphangiogram (lim **FAN** jee oh gram)	record of lymph vessels
	angi/o -graphy	lymphangiography (lim fan jee **OG** rah fee)	recording of lymph vessels
	angi/o -oma	lymphangioma (lim fan jee **OH** mah)	lymph vessel tumor
	-cyte	lymphocyte (**LIM** foh sight)	lymph cell
	-oma	lymphoma (lim **FOH** mah)	lymph tumor
	-tic	lymphatic (lim **FAT** ik)	pertaining to lymph
nucle/o	mono- -sis	mononucleosis (mon oh noo klee **OH** sis)	condition of one nucleus
path/o	-genic	pathogenic (path oh **JEN** ik)	disease producing
phag/o	-cyte	phagocyte (**FAG** oh sight)	eating cell
	macro-	macrophage (**MACK** roh fayj)	large eating (cell)
splen/o	-ectomy	splenectomy (splee **NEK** toh mee)	excision of spleen
	-megaly	splenomegaly (splee noh **MEG** ah lee)	enlarge spleen
	-pexy	splenopexy (**SPLEE** noh pek see)	surgical fixation of the spleen
thym/o	-ectomy	thymectomy (thigh **MEK** toh mee)	excision of the thymus
	-oma	thymoma (thigh **MOH** mah)	thymus tumor
tonsill/o	-ectomy	tonsillectomy (ton sih **LEK** toh mee)	excision of the tonsils
	-itis	tonsillitis (ton sil **EYE** tis)	inflammation of the tonsils

Vocabulary Relating to the Lymphatic System

allergen (AL er jin)	Antigen capable of causing a hypersensitivity or allergy in the body.
allergy (AL er jee)	Hypersensitivity to a substance in the environment or to a medication. See Figure 7.7 for an illustration of allergy testing.
anaphylaxis (an ah fih LAK sis)	Severe reaction to an antigen.
antibody (AN tih bod ee)	Protein material produced in the body as a response to the invasion of a foreign substance.
antigen (AN tih jen)	Substance that is capable of inducing the formation of an antibody. The antibody then interacts with the antigen in the antigen–antibody reaction.
antigen–antibody reaction (AN tih jen AN tih bod ee)	Combination of the antigen with its specific antibody to increase susceptibility to phagocytosis and immunity.
atypical (ay TIP ih kal)	Abnormal.
cell-mediated immunity	Immunity that results from the activation of sensitized T lymphocytes. The immune response causes antigens to be destroyed by the direct action of cells.
cytotoxic (sigh toh TOK sik) cells	T cells that are destructive to cells and can kill foreign invasion cells. Also called *T8* cells.
human immunodeficiency (im yoo noh dee FIH shen see) virus (HIV)	Virus that causes AIDS; also known as a *retrovirus* (see Figure 7.8).
humoral immunity (HYOO mor al im YOO nih tee)	Immunity that responds to antigens such as bacteria and foreign agents. It is the result of circulating antibodies.
immune response	Ability of lymphocytes to respond to specific antigens.
immunoglobulins (im yoo noh GLOB yoo linz)	Antibodies secreted by the B cells. All antibodies are immunoglobulins. They assist in protecting the body and its surfaces from the invasion of bacteria. For example, the immunoglobulin IgA in colostrum, the first milk from the mother, helps to protect the newborn from infection.
immunologist (im yoo NALL oh jist)	A physician who specializes in treating infectious diseases and other disorders of the immune system.
immunology (im yoo NALL oh jee)	Study of the immune system and infectious diseases.
inflammatory process	Nonspecific immune response that occurs as a reaction to any type of bodily injury (see Figure 7.9). The signs are redness, heat, swelling, and pain (see Figure 7.10).
lymph (LIMF)	Clear, transparent, colorless fluid found in the lymphatic vessels and the cisterna chyli.
natural killer (NK) cells	T cells that can kill by entrapping foreign cells, tumor cells, and bacteria. Also called *T8 cells*.
opportunistic infections	Infectious diseases that are associated with AIDS since they occur as a result of the lowered immune system and resistance of the body to infections and parasites.
retrovirus (REH troh vi rus)	Virus, such as HIV, in which the virus copies itself using the host's DNA.
T-helper cells	T cells that help the B cells recognize the antigens. Also called *T4 cells*.

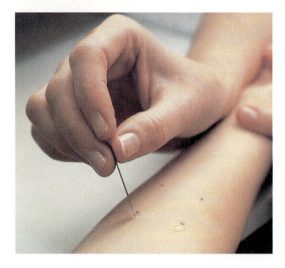

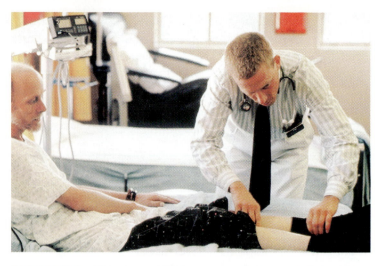

FIGURE 7.7 Allergy testing. (James King-Holmes/ Science Photo Library/Photo Researchers, Inc.)

FIGURE 7.8 HIV patient in AIDS outpatient clinic. (David Weintraub/ Science Source/Photo Researchers, Inc.)

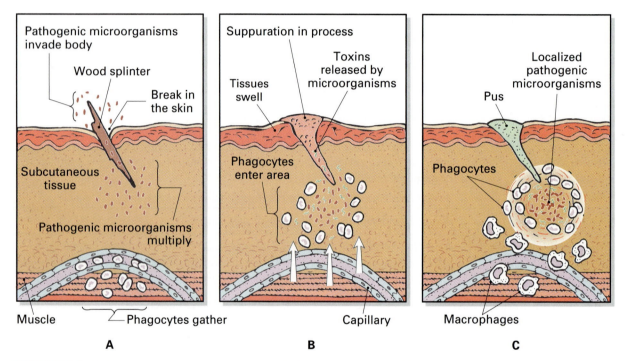

FIGURE 7.9 Inflammatory process. (A) Injury breaks the skin and introduces pathogens. (B) Inflammatory response initiated. (C) Macrophages clean up cell debris.

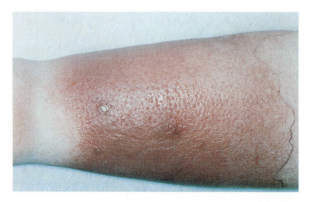

FIGURE 7.10 Cellulitis of the arm showing signs of the inflammatory process.

Pathology of the Lymphatic System

acquired immunodeficiency syndrome (acquired im yoo noh dee FIH shen see SIN drohm) (AIDS)	Disease that involves a defect in the cell-mediated immunity system. A syndrome of opportunistic infections that occur in the final stages of infection with the human immunodeficiency virus (HIV). This virus attacks T4 lymphocytes and destroys them, which reduces the person's ability to fight infection.
adenoiditis (add eh noyd EYE tis)	Inflammation of the adenoid tissue.
AIDS-related complex (ARC)	Early stage of AIDS. There is a positive test for the virus but only mild symptoms of weight loss, fatigue, skin rash, and anorexia.
anaphylactic (an ah fih LAK tik) shock	Life-threatening condition resulting from the ingestion of food or medications that produce a severe allergic response. Circulatory and respiratory problems occur, including respiratory distress, hypotension, edema, tachycardia, and convulsions.
edema (eh DEE mah)	Local condition in which the body tissues contain excessive amounts of fluid. One of the causes is lymphatic obstruction.
elephantiasis (el eh fan TYE ah sis)	Inflammation, obstruction, and destruction of the lymph vessels that results in enlarged tissues due to edema.
Epstein–Barr (EP steen BAR) virus	Virus that is believed to be the cause of infectious mononucleosis. It was discovered by Anthony Epstein, a British virologist, and Yvonne Barr, a French physician.
hepatitis (hep ah TYE tis) B	Serious, inflammatory disease of the liver caused by the hepatitis B virus. It is spread through contact with blood and body fluids. There is a vaccine that provides protection (see Figure 7.11).
Hodgkin's disease (HOJ kins dih ZEEZ)	Also called Hodgkin's lymphoma. Cancer of the lymphatic cells found in concentration in the lymph nodes (see Figure 7.12). Named after Thomas Hodgkin, a British physician, who first described it.
Kaposi's sarcoma (KAP oh seez sar KOH mah)	Form of skin cancer frequently seen in patients with acquired immunodeficiency syndrome (AIDS). It consists of brownish-purple papules that spread from the skin and metastasize to internal organs. Named for Moritz Kaposi, an Austrian dermatologist.
lymphadenitis (lim fad en EYE tis)	Inflammation of the lymph glands. Referred to as *swollen glands*.
lymphangioma (lim fan jee OH mah)	Benign mass of lymphatic vessels.
malignant lymphoma (lim FOH mah)	Cancerous tumor of lymphatic tissue; most commonly occurs in lymph nodes, the spleen, or other body sites containing large amounts of lymphatic cells.
mononucleosis (mon oh noo klee OH sis)	Acute infectious disease with a large number of atypical lymphocytes. Caused by the Epstein–Barr virus. There may be abnormal liver function.
non-Hodgkin's lymphoma (NHL)	Cancer of the lymphatic tissues other than Hodgkin's lymphoma.
peritonsillar abscess (pair ih TON sih lar AB sess)	Infection of the tissues between the tonsils and the pharynx. Also called a *quinsy sore throat*.
Pneumocystis carinii pneumonia (noo moh SIS tis kah RYE nee eye new MOH nee ah)	Pneumonia common in AIDS patients that is caused by infection with a parasite.
sarcoidosis (sar koyd OH sis)	Inflammatory disease of the lymph system in which lesions may appear in the liver, skin, lungs, lymph nodes, spleen, eyes, and small bones of the hands and feet.
splenomegaly (splee noh MEG ah lee)	Enlargement of the spleen.
systemic lupus erythematosus (sis TEM ik LOO pus air ih them ah TOH sis) (SLE)	Chronic autoimmune disorder of connective tissue that causes injury to the skin, joints, kidneys, mucous membranes, and nervous system.
thymoma (thigh MOH mah)	Malignant tumor of the thymus gland.
tonsillitis (ton sil EYE tis)	Inflammation of the tonsils.

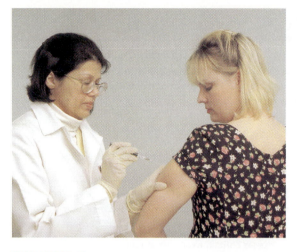

FIGURE 7.11 Adult receiving injection of hepatitis vaccine.

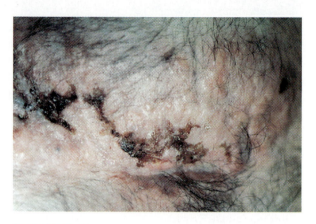

FIGURE 7.12 Late stage Hodgkin's disease with tumor eroding skin above cancerous lymph node.

Diagnostic Procedures Relating to the Lymphatic System

bone marrow aspiration (as pih RAY shun)	Removing a sample of bone marrow by syringe for microscopic examination. Useful for diagnosing such diseases as leukemia. For example, a proliferation (massive increase) of white blood cells could confirm the diagnosis of acute leukemia.
CT scan (CAT)	Use of computerized tomography to diagnose disorders of the lymphoid organs.
ELISA (enzyme-linked immunosorbent assay) (EN zym LINK'T im yoo noh sor bent ASS say)	A blood test for an antibody to the AIDS virus. A positive test means that the person has been exposed to the virus. There may be a false-positive reading and then the Western blot test would be used to verify the results.
lymphangiogram (lim FAN jee oh gram)	X-ray taken of the lymph vessels after the injection of dye into the foot. The lymph flow through the chest is traced.
Western blot	Test used as a backup to the ELISA blood test to detect the presence of the antibody to HIV (AIDS virus) in the blood.

Treatment Procedures Relating to the Lymphatic System

lymphadenectomy (lim fad eh NEK toh mee)	Excision of a lymph node. This is usually done to test for malignancy.
lymphoidectomy (lim foy DEK toh mee)	Surgical excision of lymphoid tissue.
splenopexy (SPLEE noh pek see)	Artificial fixation of a movable spleen.
tonsillectomy (ton sih LEK toh mee)	Surgical removal of the tonsils.

Abbreviations Relating to the Lymphatic System

AIDS	acquired immunodeficiency syndrome	**Ig**	immunoglobins (IgA, IgD, IgE, IgG, IgM)
ARC	AIDS-related complex	**KS**	Kaposi's sarcoma
CD4	protein on T-helper cell lymphocyte	**lymph**	lymphocyte
EBV	Epstein-Barr virus	**mono**	mononucleosis, monocyte
ELISA	enzyme-linked immunosorbent assay	**NHL**	non-Hodgkin's lymphoma
HIV	human immunodeficiency virus (causes AIDS)	**T4**	T-cell lymphocyte (destroyed by the AIDS virus)
HSV	herpes simplex virus	**T8**	T-cell lymphocyte (cytotoxic or killer cell)

Overview

PART II: The Hematic System

COMPONENTS OF THE HEMATIC SYSTEM

blood	**plasma**
erythrocytes	**platelets**
leukocytes	

COMBINING FORMS RELATING TO THE HEMATIC (BLOOD) SYSTEM

agglutin/o	clumping	**leukocyt/o**	white cell
bas/o	base	**mon/o**	one
blast/o	primitive cell	**morph/o**	shape
chrom/o	color	**myel/o**	bone marrow
coagul/o	clotting	**neutr/o**	neutral
cyt/o	cell	**nucle/o**	nucleus
eosin/o	red, rosy	**phag/o**	eat, swallow
erythr/o	red	**reticul/o**	immature, net
granul/o	granules	**sangui/o**	blood
hem/o	blood	**spher/o**	round
hemat/o	blood	**thromb/o**	clot
hemoglobin/o	hemoglobin	**thrombocyt/o**	platelet
leuk/o	white		

Suffix	Meaning	Example
-emia	blood condition	leukemia
-lytic	destruction	hemolytic
-penia	abnormal decrease	cytopenia
-phil	to have an attraction for	neutrophil
-philia	to have an attraction for	hemophilia
-poiesis	formation	erythropoiesis
-stasis	standing still	hemostasis

ANATOMY AND PHYSIOLOGY OF THE HEMATIC SYSTEM

BLOOD

formed elements	hematology
hematologist	plasma

The study of the blood is known as **hematology** (hee mah **TALL** oh jee) and a physician who specializes in this area is a **hematologist** (hee mah **TALL** oh jist). The average adult has about 6 quarts of blood, a combination of **plasma** (**PLAZ** mah) and **formed elements** or blood cells.

Plasma

amino acids	fibrinogen	prothrombin	urea
ammonia	gamma globulin	serum	uric acid
calcium	glucose	serum albumin	
cholesterol	plasma proteins	serum globulin	
creatinine	potassium	sodium	

Liquid plasma composes about 55 percent of the blood in the average adult and is 90 percent water. The remaining 10 percent portion of plasma consists of **plasma** (**PLAZ** mah) **proteins.** These include **serum albumin** (**SEE** rum al **BEW** min), **serum globulin** (**SEE** rum **GLOB** yew lin), **fibrinogen** (fye **BRIN** oh jen), and **prothrombin** (proh **THROM** bin). Fibrinogen and prothrombin are the clotting proteins. **Gamma globulin** (**GAM** ah **GLOB** yoo lin), one of the three types of globulin, is an important source of antibodies.

There are also small amounts of inorganic substances in plasma, such as **calcium** (**KAL** see um), **potassium** (poh **TASS** ee um), and **sodium.** Organic components consist of **glucose** (**GLOO** kohs), **amino** (ah **MEE** noh) **acids,** fats and **cholesterol** (koh

LES ter all), and the waste products of **urea** (yoo **REE** ah), **uric** (**YOO** rik) **acid,** **ammonia** (ah **MOHN** yah), and **creatinine** (kree **AT** in in). Plasma carries these materials to all parts of the body. **Serum** (**SEE** rum) is plasma after all the clotting proteins have been removed.

Serum is the clear fluid that remains in the test tube after a blood sample clots.

Formed Elements

erythrocytes   **platelets**

leukocytes

There are three basic types of blood cells or formed elements in the plasma: **erythrocytes** (eh **RITH** roh sights), **leukocytes** (**LOO** koh sights), and **platelets** (**PLAYT** lets).

Erythrocytes

hemoglobin (Hgb, Hb)   **nucleus**

hemorrhage   **red blood cells (RBCs)**

Erythrocytes are also called **red blood cells (RBCs).** They are biconcave disks and contain no **nucleus** (**NOO** klee us).

The shape of a cell and the presence of a nucleus are important factors when observing cells under a microscope. The red blood cell is readily apparent due to its rounded, biconcave, nonnucleated shape.

Red blood cells contain **hemoglobin** (hee moh **GLOH** bin), which is an iron-containing pigment. The function of hemoglobin is to carry oxygen from the lungs to the tissues. Therefore, hemoglobin is critical to life. A sudden decrease in red blood cells, such as occurs in a **hemorrhage** (**HEM** eh rij), can be life-threatening.

There are about five million erythrocytes per cubic millimeter of blood. The total number in an average-sized adult is thirty-five trillion, with males having more red blood cells than females. Erythrocytes, which are formed in the red bone marrow, have an average life span of 120 days and then the body needs to produce more to maintain their concentration in the blood.

Table 7.2 *Leukocyte Classification*	
Leukocyte	**Function**
Granulocytes	
Basophils (basos) (**BAY** soh fillz)	Release histamine and heparin to damaged tissues
Eosinophils (eosins) (ee oh **SIN** oh fillz)	Destroy parasites and increase during allergic reactions
Neutrophils (**NOO** troh fillz)	Important for phagocytosis; most numerous of the leukocytes
Agranulocytes	
Monocytes (monos)	Important for phagocytosis
Lymphocytes (lymphs)	Provide protection through an immunity activity

Leukocytes

agranulocytes	lymphocytes (lymphs)
basophils (basos)	monocytes (monos)
eosinophils (eosins)	neutrophils
granulocytes	white blood cells (WBCs)

Leukocytes, also referred to as **white blood cells** (**WBCs**), provide protection against the invasion of bacteria and other foreign material. They are able to leave the bloodstream and search out the foreign invaders (bacteria, virus, and toxins), where they perform phagocytosis.

They have a spherical shape with a nucleus, and number around 8,000 per cubic millimeter of blood. Leukocytes can be placed in two categories: **granulocytes** (**GRAN** yew loh sights) (with granules in the cytoplasm) and **agranulocytes** (ah **GRAN** yew loh sights) (without granules in the cytoplasm). Table 7.2 contains a list of leukocytes in each category and their functions.

Platelets

agglutinate	thrombocytes
fibrin	thrombokinase
thrombin	

Platelets is the modern term for **thrombocytes** (**THROM** boh sights). They have a round or oval disk shape or *platelike* appearance. Platelets are the smallest of all the formed blood elements. There are between 200,000 and 300,000 per cubic millimeter in the body.

Platelets play a critical part in the blood clotting process. They **agglutinate** (ah **GLOO** tih nayt) into small clusters when a blood vessel is cut or damaged. Platelets release **thrombokinase** (throm boh **KYE** nays), which, in the presence of calcium, reacts with prothrombin to form **thrombin** (**THROM** bin). Thrombin converts fibrinogen to **fibrin** (**FYE** brin), which eventually becomes the meshlike blood clot.

BLOOD GROUPINGS

ABO system   **RH factor**

blood typing

Blood grouping is also referred to as **blood typing.** The blood of one person is different from another's due to the presence of antigens on the surface of erythrocytes. These antigens, or markers on the blood cell, stimulate the production of antibodies that react with the antigen in the antigen–antibody reaction. The two most important blood groups are the **ABO system,** determined by blood antigens A and B, and **Rh factor,** determined by the Rh blood antigen.

ABO System

type A   **type O**

type AB   **universal donor**

type B   **universal recipient**

In the ABO blood system there are two possible RBC surface markers, A and B. A person with A markers has **type A** blood. The presence of B markers gives **type B** blood. The absence of either marker results in **type O** blood, and if both markers are present, the blood is **type AB.**

Because type O blood does not react with anti-A or anti-B antibodies, it is referred to as the **universal donor.** In an emergency, type O blood may be given to a person with any of the other blood types. Type AB is referred to as the **universal recipient.** A person with type AB blood can receive type AB, type A, or type B blood.

Rh Factor

agglutination   **Rh-negative (−)**

erythroblastosis fetalis   **Rh-positive (+)**

The two types of Rh factors are **Rh-positive** (+), which contains the Rh marker, and **Rh-negative (−),** which does not. Rh− blood will form antibodies against Rh+ blood but, since Rh− blood has no markers, Rh+ blood will not form anti-Rh antibodies.

The Rh blood type is important information to have when considering a blood transfusion. If a person with Rh− blood receives a transfusion of Rh+ blood, it will cause the formation of anti-Rh **agglutination** (ah gloo tih **NAY** shun). Any transfusions *after* the first one can result in serious reactions. A pregnant woman who is Rh− may become sensitized by an Rh+ fetus. In pregnancies after the first, if the fetus is Rh+, the maternal antibodies may cross the placenta and destroy fetal cells, which will lead to **erythroblastosis fetalis** (eh rith roh blass **TOH** sis fee **TAL** is).

Word Building Relating to the Hematic System

The following list contains examples of medical terms built directly from word parts. Their definitions can be determined by a straightforward translation of the word parts.

Combining Form	Combined With	Medical Term	Definition
coagul/o	anti- -ant	anticoagulant (an tih koh **AG** yoo lant)	against coagulation
cyt/o	erythro-	erythrocyte (eh **RITH** roh sight)	red (blood) cell
	leuko-	leukocyte (**LOO** koh sight)	white (blood) cell
	poly- -emia	polycythemia (pol ee sigh **THEE** mee ah)	many cells in the blood
	thrombo-	thrombocyte (**THROM** boh sight)	clotting cell
fibrin/o	-gen	fibrinogen (fye **BRIN** oh jen)	fiber producing
granul/o	a- -cyte	agranulocyte (ah **GRAN** yoo loh sight)	cell with no granules
	-cyte	granulocyte (**GRAN** yew loh sight)	cell with granules
hem/o	-globin	hemoglobin (hee moh **GLOH** bin)	blood protein
	-lysis	hemolysis (hee **MALL** ih sis)	blood destruction
	-rrhage	hemorrhage (**HEM** er rij)	rapid flow of blood
	-stasis	hemostasis (hee moh **STAY** sis)	stopping blood
hemat/o	-cyt/o -penia	hematocytopenia (hee mah toh sigh toh **PEE** nee ah)	too few blood cells
	-ologist	hematologist (hee mah **TALL** oh jist)	specialist in the blood
	-ology	hematology (hee mah **TALL** oh jee)	study of blood
	-oma	hematoma (hee mah **TOH** mah)	blood swelling
	-poiesis	hematopoiesis (hee mah toh poy **EE** sis)	blood producing
sanguin/o	-ous	sanguinous (**SANG** guih nus)	pertaining to blood

Vocabulary Relating to the Hematic System

agglutination (ah gloo tih NAY shun)	Antigen–antibody reaction in which a solid antigen clumps together with a soluble antibody. Often used to refer to the process of clumping together of blood cells.
agranulocyte (ah GRAN yew loh sight)	Nongranular leukocyte. This is one of the two types of leukocytes found in plasma that are classified as either monocytes or lymphocytes.
anticoagulant (an tih koh AG yoo lant)	Substance that prevents or delays the clotting or coagulation of blood.
antihemorrhagic (an tih hem er RAJ ik)	Substance that prevents or stops hemorrhaging.
erythrocytes (eh RITH roh sights)	Mature red blood cells.
erythropoiesis (eh rith roh poy EE sis)	The process of forming erythrocytes.
fibrin (FYE brin)	Whitish protein formed by the action of thrombin and fibrinogen, which is the basis for the clotting of blood.
fibrinogen (fye BRIN oh jen)	Blood protein that is essential for clotting to take place.
gamma globulin (GAM ah GLOB yoo lin)	Protein component of blood containing antibodies that help to resist infection.
granulocytes (GRAN yew loh sights)	Granular polymorphonuclear leukocyte. There are three types: neutrophil, eosinophil, and basophil.
hematologist (hee mah TALL oh jist)	A physician who specializes in treating diseases and conditions of the blood.
hematology (hee mah TALL oh jee)	Study of the blood, its components, and blood-forming tissues.
hemoglobin (hee moh GLOH bin) (Hg)	Iron-containing pigment of red blood cells that carries oxygen from the lungs to the tissue.
hemostasis (hee moh STAY sis)	To stop bleeding or the stagnation of the circulating blood.
leukocytes (LOO koh sights)	White blood cells (WBCs).
phagocyte (FAG oh sight)	Neutrophil component of the blood; has the ability to ingest and destroy bacteria.
plasma (PLAZ mah)	Fluid portion of the blood.
platelets (PLAYT lets)	Cells responsible for the coagulation of blood. These are also called thrombocytes and contain no hemoglobin.
prothrombin (proh THROM bin)	Protein element within the blood that interacts with calcium salts to form thrombin.
reticulocyte (reh TIK yoo loh sight)	Red blood cell containing granules or filaments in an immature stage of development.
serum (SEE rum)	Clear, sticky fluid that remains after the blood has clotted.
serum albumin (SEE rum al BEW min)	Protein in blood serum.
serum globulin (SEE rum GLOB yew lin)	Protein in the blood.

Pathology of the Hematic System

anemia **(an NEE mee ah)**	Reduction in the number of red blood cells (RBCs) or amount of hemoglobin in the blood; results in less oxygen reaching the tissues.
cytopenia **(sigh toh PEE nee ah)**	A decrease in the number of circulating cells—erythrocytes, leukocytes, platelets—in the blood.
erythroblastosis fetalis **(eh rith roh blass** **TOH sis fee TAL is)**	Condition in which antibodies in the mother's blood enter the fetus' blood and cause anemia, jaundice, edema, and enlargement of the liver and spleen. Also called *hemolytic disease of the newborn.*
hematoma **(hee mah TOH mah)**	Swelling or mass of blood caused by a break in a vessel in an organ or tissue, or beneath the skin.
hemolytic **(hee moh LIT ik)** **disease of the newborn**	Condition in which antibodies in the mother's blood enter the fetus' blood and cause anemia, jaundice, edema, and enlargement of the liver and spleen. Also called *erythroblastosis fetalis.*
hemophilia **(hee moh FILL ee ah)**	Hereditary blood disease in which there is a prolonged blood clotting time. It is transmitted by a sex-linked trait from females to males. It appears almost exclusively in males.
leukemia **(loo KEE mee ah)**	Cancer of the WBC-forming bone marrow; results in a large number of abnormal WBCs circulating in the blood.
polycythemia vera **(pol ee sigh THEE** **mee ah VAIR rah)**	Production of too many red blood cells by the bone marrow.

Diagnostic Procedures Relating to the Hematic System

bleeding time	Test to measure the amount of time it takes for blood to coagulate.
complete blood count (CBC)	Blood test that consists of five tests: red blood cell count (RBC), white blood cell count (WBC), hemoglobin (Hg), hematocrit (Hct), and white blood cell differential (see Figure 7.13).
differential **(diff er EN shal)**	Blood test to determine the number of each variety of leukocytes.
erythrocyte sedimentation rate (eh RITH roh sight sed ih men TAY shun) (ESR)	Blood test to determine the rate at which mature red blood cells settle out of the blood after the addition of an anticoagulant. An indicator of the presence of an inflammatory disease.
hematocrit (hee MAT oh krit) (HCT, Hct, crit)	Blood test to measure the volume of red blood cells (erythrocytes) within the total volume of blood.
Monospot	Test for infectious mononucleosis in which there is a nonspecific antibody called heterophile antibody.
prothrombin (proh THROM bin) time (Pro time, PT)	A measure of the blood's coagulation abilities.
red blood count (RBC)	Blood test to determine the number of erythrocytes in a volume of blood. A decrease in red blood cells may indicate anemia; an increase may indicate polycythemia.
white blood count (WBC)	Blood test to measure the number of leukocytes in a volume of blood. An increase may indicate the presence of infection or a disease such as leukemia. A decrease in WBCs is caused by X-ray therapy and chemotherapy.

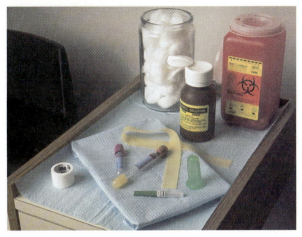

A Equipment required to draw blood.

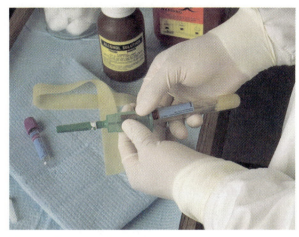

B Vacutube is placed in the syringe.

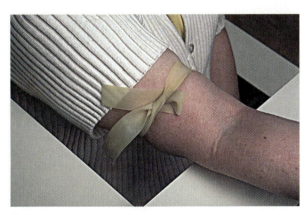

C A tourniquet is placed above the vein.

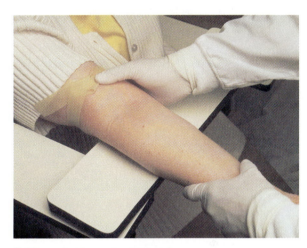

D The patient's arm is positioned.

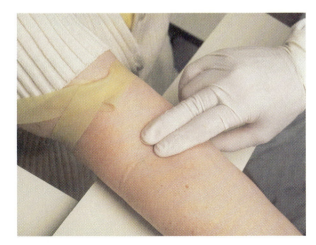

E The vein is palpated.

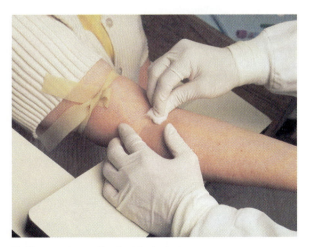

F The area is sterilized with alcohol.

FIGURE 7.13 Nurse drawing blood from a patient for a test. *(continued)*

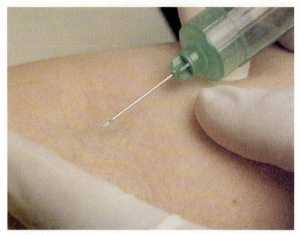

G The needle is inserted into the vein.

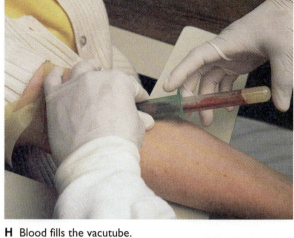

H Blood fills the vacutube.

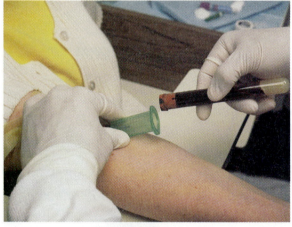

I The filled tube is removed.

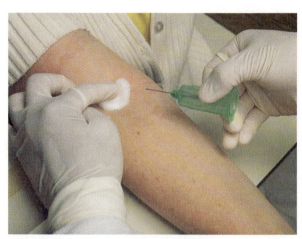

J The needle is removed.

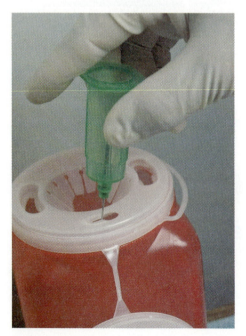

K The needle is properly disposed of.

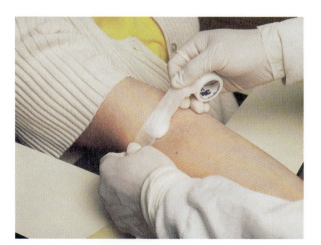

L A bandage is placed over the puncture side.

FIGURE 7.13 Nurse drawing blood from a patient for a test. *(continued)*

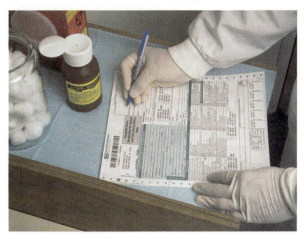

M Nurse completes proper paperwork.

FIGURE 7.13 Nurse documenting blood drawn from a patient for a test. *(continued)*

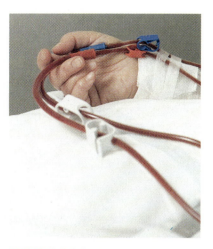

FIGURE 7.14 Blood transfusion in process. (Photo Researchers, Inc.)

Treatment Procedures Relating to the Hematic System

autohemotherapy **(aw toh hee moh THAIR ah pee)**	Treatment of using a person's own blood in a transfusion by withdrawing and injecting the blood intramuscularly.
autologous transfusion **(aw TALL oh gus trans FYOO zhun)**	Procedure for collecting and storing a patient's own blood several weeks prior to the actual need. It can then be used to replace blood lost during a surgical procedure.
homologous transfusion **(hoh MALL oh gus trans FYOO zhun)**	Replacement of blood by transfusion of blood received from another person.
transfusion (trans FYOO zhun)	Artificial transfer of blood into the bloodstream (see Figure 7.14).

UNIVERSAL PRECAUTIONS

Hospital and other health care settings contain a large number of infective microorganisms—pathogens. Patients and health care workers are exposed to each other's pathogens and sometimes become infected. An infection acquired in this manner, as a result of hospital exposure, is referred to as a nosocomial infection. Nosocomial infections can spread in several ways. Cross infection occurs when a person, either a patient or health care worker, acquires a pathogen from another patient or health care worker. Reinfection takes place when a person becomes infected again with the same pathogen that originally brought him or her to the hospital. Self-inoculation occurs when a person becomes infected in a different part of the body by a pathogen from another part of his or her own body—such as intestinal bacteria spreading to the urethra.

With the appearance of the human immunodeficiency virus (HIV) and the hepatitis B virus (HBV) in the mid-1980s, the fight against spreading infections took on even greater significance. In 1987 the Occupational Safety and Health Administration (OSHA) issued mandatory guidelines to insure that all employees at risk of exposure to body fluids are provided with personal protective equipment. These guidelines state that all human blood, tissue, and body fluids must be treated as if they were infected with HIV, HBV, or other blood-borne pathogens. These guidelines were expanded in 1992 and 1996 to encourage the fight against not just blood-borne pathogens, but all nosocomial infections spread by contact with blood, mucous membranes, nonintact skin, and all body fluids (see Table 7.3). These guidelines are commonly referred to as the Universal or Standard Precautions (see Table 7.4). According to the Universal Precautions, within 10 days of being hired all new employees at risk for exposure to body fluids must receive training in the use of appropriate personal protective equipment and be offered HBV vaccination at no charge. In addition, they must receive an update and review of their training annually.

Table 7.3	*Body Fluids*	
• Blood	• Semen
• Tissue specimens	• Amniotic fluid
• Vaginal secretions	• Pleural fluid
• Cerebrospinal fluid	• Peritoneal fluid
• Pericardial fluid	• Any other body fluid that contains visible blood
• Interstitial fluid	

Table 7.4	*Summary of Universal Precautions Guidelines*
1. Wash hands before putting on and after removing gloves and before and after working with each patient or patient equipment.
2. Wear gloves when in contact with any body fluid, mucous membrane, or nonintact skin or if you have chapped hands, a rash, or open sores.
3. Wear a nonpermeable gown or apron during procedures that are likely to expose you to any body fluid, mucous membrane, or nonintact skin.
4. Wear a mask and protective eyewear or a face shield when patients are coughing often or if body fluid droplets or splashes are likely.
5. Wear a face mask and eyewear that seal close to the face during procedures that cause body tissues to be vaporized.

Remove for proper cleaning any shared equipment—such as a thermometer, stethoscope, or blood pressure cuff—that has come into contact with body fluids, mucous membrane, or nonintact skin.

Medical Laboratory

Clinical Laboratory Scientist

Clinical laboratory scientists perform a variety of tests using laboratory equipment, microscopes, and computers. These laboratory tests include chemical analyses on body tissues, blood, and other body fluids; growing bacterial cultures; and typing and cross-matching blood for transfusions. Medical laboratory technologists play a key role in patient care because physicians study and use the results of these tests to make their diagnoses. Medical laboratories are found in acute care facilities, physician's offices, clinics, private laboratories, public health facilities, and research facilities. Medical technologists graduate from a four-year college- or university-sponsored medical technologist program and must pass a national certification exam. Students interested in medical technology might also consider becoming clinical laboratory technicians. These technicians perform tests under the supervision of clinical laboratory scientists, physicians, or other scientists who order the tests. Clinical laboratory technicians graduate from an accredited associates degree program. For more information, visit American Society for Clinical Laboratory Science's web site at www.ascls.org or American Society of Clinical Pathologists at www.ascp.org.

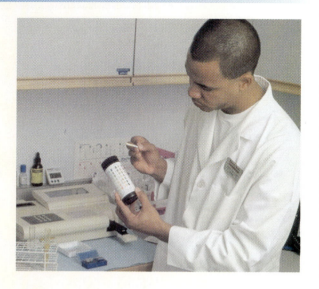

Medical Technologist (MT) or Clinical Laboratory Scientist (CLS)

- **Performs laboratory tests as ordered by a physician**
- **Graduates from a four-year college or university medical technologist program**
- **Passes a national certification exam**

Medical Laboratory Technician (MLT) or Clinical Laboratory Technician (CLT)

- **Works under the supervision of a medical technologist**
- **Graduates from a two-year laboratory technician program at a community college or vocational education program**
- **Passes a national certification exam**

Phlebotomist

- **A specialist in drawing venous blood**
- **Does not conduct laboratory tests**
- **Completes a vocational education program or on-the-job training program**
- **Certification exam is available**

Abbreviations Relating to the Hematic System

ALL	acute lymphocytic leukemia	**HCT, Hct, crit**	hematocrit
AML	acute myelogenous leukemia	**Hgb, Hb**	hemoglobin
baso	basophil	**lymph**	lymphocyte
CBC	complete blood count	**mono**	monocyte (also mononucleosis)
CGL	chronic granulocytic leukemia	**PCV**	packed cell volume (hematocrit)
CLL	chronic lymphocytic leukemia	**PMN, seg, poly**	polymorphonuclear neutrophil
diff	differential	**PT**	prothrombin time
eosin	eosinophil	**RBC**	red blood cell
ESR, SR, sed rate	erythrocyte sedimentation rate	**WBC**	white blood cell

KEY TERMS

- ABO System
- acquired immunity
- acquired immunodeficiency syndrome (AIDS)
  (acquired im yoo noh dee **FIH** shen see **SIN** drohm)
- active acquired immunity
- adenoiditis (add eh noyd **EYE** tis)
- adenoids (**ADD** eh noydz)
- agglutinate (ah **GLOO** tih nayt)
- agglutination (ah gloo tih **NAY** shun)
- agranulocytes (ah **GRAN** yew loh sights)
- AIDS-related complex (ARC)
- allergen (**AL** er jin)
- allergy (**AL** er jee)
- amino acids (ah **MEE** noh)
- ammonia (ah **MOHN** yah)
- anaphylactic shock (an ah fih **LAK** tik)
- anaphylaxis (an ah fih **LAK** sis)
- anemia (an **NEE** mee ah)
- antibody (**AN** tih bod ee)
- antibody-mediated immunity (**AN** tih bod ee **MEE** dee ay ted im **YOO** nih tee)
- anticoagulant (an tih koh **AG** yoo lant)
- antigen (**AN** tih jen)
- antigen–antibody reaction (**AN** tih jen **AN** tih bod ee)
- antihemorrhagic (an tih hem er **RAJ** ik)
- atypical (ay **TIP** ih kal)
- autohemotherapy (aw toh hee moh **THAIR** ah pee)
- autologous transfusion
  (aw **TALL** oh gus trans **FYOO** zhun)
- axillary (**AK** sih lair ee)
- bacteria (bak **TEE** ree ah)
- basophils (baso) (**BAY** soh fillz)
- B cells
- bleeding time
- blood typing
- B lymphocytes (**LIM** foh sights)
- bone marrow aspiration (as pih **RAY** shun)
- calcium (**KAL** see um)
- capillaries (**CAP** ih lair eez)
- cell-mediated immunity
- cellular immunity

- cervical (**SER** vih kal)
- cholesterol (koh **LES** ter all)
- cisterna chyli (sis **TER** nah **KYE** lee)
- complete blood count (CBC)
- creatinine (kree **AT** in in)
- CT scan (CAT) (**CAT** scan)
- cytopenia (sigh toh **PEE** nee ah)
- cytotoxic (sigh toh **TOK** sik)
- cytotoxic cells (sigh toh **TOK** sik)
- differential (diff) (diff er **EN** shal)
- edema (eh **DEE** mah)
- elephantiasis (el eh fan **TYE** ah sis)
- ELISA (enzyme-linked immunosorbent assay) (**EN** zym **LINK'T** im yoo noh sor bent **ASS** say)
- eosinophils (eosin) (ee oh **SIN** oh fillz)
- Epstein-Barr virus (**EP** steen **BAR**)
- erythroblastosis fetalis
  (eh rith roh blass **TOH** sis fee **TAL** iss)
- erythrocyte (eh **RITH** roh sight)
- erythrocyte sedimentation rate (ESR, SR, sed rate)
  (eh **RITH** roh sight sed ih men **TAY** shun)
- erythropoiesis (eh rith roh poy **EE** sis)
- fibrin (**FYE** brin)
- fibrinogen (fye **BRIN** oh jen)
- formed elements
- fungi (**FUN** jee)
- gamma globulin (**GAM** ah **GLOB** yoo lin)
- glucose (**GLOO** kohs)
- granulocyte (**GRAN** yew loh sight)
- hematocrit (HCT, Hct, crit) (hee **MAT** oh krit)
- hematocytopenia (hee mah toh sigh toh **PEE** nee ah)
- hematologist (hee mah **TALL** oh jist)
- hematology (hee mah **TALL** oh jee)
- hematoma (hee mah **TOH** mah)
- hematopoiesis (hee mah toh poy **EE** sis)
- hemoglobin (Hgb, Hb) (hee moh **GLOH** bin)
- hemolysis (hee **MALL** ih sis)
- hemolytic disease of the newborn (hee moh **LIT** ik)
- hemophilia (hee moh **FILL** ee ah)
- hemorrhage (**HEM** eh rij)
- hemostasis (hee moh **STAY** sis)

- hepatitis B (hep ah **TYE** tis)
- Hodgkin's disease (**HOJ** kins dih **ZEEZ**)
- homologous transfusion
  (hoh **MALL** oh gus trans **FYOO** zhun)
- human immunodeficiency virus (HIV)
  (im yoo noh dee **FIH** shen see)
- humoral immunity (**HYOO** mor al im **YOO** nih tee)
- immune response (im **YOON**)
- immunizations (im yoo nih **ZAY** shuns)
- immunoglobulin (im yoo noh **GLOB** yoo lin)
- immunologist (im yoo **NALL** oh jist)
- immunology (im yoo **NALL** oh jee)
- inflammatory process
- inguinal (**ING** gwih nal)
- innate immunity
- Kaposi's sarcoma (**KAP** oh seez sar **KOH** mah)
- left subclavian vein (sub **KLAY** vee an)
- leukemia (loo **KEE** mee ah)
- leukocyte (**LOO** koh sight)
- lingual tonsils (**LING** gwal **TON** sulls)
- lymph (**LIMF**)
- lymph ducts (**LIMF**)
- lymph nodes (**LIMF**)
- lymph vessels (**LIMF**)
- lymphadenectomy (lim fad eh **NEK** toh mee)
- lymphadenitis (lim fad en **EYE** tis)
- lymphadenography (lim fad eh **NOG** rah fee)
- lymphadenopathy (lim fad eh **NOP** ah thee)
- lymphangiogram (lim **FAN** jee oh gram)
- lymphangiography (lim fan jee **OG** rah fee)
- lymphangioma (lim fan jee **OH** mah)
- lymphatic (lim **FAT** ik)
- lymphatic duct (lim **FAT** ik)
- lymphocyte (lymph) (**LIM** foh sight)
- lymphoidectomy (lim foy **DEK** toh mee)
- lymphoma (lim **FOH** mah)
- macrophage (**MACK** roh fayj)
- malignant lymphoma (lim **FOH** mah)
- mediastinal (mee dee ass **TYE** nal)
- metastasized (meh **TASS** tah sized)
- microorganisms (my kroh **OR** gan izmz)
- monocytes (monos) (**MON** oh sights)
- mononucleosis (mon oh noo klee **OH** sis)
- Monospot
- natural immunity (im **YOO** nih tee)
- natural killer (NK) cells
- neutrophils (**NOO** troh fills)
- non-Hodgkin's lymphoma (NHL) (lim **FOH** mah)
- nucleus (**NOO** klee us)
- opportunistic infections
  (op or **TOON** is tik in **FEK** shuns)
- palatine tonsils (**PAL** ah tyne **TON** sulls)
- passive acquired immunity
- pathogenic (path oh **JEN** ik)
- peritonsillar abscess (pair ih **TON** sih lar **AB** sess)
- phagocyte (**FAG** oh sight)
- phagocytic cells (fag oh **SIT** ik)
- phagocytosis (fag oh sigh **TOH** sis)
- pharyngeal tonsils (fair **IN** jee al **TON** sulls)
- pharynx (**FAIR** inks)

- plasma (**PLAZ** mah)
- plasma proteins (**PLAZ** mah)
- platelets (**PLAYT** lets)
- *Pneumocystis carinii* pneumonia
  (noo moh **SIS** tis kah **RYE** nee eye new **MOH** nee ah)
- polycythemia (pol ee sigh **THEE** mee ah)
- polycythemia vera (pol ee sigh **THEE** mee ah **VAIR** ah)
- potassium (poh **TASS** ee um)
- prothrombin (proh **THROM** bin)
- prothrombin time (Pro time, PT) (proh **THROM** bin)
- protozoa (proh toh **ZOH** ah)
- red blood cells (RBCs)
- red blood count (RBC)
- reticulocyte (reh **TIK** yoo loh sight)
- retrovirus (**REH** troh vi rus)
- Rh factor
- Rh-negative
- Rh-positive
- right subclavian vein (sub **KLAY** vee an)
- sanguinous (**SANG** gwih nus)
- sarcoidosis (sar koyd **OH** sis)
- serum (**SEE** rum)
- serum albumin (**SEE** rum al **BEW** min)
- serum globulin (**SEE** rum **GLOB** yew lin)
- sodium
- spleen
- splenectomy (splee **NEK** toh mee)
- splenomegaly (splee noh **MEG** ah lee)
- splenopexy (**SPLEE** noh pek see)
- systemic lupus erythematosus (SLE)
  (sis **TEM** ik **LOO** pus air ih them ah **TOH** sis)
- T cells
- T-helper cells
- thoracic duct (tho **RASS** ik)
- thrombin (**THROM** bin)
- thrombocytes (**THROM** boh sights)
- thrombokinase (throm boh **KYE** nays)
- thymectomy (thigh **MEK** toh mee)
- thymoma (thigh **MOH** mah)
- thymosin (thigh **MOH** sin)
- thymus gland (**THIGH** mus)
- T lymphocytes (**LIM** foh sights)
- tonsillectomy (ton sih **LEK** toh mee)
- tonsillitis (ton sil **EYE** tis)
- tonsils (**TON** sulls)
- transfusion (trans **FYOO** zhun)
- type A
- type AB
- type B
- type O
- universal donor
- universal recipient
- urea (yoo **REE** ah)
- uric acid (**YOO** rik)
- vaccinations (vak sih **NAY** shuns)
- valves
- viruses
- Western blot
- white blood cells (WBCs)
- white blood count (WBC)

Case Study

DISCHARGE SUMMARY

Admitting Diagnosis: Splenomegaly, weight loss, diarrhea, fatigue, chronic cough

Final Diagnosis: Non-Hodgkin's lymphoma, primary site spleen; splenectomy

History of Present Illness: Patient is a 36-year-old businessman who was first seen in the office with complaints of feeling generally "run down," intermittent diarrhea, weight loss, and, more recently, a dry cough. He states he has been aware of these symptoms for approximately six months, but admits it may have been "coming on" for closer to one year. A screening test for mononucleosis was negative. A chest X-ray was negative for pneumonia or bronchitis, but did reveal suspicious nodules in the left thoracic cavity. In spite of a 35# weight loss, he has abdominal ascites with splenomegaly detected with abdominal palpation. He was admitted to the hospital for further evaluation and treatment.

Summary of Hospital Course: Blood tests were negative for the Epstein-Barr virus and hepatitis B. Abdominal ultrasound confirmed generalized splenomegaly and located a 1 × 3-cm encapsulated tumor. A lymphangiogram identified the thoracic nodules to be enlarged lymph glands. Biopsies taken from the spleen tumor and thoracic lymph glands confirmed the diagnosis of non-Hodgkin's lymphoma. A full body MRI failed to demonstrate any additional metastases in the liver or brain. The patient underwent splenectomy for removal of the primary tumor.

Discharge Plans: Patient was discharged home following recovery from the splenectomy. The ascites and diarrhea were resolved, but the dry cough persisted. He was referred to an oncologist for evaluation and establishment of a chemotherapy and radiation therapy protocol to treat the metastatic thoracic lympadenomas and ongoing surveillance for additional metastases.

CRITICAL THINKING QUESTIONS

1. What complaints caused the patient to go to the doctor?

2. Explain in your own words what negative, as in chest X-ray was negative for pneumonia, means.

3. This discharge summary contains four medical terms that have not been introduced yet. Describe each of these terms in your own words. Use your text as a dictionary.

   a. primary site

   b. encapsulated

   c. ascites

   d. metastases

4. What is the name of a diagnostic procedure that produces an image from high-frequency sound waves?

   The procedure is _____ .

Which of the following pathological conditions was discovered using this procedure?

   a. inflammatory liver disease

   b. an acute infection with a large number of lymphocytes

   c. a malignant tumor of the thymus gland

   d. an enlarged spleen

5. What diagnostic test failed to find any cancer in other organs of the body? Which organs are free of cancer?

6. When the patient was discharged from the hospital, which symptoms were resolved and which persisted?

   resolved:

   persisted:

Chart Note Transcription

Chart Note

The chart note below contains ten phrases that can be reworded with a medical term that you learned in this chapter. Each phrase is identified with an underline. Determine the medical term and write your answers in the space provided.

Current Complaint: Patient is a 22-year-old female referred to the specialist in treating blood disorders[1] by her internist. Her complaints include fatigue, weight loss, and easy bruising.

Past History: Patient had normal childhood diseases. She is a college student and was feeling well until symptoms gradually appeared starting approximately 3 months ago.

Signs and Symptoms: An immunoassay test for AIDS[2] was normal. The measure of the blood's coagulation abilities[3] indicated that the blood took too long to form a clot. A blood test to count all the blood cells[4] reported too few red blood cells[5] and clotting cells.[6] There were too many white blood cells,[7] but they were immature and abnormal. A sample of bone marrow[8] obtained for microscopic examination found an excessive number of immature white blood cells.

Diagnosis: Cancer of the white blood cell forming bone marrow.[9]

Treatment: Aggressive chemotherapy for the cancer of the white blood cell forming bone marrow and replacement blood from another person to replace the red blood cells[10] and clotting cells.

1 _____

2 _____

3 _____

4 _____

5 _____

6 _____

7 _____

8 _____

9 _____

10 _____

Practice Exercises

A. COMPLETE THE FOLLOWING STATEMENTS.

1. The study of the blood is called _____ .
2. The accessory organs of the lymphatic system are the _____ , _____ , and _____ .
3. The two main lymph ducts are the _____ and _____ .
4. The primary sites for lymph nodes are the _____ , _____ , _____ , and _____ regions.
5. The process whereby cells ingest and destroy bacteria within the body is _____ .

B. STATE THE TERMS DESCRIBED USING THE COMBINING FORMS PROVIDED.

The combining form splen/o refers to the spleen. Use it to write a term that means

1. enlargement of the spleen _____
2. surgical removal of the spleen _____
3. suture of the spleen _____
4. bleeding from the spleen _____
5. tumor of the spleen _____
6. destruction of splenic tissue _____
7. study of diseases of the spleen _____
8. softening of the spleen _____
9. relating to the spleen _____

The combining form lymph/o refers to the lymph. Use it to write a term that means

10. lymph cells in the blood _____
11. cancerous tumor of the lymph system _____

The combining form lymphaden/o refers to the lymph glands. Use it to write a term that means

12. disease of a lymph gland _____
13. tumor of a lymph gland _____
14. inflammation of a lymph gland _____

The combining form immun/o refers to the immune system. Use it to write a term that means

15. suppresses the body's immune response _____
16. globulin capable of acting as an antibody _____
17. deficiency in immune system _____
18. to create an immunity by artificial means _____
19. study of the immune system _____

The combining form hem/o refers to the blood. Use it to write a term that means

20. blood therapy _____
21. relating to the blood _____
22. tumor or mass of blood cells _____
23. blood formation _____

C. USE THE FOLLOWING SUFFIXES TO CREATE A MEDICAL TERM FOR THE FOLLOWING DEFINITIONS.

-blast   -penia   -stasis   -globin   -phil   -osis   -cyte

1. decrease in WBC _____
2. decrease in RBC _____
3. decrease in platelets _____
4. decrease in lymphocytes _____
5. increase in WBC _____
6. increase in RBC _____
7. increase in platelets _____
8. increase in lymphocytes in the blood _____
9. attraction to blood _____
10. attraction to red (eosin dye) _____
11. attraction to neutral (dye) _____
12. immature (primitive) red blood cell _____
13. immature single-cell _____
14. red blood cell _____
15. white blood cell _____
16. lymph cell present in the blood _____
17. one-celled blood cell _____

D. WRITE THE COMBINING FORM FOR EACH TERM AND USE IT TO FORM A MEDICAL TERM.

	Combining Form	*Medical Term*
1. shape		
2. clot		
3. blood		
4. cell		
5. white cell		
6. eat/swallow		
7. platelet		
8. immature		
9. spleen		
10. lymph		

E. IDENTIFY THE FOLLOWING ABBREVIATIONS.

1. baso _____
2. CBC _____
3. Hgb _____
4. PT _____
5. WBC _____
6. RBC _____
7. PCV _____
8. ESR _____
9. diff _____

10. lymph _____
11. AIDS _____
12. ARC _____
13. HIV _____
14. ALL _____
15. T4 _____
16. mono _____
17. KS _____

F. Match the terms in column A with the definitions in column B.

A	B
1. _____ allergy	a. abnormal
2. _____ Rh positive	b. induce antibody formation
3. _____ Rh negative	c. decreased RBCs
4. _____ atypical	d. mass of blood
5. _____ thymoma	e. hypersensitivity
6. _____ hematoma	f. absence of factor
7. _____ anemia	g. response to invasion
8. _____ antibody	h. thymus tumor
9. _____ antigen	i. presence of factor

G. Match the terms in column A with the definitions in column B.

A	B
1. _____ WBC	a. fluid portion
2. _____ RBC	b. neutrophil
3. _____ A, B, AB, O	c. clotting time
4. _____ plasma	d. blood type
5. _____ serum	e. necessary for clotting
6. _____ phagocyte	f. leukocyte
7. _____ hematocrit	g. RBCs in total volume
8. _____ prothrombin time	h. erythrocyte
9. _____ reticulocyte	i. clear fluid (absence of clotting factor)
10. _____ fibrinogen	j. immature stage

H. Use the following terms in the sentences below.

Kaposi's sarcoma
polycythemia vera
Pneumocystis carinii
mononucleosis
anaphylactic shock
HIV
Hodgkin's disease
AIDS
peritonsillar abscess

1. The production of too many red blood cells is called _____ .

2. The Epstein–Barr virus is thought to be responsible for what infectious disease? _____

3. A life-threatening reaction as the result of an allergy is _____ .

4. The virus responsible for causing AIDS is _____ .

5. A sarcoma that is seen frequently in AIDS patients is _____ .

6. An autoimmune disease in which T cells are destroyed is _____ .

7. Malignant tumors can appear in any lymphoid tissue with this disease. _____

8. A type of pneumonia seen in AIDS patients is _____ .

9. _____ is also known as quinsy sore throat.

Getting Connected

Multimedia Extension Activities

CD-ROM

Use the CD-ROM enclosed with your textbook to gain additional reinforcement through interactive word building exercises, spelling games, labeling activities, and additional quizzes.

www.prenhall.com/fremgen

Use the above address to access the free, interactive Companion Website created for this textbook. Get hints, instant feedback, and textbook references to chapter-related multiple choice questions, and labeling and matching exercises. In addition, you will find an audio glossary, case studies, Internet exploration exercises, flashcards, and a comprehensive exam.

Answers

CASE STUDY (CRITICAL THINKING QUESTIONS)

1. feeling "run down," intermittent diarrhea, weight loss, dry cough   2. negative means absence; there was no evidence of pneumonia in the X-ray   3. a — the original or critical reaction; b — contained within a capsule; c — fluid collecting within the abdominal cavity; d — spread to a distant site   4. ultrasound; d — an enlarged spleen (splenomegaly)   5. magnetic resonance image (MRI); brain, liver   6. resolved: ascites, diarrhea; persisted: dry cough

CHART NOTE TRANSCRIPTION

1. hematologist — specialist in treating blood disorders   2. ELISA — immunoassay test for AIDS   3. prothrombin time — measure of the blood's coagulation abilities   4. complete blood count (CBC) — blood test to count all the blood cells   5. erythrocyte (RBC) — red blood cell   6. thrombocyte or platelet — clotting cell   7. leukocyte (WBC) — white blood cell   8. bone marrow aspiration — sample of bone marrow obtained for microscopic examination   9. leukemia — cancer of the white blood cell forming bone marrow   10. homologous transfusion — replacement blood from another person

PRACTICE EXERCISES

A. 1. hematology   2. spleen, tonsils, thymus   3. thoracic duct, lymphatic duct   4. axillary, cervical, mediastinal, inguinal   5. phagocytosis

B. 1. splenomegaly   2. splenectomy   3. splenorrhaphy   4. splenorrhagia   5. splenoma   6. splenolysis   7. splenology   8. splenomalacia   9. splenic   10. lymphocytes   11. malignant lymphoma   12. lymphoadenopathy   13. lymphadenoma   14. lymphadenitis   15. immunosuppressant   16. immunoglobin   17. immunodeficiency   18. immunization   19. immunology   20. hematherapy   21. hematic   22. hematoma   23. hemapoiesis

C. 1. leukocytopenia   2. erythrocytopenia   3. thrombocytopenia   4. lymphocytopenia   5. leukocytosis   6. erythrocytosis   7. thrombocytosis   8. lymphocytosis   9. hematophil   10. eosinophil   11. neutrophil   12. erythroblast   13. monoblast   14. erythrocyte   15. leukocyte   16. lymphocyte   17. monocyte

D. 1. morph/o   2. thromb/o   3. sangui/o   4. cyt/o   5. leukocyt/o   6. phag/o   7. thrombocyt/o   8. reticul/o   9. splen/o   10. lymph/o

E. 1. basophil   2. complete blood count   3. hemaglobin   4. prothrombin time   5. white blood count   6. red blood count   7. packed cell volume   8. erythrocyte sedimentation rate   9. differential   10. lymphocyte   11. acquired immune deficiency syndrome   12. AIDS-related complex   13. human immunodeficiency virus   14. acute lymphocytic leukemia   15. T-cell lymphocyte destroyed by AIDS virus   16. mononucleosis   17. Kaposi's sarcoma

F. 1. e   2. i   3. f   4. a   5. h   6. d   7. c   8. g   9. b

G. 1. f   2. h   3. d   4. a   5. i   6. b   7. g   8. c   9. j   10. e

H. 1. polycythemia vera   2. mononucleosis   3. anaphylactic shock   4. HIV   5. Kaposi's sarcoma   6. AIDS   7. Hodgkin's disease   8. *Pneumocystis carinii*   9. peritonsillar abscess

Chapter 8

RESPIRATORY SYSTEM

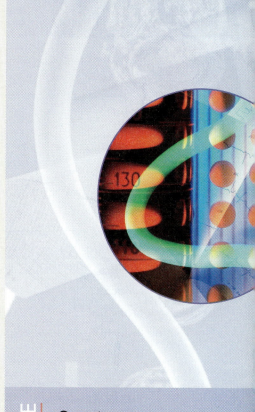

LEARNING OBJECTIVES

Upon completion of this chapter, you will be able to:

- Recognize the combining forms and suffixes introduced in this chapter.

- Gain the ability to pronounce medical terms and major anatomical structures.

- List the major organs of the respiratory system and their functions.

- Discuss the process of respiration.

- Build respiratory system medical terms from word parts.

- Define vocabulary, pathology, diagnostic, and therapeutic medical terms relating to the respiratory system.

- Interpret abbreviations associated with the respiratory system.

ORGANS OF THE RESPIRATORY SYSTEM

bronchi	nose
larynx	pharynx
lungs	trachea

COMBINING FORMS RELATING TO THE RESPIRATORY SYSTEM

adenoid/o	adenoids	pharyng/o	pharynx
alveol/o	alveolus; air sac	phon/o	voice
bronch/i	bronchus	phren/o	diaphragm
bronch/o	bronchus	pleur/o	pleura, side
bronchi/o	bronchiole	pneum/o	lung, air
bronchiol/o	bronchiole	pneumat/o	lung, air
cyan/o	blue	pneumon/o	lung, air
diaphragmat/o	diaphragm	pulmon/o	lung
epiglott/o	epiglottis	rhin/o	nose
laryng/o	larynx	sinus/o	sinus, cavity
lob/o	lobe	spir/o	breathing
mediastin/o	mediastinum	steth/o	chest
nas/o	nose	tonsil/o	tonsils
orth/o	straight, upright	trache/o	trachea, windpipe
ox/o	oxygen	thorac/o	chest
pector/o	chest		

SUFFIXES RELATING TO THE RESPIRATORY SYSTEM

Suffix	Meaning	Example
-centesis	surgical puncture to withdraw fluid	thoracocentesis
-ectasis	dilated, expansion	bronchiectasis
-itis	inflammation	bronchitis
-otomy	to cut into	tracheotomy
-rrhagia	excessive flow of blood	rhinorrhagia
-rrhea	flow	rhinorrhea
-scopy	visual examination	bronchoscopy
-thorax	chest	hemothorax

ANATOMY AND PHYSIOLOGY OF THE RESPIRATORY SYSTEM

bronchi	internists	pharynx
carbon dioxide (CO_2)	larynx	pulmonary medicine
exhalation	lungs	pulmonologists
expiration	metabolism	thoracic medicine
inhalation	nose	thoracic surgeons
inspiration	oxygen (O_2)	trachea

The respiratory system is a combination of organs that function together to perform the mechanical and, for the most part, unconscious mechanism of respiration (see Figure 8.1). The study of the respiratory system is called **pulmonary** (**PULL** mon air ee) or **thoracic** (tho **RASS** ik) **medicine.** Physicians who specialize in the diagnosis and

FIGURE 8.1 The respiratory system.

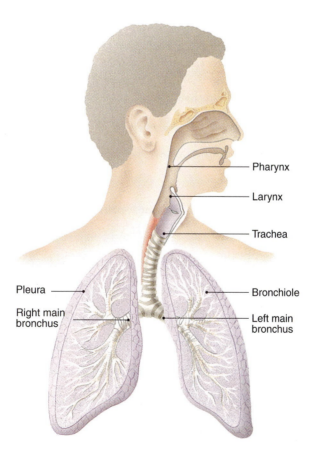

Pharynx

Larynx

Trachea

Pleura

Right main bronchus

Bronchiole

Left main bronchus

treatment of diseases of this system are called **pulmonologists** (pull mon **ALL** oh gists), **thoracic** (tho **RASS** ik) **surgeons,** or **internists** (in **TUR** nists).

Respiration consists of two distinct phases: **inspiration** (in spih **RAY** shun) and **expiration** (ek spih **RAY** shun). This process allows for the exchange of **oxygen (O_2)** (**OK** sih jen) and **carbon dioxide (CO_2).** Oxygen is necessary for the body cells' **metabolism** (meh **TAB** oh lizm), all the physical and chemical changes within the body that are necessary for life. The by-product of metabolism is the formation of a waste product; carbon dioxide. The body cells require a constant exchange of fresh oxygen and the removal of carbon dioxide. The respiratory system has to work in conjunction with the cardiovascular system, which includes the heart and blood vessels, for this exchange to take place in body cells. The process of respiration must be continuous; interruption for even a few minutes can result in brain damage and/or death.

MED TERM TIP

The terms **inspiration** and **inhalation** (in hah **LAY** shun) can be used interchangeably. Similarly, the terms **expiration** and **exhalation** (eks hah **LAY** shun) are interchangeable.

The respiratory system consists of six major organs: **nose, pharynx** (**FAIR** inks), **larynx** (**LAIR** inks), **trachea** (**TRAY** kee ah), **bronchi** (**BRONG** kigh), and **lungs.**

The process of respiration is both internal and external. The external component of respiration refers to the exchange of O_2 and CO_2 that takes place in the lungs. Internal respiration is the process of the oxygen and carbon dioxide exchange at the cellular level. The exchange is between the blood in the capillaries and the cells in the body. This process is referred to as *tissue breathing* since the cells within the body also must *breathe* fresh oxygen or, in other words, have a fresh supply of oxygen to maintain life. Carbon dioxide, formed as the waste product by the cells, is eventually expelled by the lungs.

NOSE

cilia	nasal septum
epistaxis	palate
mucous membrane	sinuses
nasal cavity	

The process of respiration requires a coordination of several organs. The first of these is the nose. Air passes through the nasal cavities, which are separated by the **nasal** (**NAY** zl) **septum.** The **palate** (**PAL** at) in the roof of the mouth separates the mouth from the **nasal** (**NAY** zl) **cavity.**

The walls of the nasal cavity and the nasal septum are made up of flexible cartilage covered with **mucous** (**MYOO** kus) **membrane.** In fact, much of the respiratory tract is covered with mucous membrane, which cleanses, warms, and moisturizes the air and allows for its smooth passage. Unfortunately, mucous membranes also serve as hosts for bacteria and virus infections. Very small hairs or **cilia** (**SIL** ee ah) line the opening to the nose, and these filter out large dirt particles before they can enter the nostrils.

Capillaries in the mucous membranes warm inhaled air as it passes through the nasal cavities. The capillaries or small blood vessels cause the temperature to rise and bring the inhaled air to body temperature.

In addition, numerous **sinuses** (**SIGH** nus es) or air-filled cavities are located within the facial bones. These produce mucous fluids, which are routed, in part, into the nasal cavity. The sinuses also play a role in sound production.

PHARYNX

adenoidectomy	**nasopharynx**	**T & A**
adenoids	**oropharynx**	**tonsillectomy**
laryngopharynx	**palatine tonsils**	**tonsils**
lingual tonsils	**pharyngeal tonsils**	

Air next enters the pharynx, also called the *throat,* which is used by both the respiratory system and the digestive system. The pharynx is critical for the respiratory system since it allows air to pass directly from the nasal cavity and mouth into the larynx without entering the stomach.

The pharynx is about 5 inches long and consists of three parts: the **nasopharynx** (nay zoh **FAIR** inks), **oropharynx** (or oh **FAIR** inks), and **laryngopharynx** (lair ring goh **FAIR** inks) (see Figure 8.2). Three pairs of **tonsils** (**TON** sulls), which are composed of lymphatic tissue, are located in the pharynx. Tonsils are strategically placed to help keep infection from entering the body's system. The nasopharynx, behind the nose, contains the **adenoids** (**ADD** eh noydz) or **pharyngeal tonsils** (fair **IN** jee al **TON** sulls). The oropharynx, behind the mouth, contains the **palatine tonsils** (**PAL** ah tine **TON** sulls) and the **lingual tonsils** (**LING** gwal **TON** sulls). Tonsils are considered a part of the lymphatic system.

FIGURE 8.2 Anatomy of upper airway.

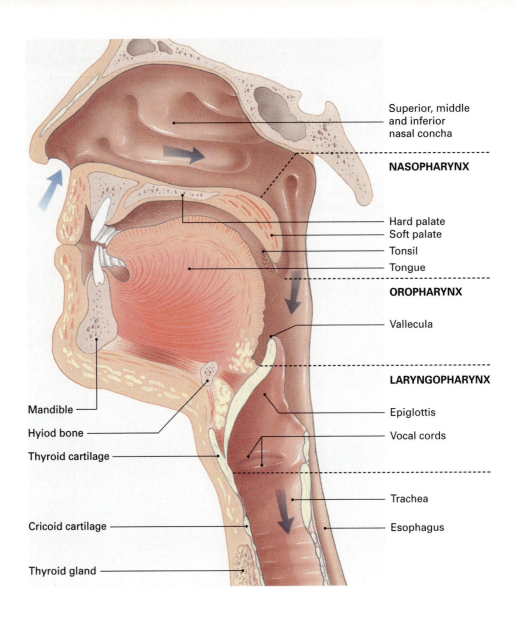

Superior, middle and inferior nasal concha

NASOPHARYNX

Hard palate
Soft palate
Tonsil
Tongue

OROPHARYNX

Vallecula

LARYNGOPHARYNX

Epiglottis
Vocal cords

Trachea
Esophagus

Mandible
Hyiod bone
Thyroid cartilage

Cricoid cartilage

Thyroid gland

FIGURE 8.3 Examination of child's tonsils.

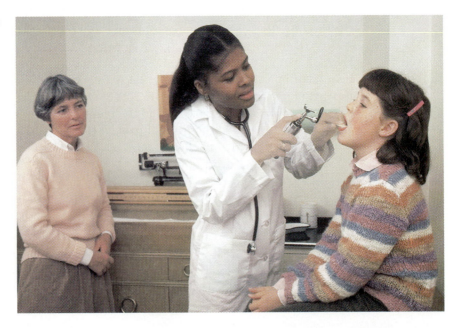

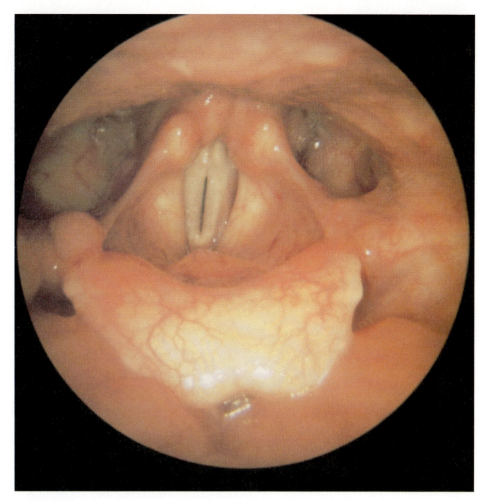

FIGURE 8.4 Vocal cords. (CNRI/Phototake NYC)

LARYNX

epiglottis   thyroid cartilage

glottis   vocal cords

The larynx or *voice box* is a muscular structure located between the pharynx and the trachea (see Figure 8.1). It contains the **vocal cords** (see Figure 8.4).

Stuttering may actually result from faulty neuromuscular control of the larynx. Some stutterers can sing or whisper without difficulty. Both singing and whispering involve movements of the larynx that differ from those required for normal speech.

The space between the two vocal cords is called the **glottis** (**GLOT** iss), and the small flap of tissue covering this opening is the **epiglottis** (ep ih **GLOT** iss). The epiglottis provides protection against food and liquid being inhaled into the lungs since it covers the larynx and trachea during swallowing. This shunts food and liquid from the pharynx into the esophagus.

The larynx has several rings of cartilage plates held together with ligaments and muscles. One of these cartilages, the **thyroid cartilage** (**THIGH** royd **CAR** tih lij), forms what is known as the *Adam's apple*. The thyroid cartilage is generally larger in the male than in the female and helps to form the deeper voice of the male.

TRACHEA

The trachea, also called the *windpipe,* is the passageway for air that extends from the pharynx and larynx down to the main bronchi. It measures approximately 4 inches in length and is composed of smooth muscle and cartilage rings. Foreign material is removed from the trachea by means of cilia located in mucous membranes.

BRONCHI

alveoli   bronchus

bronchial tree   capillaries

bronchioles

The distal end of the trachea divides to form the left and right main bronchi. Each **bronchus** (**BRONG** kus) enters one of the lungs and branches repeatedly to form secondary bronchi. Each branch becomes more narrow until the most narrow branches, the **bronchioles** (**BRONG** key ohlz), are formed. Each bronchiole terminates in a small group of air sacs, called the **alveoli** (al **VEE** oh lye). There are approximately 150 million alveoli in each lung (see Figure 8.5). A network of **capillaries** (**CAP** ih lair eez) from the pulmonary blood vessels tightly encases each alveolus. Exchange of oxygen (O_2) and carbon dioxide (CO_2) between the air within the alveolus and the blood inside the capillary takes place across the alveolar and capillary walls.

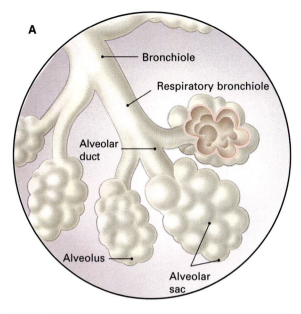

A

- Bronchiole
- Respiratory bronchiole
- Alveolar duct
- Alveolus
- Alveolar sac

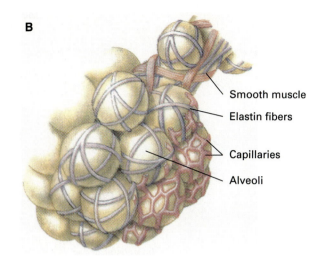

B

- Smooth muscle
- Elastin fibers
- Capillaries
- Alveoli

FIGURE 8.5 (A) Alveolar sac; (B) alveoli.

LUNGS

mediastinum	**pleurisy**	**visceral layer**
parietal layer	**serous**	
pleura	**stethoscope**	

Respiration actually occurs within the lungs, where the main function is to bring air into contact with blood so that oxygen (O_2) and carbon dioxide (CO_2) can be exchanged in the alveoli. The lungs are protected by a double membrane called the **pleura** (**PLOO** rah). The pleura's outer membrane is the **parietal** (pah **RYE** eh tal) **layer,** which also lines the wall of the chest cavity. The inner membrane or **visceral** (**VISS** er al) **layer** adheres to the lungs. There is normally a **serous** (**SEER** us) fluid between the two layers that allows for friction-free movement when the two layers rub together during respiration. See Figure 8.6 for illustration of the chest cavity.

MED TERM TIP

Some of the abnormal lung sounds heard with a **stethoscope** (**STETH** oh scope), such as crackling and rubbing, are made when the pleural and visceral membranes become inflamed, contain exudate or fluid, and rub against one another. **Pleurisy** (**PLOOR** ih see), an inflammation of the parietal pleura, is an extremely painful condition that can be caused by a variety of problems, such as pneumonia, abscesses, or tuberculosis.

The lungs contain divisions or lobes. There are three lobes in the larger right lung and two in the left lung. The lungs within the thoracic cavity are protected from puncture and damage by the ribs. The area between the right and left lung is called the **mediastinum** (mee dee ass **TYE** num). The mediastinum contains the heart, aorta, esophagus, and bronchi.

CHEST CAVITY

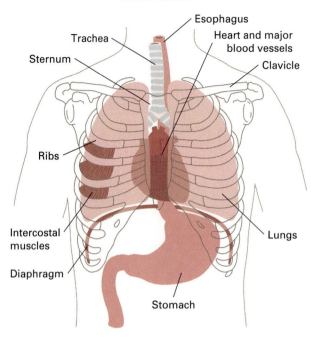

FIGURE 8.6 Chest cavity.

RESPIRATION

diaphragm	**emphysema**	**inhalation**
diaphragmatic breathing	**exhalation**	**intercostal muscles**

The lungs are able to fill with air and expel air due to the difference between the atmospheric pressure and the pressure within the chest cavity. Actually, the **diaphragm** (**DYE** ah fram), which is the muscle separating the abdomen from the thoracic cavity, is able to produce the necessary difference in pressure. To do this the diaphragm contracts and moves down into the abdominal cavity, which causes a decrease of pressure, or negative thoracic pressure, within the chest cavity. Air can then enter the lungs to equalize the pressure during what is called **inhalation** (in hah **LAY** shun). The **intercostal** (in ter **COS** tal) **muscles** between the ribs assist in inhalation by raising the rib cage to enlarge the thoracic cavity. The diaphragm then relaxes and moves back up into the chest or thoracic cavity. When this happens, pressure within the cavity increases and air can be pushed out of the lungs; **exhalation** (eks hah **LAY** shun) then takes place. See Figure 8.7 for an illustration of the mechanism of breathing.

MED TERM TIP

Diaphragmatic (dye ah frag **MAT** ik) **breathing,** or correct breathing, is taught to singers and public speakers. You can practice this type of breathing by allowing your abdomen to expand during inspiration and contract during expiration while your shoulders remain motionless.

When an injury occurs to the chest that allows air to enter the pleural cavity, the lung may collapse. This type of injury is called a sucking chest wound (see Figure 8.8).

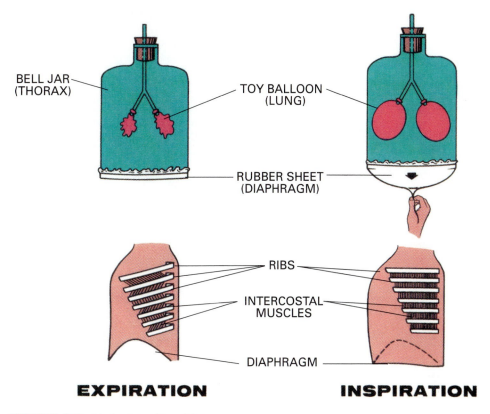

BELL JAR (THORAX)

TOY BALLOON (LUNG)

RUBBER SHEET (DIAPHRAGM)

RIBS

INTERCOSTAL MUSCLES

DIAPHRAGM

EXPIRATION

INSPIRATION

FIGURE 8.7 Mechanism of breathing.

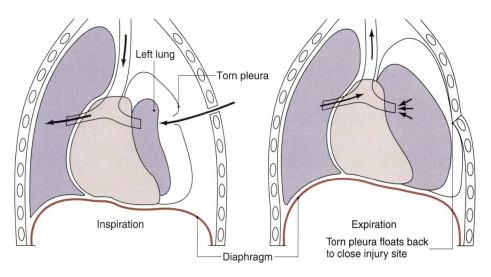

Left lung

Torn pleura

Inspiration

Diaphragm

Expiration

Torn pleura floats back to close injury site

FIGURE 8.8 Sucking chest wound (pneumothorax).

For some types of medical conditions, such as **emphysema** (em fih **SEE** mah), it is important to know the lung capacity and the volume of air that is actually flowing in and out of the lungs (see Figure 8.9). The actual volume of air exchanged in breathing is measured by respiratory specialists to aid in determining the functioning level of the respiratory system. Terminology relating to this measurement is listed in Table 8.1. This volume is measured with pulmonary function equipment.

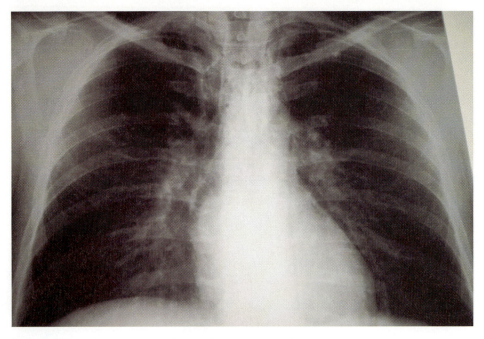

FIGURE 8.9 Normal chest X-ray. (Charles Stewart and Associates)

Table 8.1	Terminology Relating to Measurement of Volume of Air Exchanged
Term	**Definition**
Complemental air	The air that can be *forcibly* inspired after a normal respiration has taken place. Also called the inspiratory reserve volume (IRV); generally measures around 3,000 cc.*
Functional residual capacity (FRC)	The air that remains in the lungs after a normal expiration has taken place.
Residual air	The air remaining in the lungs after a forced expiration; about 1,500 cc* in the adult.
Supplemental air	The amount of air that can be *forcibly* expelled after a normal quiet respiration. This is also called the expiratory reserve volume (ERV) and is about 1,000 cc.*
Tidal volume (TV)	The amount of air that enters the lungs in a single inspiration or leaves the lungs in a single expiration of quiet breathing. In an adult this is normally 500 cc.*
Total lung capacity (TLC)	The volume of air in the lungs after a maximal inhalation or inspiration.
Vital capacity (VC)	The total volume of air that can be exhaled after a maximum inspiration. This amount will be equal to the sum of tidal air, complemental air, and supplemental air.

*There is a normal range for measurements of the volume of air exchanged. The numbers given are for the average measurement.

MED TERM TIP

Many disorders of the respiratory system are self-induced. Smoking is responsible for conditions such as cancer and emphysema. Smoking low-tar cigarettes may not be the solution to preventing these diseases. According to research studies, since low-tar cigarettes are milder, people tend to inhale more deeply. In addition, the combination of smoking while drinking alcohol is even more deadly than when done singly. The chemical ethyl nitrite is formed when both cigarette smoke and alcohol are in the mouth at the same time. This chemical is a carcinogen, or capable of producing cancer (see Figure 8.10).

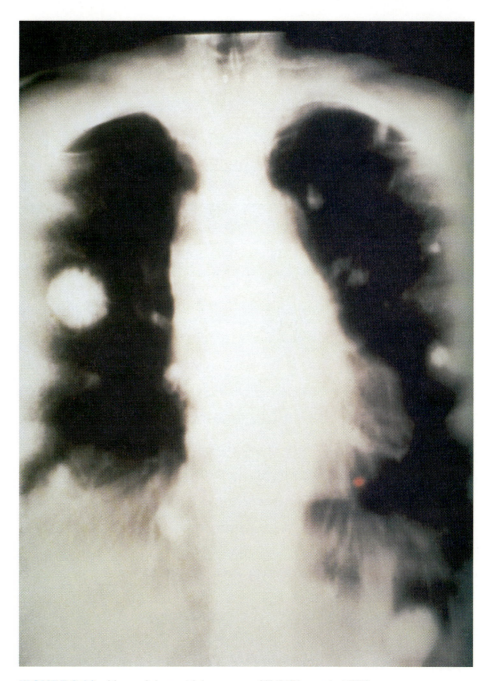

FIGURE 8.10 X-ray of chest with lung cancer. (CNRI/Phototake NYC)

Respiratory Rate

The respiratory rate is considered one of our vital signs. This rate is usually taken along with the pulse and temperature. Respiratory rate is dependent on the level of CO_2 in the blood. When the CO_2 level is high, we breathe more rapidly to expel the excess. On the other hand, if CO_2 levels drop, our respiratory rate will also drop. When a respiratory rate falls outside the range of normal, it could indicate an illness or medical condition. For example, when a patient is running an elevated temperature and has shortness of breath (SOB) due to pneumonia, the respiratory rate may increase dramatically. On the other hand, some medications, pain medications in particular, can cause a decrease in the respiratory rate. See Table 8.2 for respiratory rate ranges for different age groups.

Table 8.2	Respiratory Rates for Different Age Groups	
Age	**Respirations per Minute**	
Newborn	30–60	
1-year-old	18–30	
16-year-old	16–20	
Adult	12–20	

Word Building Relating to the Respiratory System

The following list contains examples of medical terms built directly from word parts. The definition for these terms can be determined by a straightforward translation of the word parts.

Combining Form	Combined With	Medical Term	Definition
adenoid/o	-ectomy	adenoidectomy (add eh noyd **EK** toh mee)	excision of adenoids
	-itis	adenoiditis (add eh noyd **EYE** tis)	inflammation of adenoids
bronch/i or	-ectasis	bronchiectasis (brong key **EK** tah sis)	dilated bronchi
bronch/o	-gram	bronchogram (**BRONG** koh gram)	record of the bronchus
	-graphy	bronchography (brong **KOG** rah fee)	process of recording a bronchus
	-itis	bronchitis (brong **KIGH** tis)	inflammation of a bronchus
	-plasty	bronchoplasty (**BRONG** koh plas tee)	surgical repair of a bronchus
	-scope	bronchoscope (**BRONG** koh scope)	instrument to view inside bronchus
	-scopy	bronchoscopy (brong **KOSS** koh pee)	procedure for viewing inside bronchi
	-spasm	bronchospasm (**BRONG** koh spazm)	involuntary muscle spasm of bronchi
diaphragmat/o	-cele	diaphragmatocele (dye ah frag **MAT** oh seel)	diaphragm hernia
hem/o	-thorax	hemothorax (hee moh **THOH** raks)	blood in the chest
laryng/o	-ectomy	laryngectomy (lair in **JEK** toh mee)	excision of the voice box
	-itis	laryngitis (lair in **JYE** tis)	inflammation of the voice box
	-ostomy	laryngostomy (lair in **GOSS** toh mee)	create an opening in the voice box
	-plasty	laryngoplasty (lair **RING** goh plas tee)	surgical repair of the voice box
	-scope	laryngoscope (lair **RING** goh scope)	instrument to view voice box
	-scopy	laryngoscopy (lair in **GOSS** koh pee)	procedure of viewing voice box

lob/o	-ectomy	lobectomy (loh **BEK** toh mee)	excision of a (lung) lobe
ox/o	an- -ia	anoxia (ah **NOK** see ah)	condition of no oxygen
	hypo- -emia	hypoxemia (high pox **EE** mee ah)	insufficient oxygen in the blood
	hypo- -ia	hypoxia (high **POX** ee ah)	insufficient oxygen
pleur/o	-centesis	pleurocentesis (ploor oh sen **TEE** sis)	puncture of the pleura
	-pexy	pleuropexy (**PLOOR** oh pek see)	surgical fixation of the pleura
py/o	-thorax	pyothorax (pye oh **THOH** raks)	pus in the chest
rhin/o	-itis	rhinitis (rye **NYE** tis)	inflammation of the nose
	myc/o -osis	rhinomycosis (rye noh my **KOH** sis)	abnormal condition of nose fungus
	-plasty	rhinoplasty (**RYE** noh plas tee)	surgical repair of the nose
	-rrhagia	rhinorrhagia (rye noh **RAH** jee ah)	rapid flow (of blood) from the nose
	-rrhea	rhinorrhea (rye noh **REE** ah)	nose discharge
sept/o	-plasty	septoplasty (**SEP** toh plas tee)	surgical repair of the septum
sinus/o	pan- -itis	pansinusitis (pan sigh nus **EYE** tis)	inflammation of all the sinuses
thorac/o	-algia	thoracalgia (thor ah **KAL** jee ah)	chest pain
	-ic	thoracic (tho **RASS** ik)	pertaining to the chest
	-otomy	thoracotomy (thor ah **KOT** oh mee)	incision into the chest
trache/o	endo- -al	endotracheal (en doh **TRAY** kee al)	pertaining to inside the trachea
	-ostomy	tracheostomy (tray kee **OSS** toh mee)	create an opening in the trachea
	-otomy	tracheotomy (tray kee **OTT** oh mee)	incision into the trachea
	-stenosis	tracheostenosis (tray kee oh steh **NOH** sis)	narrowing of the trachea

The word ending -*pnea* stands for *breathing* (air or gas). When added to any one of several prefixes, it will create many commonly used terms.

Prefix	Suffix	Medical Term	Definition
a-	-pnea	apnea (**AP** nee ah)	not breathing
dys-		dyspnea (**DISP** nee ah)	difficult, labored breathing
eu-		eupnea (yoop **NEE** ah)	normal breathing
hyper-		hyperpnea (high per **NEE** ah)	excessive (deep) breathing
hypo-		hypopnea (high **POP** nee ah)	insufficient (shallow) breathing
ortho-		orthopnea (or **THOP** nee ah)	(sitting) straight breathing
tachy-		tachypnea (tak ip **NEE** ah)	rapid breathing

Vocabulary Relating to the Respiratory System

anoxemia (ah nok **SEE** mee ah)	Absence of oxygen in the blood.
anoxia (ah **NOK** see ah)	Lack of oxygen.
asphyxia (as **FIK** see ah)	Lack of oxygen that can lead to unconsciousness and death if not corrected immediately. Some of the common causes are drowning, foreign body in the respiratory tract, poisoning, and electric shock.
auscultation (oss kull **TAY** shun)	Process of listening for sounds within the body. Generally performed with an instrument to amplify sounds, such as a stethoscope.
hemoptysis (hee **MOP** tih sis)	Coughing up blood or blood-stained sputum.
hypoxemia (high pox **EE** mee ah)	Deficiency of oxygen in the blood.
hypoxia (high **POX** ee ah)	Absence of oxygen in the tissues.
internist (in TUR nist)	A physician specialized in treating diseases and conditions of internal organs such as the respiratory system.
intubation (in too **BAY** shun)	Insertion of a tube into the larynx or trachea through the glottis to allow for air to enter the lungs (see Figure 8.11).
patent (PAY tent)	Open or unblocked, such as a patent airway.
percussion (per **KUH** shun)	Using the fingertips to tap on a surface to determine the condition beneath the surface. Determined in part by the feel of the surface as it is tapped and the sound generated.
phlegm (FLEM)	Thick mucus secreted by the membranes that line the respiratory tract. When phlegm is coughed through the mouth, it is called *sputum*. Phlegm is examined for color, odor, and consistency.
pleural (**PLOO** ral) **rub**	Grating sound made when two surfaces, such as the pleura surfaces, rub together during respiration. It is caused when one of the surfaces becomes thicker as a result of inflammation or other disease conditions. This rub can be felt through the fingertips when they are placed on the chest wall or heard through the stethoscope.
pulmonary (PULL mon air ee) medicine	The study of diseases of the respiratory system. Also called *thoracic medicine*.
pulmonologist (pull mon **ALL** oh jist)	A physician specialized in treating diseases and disorders of the respiratory system.
purulent (**PEWR** yoo lent)	Pus-filled sputum that can be the result of infection.
sputum (SPEW tum)	Mucus or phlegm that is coughed up from the lining of the respiratory tract. Tested to determine what type of bacteria or virus is present as an aid in selecting the proper antibiotic treatment.
thoracic (tho RASS ik) surgeon	A physician specialized in treating conditions and diseases of the respiratory system by surgical means.

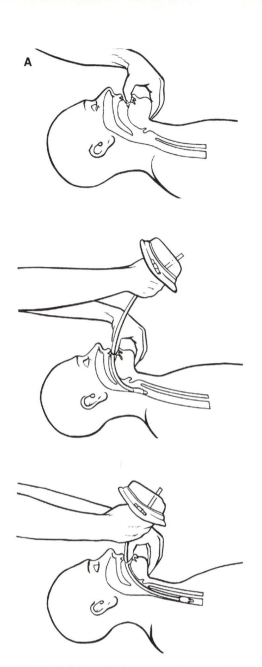

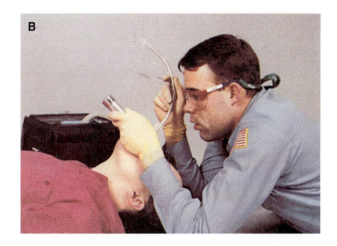

FIGURE 8.11   (A) Insertion of esophageal airway; (B) intubation into the trachea to ensure an airway.

Pathology of the Respiratory System

adult respiratory (RES pih rah tor ee) distress syndrome (ARDS)	Acute respiratory failure in adults characterized by tachypnea, dyspnea, cyanosis, tachycardia, and hypoxemia.
asthma (AZ mah)	Disease caused by various conditions, such as allergens, and resulting in constriction of the bronchial airways and labored respirations. Can cause violent spasms of the bronchi (bronchospasms) but is generally not a life-threatening condition. Medication can be very effective.
atelectasis (at eh LEK tah sis)	Condition in which lung tissue collapses, which prevents the respiratory exchange of oxygen and carbon dioxide. Can be caused by a variety of conditions, including pressure upon the lung from a tumor or other object.
bronchiectasis (brong key EK tah sis)	Results from a dilation of a bronchus or the bronchi, and can be the result of infection. This abnormal stretching can be irreversible and result in destruction of the bronchial walls. The major symptom is a large amount of purulent (pus-filled) sputum. Rales (bubbling chest sound) and hemoptysis may be present.
bronchitis (brong KIGH tis)	Inflammation of the bronchial tubes.
bronchogenic carcinoma (brong koh JEN ik car sin OH mah)	Malignant lung tumor that originates in the bronchi. Usually associated with a history of cigarette smoking.
Cheyne–Stokes (CHAIN STOHKS) respiration	Abnormal breathing pattern in which there are long periods (10 to 60 seconds) of apnea followed by deeper, more rapid breathing. Named for John Cheyne, a Scottish physician, and Sir William Stokes, an Irish surgeon.
chronic obstructive pulmonary (PULL mon air ee) disease (COPD)	Progressive, chronic, and usually irreversible condition in which the lungs have a diminished capacity for inspiration (inhalation) and expiration (exhalation). The person may have difficulty breathing upon exertion (dyspnea) and a cough. Also called *chronic obstructive lung disease (COLD)*.
cor pulmonale (KOR pull moh NAY lee)	Hypertrophy of the right ventricle of the heart as a result of lung disease.
croup (KROOP)	Acute respiratory condition found in infants and children which is characterized by a barking type of cough or stridor.
cystic fibrosis (SIS tik fye BROH sis)	Hereditary condition that causes the exocrine glands to malfunction. The patient produces very thick mucous that causes severe congestion within the lungs and digestive system. Through more advanced treatment, many children are now living into adulthood with this disease.
emphysema (em fih SEE mah)	Pulmonary condition that can occur as a result of long-term heavy smoking. Air pollution also worsens this disease. The patient may not be able to breathe except in a sitting or standing position.
empyema (em pye EE mah)	Pus within the pleural space, usually the result of infection.
epistaxis (ep ih STAKS is)	Nosebleed.
histoplasmosis (his toh plaz MOH sis)	Pulmonary disease caused by a fungus in dust in the droppings of pigeons and chickens.
hyaline (HIGH ah leen) membrane disease (HMD)	Condition seen in premature infants whose lungs have not had time to develop properly. The lungs are not able to expand fully and a membrane (hyaline membrane) actually forms that causes extreme difficulty in breathing and may result in death. Also known as *infant respiratory distress syndrome (IRDS)*.
laryngitis (lair in JYE tis)	Inflammation of the larynx causing difficulty in speaking.
Legionnaire's (lee jen AYRZ) disease	Severe, often fatal disease characterized by pneumonia and gastrointestinal symptoms. Caused by a gram-negative bacillus and named after people who came down with it at an American Legion Convention in 1976.
paroxysmal nocturnal dyspnea (pah rok SIZ mal nok TUR nal disp NEE ah) (PND)	Attacks of shortness of breath (SOB) that only occur at night and awaken the patient.

pertussis (per TUH is)	Commonly called *whooping cough,* due to the *whoop* sound made when coughing. An infectious disease that children receive immunization against as part of their DPT shots.
pharyngitis (fair in JYE tis)	Inflammation of the mucous membrane of the pharynx; usually caused by a viral or bacterial infection; commonly called a sore throat.
pleural effusion (PLOO ral eh FYOO zhun)	Abnormal presence of fluid or gas in the pleural cavity. Physicians can detect the presence of fluid by tapping the chest (percussion) or listening with a stethoscope (auscultation).
pleurisy (PLOOR ih see)	Inflammation of the pleura.
pneumoconiosis (noo moh koh nee OH sis)	Condition that is the result of inhaling environmental particles that become toxic. Can be the result of inhaling coal dust (anthracosis), or asbestos (asbestosis).
***Pneumocystis carinii* pneumonia (noo moh SIS tis kah RYE nee eye new MOH nee ah) (PCP)**	Pneumonia with a nonproductive cough, very little fever, and dyspnea. Seen in persons with weakened immune systems, such as AIDS patients.
pneumonia (new MOH nee ah)	Inflammatory condition of the lung that can be caused by bacterial and viral infections, diseases, and chemicals.
pneumonomycosis (noo moh noh my KOH sis)	Disease of the lungs caused by a fungus.
pneumothorax (new moh THOH raks)	Collection of air or gas in the pleural cavity, which may result in collapse of the lung (see Figure 8.12).
pulmonary edema (PULL mon air ee eh DEE mah)	Condition in which lung tissue retains an excessive amount of fluid. Results in labored breathing.
pulmonary embolism (PULL mon air ee EM boh lizm)	Blood clot or air bubble in the pulmonary artery or one of its branches.
rales (RALZ)	Abnormal *crackling* sound made during inspiration. Usually indicates the presence of moisture and can indicate a pneumonia condition.
rhinorrhagia (rye noh RAJ jee ah)	Rapid and excessive flow of blood from the nose.
rhinorrhea (rye noh REE ah)	Watery discharge from the nose, especially with allergies or a cold, *runny nose.*
rhonchi (RONG kigh)	Somewhat musical sound during expiration, often found in asthma or infection. Caused by spasms of the bronchial tubes. Also called *wheezing.*
shortness of breath (SOB)	Term used to indicate that a patient is having some difficulty breathing. The causes can range from mild SOB after exercise to SOB associated with heart disease. See Figure 8.13 for illustration of patient receiving oxygen for SOB.
silicosis (sil ih KOH sis)	Form of respiratory disease resulting from the inhalation of silica (quartz) dust. Considered an occupational disease.
stridor (STRIGH dor)	Harsh, high-pitched, noisy breathing sound that is made when there is an obstruction of the bronchus or larynx. Found in conditions such as croup in children.
sudden infant death syndrome (SIDS)	Unexpected and unexplained death of an apparently well infant.
tracheostenosis (tray kee oh steh NOH sis)	Narrowing and stenosis of the lumen or opening into the trachea.
tuberculosis (TB) (too ber kyoo LOH sis)	Infectious disease caused by the tubercle bacillus, *Mycobacterium tuberculosis.* Most commonly affects the respiratory system and causes inflammation and calcification of the system. Tuberculosis is again on the uprise and is seen in many patients who have AIDS.

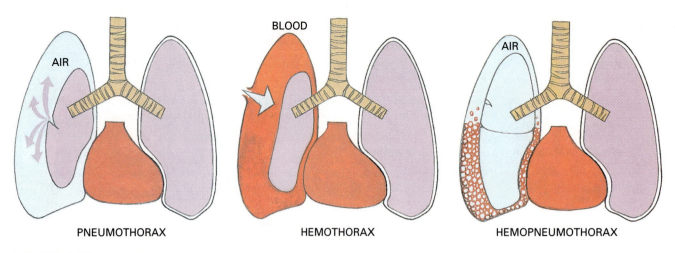

AIR

BLOOD

AIR

PNEUMOTHORAX

HEMOTHORAX

HEMOPNEUMOTHORAX

FIGURE 8.12 Chest injuries.

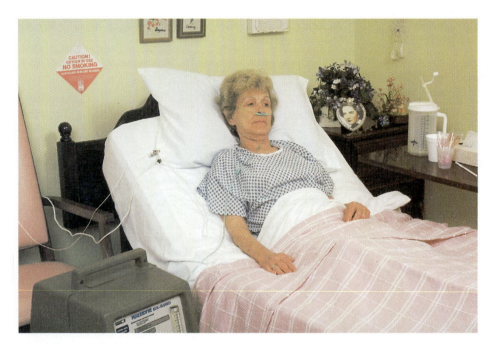

FIGURE 8.13 Residential oxygen container with nasal cannula.

Diagnostic Procedures Relating to the Respiratory System

arterial (ar TEE ree al) blood gases (ABG)	Testing for the gases present in the blood. Generally used to assist in determining the levels of oxygen (O_2) and carbon dioxide (CO_2) in the blood.
bronchography (brong KOG rah fee)	X-ray of the lung after a radiopaque substance has been inserted into the trachea or bronchial tube.
bronchoscopy (Broncho) (brong KOSS koh pee)	Using a bronchoscope to visualize the bronchi (see Figure 8.14).
chest X-ray (CXR)	Taking a radiographic picture of the lungs and heart from the back and sides (see Figure 8.15).
computerized tomography (toh MOG rah fee) of the bronchial tree (CT scan)	Taking films that allow for an X-ray slicing of the chest to aid in diagnosing tumors and other conditions.
laryngoscopy (lair in GOSS koh pee)	Examination of the interior of the larynx with a lighted instrument.
pulmonary (PULL mon air ee) function test (PFT)	Breathing equipment used to determine respiratory function and measure lung volumes and gas exchange.
pulmonary angiography (PULL mon air ee an jee OG rah fee)	Injecting dye into a blood vessel for the purpose of taking an X-ray of the arteries and veins of the lungs.
sinus (SIGH nus) X-ray	Taking an X-ray view of the sinus cavity from the front of the head.
spirometer (spy ROM eh er)	Instrument consisting of a container into which a patient can exhale for the purpose of measuring the air capacity of the lungs.
spirometry (spy ROM eh tree)	Using a device to measure the breathing capacity of the lungs.
sputum (SPEW tum) culture and sensitivity (CS)	Testing sputum by placing it on a culture medium and observing any bacterial growth. The specimen is then tested to determine antibiotic effectiveness.
sputum cytology (SPEW tum sigh TALL oh jee)	Testing for malignant cells in sputum.
throat culture	Removing a small sample of tissue or material from the pharynx and placing it upon a culture medium to determine bacterial growth.
tuberculin (too BER kyoo lin) skin tests (TB test)	Applying a chemical agent (Tine or Mantoux tests) under the surface of the skin to determine if the patient has been exposed to tuberculosis.

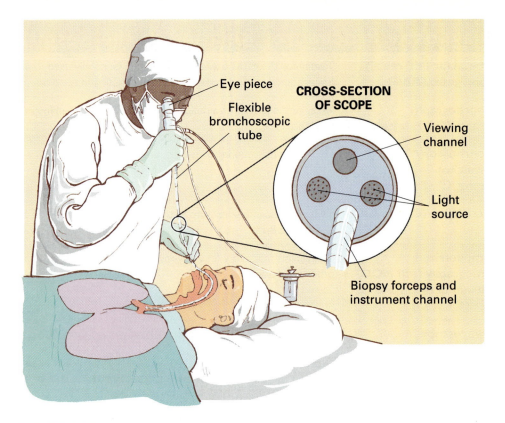

Eye piece

Flexible
bronchoscopic
tube

**CROSS-SECTION
OF SCOPE**

Viewing
channel

Light
source

Biopsy forceps and
instrument channel

FIGURE 8.14   Bronchoscopy.

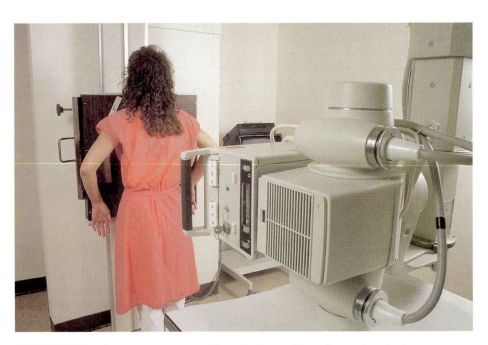

FIGURE 8.15   Patient receiving chest X-ray. (Bachmann/Photo Researchers, Inc.)

Treatment Procedures Relating to the Respiratory System

bronchoplasty (**BRONG** koh plas tee)	Surgical repair of a bronchial defect.
bronchoscopy (Broncho) (brong **KOSS** koh pee)	Using the bronchoscope to visualize the bronchi. The instrument can also be used to obtain tissue for biopsy and remove foreign objects (see Figure 8.14).
bronchotomy (brong **KOT** oh mee)	Surgical incision of a bronchus, larynx, or trachea.
cardiopulmonary resuscitation (car dee oh **PULL** mon air ee ree suss ih **TAY** shun) (CPR)	Emergency treatment provided by persons trained in CPR and given to patients when their respirations and heart stop. CPR provides oxygen to the brain, heart, and other vital organs until medical treatment can restore a normal heart and pulmonary function.
endotracheal intubation (en doh **TRAY** kee al in too **BAY** shun)	Placing a tube through the mouth to create an airway.
Heimlich (**HYME** lik) **maneuver**	Technique for removing a foreign body from the trachea or pharynx by exerting diaphragmatic pressure. Named for Harry Heimlich, an American thoracic surgeon.
hyperbaric (high per **BAR** ik) **oxygen therapy**	Use of oxygen under greater than normal pressure to treat cases of smoke inhalation, carbon monoxide poisoning, and other conditions. In some cases the patient is placed in a hyperbaric oxygen chamber for this treatment.
intermittent positive pressure breathing (IPPB)	Method for assisting patients in breathing using a mask that is connected to a machine that produces an increased pressure.
laryngectomy (lair in **JEK** toh mee)	Surgical removal of the larynx. This procedure is most frequently performed for excision of cancer.
laryngoplasty (lair **RING** goh plas tee)	Surgical repair of the larynx.
lobectomy (loh **BEK** toh mee)	Surgical removal of a lobe of the lung. Often the treatment of choice for lung cancer (see Figure 8.16).
pneumonectomy (noo moh **NEK** toh mee)	Surgical removal of lung tissue (see Figure 8.16).
postural drainage	Drainage of secretions from the bronchi by placing the patient in a position that uses gravity to promote drainage. Used for the treatment of cystic fibrosis, bronchiectasis, and before lobectomy surgery.
rhinoplasty (**RYE** noh plas tee)	Plastic surgery of the nose.
thoracocentesis (thor ah co sen **TEE** sis)	Surgical puncture of the chest wall for the removal of fluids (see Figure 8.17).
thoracostomy (thor ah **KOS** toh mee)	Insertion of a tube into the chest for the purpose of draining off fluid or air.
tracheostomy (tray kee **OSS** toh mee)	Surgical procedure used to create an opening in the trachea to create an airway. A tracheostomy tube can be inserted to keep the opening patent (see Figure 8.18).
tracheotomy (tray kee **OTT** oh mee)	Surgical incision into the trachea to provide an airway.

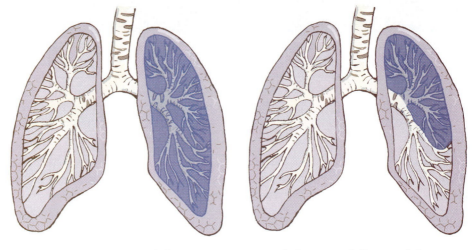

Pneumonectomy–left   Lobectomy–left upper lobe

FIGURE 8.16 Lung resection: pneumonectomy and lobectomy.

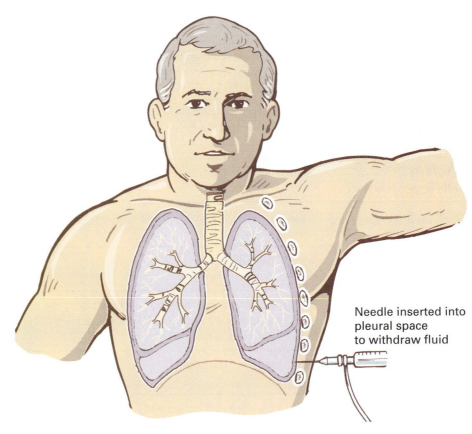

Needle inserted into
pleural space
to withdraw fluid

FIGURE 8.17 Thoracentesis.

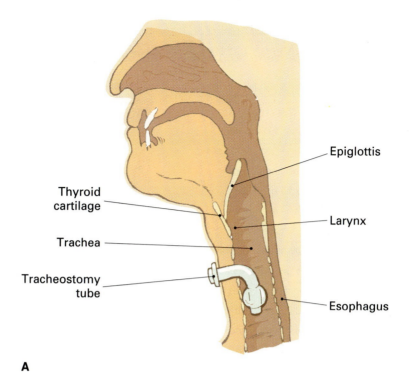

Thyroid cartilage

Trachea

Tracheostomy tube

Epiglottis

Larynx

Esophagus

A

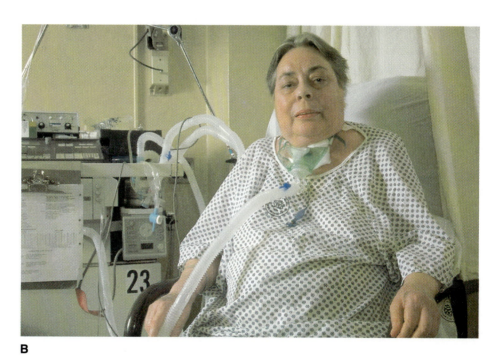

B

FIGURE 8.18 (A) Tracheostomy tube in place; (B) patient with tracheostomy tube in place receiving oxygen through mask placed over ostomy opening. (Ansell Horn/Phototake NYC)

Respiratory Therapist

Respiratory therapists assist patients/clients with breathing and lung problems. They carry out a wide variety of duties that include performing tests to assess pulmonary function, monitoring oxygen and carbon dioxide levels in the blood, administering breathing treatments, and educating the public on respiratory issues. Often, respiratory therapists are called in to handle emergency situations. They may be responsible for treating victims in distress such as premature babies and drowning victims. Respiratory therapy services are found in acute and long-term care facilities, health maintenance organizations, and home health agencies. To become a Registered Respiratory Therapist (RRT), students must attend an accredited two-year associates or four-year bachelors degree program and must pass an examination given by the National Board of Respiratory Therapy. To learn more about a career in respiratory therapy, visit the American Association for Respiratory Care's web site at www.aarc.org.

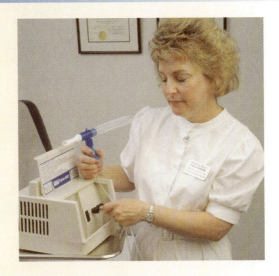

Registered Respiratory Therapist (RRT)

- **Provides respiratory therapy as ordered by a physician**
- **Graduates from an accredited two-year associate or four-year bachelor's degree respiratory therapy program**

- **Completes two years of work experience**
- **Passes the national registry examination**

Certified Respiratory Therapy Technician (CRTT)

- **Works under the supervision of a physician or Registered Respiratory Therapist**
- **Completes an approved two-year respiratory technician program**
- **Completes one year of work experience**
- **Passes the national technician certification examination**

Abbreviations Relating to the Respiratory System

A&P	auscultation and percussion	**COPD**	chronic obstructive pulmonary disease
ABG	arterial blood gases	**CPR**	cardiopulmonary resuscitation
AP view	anteroposterior view in radiology	**CS**	sputum culture and sensitivity
ARD	acute respiratory disease	**CT scan**	computerized tomography of the bronchial tree
ARDS	adult respiratory distress syndrome	**CTA**	clear to auscultation
ARF	acute respiratory failure	**CXR**	chest X-ray
Broncho	bronchoscopy	**DOE**	dyspnea upon exertion
BS	breath sounds	**DPT**	diphtheria, pertussis, tetanus injection
CO$_2$	carbon dioxide	**ENT**	ear, nose, and throat
COLD	chronic obstructive lung disease	**ERV**	expiratory reserve volume

ET	endotracheal	**PND**	paroxysmal nocturnal dyspnea (also postnasal drip)
FEF	forced expiratory flow	**PPD**	purified protein derivative (tuberculin test)
FEV	forced expiratory volume	**R**	respiration, right
FRC	functional residual capacity	**RD**	respiratory disease
FVC	forced vital capacity	**RDS**	respiratory distress syndrome
HBOT	hyperberic oxygen therapy	**RLL**	right lower lobe
HMD	hyaline membrane disease	**RML**	right middle lobe
IPPB	intermittent positive pressure breathing	**RRV**	respiratory reserve volume
IRDS	infant respiratory distress syndrome	**RUL**	right upper lobe
IRV	inspiratory reserve volume	**SIDS**	sudden infant death syndrome
L	left	**SOB**	shortness of breath
LLL	left lower lobe	**STAT**	immediately
LUL	left upper lobe	**T&A**	tonsillectomy and adenoidectomy
MBC	maximal breathing capacity	**TB**	tuberculosis
MV	minute volume	**TLC**	total lung capacity
MVV	maximal voluntary ventilation	**TPR**	temperature, pulse, and respiration
O₂	oxygen	**TV**	tidal volume
PCP	*Pneumocystis carinii* pneumonia	**URI**	upper respiratory infection
PFT	pulmonary function test	**VC**	vital capacity

KEY TERMS

- adenoidectomy (add eh noyd **EK** toh mee)
- adenoiditis (add eh noyd **EYE** tis)
- adenoids (**ADD** eh noydz)
- adult respiratory distress syndrome (ARDS) (**RES** pih rah tor ee)
- alveoli (al **VEE** oh lye)
- anoxemia (an ok **SEE** me ah)
- anoxia (ah **NOK** see ah)
- apnea (**AP** nee ah)
- arterial blood gases (ABG) (ar **TEE** ree al)
- asphyxia (as **FIK** see ah)
- asthma (**AZ** mah)
- atelectasis (at eh **LEK** tah sis)
- auscultation (oss kull **TAY** shun)
- bronchi (**BRONG** kigh)
- bronchial tree (**BRONG** kee al)
- bronchiectasis (brong key **EK** tah sis)
- bronchioles (**BRONG** key ohlz)
- bronchitis (brong **KIGH** tis)
- bronchogenic carcinoma (brong koh **JEN** ik car sin **OH** mah)
- bronchogram (**BRONG** koh gram)
- bronchography (brong **KOG** rah fee)
- bronchoplasty (**BRONG** koh plas tee)
- bronchoscope (**BRONG** koh scope)
- bronchoscopy (Broncho) (brong **KOSS** koh pee)
- bronchospasm (**BRONG** koh spazm)
- bronchotomy (brong **KOT** oh mee)

- bronchus (**BRONG** kus)
- capillaries (**CAP** ih lair eez)
- carbon dioxide (CO₂)
- cardiopulmonary resuscitation (CPR) (car dee oh **PULL** mon air ee ree suss ih **TAY** shun)
- chest X-ray (CXR)
- Cheyne-Stokes respiration (**CHAIN STOHKS** res pir **AY** shun)
- chronic obstructive pulmonary disease (COPD) (**PULL** mon air ee)
- cilia (**SIL** ee ah)
- computerized tomography of the bronchial tree (CT scan) (toh **MOG** rah fee)
- cor pulmonale (**KOR** pull moh **NAY** lee)
- croup (**KROOP**)
- cystic fibrosis (**SIS** tik fye **BROH** sis)
- diaphragm (**DYE** ah fram)
- diaphragmatic breathing (dye ah frag **MAT** ik)
- diaphragmatocele (dye ah frag **MAT** oh seel)
- dyspnea (**DISP** nee ah)
- emphysema (em fih **SEE** mah)
- empyema (em pye **EE** mah)
- endotracheal (ET) (en doh **TRAY** kee al)
- endotracheal intubation (en doh **TRAY** kee al in too **BAY** shun)
- epiglottis (ep ih **GLOT** iss)
- epistaxis (ep ih **STAKS** is)
- eupnea (yoop **NEE** ah)

- exhalation (eks hah **LAY** shun)
- expiration (ek spih **RAY** shun)
- glottis (**GLOT** iss)
- Heimlich maneuver (**HYME** lik)
- hemoptysis (hee **MOP** tih sis)
- hemothorax (hee moh **THOH** raks)
- histoplasmosis (his toh plaz **MOH** sis)
- hyaline membrane disease (HMD) (**HIGH** ah leen)
- hyperbaric oxygen therapy (high per **BAR** ik)
- hyperpnea (high per **NEE** ah)
- hypopnea (high **POP** nee ah)
- hypoxemia (high pox **EE** mee ah)
- hypoxia (high **POX** ee ah)
- inhalation (in hah **LAY** shun)
- inspiration (in spih **RAY** shun)
- intercostal muscles (in ter **COS** tal)
- intermittent positive pressure breathing (IPPB)
- internist (in **TUR** nist)
- intubation (in too **BAY** shun)
- laryngectomy (lair in **JEK** toh mee)
- laryngitis (lair in **JYE** tis)
- laryngopharynx (lair ring goh **FAIR** inks)
- laryngoplasty (lair **RING** goh plas tee)
- laryngoscope (lair **RING** goh scope)
- laryngoscopy (lair in **GOSS** koh pee)
- laryngostomy (lair in **GOSS** toh mee)
- larynx (**LAIR** inks)
- Legionnaire's disease (lee jen **AYRZ**)
- lingual tonsils (**LING** gwal **TON** sulls)
- lobectomy (loh **BEK** toh mee)
- lungs
- mediastinum (mee dee ass **TYE** num)
- metabolism (meh **TAB** oh lizm)
- mucous membrane (**MYOO** kus)
- nasal cavity (**NAY** zl)
- nasal septum (**NAY** zl)
- nasopharynx (nay zoh **FAIR** inks)
- nose
- oropharynx (or oh **FAIR** inks)
- orthopnea (or **THOP** nee ah)
- oxygen (O₂) (**OK** sih jen)
- palate (**PAL** at)
- palatine tonsils (**PAL** ah tine **TON** sulls)
- pansinusitis (pan sigh nus **EYE** tis)
- parietal layer (pah **RYE** eh tal)
- paroxysmal nocturnal dyspnea (PND) (pah rok **SIZ** mal nok **TUR** nal disp **NEE** ah)
- patent (**PAY** tent)
- percussion (per **KUH** shun)
- pertussis (per **TUH** sis)
- pharyngeal tonsils (fair **IN** jee al **TON** sulls)
- pharyngitis (fair in **JYE** tis)
- pharynx (**FAIR** inks)
- phlegm (**FLEM**)
- pleura (**PLOO** rah)
- pleural effusion (**PLOO** ral eh **FYOO** zhun)
- pleural rub (**PLOO** ral)
- pleurisy (**PLOOR** ih see)
- pleurocentesis (ploor oh sen **TEE** sis)
- pleuropexy (**PLOOR** oh pek see)

- pneumoconiosis (noo moh koh nee **OH** sis)
- *Pneumocystis carinii* pneumonia (noo moh **SIS** tis kah **RYE** nee eye new **MOH** nee ah)
- pneumonectomy (noo moh **NEK** toh mee)
- pneumonia (new **MOH** nee ah)
- pneumonomycosis (noo moh noh my **KOH** sis)
- pneumothorax (new moh **THOH** raks)
- postural drainage
- pulmonary angiography (**PULL** mon air ee an jee **OG** rah fee)
- pulmonary edema (**PULL** mon air ee eh **DEE** mah)
- pulmonary embolism (**PULL** mon air ee **EM** boh lizm)
- pulmonary function test (PFT) (**PULL** mon air ee)
- pulmonary medicine (**PULL** mon air ee)
- pulmonologist (pull mon **ALL** oh jist)
- purulent (**PEWR** yoo lent)
- pyothorax (pye oh **THOH** raks)
- rales (**RALZ**)
- rhinitis (rye **NYE** tis)
- rhinomycosis (rye noh my **KOH** sis)
- rhinoplasty (**RYE** noh plas tee)
- rhinorrhagia (rye noh **RAH** jee ah)
- rhinorrhea (rye noh **REE** ah)
- rhonchi (**RONG** kigh)
- septoplasty (**SEP** toh plas tee)
- serous (**SEER** us)
- shortness of breath (SOB)
- silicosis (sill ih **KOH** sis)
- sinus X-ray (**SIGH** nus)
- sinuses (**SIGH** nus es)
- spirometer (spy **ROM** eh ter)
- spirometry (spy **ROM** eh tree)
- sputum (**SPEW** tum)
- sputum culture and sensitivity (CS) (**SPEW** tum)
- sputum cytology (**SPEW** tum sigh **TALL** oh jee)
- stethoscope (**STETH** oh scope)
- stridor (**STRIGH** dor)
- sudden infant death syndrome (SIDS)
- tachypnea (tak ip **NEE** ah)
- thoracalgia (thor ah **KAL** jee ah)
- thoracic (tho **RASS** ik)
- thoracic medicine (tho **RASS** ik)
- thoracic surgeon (tho **RASS** ik)
- thoracocentesis (thor ah co sen **TEE** sis)
- thoracostomy (thor ah **KOS** toh mee)
- thoracotomy (thor ah **KOT** oh mee)
- throat culture
- thyroid cartilage (**THIGH** royd)
- tonsillectomy (ton sih **LEK** toh mee)
- tonsillectomy and adenoidectomy (T & A) (ton sih **LEK** toh mee and add eh noyd **EK** toh mee)
- tonsils (**TON** sulls)
- trachea (**TRAY** kee ah)
- tracheostenosis (tray kee oh steh **NOH** sis)
- tracheostomy (tray kee **OSS** toh mee)
- tracheotomy (tray kee **OTT** oh mee)
- tuberculin skin tests (TB test) (too **BER** kyoo lin)
- tuberculosis (TB) (too ber kyoo **LOH** sis)
- visceral layer (**VISS** er al)
- vocal cords

Case Study

PULMONOLOGY CONSULTATION REPORT

Reason for Consultation: Evaluation of increasingly severe asthma.

History of Present Illness: Patient is currently a 10-year-old male who first presented to the Emergency Room with dyspnea, coughing, and wheezing at 7 years of age. Paroxysmal attacks are increasing in frequency and there does not appear to be any precipitating factors such as exercise. No other family members are asthmatics.

Results of Physical Examination: Patient is currently in the ER with a paroxysmal attack with marked dyspnea, cyanosis around the lips, prolonged expiration, and a hacking cough producing thick, non-purulent phlegm. Thoracic auscultation with stethoscope revealed rhonchi throughout bilateral lung fields. Chest X-ray shows poor pulmonary expansion, with hypoxemia indicated by ABG. A STAT pulmonary function test reveals moderately severe airway obstruction during expiration. This attack responded to oxygen therapy and IV Alupent and steroids, and he is beginning to cough less and breathe with less effort.

Assessment: Acute asthma attack with severe airway obstruction. There is no evidence of pulmonary infection. In view of increasing severity and frequency of attacks, all his medications should be reevaluated for effectiveness and all attempts to identify precipitating factors should be made.

Recommendations: Patient is to continue to use Alupent for relief of bronchospasms and steroids to reduce general inflammation. Instructions for taking medications and controlling severity of asthma attacks were carefully reviewed with the patient and his family. A referral to an allergist was made to evaluate this young man for presence of environmental allergies.

CRITICAL THINKING QUESTIONS

1. What does the medical term *paroxysmal* mean?

2. What do the following abbreviations stand for?

   a. IV

   b. STAT

   c. ABG

3. The patient was discharged and sent home with two medications. Explain in your own words the purpose of each of these medications.

4. What important information regarding this young man's asthma is unknown to the physicians? What does this consulting physician recommend to address this problem?

5. Describe the characteristics related to this patient's cough in your own words.

6. Which of the following is not one of the symptoms seen in the emergency room?

   a. crackling lung sounds

   b. bluish skin

   c. difficulty breathing

   d. extended breathing out time

Chart Note Transcription

Chart Note

The chart note below contains ten phrases that can be reworded with a medical term that you learned in this chapter. Each phrase is identified with an underline. Determine the medical term and write your answers in the space provided.

Current Complaint: A 43-year-old female was brought to the Emergency Room by her family. She complained of painful and labored breathing,[1] rapid breathing,[2] and fever. Symptoms began 3 days ago, but have become much worse over the past 12 hours.

Past History: Patient is a mother of three and a business executive. She has had no surgeries or previous serious illnesses.

Signs and Symptoms: Temperature is 103° F, respiratory rate is 20 breaths/minute, blood pressure is 165/98, and heart rate is 90/minute. A blood test to measure the levels of oxygen in the blood[3] indicate marked low level of oxygen in the blood.[4] The process of listening to body sounds[5] of the lungs revealed abnormal crackling sounds over the left lower chest.[6] She is producing large amounts of pus-filled[7] mucus coughed up from the respiratory tract[8] and a back-to-front chest X-ray[9] shows a large cloudy patch in the lower lobe of the left lung.

Diagnosis: Left lower lobe inflammatory condition of the lungs caused by bacterial infection.[10]

Treatment: Patient was started on intravenous antibiotics. She also required a tube placed through the mouth to create an airway for 3 days.

1 _____

2 _____

3 _____

4 _____

5 _____

6 _____

7 _____

8 _____

9 _____

10 _____

Practice Exercises

A. COMPLETE THE FOLLOWING STATEMENTS.

1. The primary function of the respiratory system is _____ .
2. Define external respiration._____
3. Define internal respiration. _____
4. The organs of the respiratory system are _____ , _____ , _____ , _____ , _____ , and _____ .
5. The passageway for food, liquids, and air is the _____ .
6. The _____ helps to keep food out of the respiratory tract.
7. The function of the cilia in the nose is to _____ .
8. The musculomembranous wall that divides the thoracic cavity from the abdominal cavity is the _____ .
9. The respiratory rate for an adult is _____ to _____ respirations per minute.
10. The respiratory rate for a newborn is _____ to _____ respirations per minute.
11. The right lung has _____ lobes; the left lung has _____ lobes.
12. The air sacs at the ends of the bronchial tree are called _____ .
13. The term for the lining of the lungs is _____ .
14. The nasal cavity is separated from the mouth with the _____ .
15. The small branches of the bronchi are the _____ .

B. STATE THE TERMS DESCRIBED USING THE COMBINING FORMS PROVIDED.

The combining form rhin/o refers to the nose. Use it to write a term that means
1. inflammation of the mucous membranes in the nasal cavity _____
2. pertaining to the nose _____
3. discharge from the nose _____
4. surgical repair of the nose _____

The combining forms pulmon/o, pneumon/o, and pneum/o all refer to the lungs. Use them to write a term that means
5. inflammation of the lungs _____
6. pertaining to the lungs _____
7. excision of a lung _____
8. suture of the lung _____
9. surgical puncture of the chest _____
10. excision of one lobe of a lung _____

The combining form laryng/o refers to the larynx or voice box. Use it to write a term that means
11. inflammation of the larynx _____
12. spasm of the larynx _____
13. visual examination of the larynx using an instrument _____
14. pertaining to the larynx _____
15. incision of the larynx _____
16. excision of the larynx _____
17. surgical repair of the larynx _____
18. paralysis of the larynx _____

The combining forms bronch/o and bronchi/o refer to the bronchus. Use them to write a term that means

19. bronchial hemorrhage _____

20. inflammation of the bronchus _____

21. instrument to visually examine the interior of the bronchus _____

22. pathological condition of the bronchus _____

23. spasm of the bronchus _____

The combining form thorac/o refers to the chest, and my/o refers to muscle. Use these combining forms to write a term that means

24. plastic surgery _____

25. incision into _____

26. surgical puncture _____

27. chest muscle pain _____

28. examination with an instrument _____

The combining form trache/o refers to the trachea. Use it to write a term that means

29. cutting into _____

30. plastic surgery _____

31. narrowing _____

32. disease _____

33. suture _____

34. inflammation _____

35. forming an artificial opening into the trachea _____

C. DEFINE THE FOLLOWING COMBINING FORMS.

1. trache/o _____

2. laryng/o _____

3. bronch/o _____

4. sten/o _____

5. pneumon/o _____

6. rhin/o _____

7. py/o _____

8. hem/o _____

9. pleur/o _____

10. epiglott/o _____

11. cyan/o _____

12. alveoli _____

13. pulmon/o _____

14. tonsill/o _____

15. sinus _____

16. lob/o _____

17. pector/o _____

18. nas/o _____

D. DEFINE EACH SUFFIX AND USE IT TO FORM A TERM FROM THE RESPIRATORY SYSTEM.

	Meaning	*Respiratory Term*
1. -centesis		
2. -ectasis		
3. -pnea		
4. -plasty		
5. -ia		
6. -cele		
7. -ectomy		
8. -osis		
9. -rrhagia		

E. THE SUFFIX -PNEA MEANS BREATHING. USE THIS SUFFIX TO WRITE A MEDICAL TERM THAT MEANS

1. normal breathing _____
2. difficult or labored breathing _____
3. rapid breathing _____
4. only can breath in an upright position _____
5. infrequent breathing _____

F. DEFINE THE FOLLOWING TERMS.

1. total lung capacity _____
2. tidal volume _____
3. residual volume _____

G. WRITE THE MEDICAL TERM FOR EACH DEFINITION.

1. the process of breathing in _____
2. spitting up of blood _____
3. any disease of the lung _____
4. inflammation of a sinus _____
5. difficulty in speaking due to dry throat and hoarseness _____
6. air in the pleural cavity _____
7. paralysis of the bronchi _____
8. incision into the pleura _____
9. pain in the pleural region _____
10. herniation of lung tissue or pleura _____

H. CHANGE THE FOLLOWING SINGULAR TERMS TO PLURAL TERMS.

1. bronchus _____
2. sputum _____
3. lumen _____
4. alveolus _____

I. WRITE THE ABBREVIATIONS FOR THE FOLLOWING TERMS.

1. auscultation and percussion   _____
2. pulmonary function test   _____
3. left lower lobe   _____
4. oxygen   _____
5. carbon dioxide   _____
6. intermittent positive pressure breathing   _____
7. chronic obstructive lung disease   _____
8. bronchoscopy   _____
9. total lung capacity   _____
10. tuberculosis   _____
11. paroxysmal nocturnal dyspnea   _____

J. IDENTIFY THE FOLLOWING ABBREVIATIONS.

1. URI _____
2. AP View _____
3. TPR _____
4. COPD _____
5. RD _____
6. RUL _____

7. SIDS _____
8. TLC _____
9. ARDS _____
10. HBOT _____
11. PA view _____
12. PFT _____

Getting Connected

Multimedia Extension Activities

CD-ROM

Use the CD-ROM enclosed with your textbook to gain additional reinforcement through interactive word building exercises, spelling games, labeling activities, and additional quizzes.

www.prenhall.com/fremgen

Use the above address to access the free, interactive Companion Website created for this textbook. Get hints, instant feedback, and textbook references to chapter-related multiple choice questions, and labeling and matching exercises. In addition, you will find an audio glossary, case studies, Internet exploration exercises, flashcards, and a comprehensive exam.

Answers

CASE STUDY (CRITICAL THINKING)

1. sudden attack   2. intravenous, immediately, arterial blood gases   3. steroid to reduce inflammation; Alupent to relax bronchospasms   4. what triggers his attacks; referred patient to an allergist   5. hacking and producing thick, non-purulent phlegm   6. a—crackling lung sounds

CHART NOTE

1. dyspnea—painful and labored breathing   2. tachypnea—rapid breathing   3. arterial blood gases (ABG)—a blood test to measure the levels of oxygen in the blood   4. hypoxemia—low level of oxygen in the blood   5. auscultation—process of listening to body sounds   6. rales—abnormal crackling sounds   7. purulent—pus-filled   8. sputum—mucus coughed up from the respiratory tract   9. posteroanterior view (PA)—back-to-front   10. pneumonia—inflammatory condition of the lungs caused by bacterial infection   11. endotracheal intubation—a tube placed through the mouth to create an airway

PRACTICE EXERCISES

A. 1. exchange of O_2 and CO_2 2. exchange of O_2 and CO_2 in the lungs   3. exchange of O_2 and CO_2 at cellular level   4. nose, pharynx, larynx, trachea, bronchus, lungs   5. pharynx   6. epiglottis   7. filter out dust   8. diaphragm   9. 12–20   10. 30–60   11. 3/2   12. alveoli   13. pleura   14. palate   15. bronchioles

B. 1. rhinitis   2. rhinal   3. rhinorrhea   4. rhinoplasty   5. pneumonitis   6. pulmonary   7. pneumonectomy   8. pneumorrhaphy   9. pneumocentesis   10. lobectomy   11. laryngitis   12. laryngospasm   13. laryngoscopy   14. laryngeal   15. laryngotomy   16. laryngectomy   17. laryngoplasty   18. laryngoplegia   19. bronchorrhagia   20. bronchitis   21. bronchoscope   22. bronchopathy   23. bronchospasm   24. thoracoplasty   25. thoracotomy   26. thoracocentesis   27. thoracomyodynia   28. thoracoscopy   29. tracheotomy   30. tracheoplasty   31. tracheostenosis   32. tracheopathy   33. tracheorrhaphy   34. tracheitis   35. tracheostomy

C. 1. trachea   2. larynx   3. bronchus   4. stricture   5. lung   6. nose   7. pus   8. blood   9. pleura, side   10. epiglottis   11. blue   12. alveolus   13. lung   14. tonsil   15. sinus   16. lobe   17. chest   18. nose

D. 1. surgical puncture   2. dilation   3. breathing   4. repair   5. pertaining to   6. swelling, hernia   7. removal of   8. condition of   9. hemorrhage

E. 1. eupnea   2. dyspnea   3. hyperpnea   4. orthopnea   5. oligopnea

F. 1. Volume of air in the lungs after a maximal inhalation or inspiration.   2. Amount of air entering lungs in a single inspiration or leaving air in single expiration of quiet breathing.   3. Air remaining in the lungs after a forced expiration.

G. 1. inhalation or inspiration   2. hemoptysis   3. pneumopathy   4. sinusitis   5. laryngitis   6. pneumothorax   7. bronchoplegia   8. pleurotomy   9. pleurisy or pleuralgia   10. pneumocele or pleurocele

H. 1. bronchi   2. sputa   3. lumina   4. alveoli

I. 1. A&P   2. PFT   3. LLL   4. O_2 5. CO_2 6. IPPB   7. COLD   8. Broncho   9. TLC   10. TB   11. PND

J. 1. upper respiratory infection   2. anteroposterior view   3. temperature, pulse, respirations   4. chronic obstructive pulmonary disease   5. respiratory disease   6. right upper lobe   7. sudden infant death syndrome   8. total lung capacity   9. adult respiratory distress syndrome   10. hyperbaric oxygen therapy   11. posteroanterior view   12. pulmonary function test

Chapter 9

DIGESTIVE SYSTEM

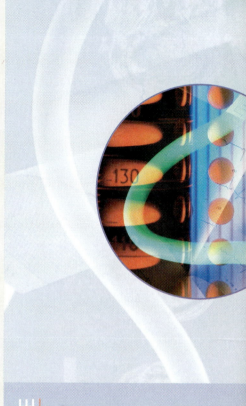

LEARNING OBJECTIVES

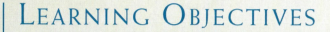

Upon completion of this chapter, you will be able to:

- Recognize the combining forms and suffixes introduced in this chapter.

- Gain the ability to pronounce medical terms and major anatomical structures.

- List the major organs of the alimentary canal and their functions.

- Describe the function of the accessory organs of the digestive system.

- Identify the shape and function of each type of tooth.

- Build digestive system medical terms from word parts.

- Define vocabulary, pathology, diagnostic, and therapeutic medical terms relating to the digestive system.

- Interpret abbreviations associated with the digestive system.

Overview

ORGANS OF THE DIGESTIVE SYSTEM

anus	gallbladder (GB)	pancreas	salivary glands
colon	liver	pharynx	small intestine
esophagus	mouth	rectum	stomach

COMBINING FORMS RELATING TO THE DIGESTIVE SYSTEM

abdomin/o	abdomen	gluc/o	sugar
aliment/o	nourish	glyc/o	sugar
amyl/o	starch	glycogen/o	glycogen
an/o	anus	hepat/o	liver
append/o	appendix	herni/o	hernia
appendic/o	appendix	ile/o	ileum
bil/i	bile, gall	intestin/o	intestine
bilirubin/o	bilirubin	jejun/o	jejunum
bucc/o	cheek	labi/o	lip
cec/o	cecum	lapar/o	abdomen
celi/o	abdomen	lingu/o	tongue
cheil/o	lip	lip/o	fat, lipid
chol/e	bile, gall	lith/o	stone
chol/o	bile, gall	odont/o	tooth
cholangi/o	bile duct	or/o	mouth
cholecyst/o	gallbladder	palat/o	palate
choledoch/o	common bile duct	pancreat/o	pancreas
col/o	colon	peritone/o	peritoneum
colon/o	colon	phag/o	to eat
cyst/o	cyst, sac	polyp/o	polyp
dent/i, dent/o	tooth	proct/o	anus and rectum
diverticul/o	diverticulum, blind pouch	pylor/o	pylorus
duoden/o	duodenum	rect/o	rectum
enter/o	small intestine	sial/o	saliva, salivary gland
esophag/o	esophagus	sigmoid/o	sigmoid colon
gastr/o	stomach	steat/o	fat
gingiv/o	gums	stomat/o	mouth
gloss/o	tongue	uvul/o	uvula

Suffix	Meaning	Example
-emesis	vomit	hematemesis
-iasis	abdominal condition	chlelithiasis
-lith	stone	lithotripsy
-pepsia	digestion	dyspensia
-phagia	eat, swallow	polyphagia
-prandial	pertaining to a meal	postprandial
-rrhea	flow, discharge	diarrhea

ANATOMY AND PHYSIOLOGY OF THE DIGESTIVE SYSTEM

accessory organs	**inflammatory bowel disease (IBD)**
alimentary canal	**irritable bowel syndrome (IBS)**
bacterium	**peptic ulcers**
feces	

The digestive system, also known as the gastrointestinal system, includes 30 feet of intestinal tubing that covers the area between the mouth and the anus and has a wide range of functions. This system serves to store and digest food, absorb nutrients, and eliminate waste (see Figure 9.1). Terminology for this system includes all terms relating to digestion, absorption, and elimination.

Perhaps more than any other system in the body, this system gives us clear indications of when it is working well and when it needs attention. Two of the most important messages are hunger and the need to have a bowel movement (BM).

This system depends on many other systems, including the immune and nervous systems, to function fully. While there are organs that are directly related to this system, such as the mouth and stomach, there are also **accessory organs** of digestion, which include the liver, pancreas, gallbladder, and salivary glands. The nervous, hormonal, and endocrine systems also contribute to digestion. In addition, the psychological health or mental status of the person can aid in digestion.

The organs of digestion—mouth or oral cavity, pharynx, esophagus, stomach, small intestine, colon, rectum, and anus—are referred to as the **alimentary canal** (al ih **MEN** tar ree can **NAL**).

MED TERM TIP

It is still believed that digestive disorders such as **peptic ulcers** (**PEP** tik **ULL** sirs), indigestion, **inflammatory bowel disease** (in **FLAM** ah tor ee **BOW** el dih **ZEEZ**), and **irritable bowel syndrome (IBS)** (**EAR** it ah b'l **BOW** el **SIN** drohm) **(IBS)** can be due, at least partly, to psychological problems. This demonstrates a need for psychological as well as physical intervention. However, some gastric ulcer conditions, which previously were considered emotional in origin, are now being treated effectively with medications such as antibiotics to treat the **bacterium** (bak **TEE** ree um) causing the ulcer.

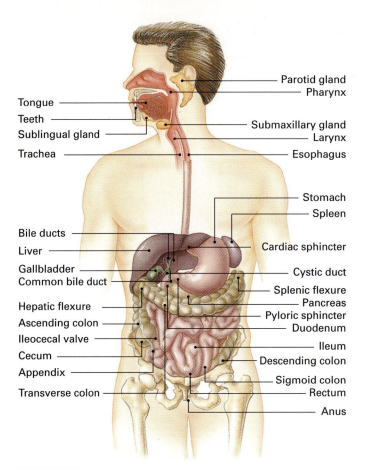

Tongue
Teeth
Sublingual gland
Trachea

Parotid gland
Pharynx
Submaxillary gland
Larynx
Esophagus

Bile ducts
Liver
Gallbladder
Common bile duct
Hepatic flexure
Ascending colon
Ileocecal valve
Cecum
Appendix
Transverse colon

Stomach
Spleen
Cardiac sphincter
Cystic duct
Splenic flexure
Pancreas
Pyloric sphincter
Duodenum
Ileum
Descending colon
Sigmoid colon
Rectum
Anus

FIGURE 9.1   Organs of the digestive system.

The actual function of the digestive system is the physical and chemical breakdown of food. The body needs the nutrients from food for growth and repair of organs and tissues. Ultimately, food is digested in minute nutrient molecules that are absorbed from the intestines and circulated throughout the body in the blood system. Any food that cannot be digested becomes a waste product and is expelled or defecated as **feces** (**FEE** ceez).

ORAL CAVITY

bicuspids	**enamel**	**papillae**
canines	**incisors**	**permanent teeth**
cuspids	**molars**	**premolars**
deciduous teeth	**orthodontics**	**tongue**
dentin	**palate**	

The digestive process begins when food enters the mouth and is broken up by the chewing movements of the teeth. The **tongue,** with its muscular action, actually moves the food within the mouth also known as the oral cavity (see Figure 9.2). Mucous membrane lines the oral cavity. Taste buds, or **papillae** (pah **PILL** ay), are raised projections on the surface of the tongue that distinguish bitterness, sweetness, sourness, and saltiness in our food (see Figure 9.3 for a sagittal view of the oral cavity).

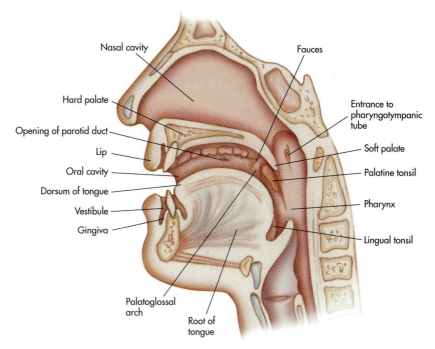

FIGURE 9.2 The oral cavity.

Teeth are important for the first stage of digestion. The smaller teeth in the front of the mouth are called **canines** (**KAY** nines) or **cuspids** (**CUSS** pids) and **incisors** (in **SIGH** zors) (see Figure 9.4). They can tear and cut food into smaller pieces. The **bicuspids** (bye **CUSS** pids) or **premolars** (pre **MOH** lars) and large **molars** (**MOH** lars) located at the back of the mouth can crush and grind down the food into even finer pieces. Teeth are

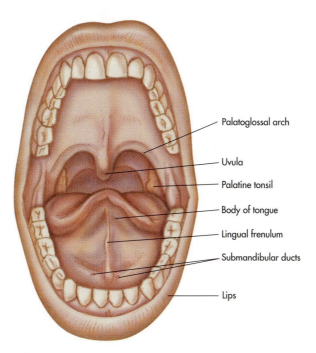

FIGURE 9.3 Mouth: Sagittal view.

FIGURE 9.4 Adult teeth.

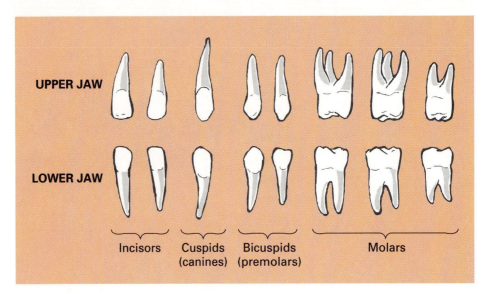

covered with a hard surface called **enamel** (en **AM** el). Enamel covers the **dentin** (**DEN** tin) of the tooth, which is actually the main part of the tooth (see Figure 9.5).

Types of Teeth

Bicuspid: Premolar permanent tooth having two cusps or projections that assist in grinding food.

Canines or cuspids: The eyeteeth, which are located between the incisors and the molars.

FIGURE 9.5 Cross-section of a tooth.

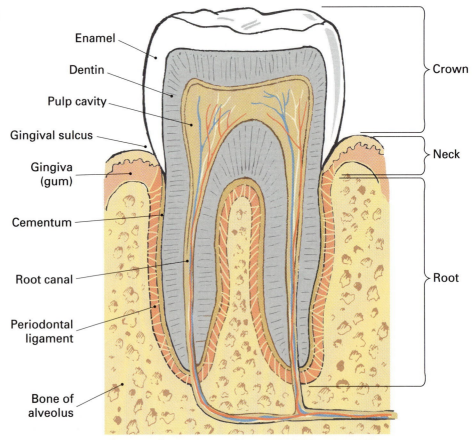

FIGURE 9.6 Full mouth X-rays. (Vanessa Vick/Photo Researchers, Inc.)

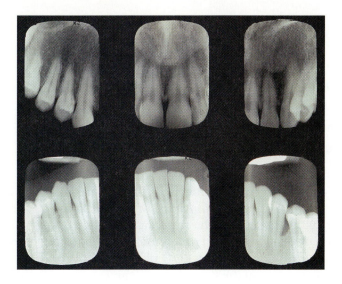

Deciduous (dee **SID** yoo us) **teeth:** The twenty teeth that begin to erupt around the age of six months. They are eventually pushed out by the permanent teeth.

Incisor: One of the four front cutting teeth in the adult.

Molar: One of three back teeth on each side of the jaw used for grinding.

Permanent teeth: The 32 permanent teeth begin to erupt at about the age of six and are generally complete by the age of 16.

See Figure 9.6 for a photo of dental X-rays.

MED TERM TIP

The combining term *dent/o* means *teeth.* Hence we have terms such as *dentist* and *dental* care. When the term *ortho*, which means *straight*, is combined with *dent/o*, we have the specialty of **orthodontics** (or thoh **DON** tiks), or straightening teeth.

The roof of the mouth is known as the **palate** (**PAL** at). The mouth contains both a hard or bony portion and a soft palate or flexible portion. The oral cavity is lined with mucous membrane.

PHARYNX

epiglottis   trachea

larynx

After food has left the mouth, it travels down the pharynx, or throat, into the esophagus. The **epiglottis** (ep ih **GLOT** is), a small piece of tissue at the back of the pharynx, covers the **larynx** (**LAIR** inks) and **trachea** (**TRAY** kee ah) so that food cannot enter the lungs. The pharynx carries the food down into the esophagus.

ESOPHAGUS

peristalsis

The esophagus is actually a thick-walled muscle that is about 10 inches long in most adults. It connects the pharynx with the stomach. The food is propelled along the esophagus by wavelike muscular movements called **peristalsis** (pair ih **STALL** sis).

STOMACH

antrum	emesis	pyloric sphincter
body	fundus	pyloric stenosis
cardiac sphincter	hydrochloric acid (HCl)	regurgitation
chyme	lower esophageal sphincter	rugae
duodenum	mucosa	sphincters

The stomach is a J-shaped muscular organ that acts as a bag or sac to collect, churn, digest, and store food. It is composed of three parts: the **fundus** (**FUN** dus) or upper region, the **body** or main portion, and the **antrum** (**AN** trum) or lower region (see Figure 9.7). The folds in the **mucosa** (myoo **KOH** sah) lining the stomach are called **rugae** (**ROO** gay). When the stomach is filled with food, the rugae disappear. **Hydrochloric** (high droh **KLOH** rik) **acid (HCl)** is secreted by glands in the mucous membrane lining of the stomach. Food mixes with HC1 and other gastric juices to form a semisoft mixture called **chyme** (**KIGHM**), which can then pass through the remaining portion of the digestive system.

The stomach contains muscular valves called **sphincters** (**SFINGK** ters) that control the flow of food in one direction only. The **cardiac sphincter** (**CAR** dee ak **SFINGK** ter), named after its location near the heart, is located at the distal or lower end of the esophagus. It is also called the **lower esophageal sphincter** (eh soff ah **JEE** al **SFINGK** ter) (LES). This valve keeps food from backing up into the esophagus, which is called **regurgitation** (ree gur jih **TAY** shun).

The **pyloric sphincter** (pigh **LOR** ik **SFINGK** ter) is located at the distal or lower end of the stomach and controls the passage of food into the **duodenum** (doo oh **DEE** num or doo **OD** eh num) of the small intestine. The pyloric sphincter keeps food in the stomach while it is being mixed with gastric juices that aid digestion.

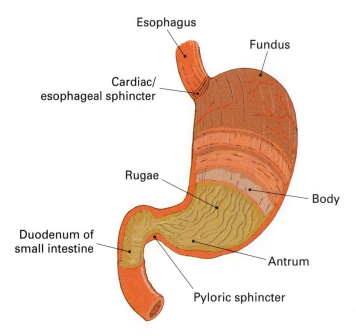

FIGURE 9.7 Stomach.

When the pyloric sphincter becomes abnormally narrow, a condition called **pyloric stenosis** (pigh **LOR** ik steh **NOH** sis) results in which food is unable to pass from the stomach to the small intestines. **Emesis** (**EM** eh sis) or vomiting is the main symptom. The pyloric sphincter is mentioned in surgical reports and patient reports. It is easier to remember when you note that *pylor/o* means *gatekeeper*. This gatekeeper helps food move forward.

SMALL INTESTINE

cecum	ileocecal valve	jejunoileostomy
Crohn's disease	ileostomy	jejunostomy
duodenum	ileum	jejunum

The small intestine, or small bowel, is considered to be the major organ of digestion and absorption of nutrients from food during the digestive process (see Figure 9.8). It is located between the pyloric sphincter and the large intestine. The small intestine contains an average of 20 feet of intestine, making it the longest portion of the alimentary canal. There are three sections to the small intestine.

- The **duodenum,** which extends from the pylorus of the stomach to the **jejunum** (jee **JOO** num), is about 10 to 12 inches long. Digestion is completed in the duodenum after the partly digested food mixes with digestive juices from the pancreas and gallbladder.

- The **jejunum** or middle portion extends from the middle of the small intestine to the **ileum** (**ILL** ee um) and is about 8 feet long.

- The **ileum** is the last portion of the small intestine and extends from the jejunum to the **cecum** (**SEE** kum) of the large intestine. At 12 feet in length, it is the longest portion of the small intestine. The ileum comes together with the large intestine at the **ileocecal** (ill ee oh **SEE** kal) **valve.**

FIGURE 9.8 Small intestine.

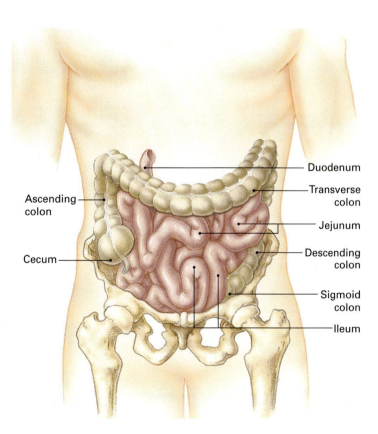

Ascending colon

Cecum

Duodenum

Transverse colon

Jejunum

Descending colon

Sigmoid colon

Ileum

MED
TERM
TIP

We can live without a portion of the small intestine. In cases of carcinoma or a condition such as **Crohn's disease** (**KROHNZ** dih **ZEEZ**), the entire intestine may have to be removed. An opening is created between the remaining intestine and the abdominal wall. This is called an **ileostomy** (ill ee **OSS** toh me) since it is an opening from the ileum (see Figure 9.9).

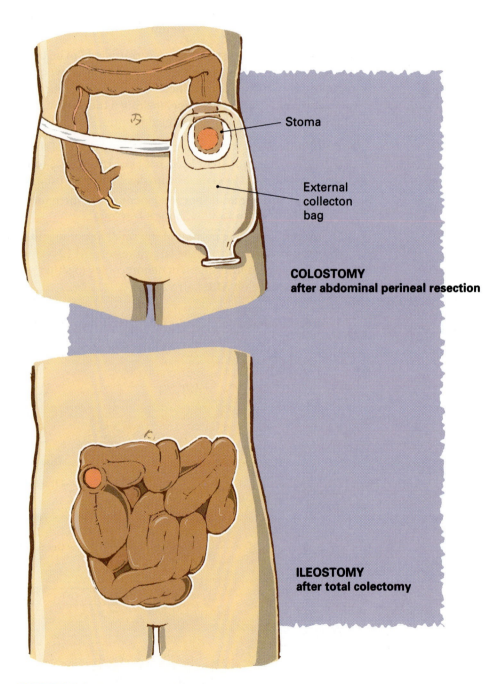

Stoma

External
collecton
bag

COLOSTOMY
after abdominal perineal resection

ILEOSTOMY
after total colectomy

FIGURE 9.9 Colostomy and ileostomy.

When you have an understanding of the location for the duodenum, jejunum, and ileum, it is then possible to decipher the terms relating to this area. For instance, the term **jejunostomy** (jee joo **NOSS** toh mee) indicates a surgical opening into the jejunum. When we build on that term and see the word **jejunoileostomy** (jee joo noh ill ee **OSS** toh mee), we know that it is creating an opening or passage between the jejunum and the ileum. If a patient is diagnosed with a duodenal ulcer, you will be able to picture where this lesion is located.

Since the small intestine is concerned with absorption of food products, an abnormality in this organ can cause malnutrition or a state of poor nutrition. Digestive secretions from the accessory organs enter the duodenum for final breakdown.

LARGE INTESTINE

anal sphincter	**cecum**	**feces**
anus	**colectomy**	**prophylactic**
appendicitis	**colon**	**rectum**
appendix	**colostomy**	**sigmoid colon**
ascending colon	**descending colon**	**transverse colon**

Fluid that remains as a result of the food breakdown in the small intestine enters the large intestine, which is also called the **colon** (**COH** lon) (see Figure 9.10).

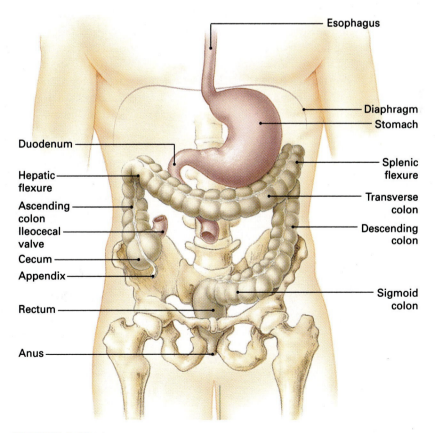

FIGURE 9.10 Large intestine.

MED TERM TIP

The term *colon* refers to the large intestine. However, you should be aware that many people use it as a general term referring to the entire intestinal system, both small and large intestines. This is incorrect.

Most of the fluid is absorbed and retained by the body. The material that remains after absorption is solid waste called feces. This is the product evacuated in bowel movements (BM).

The large intestine is approximately 5 feet long and extends from the ileocecal valve of the small intestine to the **anus** (**AY** nus). The **cecum** is a pouch or saclike area in the first 2 to 3 inches at the beginning of the large intestine. The **appendix** (ah **PEN** diks) is a small wormlike outgrowth at the end of the cecum.

MED TERM TIP

The appendix appears to have no function or purpose within the body. It can be thought of as an appendage. Unfortunately, it can cause a problem when it becomes inflamed and infected. **Appendicitis** (ah pen dih **SIGH** tis) most often occurs in young males between 15 and 25 years of age. Even if it is not infected, the appendix is frequently removed, with the consent of the patient, during other surgical procedures as a **prophylactic** (proh fih **LAK** tik) measure.

The colon consists of the **ascending** (ah **SEND** ing), **transverse** (trans **VERS**), **descending** (dee **SEND** ing), and **sigmoid colon** (**SIG** moyd **COH** lon). The ascending colon on the right side extends from the cecum to the lower border of the liver. The transverse colon begins where the ascending colon leaves off and moves horizontally across the upper abdomen toward the spleen. The descending colon then travels down the left side of the body where the sigmoid colon begins.

The sigmoid colon is connected above to the descending colon and below to the **rectum** (**REK** tum). The rectum is the area for storage of solid waste (feces). The rectum leads into the anus, which contains the **anal sphincter** (**AY** nal **SFINGK** ter). This sphincter is controlled by muscles that assist in the evacuation of feces.

MED TERM TIP

When the large intestine has to be removed due to a disease or disorder, it is called a **colectomy** (koh **LEK** toh mee). The surgeon will make an opening between the colon and the abdominal wall and create a **colostomy** (koh **LOSS** toh mee). This allows the bowel contents to empty into an appliance or bag worn on the outside of the body. Patients can lead active lives after receiving a colostomy (see Figure 9.9).

ACCESSORY ORGANS: SALIVARY GLANDS, LIVER, GALLBLADDER, AND PANCREAS

Salivary Glands

bolus	**sublingual glands**
parotid glands	**submandibular glands**

Salivary glands in the oral cavity produce a fluid that allows food to be swallowed with less danger of choking. When saliva mixes with food, a **bolus** (**BOH** lus) is formed,

FIGURE 9.11 Salivary glands.

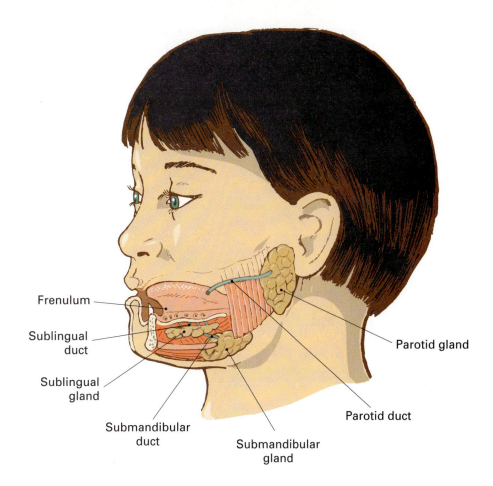

Frenulum

Sublingual duct

Sublingual gland

Submandibular duct

Submandibular gland

Parotid gland

Parotid duct

which is then ready to be swallowed. There are three pairs of salivary glands. The **parotid** (pah **ROT** id) **glands** are in front of the ears. The **submandibular** (sub man **DIB** yoo lar) **glands** and **sublingual** (sub **LING** gwal) **glands** are in the floor of the mouth (see Figure 9.11).

Liver

bile

This large organ, located in the right upper quadrant of the abdomen, processes the absorbed nutrients, aids in detoxifying harmful materials, and produces **bile** (**BYE** al) (see Figure 9.12).

MED TERM *TIP*

The liver weighs about four pounds and has so many important functions that people cannot live without it. It has become a major transplant organ.

Gallbladder

cholesterol (chol)   **gallstones**

common bile duct (CBD)

The bile produced by the liver is stored in the gallbladder (GB). Bile, necessary for the digestive process, is released into the duodenum through the **common bile duct (CBD)** (see also Figure 9.12). **Gallstones** form when the bile contains an excessive amount of **cholesterol** (koh **LES** ter all) **(chol).** The cholesterol then becomes compacted into gallstones (see Figure 9.13). There is a higher incidence of stone formation in women than in men, with obesity increasing the risk.

FIGURE 9.12 Gallbladder, liver, and pancreas.

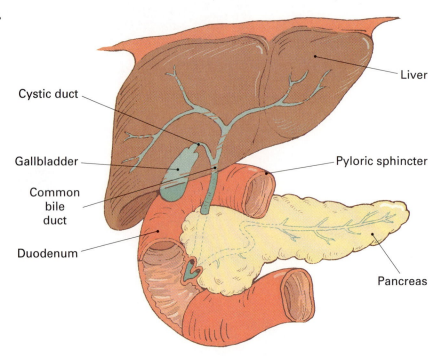

FIGURE 9.13 Common sites for cholelithiasis.

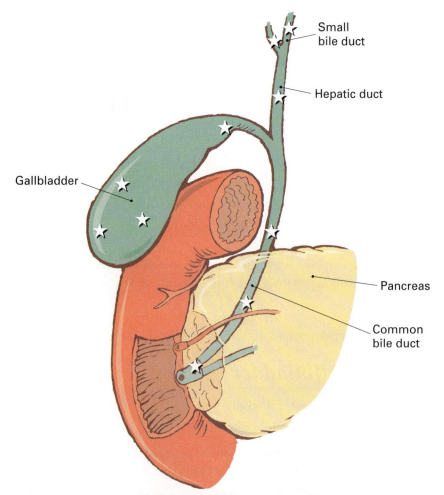

Pancreas

pancreatic enzymes

The pancreas produces **pancreatic enzymes** (pan kree **AT** ik **EN** zimes) that emulsify or break down food so it can be absorbed by the body (see also Figure 9.12). The pancreas is an endocrine gland that is studied more fully in Chapter 5.

Word Building Relating to the Digestive System

The following list contains examples of medical terms built directly from word parts. The definitions for these terms can be determined by a straightforward translation of the word parts.

Combining Form	Combined With	Medical Term	Definition
abdomin/o	-al	abdominal (ab **DOM** ih nal)	pertaining to the abdomen
	-plasty	abdominoplasty (ab dom ih noh **PLASS** tee)	surgical repair of the abdomen
appendic/o	-ectomy	appendectomy (ap en **DEK** toh mee)	excision of the appendix
	-itis	appendicitis (ah pen dih **SIGH** tis)	inflammation of the appendix
celi/o	-otomy	celiotomy (see lee **OTT** oh mee)	incision into the abdomen
cheil/o	-rrhaphy	cheilorrhaphy (kigh **LOR** ah fee)	suture the lip
chol/e	cyst/o -ectomy	cholecystectomy (koh lee sis **TEK** toh mee)	excision of the gallbladder
	cyst/o -gram	cholecystogram (koh lee **SIS** toh gram)	record of the gallbladder
	cyst/o -itis	cholecystitis (koh lee sis **TYE** tis)	inflammation of the gallbladder
	lith/o -iasis	cholelithiasis (koh lee lih **THIGH** ah sis)	abnormal condition of gallstones
col/o	-ectomy	colectomy (koh **LEK** toh mee)	excision of the colon
	-ostomy	colostomy (koh **LOSS** toh mee)	create an opening in the colon
colon/o	-scope	colonoscope (koh **LON** oh scope)	instrument to view colon
	-scopy	colonscopy (koh lon **OSS** koh pee)	procedure to view colon
dent/o	-al	dental (**DENT** al)	pertaining to teeth
diverticul/o	-itis	diverticulitis (dye ver tik yoo **LYE** tis)	inflammation of a blind pouch
	-osis	diverticulosis (Dye ver tik you **LOH** sis)	abnormal condition of having blind pouches
enter/o	-rrhaphy	enterorrhaphy (en ter **OR** ah fee)	suture small intestines
gastro/o	-dynia	gastrodynia (gas troh **DIN** ee ah)	stomach pain
	enter/o -itis	gastroenteritis (gas troh en ter **EYE** tis)	inflammation of stomach and small intestines
	enter/o -ologist	gastroenterologist (gas troh en ter **ALL** oh jist)	specialist in the stomach and small intestines (digestive system)
	enter/o -ology	gastroenterology (gas troh en ter **ALL** oh jee)	study of the stomach and small intestines (digestive system)
	-malacia	gastromalacia (gas troh mah **LAY** she ah)	softening of the stomach
	nas/o -ic	nasogastric (nay zoh **GAS** trik)	pertaining to the nose and stomach
	-ostomy	gastrostomy (gas **TROSS** toh mee)	create an opening in the stomach
	-scope	gastroscope (**GAS** troh scope)	instrument to view inside the stomach

(continued)

Combining Form	Combined With	Medical Term	Definition
gingiv/o	-ectomy	gingivectomy (jim gih **VEK** toh mee)	excision of the gums
	-itis	gingivitis (jin jih **VIGH** tis)	inflammation of the gums
hepat/o	-itis	hepatitis (hep ah **TYE** tis)	inflammation of the liver
	-oma	hepatoma (hep ah **TOH** mah)	liver tumor
herni/o	-rrhaphy	herniorrhaphy (hern nee **OR** ah fee)	suture a hernia
lapar/o	-otomy	laparotomy (lap ah **ROT** oh mee)	incision into the abdomen
	-scope	laparoscope (**LAP** ah roh scope)	instrument to view inside the abdomen
	-scopy	laparoscopy (lap ar **OSS** koh pee)	procedure to view the abdomen
lingu/o	sub- -al	sublingual (sub **LING** gwal)	pertaining to under the tongue
odont/o	orth/o tic	orthodontic (or thoh **DON** tik)	pertaining to straight teeth
or/o	-al	oral (**OR** ral)	pertaining to the mouth
pancreat/o	-itis	pancreatitis (pan kree ah **TYE** tis)	inflammation of the pancreas
polyp/o	-osis	polyposis (pall ee **POH** sis)	abnormal condition of polyps
proct/o	-ptosis	proctoptosis (prok top **TOH** sis)	drooping rectum
	-scopy	proctoscopy (prok **TOSS** koh pee)	procedure to view the rectum
sial/o	-lith	sialolith (sigh **AL** oh lith)	salivary (gland) stone
sigmoid/o	-scope	sigmoidoscope (sig **MOYD** oh scope)	instrument to view inside the sigmoid colon

Prefix	Suffix	Medical Term	Definition
a-	-phagia	aphagia (ah **FAY** jee ah)	not eating
brady-	-pepsia	bradypepsia (brad ee **PEP** see ah)	slow digestion
dys-		dyspepsia (dis **PEP** see ah)	difficult digestion
dys-		dysphagia (dis **FAY** jee ah)	difficulty eating
poly-		polyphagia (pall ee **FAY** jee ah)	many (excessive) eating

Vocabulary Relating to the Digestive System

ascites (ah SIGH teez)	Collection or accumulation of fluid in the peritoneal cavity.
bridge	Dental appliance that is attached to adjacent teeth for support to replace missing teeth.
caries (KAIR eez)	Gradual decay and disintegration of teeth that can result in inflamed tissue and abscessed teeth.
constipation (kon stih PAY shun)	Experiencing difficulty in defecation or infrequent defecation.
crown	Portion of a tooth that is covered by enamel. Also an artificial covering for the tooth created to replace the original enamel.
deciduous (dee SID yoo us) teeth	The twenty teeth that begin to erupt around the age of six months. Eventually pushed out by the permanent teeth.
dentist (DEN tist)	Person who is authorized, based on education, training, and licensure, to practice dentistry.
denture (DEN chur)	Partial or complete set of artificial teeth that are set in plastic materials. Act as a substitute for the natural teeth and related structures.

diarrhea (dye ah REE ah)	Passing of frequent, watery bowel movements. Usually accompanies gastrointestinal (GI) disorders.
dyspepsia (dis PEP ses ah)	Indigestion.
emesis (EM eh sis)	Vomiting, usually with some force.
fistula (FIH styoo lah)	Abnormal tubelike passage from one body cavity to another.
gastroenterologist (gas troh en ter **ALL oh jist)**	A physician specialized in treating diseases and conditions of the gastrointestinal tract.
gastroenterology (gas troh en ter **ALL oh jee)**	The study of diseases of the gastrointestinal tract.
halitosis (hal ih TOH sis)	Bad or offensive breath, which can often be a sign of disease.
hematemesis (hee mah **TEM** eh sis)	To vomit blood from the gastrointestinal tract, often looks like coffee grounds.
implant (IM plant)	Prosthetic device placed in the jaw to which a tooth or denture may be anchored.
jaundice (JAWN diss)	Yellow cast to the skin, mucous membranes, and the whites of the eyes caused by the deposit of bile pigment from too much *bilirubin* in the blood. Bilirubin is a waste product produced when worn-out red blood cells are broken down. May be a symptom of a disorder such as gallstones blocking the common bile duct or carcinoma of the liver.
oral surgeon	Dentist specializing in surgical treatment of the teeth and surrounding tissues.
orthodontist (or thoh **DON** tist)	Dentist who is an expert in orthodontia, which is straightening teeth.
permanent teeth	The thirty-two permanent teeth begin to erupt at about the age of six. Generally complete by the age of sixteen.
plaque (PLAK)	Gummy mass of microorganisms that grows on the crowns of teeth and spreads along the roots. It is colorless and transparent.
polyphagia (pall ee **FAY** jee ah)	To eat excessively.
postprandial (post **PRAN** dee al)	Pertaining to after a meal.
prophylactic (proh fih **LAK** tik) **measure**	Procedure performed to prevent something else from happening. For example, even if the appendix is normal, it is sometimes removed during abdominal operations to prevent a future attack of appendicitis.
regurgitation (ree gur jih **TAY** shun)	Return of fluids and solids from the stomach into the mouth. Similar to *emesis* but without the force.

MED TERM *Tip*

Our teeth are as unique to us as our fingerprints. The field of **forensic dentistry** (foh **REN** zik **DEN** tis tree) assists in identifying unknown deceased persons by their teeth.

abscess (AB sess)	Swelling of soft tissues of the jaw as a result of infection.
anorexia (an oh REK see ah)	Loss of appetite that can accompany other conditions such as a gastrointestinal (GI) upset (see Figure 9.14).
bulimia (boo LIM ee ah)	Eating disorder that is characterized by recurrent binge eating and then purging of the food with laxatives and vomiting.
cholecystitis (koh lee sis TYE tis)	Inflammation of the gallbladder.
cholelithiasis (koh lee lih THIGH ah sis)	Formation or presence of stones or calculi in the gallbladder or common bile duct (see Figure 9.15).
cirrhosis (sih ROH sis)	Chronic disease of the liver.
cleft (CLEFT) lip	Congenital anomaly in which the upper lip fails to come together. Often seen along with a cleft palate. Corrected with surgery.
cleft palate (CLEFT PAL at)	Congenital anomaly in which the roof of the mouth has a split or fissure. Corrected with surgery.
Crohn's disease (KROHNZ dih ZEEZ)	Form of chronic inflammatory bowel disease affecting the ileum and/or colon. Also called *regional ileitis*. Named for Burrill Crohn, an American gastroenterologist.
diverticulitis (dye ver tik yoo LYE tis)	Inflammation of a diverticulum or sac in the intestinal tract, especially in the colon (see Figure 9.16).
enteritis (en ter EYE tis)	Inflammation of only the small intestine.
esophageal stricture (eh soff ah JEE al STRIK chur)	Narrowing of the esophagus that makes the flow of fluids and food difficult.
esophageal varices (eh soff ah JEE al VAIR ih seez)	Enlarged and swollen veins in the lower end of the esophagus; they can rupture and result in serious hemorrhage.
fissure (FISH er)	Cracklike split in the rectum or anal canal.
gastritis (gas TRY tis)	Inflammation of the stomach that can result in pain, tenderness, nausea, and vomiting.
gastroenteritis (gas troh en ter EYE tis)	Inflammation of the stomach and small intestines.
gingivitis (jin jih VIGH tis)	Inflammation of the gums that is characterized by swelling, redness, and a tendency to bleed.
gum disease	Inflammation of the gums, leading to tooth loss, which is generally due to poor dental hygiene.
hemorrhoids (HEM oh roydz)	Varicose veins in the rectum.
hepatitis (hep ah TYE tis)	Inflammation of the liver.

(continued)

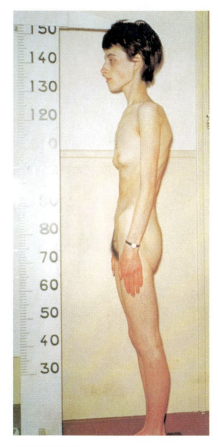

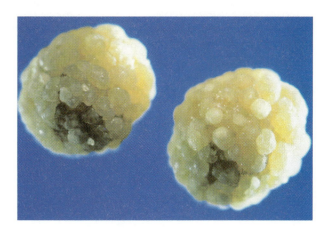

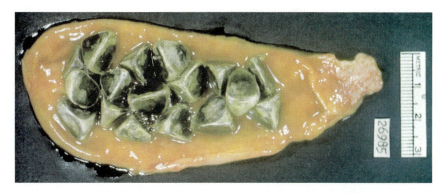

FIGURE 9.14 Anorexia in young woman. (CNRI/Phototake NYC)

FIGURE 9.15 Gallbladder with gallstones. (Martin Rotker/Phototake NYC)

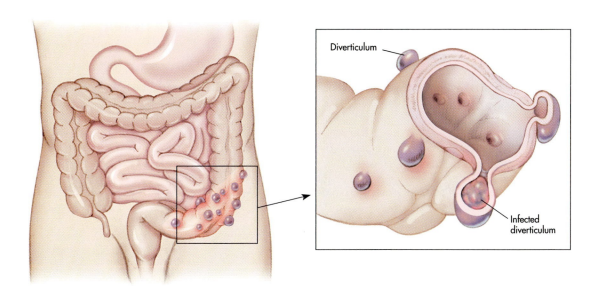

Diverticulum

Infected diverticulum

FIGURE 9.16 Diverticulitis.

hiatal hernia (high AY tal HER nee ah)	Protrusion of the stomach through the diaphragm and extending into the thoracic cavity; reflux esophagitis is a common symptom.
ileitis (ill ee EYE tis)	Inflammation of the ileum.
impacted (im PAK ted) **wisdom tooth**	Wisdom tooth that is tightly wedged into the jaw bone so that it is unable to erupt (see Figure 9.17).
inflammatory bowel disease (IBD) (in FLAM ah tor ee BOW el dih ZEEZ)	Ulceration of the mucous membranes of the colon of unknown origin. Also known as *ulcerative colitis*.
inguinal hernia (ING gwi nal HER nee ah)	Hernia or outpouching of intestines into the inguinal region of the body (see Figure 9.18).
intussusception (in tuh suh SEP shun)	Result of the intestine slipping or telescoping into another section of intestine just below it. More common in children (see Figure 9.19).
irritable bowel syndrome (IBS) (EAR it ah b'l BOW el SIN drohm)	Disturbance in the functions of the intestine from unknown causes. Symptoms generally include abdominal discomfort and an alteration in bowel activity.
malabsorption syndrome (mal ab SORP shun SIN drohm)	Inadequate absorption of nutrients from the intestinal tract. May be caused by a variety of diseases and disorders, such as infections and pancreatic deficiency.
peptic ulcer (PEP tik ULL sir)	Ulcer occurring in the lower portion of the esophagus, stomach, and duodenum thought to be caused by the acid of gastric juices (see Figure 9.20).
periodontal disease (pair ee oh DON tal dih ZEEZ)	Disease of the supporting structures of the teeth, including the gums and bones.
pilonidal cyst (pye loh NYE dal SIST)	Cyst in the sacrococcygeal region due to tissue being trapped below the skin.
polyposis (pall ee POH sis)	Small tumors that contain a pedicle or footlike attachment in the mucous membranes of the large intestine (colon).
pyorrhea (pye oh REE ah)	Discharge of purulent material from dental tissue.
reflux esophagitis (REE fluks eh soff ah JIGH tis)	Acid from the stomach backs up into the esophagus causing inflammation and pain.
ulcerative colitis (ULL sir ah tiv koh LYE tis)	Ulceration of the mucous membranes of the colon of unknown origin. Also known as *inflammatory bowel disease (IBD)*.
volvulus (VOL vyoo lus)	Condition in which the bowel twists upon itself and causes an obstruction. Painful and requires immediate surgery.

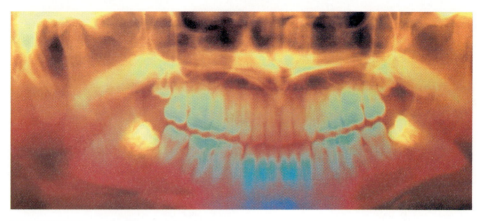

FIGURE 9.17 Enhanced color X-ray showing impacted wisdom teeth highlighted in yellow. (Science Photo Library/Photo Researchers, Inc.)

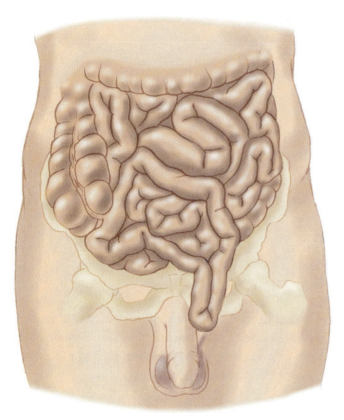

FIGURE 9.18 Inguinal hernia.

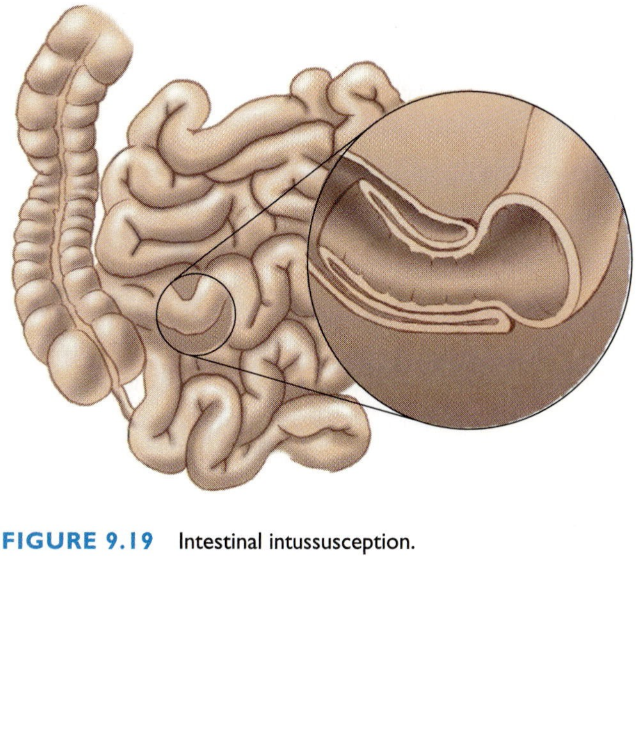

FIGURE 9.19 Intestinal intussusception.

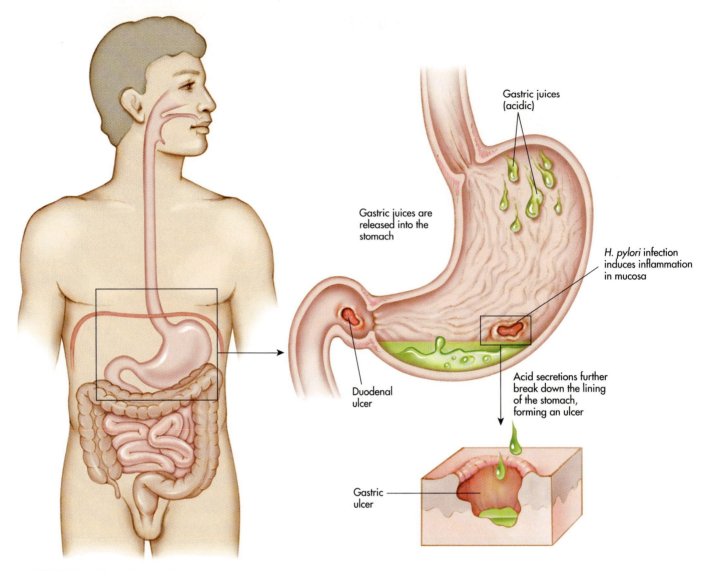

FIGURE 9.20 Peptic ulcer disease (PUD).

MED TERM TIP

Today one of the most valuable means of determining stomach and intestinal disorders is through the introduction of the **endoscope** (**EN** doh scope). The use of this viewing instrument means that physicians can now examine internal organs, such as the esophagus, stomach, and colon, without having the patient undergo surgery.

Diagnostic Procedures Relating to the Digestive System

abdominal ultrasonography (ab **DOM** ih nal ull trah sun **OG** rah fee)	Using ultrasound equipment for producing sound waves to create an image of the abdominal organs.
air contrast barium enema (**BAH** ree um **EN** eh mah)	Using both barium and air to visualize the colon.
barium enema (**BE, lower GI series**) (bah ree um **EN** eh mah)	Radiographic examination of the small intestine, large intestine, or colon in which an enema containing barium (Ba) is administered to the patient while the X-ray pictures are taken (see Figure 9.21).

barium swallow (upper GI series) (BAH ree um)	A barium (Ba) mixture swallowed while X-ray pictures are taken of the esophagus, stomach, and duodenum used to visualize the upper gastrointestinal tract (upper GI) (see Figure 9.22).
bite-wing X-ray	X-ray taken with a part of the film holder held between the teeth and parallel to the teeth.
cholecystogram (koh lee SIS toh gram)	Dye given orally to the patient is absorbed and enters the gallbladder. An X-ray is then taken.
colonoscopy (koh lon OSS koh pee)	A flexible fiberscope passed through the anus, rectum, and colon is used to examine the upper portion of the colon. Polyps and small growths can be removed during this procedure (see Figure 9.23).
endoscopic retrograde cholangiopancreatography (ERCP) (en doh SKOP ik RET roh grayd koh lan jee oh pan kree ah TOG rah fee)	Using an endoscope to X-ray the bile and pancreatic ducts.
endoscopy (en DOSS koh pee)	A general term for a procedure to visually examine the inside of a body cavity or a hollow organ using an instrument called an endoscope. Specific examples of endoscopy relating to the digestive system include colonoscopy, esophagoscopy, gastrointestinal endoscopy, and gastroscopy.
esophagoscopy and biopsy (eh soff ah GOS koh pee and BYE op see)	The esophagus is visualized by passing an instrument down the esophagus. A tissue sample for biopsy may be taken.
gastrointestinal endoscopy (gas troh in TESS tih nal en DOSS koh pee)	A flexible instrument or scope is passed either through the mouth or anus to facilitate visualization of the gastrointestinal (GI) tract.
intravenous cholangiogram (IVC) (in trah VEE nus koh LAN jee oh gram)	A dye is administered intravenously to the patient that allows for X-ray visualization of the bile vessels.
intravenous cholecystography (in trah VEE nus koh lee sis TOG rah fee)	A dye is administered intravenously to the patient that allows for X-ray visualization of the gallbladder.
laparoscopy (lap ar OSS koh pee)	An instrument or scope is passed into the abdominal wall through a small incision. The abdominal cavity is then examined for tumors and other conditions with this lighted instrument. Also called *peritoneoscopy*.
liver biopsy (LIV er BYE op see)	Excision of a small piece of liver tissue for microscopic examination. Generally used to determine if cancer is present.
liver (LIV er) scan	A radioactive substance is administered to the patient by an intravenous (IV) route. This substance enters the liver cells, and this organ can then be visualized. This is used to detect tumors, abscesses, and other pathologies that result in hepatomegaly (an enlarged liver).
occult (uh CULT) blood test	Self-administered test on the feces to determine if blood is present.
oral cholecystography (OR al kohlee sis TOG rah fee)	The patient swallows a radiopaque dye so X-ray pictures can be taken that allow visualization of the gallbladder and its components.
ova and parasites (OH vah and PAR ah sights)	Laboratory examination of feces with a microscope for the presence of parasites or their eggs.
percutaneous transhepatic cholangiography (PTC) (per kyoo TAY nee us trans heh PAT ik koh lan jee OG rah fee)	A contrast medium is injected directly into the liver to visualize the bile ducts. Used to detect obstructions.
proctoscopy (prok TOSS koh pee)	Examination of the anus and rectum with an endoscope inserted through the rectum.
spleen scan	A radioactive material injected into the patient through an intravenous (IV) route enters the spleen for visualization of this organ. Used to detect tumors, cysts, abscesses, and other splenomegaly.
upper gastrointestinal (gas troh in TESS tih nal) (UGI) series	Administering a barium contrast material orally and then taking an X-ray to visualize the esophagus, stomach, and duodenum.

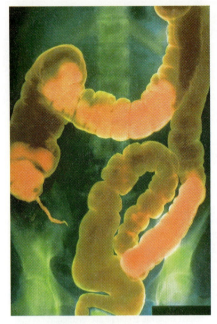

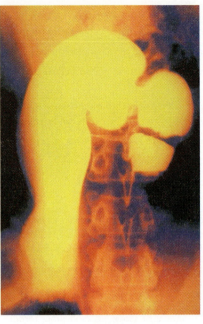

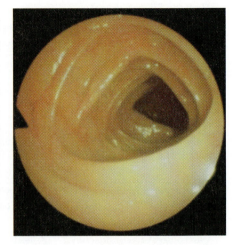

FIGURE 9.21 Enhanced color X-ray of large and small intestine during barium enema exam. (CNRI/Science Photo Library/Photo Researchers, Inc.)

FIGURE 9.22 Enhanced color X-ray of barium enema swallow.

FIGURE 9.23 Colonoscopy examination of the transverse colon. (CNRI/Science Photo Library/Photo Researchers, Inc.)

Treatment Procedures Relating to the Digestive System

anastomosis (ah nas toh **MOH** sis)	Creating a passageway or opening between two organs or vessels.
appendectomy (ap en **DEK** toh me)	Surgical removal of the appendix.
cholecystectomy (koh lee sis **TEK** toh mee)	Surgical excision of the gallbladder. Removal of the gallbladder through the laparoscope is a newer procedure with fewer complications than the more invasive abdominal surgery. The laparoscope requires a small incision into the abdominal cavity (see Figure 9.24).
choledocholithotomy (koh led uh koh lih **THOT** oh mee)	Removal of a gallstone through an incision into the bile duct.
choledocholithotripsy (koh led oh koh **LITH** oh trip see)	Crushing of a gallstone in the common bile duct.
colectomy (koh **LEK** toh mee)	Surgical removal of the colon.
colostomy (koh **LOSS** toh mee)	Surgical creation of an opening of some portion of the colon through the abdominal wall to the outside surface. The fecal material (stool) drains into a bag worn on the abdomen.
diverticulectomy (dye ver tik yoo **LEK** toh mee)	Surgical removal of a diverticulum.
esophagogastrostomy (eh soff ah goh gas **TROS** toh mee)	Surgical creation of an opening between the esophagus and the stomach.
esophagostomy (eh soff ah **GOS** toh mee)	Surgical creation of an opening into the esophagus.
exploratory laparotomy (ek **SPLOR** ah tor ee lap ah **ROT** oh mee)	Abdominal operation for the purpose of examining the abdominal organs and tissues for signs of disease or other abnormalities.

fistulectomy (fis tyoo **LEK** toh mee)	Excision of a fistula.
gastrectomy (gas **TREK** toh mee)	Surgical removal of a part or the whole of the stomach.
gastrostomy (gas **TROSS** toh mee)	Surgical creation of a gastric fistula or opening through the abdominal wall. The opening is used to place food into the stomach when the esophagus is not entirely open (esophageal stricture).
glossectomy (glos **SEK** toh mee)	Complete or partial removal of the tongue.
hemorrhoidectomy (hem oh royd **EK** toh mee)	Surgical excision of hemorrhoids from the anorectal area.
hepatic lobectomy (heh **PAT** ik loh **BEK** toh mee)	Surgical removal of a lobe of the liver.
ileostomy (ill ee **OSS** toh mee)	Surgical creation of a passage through the abdominal wall into the ileum.
jejunoileostomy (jee joo noh ill ee **OSS** toh mee)	Formation of a passage between the jejunum and the ileum.
jejunostomy (jee joo **NOSS** toh mee)	Surgical creation of a permanent opening into the jejunum.
lithotripsy (**LITH** oh trip see)	Crushing of a stone.
proctoplasty (**PROK** toh plas tee)	Plastic surgery of the anus and rectum.
root canal	Dental treatment involving the pulp cavity of the root of a tooth. Procedure is used to save a tooth that is badly infected or abscessed.
splenectomy (splee **NEK** toh mee)	Surgical removal of the spleen.
vagotomy (vah **GOT** oh mee)	Surgical resection of the vagus nerve in an attempt to decrease the amount of acid secretion into the stomach. Used as a method of treatment for ulcer patients.

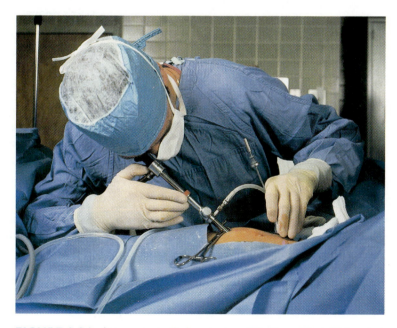

FIGURE 9.24 Laparoscopic cholecystectomy. (Southern Illinois University/ Photo Researchers, Inc.)

Dental Care

Dental care workers provide care for patients' teeth and gums. Their services include treating tooth and gum disease; fabricating and fitting crowns, bridges, and dentures; providing preventative care such as teeth cleaning and polishing; and educating the public in good oral hygiene practices. Dental care workers are found in private offices, hospital dental departments, health maintenance organizations, clinics, and public health facilities.

Dental Assistants

Dental assistants provide care for the patient's teeth and gums in conjunction with the dentist. They are responsible for maintaining and sterilizing the dental instruments, preparing the materials used in fabricating crowns, bridges, and dentures; and taking and developing X-rays. Dental assistants may also be in charge of the day-to-day operation of the dental office. They may make appointments, handle insurance claims, and maintain patients' records. Job opportunities for dental assistants can be found in private offices, hospital dental departments, clinics, and public health facilities. To become dental assistants, students must complete on-the-job-training, or a community college or vocational training program. The dental assistant then has the option of completing a certification examination administered by the Certifying Board of the Dental Assisting National Board. For more information regarding a career in dental assisting, visit the American Dental Association's web site at www.ada.org.

Dentist (DDS or DMD)

- **Completes prerequisites for dental school at a four-year college or university**
- **Graduates from an accredited four-year dental college**

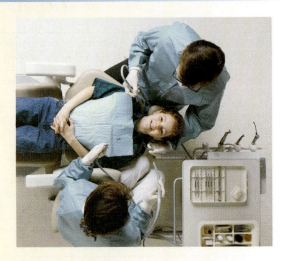

- **Receives either a Doctor of Dental Surgery (DDS) or Doctor of Dental Medicine (DMD) degree**
- **Licensed by the state of employment after passing the National Board of Dentistry examination**

Dental Hygienist

- **Works under the supervision of a dentist**
- **Specializes in cleaning teeth and taking X-rays**
- **Graduates from an accredited dental hygiene program with a two-year associate, a four-year bachelor's, or a five-year master's degree**
- **Licensed by the state of employment after passing a national examination**

Dental Laboratory Technician

- **Specialist in fabricating dental prosthetics such as crowns, bridges, and dentures as prescribed by a dentist**
- **Completes a two-year vocational program or receives three to four years of on-the-job training**
- **May choose to become certified by passing a national examination**

Abbreviations Relating to the Digestive System

Ba	barium	IBD	inflammatory bowel disease
BE	barium enema	IBS	irritable bowel syndrome
BM	bowel movement	IV	intravenous
BS	bowel sounds	IVC	intravenous cholangiogram
CBD	common bile duct	n&v	nausea and vomiting
CHO	carbohydrate	NG	nasogastric (tube)
chol	cholesterol	NPO	nothing by mouth
CUC	chronic ulcerative colitis	O&P	ova and parasites
E. coli	*Escherichia coli*	OCG	oral cholecystography
EGD	esophagogastroduodenoscopy	PEG	percutaneous endoscopic gastrostomy
ERCP	endoscopic retrograde cholangiopancreatography	P.O.	per os (by mouth)
GB	gallbladder	PP	postprandial (after meals)
GI	gastrointestinal	PTC	percutaneous transhepatic cholangiography
HAA	hepatitis-associated antigen	RDA	recommended daily allowance (dietary allowance)
HAV	hepatitis A virus		
HBIG	hepatitis B immune globulin	SBFT	small bowel follow-through
HBV	hepatitis B virus	TPN	total parenteral nutrition
HCV	hepatitis C virus	UGI	upper gastrointestinal (X-ray) series

KEY TERMS

- abdominal (ab **DOM** ih nal)
- abdominal ultrasonography
  (ab **DOM** ih nal ull trah sun **OG** rah fee)
- abdominoplasty (ab dom ih noh **PLASS** tee)
- abscess (**AB** sess)
- accessory organs
- air contrast barium enema
  (**BAH** ree um **EN** eh mah)
- alimentary canal (al ih **MEN** tar ree can **NAL**)
- anal sphincter (**AY** nal **SFINGK** ter)
- anastomosis (ah nas toh **MOH** sis)
- anorexia (an oh **REK** see ah)
- antrum (**AN** trum)
- anus (**AY** nus)
- aphagia (ah **FAY** jee ah)
- appendectomy (ap en **DEK** toh mee)
- appendicitis (ah pen dih **SIGH** tis)
- appendix (ah **PEN** diks)
- ascending colon (ah **SEND** ing **COH** lon)
- ascites (ah **SIGH** teez)
- bacterium (bak **TEE** ree um)
- barium enema (BE) (**BAH** ree um **EN** eh mah)
- barium swallow (**BAH** ree um)
- bicuspids (bye **CUSS** pids)
- bile (**BYE** al)
- bite-wing X-ray
- body
- bolus (**BOH** lus)
- bradypepsia (brad ee **PEP** see ah)
- bridge
- bulimia (boo **LIM** ee ah)
- canines (**KAY** nines)
- cardiac sphincter (**CAR** dee ak **SFINGK** ter)
- caries (**KAIR** eez)
- cecum (**SEE** kum)
- celiotomy (see lee **OT** oh mee)
- cheilorrhaphy (kigh **LOR** ah fee)
- cholecystectomy (koh lee sis **TEK** toh mee)

- cholecystitis (koh lee sis **TYE** tis)
- cholecystogram (koh lee **SIS** toh gram)
- choledocholithotomy
  (koh led uh koh lih **THOT** oh mee)
- choledocholithotripsy
  (koh led oh koh **LITH** oh trip see)
- cholelithiasis (koh lee lih **THIGH** ah sis)
- cholesterol (koh **LES** ter all)
- chyme (**KIGHM**)
- cirrhosis (sih **ROH** sis)
- cleft lip (**CLEFT**)
- cleft palate (**CLEFT PAL** at)
- colectomy (koh **LEK** toh mee)
- colon (**COH** lon)
- colonoscope (koh **LON** oh scope)
- colonoscopy (koh lon **OSS** koh pee)
- colostomy (koh **LOSS** toh mee)
- common bile duct
- constipation (kon stih **PAY** shun)
- Crohn's disease (**KROHNZ** dih **ZEEZ**)
- crown
- cuspids (**CUSS** pids)
- deciduous teeth (dee **SID** yoo us)
- dental (**DEN** tal)
- dentin (**DEN** tin)
- dentist (**DEN** tist)
- denture (**DEN** chur)
- descending colon (dee **SEND** ing **COH** lon)
- diarrhea (dye ah **REE** ah)
- diverticulectomy (dye ver tik yoo **LEK** toh mee)
- diverticulitis (dye ver tik yoo **LYE** tis)
- diverticulosis (dye ver tik yoo **LOH** sis)
- duodenum (doo oh **DEE** num or doo **OD** eh num)
- dyspepsia (dis **PEP** see ah)
- dysphagia (dis **FAY** jee ah)
- emesis (**EM** eh sis)
- enamel (en **AM** el)
- endoscope (**EN** doh scope)
- endoscopic retrograde cholangiopancreatography
  (ERCP) (en doh **SKOP** ik **RET** roh grayd koh lan
  jee oh pan kree ah **TOG** rah fee)
- endoscopy (en **DOSS** koh pee)
- enteritis (en ter **EYE** tis)
- enterorrhaphy (en ter **OR** rah fee)
- epiglottis (ep ih **GLOT** iss)
- esophageal stricture
  (eh soff ah **JEE** al **STRIK** chur)
- esophageal varices
  (eh soff ah **JEE** al **VAIR** ih seez)
- esophagogastrostomy
  (eh soff ah goh gas **TROS** toh mee)

- esophagoscopy and biopsy
  (eh soff ah **GOS** koh pee and **BYE** op see)
- esophagostomy (eh soff ah **GOS** toh mee)
- esophagus (eh **SOFF** ah gus)
- exploratory laparotomy
  (ek **SPLOR** ah tor ee lap ah **ROT** oh mee)
- feces (**FEE** seez)
- fissure (**FISH** er)
- fistula (**FIH** styoo lah)
- fistulectomy (fis tyoo **LEK** toh mee)
- forensic dentistry (foh **REN** zik **DEN** tis tree)
- fundus (**FUN** dus)
- gallbladder (**GALL** blad er)
- gallstones
- gastrectomy (gas **TREK** toh mee)
- gastritis (gas **TRY** tis)
- gastrodynia (gas troh **DIN** ee ah)
- gastroenteritis (gas troh en ter **EYE** tis)
- gastroenterologist
  (gas troh en ter **ALL** oh jist)
- gastroenterology (gas troh en ter **ALL** oh jee)
- gastrointestinal endoscopy
  (gas troh in **TESS** tih nal en **DOSS** koh pee)
- gastromalacia (gas troh mah **LAY** she ah)
- gastroscope (**GAS** troh scope)
- gastrostomy (gas **TROSS** toh mee)
- gingivectomy (jin gih **VEK** toh mee)
- gingivitis (jin jih **VIGH** tis)
- glossectomy (glos **SEK** toh mee)
- gum disease
- halitosis (hal ih **TOH** sis)
- hematemesis (hee mah **TEM** eh sis)
- hemorrhoidectomy (hem oh royd **EK** toh mee)
- hemorrhoids (**HEM** oh roydz)
- hepatic lobectomy
  (heh **PAT** tik loh **BEK** toh mee)
- hepatitis (hep ah **TYE** tis)
- hepatoma (hep ah **TOH** mah)
- herniorrhaphy (her nee **OR** ah fee)
- hiatal hernia (high **AY** tal **HER** nee ah)
- hydrochloric acid (HCl) (high droh **KLOH** rik)
- ileitis (ill ee **EYE** tis)
- ileocecal valve (ill ee oh **SEE** kal)
- ileostomy (ill ee **OSS** toh mee)
- ileum (**ILL** ee um)
- impacted wisdom tooth (im **PAK** ted)
- implant (**IM** plant)
- incisors (in **SIGH** zors)
- inflammatory bowel disease (IBD)
  (in **FLAM** ah tor ee **BOW** el dih **ZEEZ**)
- inguinal hernia (**ING** gwih nal **HER** nee ah)

- intravenous cholangiogram (IVC)
  (in trah **VEE** nus koh **LAN** jee oh gram)
- intravenous cholecystography
  (in trah **VEE** nus koh lee sis **TOG** rah fee)
- intussusception (in tuh suh **SEP** shun)
- irritable bowel syndrome (IBS)
  (**EAR** it ah b'l **BOW** el **SIN** drohm)
- jaundice (**JAWN** diss)
- jejunoileostomy (jee joo noh ill ee **OSS** toh mee)
- jejunostomy (jee joo **NOSS** toh mee)
- jejunum (jee **JOO** num)
- laparoscope (**LAP** ah roh scope)
- laparoscopy (lap ar **OSS** koh pe)
- laparotomy (lap ah **ROT** oh mee)
- larynx (**LAIR** inks)
- lithotripsy (**LITH** oh trip see)
- liver (**LIV** er)
- liver biopsy (**LIV** er **BYE** op see)
- liver scan (**LIV** er)
- lower esophageal sphincter (LES)
  (eh soff ah **JEE** al **SFINGK** ter)
- malabsorption syndrome
  (mal ab **SORP** shun **SIN** drohm)
- molars (**MOH** lars)
- mouth
- mucosa (myoo **KOH** sah)
- nasogastric (nay zoh **GAS** trik)
- occult blood test (uh **CULT**)
- oral (**OR** al)
- oral cholecystography
  (**OR** al koh lee sis **TOG** rah fee)
- oral surgeon
- orthodontics (or thoh **DON** tiks)
- orthodontist (or thoh **DON** tist)
- ova and parasites (**OH** vah and **PAR** ah sights)
- palate (**PAL** at)
- pancreas (**PAN** kree ass)
- pancreatic enzymes (pan kree **AT** ik **EN** zimes)
- pancreatitis (pan kree ah **TYE** tis)
- papillae (pah **PILL** ay)
- parotid glands (pah **ROT** id)
- peptic ulcers (**PEP** tik **ULL** sirs)
- percutaneous transhepatic cholangiography (PTC)
  (per kyoo **TAY** nee us rans heh **PAT** ik koh lan jee
  OG rah fee)
- periodontal disease
  (pair ee oh **DON** tal dih **ZEEZ**)
- peristalsis (pair ih **STALL** sis)
- permanent teeth
- pharynx (**FAIR** inks)
- pilonidal cyst (pye loh **NYE** dal **SIST**)
- plaque (**PLAK**)
- polyphagia (pall ee **FAY** jee ah)
- polyposis (pall ee **POH** sis)
- postprandial (post **PRAN** dee al)
- premolar (pree **MOH** lar)
- proctoplasty (**PROK** toh plas tee)
- proctoptosis (prok top **TOH** sis)
- proctoscopy (prok **TOSS** koh pee)
- prophylactic (proh fih **LAK** tik)
- pyloric sphincter (pigh **LOR** ik **SFINGK** ter)
- pyloric stenosis (pigh **LOR** ik steh **NOH** sis)
- pyorrhea (pye oh **REE** ah)
- rectum (**REK** tum)
- reflux esophagitis
  (**REE** fluks eh soff ah **JIGH** tis)
- regurgitation (ree gur jih **TAY** shun)
- root canal
- rugae (**ROO** gay)
- salivary glands (**SAL** ih vair ee)
- sialolith (sigh **AL** oh lith)
- sigmoid colon (**SIG** moyd **COH** lon)
- sigmoidoscope (sig **MOYD** oh scope)
- small intestine
- sphincters (**SFINGK** ters)
- spleen scan
- splenectomy (splee **NEK** toh mee)
- stomach (**STUM** ak)
- sublingual (sub **LING** gwal)
- sublingual glands (sub **LING** gwal)
- submandibular glands
  (sub man **DIB** yoo lar)
- tongue
- trachea (**TRAY** kee ah)
- transverse colon (trans **VERS COH** lon)
- ulcerative colitis (**ULL** sir ah tiv koh **LYE** tis)
- upper gastrointestinal series (UGI)
  (gas troh in **TESS** tih nal)
- vagotomy (vah **GOT** oh mee)
- volvulus (**VOL** vyoo lus)

Case Study

GASTROENTEROLOGY CONSULTATION REPORT

Reason for Consultation: Evaluation of recurrent epigastric and LUQ pain with anemia.

History of Present Illness: Patient is a 56-year-old male. He reports a long history of mild dyspepsia characterized by burning epigastric pain, especially when his stomach is empty. This pain has been relieved by over-the-counter antacids. Approximately two weeks ago, the pain became significantly worse and he is also nauseated and has vomited several times.

Past Medical History: Patient's history is not significant for other digestive system disorders. He had a tonsillectomy at age 8. He sustained a compound fracture of the left ankle in a bicycle accident at age 11 that required surgical fixation. More recently he has been diagnosed with an enlarged prostate gland and surgery has been recommended. However, he would like to resolve this epigastric pain before going forward with the TUR.

Results of Physical Examination: CBC indicates anemia and an occult blood test is positive for blood in the feces. A blood test for *Helicobacter pylori* is positive. An erosion in the gastric lining was visualized on an upper GI. Follow-up gastroscopy found evidence of mild reflux esophagitis and an ulcerated lesion in the lining of the pyloric section of the stomach. This ulcer is 1.5 cm in diameter and deep. There is evidence of active bleeding from the ulcer. Multiple biopsies were taken and they were negative for gastric cancer. IV Tagamet relieved the painful symptoms in two days.

Assessment: Peptic ulcer. Gastric cancer has been ruled out in light of the negative biopsies.

Recommendations: A gastrectomy to remove ulcerated portion of stomach is indicated because ulcer is already bleeding. Patient should continue on Tagamet to reduce stomach acid. Two medications will be added, Keflex to treat the bacterial infection and iron pills to reverse the anemia. Patient was instructed to eat frequent small meals and avoid alcohol and irritating foods.

CRITICAL THINKING QUESTIONS

1. This patient reports LUQ pain. What does LUQ stand for and what organs do you find there?

2. This patient had two diagnostic tests that indicated he was losing blood. Name these two tests and then describe them in your own words.

3. This patient had a procedure to visually examine the ulcer. Name the procedure and then describe in your own words what the physician observed.

4. Name the serious pathological condition that was ruled out.

5. Which of the following is NOT a recommendation of the consulting physician?

    a. medication to reduce stomach acid

    b. surgical removal of a portion of the stomach

    c. an antibiotic

    d. a blood transfusion

6. Briefly describe this patient's past medical history in your own words.

Chart Note Transcription

Chart Note

The chart note below contains twelve phrases that can be reworded with a medical term that you learned in this chapter. Each phrase is identified with an underline. Determine the medical term and write your answers in the space provided.

Current Complaint: Patient is a 74-year-old female seen by a physician who specializes in the treatment of the gastrointestinal tract[1] with complaints of severe lower abdominal pain and extreme difficulty with having a bowel movement.[2]

Past History: Patient has a history of the presence of gallstones[3] requiring a surgical removal of the gallbladder[4] 10 years ago and chronic acid backing up from the stomach into the esophagus.[5]

Signs and Symptoms: The patient's abdomen is distended with fluid collecting in the abdominal cavity.[6] X-ray of the colon after inserting barium dye[7] with an enema revealed the presence of multiple small tumors growing on a stalk[8] throughout the colon. Visual examination of the colon by a fiberscope inserted through the rectum[9] was performed, and biopsies taken for microscopic examination located a tumor.

Diagnosis: Carcinoma of the section of colon between the descending colon and the rectum[10]

Treatment: Surgical removal of the colon[11] between the descending colon and the rectum with the surgical creation of an opening of the colon through the abdominal wall.[12]

1 _____

2 _____

3 _____

4 _____

5 _____

6 _____

7 _____

8 _____

9 _____

10 _____

11 _____

12 _____

Practice Exercises

A. DEFINE EACH COMBINING FORM AND PROVIDE AN EXAMPLE OF ITS USE.

		Definition	Example
1.	esophag/o		
2.	hepat/o		
3.	ile/o		
4.	proct/o		
5.	gloss/o		
6.	labi/o		
7.	jejun/o		
8.	sigmoid/o		
9.	rect/o		
10.	gingiv/o		
11.	cholecyst/o		
12.	duoden/o		
13.	an/o		
14.	enter/o		
15.	dent/o		

B. STATE THE TERMS DESCRIBED USING THE COMBINING FORMS PROVIDED.

The combining form gastr/o refers to the stomach. Use it to write a term that means

1. inflammation of the stomach _____
2. study of the stomach and intestines _____
3. excision (removal) of the stomach _____
4. downward displacement of the stomach _____
5. suture of the stomach _____
6. enlargement of the stomach _____
7. narrowing (shrinking) of the stomach _____

The combining form esophag/o refers to the esophagus. Use it to write a term that means

8. inflammation of the esophagus _____
9. endoscopic examination of the esophagus _____
10. surgical repair of the esophagus _____
11. pain in the esophagus _____
12. excision of part of the esophagus _____

The combining forms proct/o and rect/o refer to the rectum. Use them to write a term that means

13. narrowing or constriction of the rectum _____
14. prolapse of the rectum _____
15. inflammation of the rectum _____
16. pain in the rectum _____

The combining forms chol/o, cholecyst/o, and choledoch/o refer to the gallbladder. Use them to write a term that means

17. excision of part of the common bile duct _____

18. pertaining to the bile duct _____

19. crushing of a gallstone _____

20. vomiting bile _____

21. stones or calculus in the gallbladder _____

22. stones or calculus in the common bile duct _____

23. the gallbladder _____

The combining form hepat/o refers to the liver. Use it to write a term that means

24. liver tumor _____

25. enlargement of the liver _____

26. pain in the liver _____

27. cirrhosis of the liver _____

The combining form pancreat/o refers to the pancreas. Use it to write a term that means

28. inflammation of the pancreas _____

29. pertaining to the pancreas _____

The combining form col/o refers to the colon. Use it to write a term that means

30. disease or disorder of the colon _____

31. inflammation of the colon and rectum _____

32. visual examination of the colon _____

33. inflammation of the colon _____

The combining form duoden/o refers to the duodenum. Use it to write a term that means

34. inflammation of the duodenum _____

35. pertaining to the duodenum _____

C. USE THE FOLLOWING SUFFIXES TO CREATE A MEDICAL TERM FOR EACH DEFINITION RELATING TO THE DIGESTIVE SYSTEM.

-rrhea	-phagia	-iasis
-emesis	-lith	-prandial

1. taken after meals _____

2. formation of gallstones _____

3. discharge of watery feces _____

4. difficulty swallowing _____

5. vomiting blood _____

6. a gallstone _____

D. Identify the Following Abbreviations

1. BM _____
2. UGI _____
3. BE _____
4. BS _____
5. RDA _____
6. O&P _____
7. PO _____
8. CBD _____
9. NPO _____
10. PP _____
11. NG _____
12. G _____
13. HBV _____
14. OCG _____
15. IBD _____

E. Break Apart the Medical Term *CHOLANGIOPANCREATOGRAPHY* into its Combining Forms and Suffix. Define the Term.

1. Combining forms: (a) _____ (b) _____
2. Suffix: _____
3. Definition: _____

F. Match the Terms in Column A with the Definitions in Column B.

A		B
1. _____ bulimia		a. indigestion
2. _____ anorexia		b. chronic liver disease
3. _____ hematemesis		c. bad breath
4. _____ halitosis		d. small colon tumors
5. _____ dyspepsia		e. fluid accumulation in abdominal cavity
6. _____ constipation		f. vomit blood
7. _____ polyphagia		g. bowel twists on self
8. _____ ascites		h. binge and purge
9. _____ cirrhosis		i. loss of appetite
10. _____ fissure		j. difficulty having BM
11. _____ polyposis		k. crack in rectum
12. _____ volvulus		l. excessive eating

G. Use the Following Terms in the Sentences that Follow.

spleen scan	occult blood test	liver scan
cholangiogram	gastrointestinal endoscopy	peptic ulcer
colonoscopy	barium swallow	lower GI
gastrectomy	colostomy	colectomy
anastomosis	lithotripsy	liver biopsy
ileostomy	pilonidal cyst	

1. Excising a small piece of hepatic tissue for microscopic examination is called a(n) _____ .
2. Mr. Rohr has a cyst that causes discomfort when he sits or puts weight on his sacrococcygeal area. He may have a(n) _____

3. When a surgeon performs a total or partial colectomy for cancer, she may have to create an opening on the surface of the skin for fecal matter to leave the body. This opening is called a(n) _____ .

4. Visualizing the spleen by injecting a radioactive material into a vein is called a(n) _____ .

5. Another name for an esophagram is a(n) _____ .

6. Mr. White has had a radioactive material placed into his large bowel by means of an enema for the purpose of viewing his colon. This procedure is called a(n) _____ .

7. A(n) _____ is the surgical removal of the colon.

8. Jessica has been on a red-meat-free diet in preparation for a test of her feces for the presence of hidden blood. This test is called a(n) _____ .

9. Dr. Mendez uses equipment to crush gallstones. This procedure is called _____ .

10. The opening or passageway created surgically between two organs is called a(n) _____ .

11. Removing all or part of the stomach is a(n) _____ .

12. Visualizing the bile ducts by injecting a dye into the patient's arm is called an IV _____ .

13. Passing an instrument into the anus and rectum to see the colon is called a(n) _____ .

14. Ms. Fayne suffers from Crohn's disease, which has necessitated the removal of much of her small intestine. She has had a surgical passage created for the external disposal of waste material from the ileum. This is called a(n) _____ .

H. MATCH THE TERMS IN COLUMN A WITH THE DEFINITIONS IN COLUMN B.

A	B
1. _____ plaque	a. decay
2. _____ pyorrhea	b. prosthetic device used to anchor
3. _____ root canal	c. inflammation of the gums
4. _____ crown	d. gummy mass of material
5. _____ bridge	e. enamel covering
6. _____ implant	f. replace missing teeth
7. _____ gingivitis	g. purulent material
8. _____ caries	h. surgery of pulp

Getting Connected

Multimedia Extension Activities

CD-ROM

Use the CD-ROM enclosed with your textbook to gain additional reinforcement through interactive word building exercises, spelling games, labeling activities, and additional quizzes.

www.prenhall.com/fremgen

Use the above address to access the free, interactive Companion Website created for this textbook. Get hints, instant feedback, and textbook references to chapter-related multiple choice questions, and labeling and matching exercises. In addition, you will find an audio glossary, case studies, Internet exploration exercises, flashcards, and a comprehensive exam.

Answers

CASE STUDY (CRITICAL THINKING QUESTIONS)

1. left upper quadrant, stomach, spleen   2. complete blood count (CBC), occult blood test   3. gastroscopy; a deep ulcer 1.5 cm in diameter, evidence of bleeding   4. gastric carcinoma   5. d—a blood transfusion   6. tonsillectomy, compound fracture, BPH, and TUR

CHART NOTE

1. gastroenterologist—physician who specializes in the treatment of the gastrointestinal tract   2. constipation—difficulty with having a bowel movement   3. cholelithiasis—the presence of gallstones   4. cholecystectomy—surgical removal of the gallbladder   5. reflux esophagitis—acid backing up from the stomach into the esophagus   6. ascites—fluid collecting in the abdominal cavity   7. barium enema—X-ray of the colon after inserting barium dye with an enema   8. polyposis—presence of multiple small tumors growing on a stalk   9. colonoscopy—visual examination of the colon by a fiberscope inserted through the rectum   10. sigmoid colon—section of colon between the descending colon and the rectum   11. colectomy—surgical removal of the colon   12. colostomy—the surgical creation of an opening of the colon through the abdominal wall

PRACTICE EXERCISES

A. 1. esophagus   2. liver   3. ileum   4. rectum   5. tongue   6. lip   7. jejunum   8. sigmoid colon   9. rectum   10. gum   11. gallbladder   12. duodenum   13. anus   14. intestine   15. teeth

B. 1. gastritis   2. gastroenterology   3. gastrectomy   4. gastroptosis   5. gastrorrhaphy   6. gastromegaly   7. gastrostenosis   8. esophagitis   9. esophagoscopy   10. esophagoplasty   11. esophagalgia   12. esophagectomy   13. rectostenosis   14. proctoptosis   15. proctitis   16. rectodynia, rectalgia   17. choledochectomy   18. choledochal   19. choledocholithrotripsy   20. cholemesis   21. cholecystolithiasis   22. cholelithiasis   23. cholecyst   24. hepatoma   25. hepatomegaly   26. hepatodynia, hepatalgia   27. hepatocirrhosis   28. pancreatitis   29. pancreatic   30. colopathy, colonopathy   31. colorectitis   32. colonoscopy   33. colitis   34. duodenitis   35. duodenal

C. 1. postprandial   2. cholelithiasis   3. diarrhea   4. dysphagia   5. hematemesis   6. cholelith

D. 1. bowel movement   2. upper gastrointestinal series   3. barium enema   4. bowel sounds   5. recommended daily allowance   6. ova and parasites   7. by mouth   8. common bile duct   9. nothing by mouth   10. postprandial (after meals)   11. nasogastric tube   12. gastrointestinal   13. hepatitis B virus   14. oral cholecystography   15. inflammatory bowel disease

E. 1. Cholangi/o - bile duct   pancreat/o - pancreas   2. graphy film or picture   3. Process of making an X-ray recording of bile duct and pancreas

F. 1. h   2. i   3. f   4. c   5. a   6. j   7. l   8 e   9. b   10. k   11. d   12. g

G. 1. liver biopsy   2. pilonidal cyst   3. colostomy   4. spleen scan   5. barium swallow   6. lower GI   7. colectomy   8. occult blood test   9. lithotripsy   10. anastomosis   11. gastrectomy   12. cholangiogram   13. colonoscopy   14. ileostomy

H. 1. d   2. g   3. h   4. e   5. f   6. b   7. c   8. a

Chapter 10

URINARY SYSTEM

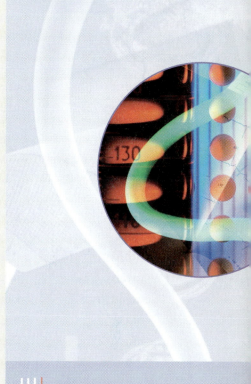

LEARNING OBJECTIVES

Upon completion of this chapter, you will be able to:

- Recognize the combining forms and suffixes introduced in this chapter.

- Gain the ability to pronounce medical terms and major anatomical structures.

- List the major organs of the urinary system and their functions.

- Describe the nephron and the mechanisms of urine production.

- Identify the characteristics of urine and a urinalysis.

- Build urinary system medical terms from word parts.

- Define vocabulary, pathology, diagnostic, and therapeutic medical terms relating to the urinary system.

- Interpret abbreviations associated with the urinary system.

Overview

ORGANS OF THE URINARY SYSTEM

kidneys (2)   urethra

ureters (2)   urinary bladder

COMBINING FORMS RELATING TO THE URINARY SYSTEM

cyst/o	bladder	**pyel/o**	renal (kidney) pelvis
glomerul/o	glomerulus	**ren/o**	kidney
glycos/o	sugar, glucose	**ur/o**	urine
lith/o	stone	**ureter/o**	ureter; urinary tube
meat/o	meatus	**urethr/o**	urethra
nephr/o	kidney	**urin/o**	urine
noct/i	night	**vesic/o**	bladder
olig/o	scanty		

SUFFIXES RELATING TO THE URINARY SYSTEM

Suffix	Meaning	Example
-megaly	enlarged	nephromegaly
-ptosis	drooping	nephroptosis
-tripsy	surgical crushing	lithotripsy
-uria	condition of the urine	hematuria

ANATOMY AND PHYSIOLOGY OF THE URINARY SYSTEM

aldosterone	nephrologists	urethra
antidiuretic hormone (ADH)	nephrology	urinary bladder
genital tract	nephrons	urinary meatus
genitourinary (GI)	nephrosis	urine
kidneys	uremia	
micturition	ureters	

You might think of the urinary system, sometimes referred to as the **genitourinary (GU)** (jen ih toh **YOO** rih nair ee) system, as similar to a water filtration plant. Its main function is to filter and remove waste products from the blood. These waste materials result in the production and excretion of **urine** (**YOO** rin) from the body (see Figure 10.1).

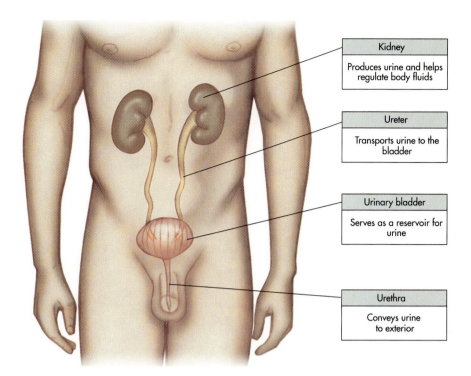

FIGURE 10.1 The organs of the urinary system with major functions.

The urinary system is one of the hardest-working systems of the body. The conversion of food and other elements and gases into energy results in the production of waste products. These waste products are a natural part of all life processes. They quickly become toxic if they stay in the body and they could result in a condition called **uremia** (yoo **REE** mee ah). The urinary system consists of two **kidneys,** two **ureters (UR** re terz), a **urinary (YOO** rih nair ee) **bladder,** and the **urethra** (yoo **REE** thrah). See Figure 10.2 for a posterior view.

Waste products in the body are removed through a very complicated system of blood vessels and tubules. The actual filtration or sifting of the waste products takes place in the **nephrons (NEF** ronz), which are in the outer layer of each kidney.

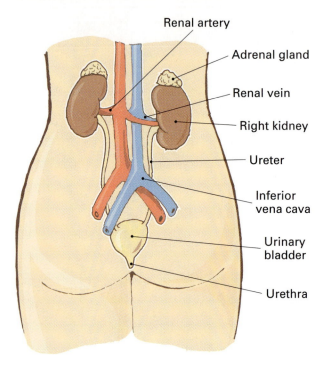

Renal artery

Adrenal gland

Renal vein

Right kidney

Ureter

Inferior
vena cava

Urinary
bladder

Urethra

FIGURE 10.2 Renal anatomy; posterior view.

Urine is actually produced by the kidneys and held in a muscular container or sac called the bladder. We are constantly producing urine and our bladders can hold about one quart of this liquid. However, the amount of time before the brain tells us that it is time to empty our bladder varies from one person to another.

Urine moves from the kidneys to the bladder via the two ureters. It then moves from the bladder down the urethra to the outside of the body and is excreted through an opening called the **urinary meatus** (**YOO** rih nair ee mee **AY** tus). In addition to waste removal, the urinary system regulates the amount of water and other fluids in our bodies and maintains the correct chemical balance.

MED
TERM
TIP

Terms such as **micturition** (mik too **RIH** shun), *voiding*, and *urination* all mean basically the same thing—the process of releasing urine from the body.

Urine formation in the body is the result of three processes: (1) filtration, (2) reabsorption, and (3) secretion. This all occurs in microscopic units called nephrons within the kidneys. The hormones **antidiuretic hormone** (an tye dye yoo **RET** ik **HOR** mohn) **(ADH)** and **aldosterone** (al **DOSS** ter ohn) control the amount of urine that the nephrons produce.

Blood is filtered in the kidneys with most of the minerals and selected fluids reabsorbed. Any remaining wastes are collected in the bladder and passed to the outside of the body through the urethra.

This system also includes some of the male and female organs of reproduction (or genitalia). Hence the term genitourinary (GI) is sometimes used to describe the urinary system. The male and female reproductive processes are discussed in Chapter 11.

KIDNEYS

calyx	hilum	peritoneum	renal pelvis
cortex	medulla	pyramids	renal vein
fascia	papilla	renal artery	retroperitoneal

The kidneys are considered vital organs, which means that they are necessary for life. It is, however, possible to live with only one functioning kidney.

The two kidneys are located in the lumbar region of the back behind the **peritoneum** (pair ih toh **NEE** um), which is the membrane lining the abdominal cavity. The term for this location is **retroperitoneal** (ret roh pair ih toh **NEE** al). They are under the muscles of the back, just a little above the waist. Since they are located behind the peritoneum, the surgeon can operate on a kidney without entering the peritoneum.

MED TERM TIP

The kidney actually resembles a kidney bean in shape. Each weighs 4 to 6 ounces, is 2 to 3 inches wide and approximately 1 inch thick, and is about the size of your fist. In most people the left kidney is slightly higher and larger than the right kidney.

Each kidney has a concave or depressed area on the edge toward the center that gives the kidney its bean shape (see Figure 10.3). The center of this concave area is called the **hilum** (**HIGH** lum). The hilum is an important landmark in the kidney and provides an important function. The hilum is where the **renal artery** (**REE** nal **AR** teh ree) enters the kidney and the **renal** (**REE** nal) **vein** leaves it. These are extremely important blood vessels since they provide a large supply of blood to the kidneys. The renal artery

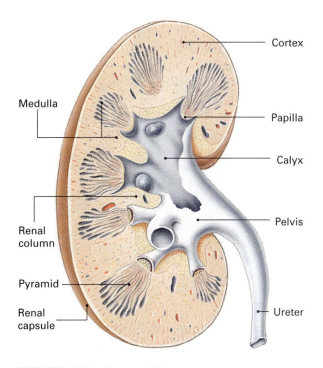

FIGURE 10.3   Sectioned kidney.

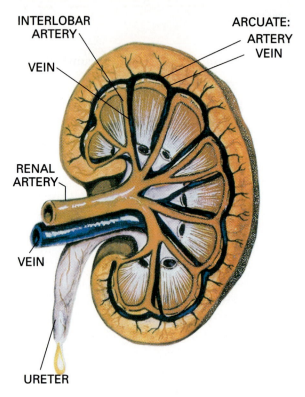

INTERLOBAR ARTERY

VEIN

ARCUATE:
ARTERY
VEIN

RENAL ARTERY

VEIN

URETER

FIGURE 10.4 Renal artery and vein.

delivers the blood that is full of waste products to the filtering tubules in the kidney (see Figure 10.4). Near the hilum the ureters leave the kidneys. The ureters are narrow tubes that lead from the kidneys to the bladder.

Strong fibrous tissue or renal **fascia** (**FASH** ee ah) holds the kidneys in place. A layer of fat covers and protects these vital organs.

When the surgeon cuts into the kidney, several structures or areas are visible. The outer portion is called the **cortex** (**KOR** teks). The cortex is much like a shell for the kidney. The inner area is called the **medulla** (meh **DULL** ah). Within the medulla are a dozen or so triangular structures called the **pyramids** (**PEER** ah mids) that resemble their namesake, the Egyptian Pyramids. The tip of each pyramid points inward toward the hilum. At its tip, called the **papilla** (pah **PILL** ah), each pyramid connects with a **calyx** (**KAY** liks) (plural is *calyces*), which is a duct that joins the **renal pelvis** (**REE** nal **PELL** vis). Between the pyramids in the medulla are sections of tissue called *renal columns*. These columns are continuous with the cortex and are made of the same type of tissue as the cortex.

The renal pelvis serves the important function of being the collection point for urine as it is formed. The ureter for each kidney is attached to the renal pelvis.

MED TERM TIP

Think of the parts of the kidney moving in an inward fashion from the cortex to medulla to pyramids to papilla to calyx, and finally to the renal pelvis. All these special components play a role in urine formation.

afferent arteriole	glomerular filtrate
Bowman's capsule	glomerulus
collecting tubule	homeostasis
diabetes mellitus	loop of Henle
distal convoluted tubule	proximal convoluted tubule
efferent arteriole	renal corpuscle
electrolytes	renal tubule
glomerular capsule	

The functional or working unit of the kidney is the nephron. You have to examine a small portion of the kidney under a microscope to see these microscopic units. There are more than one million nephrons in each human kidney.

These little nephrons are responsible for maintaining the **homeostasis** (hoh mee oh **STAY** sis) or balance in your body. They continually adjust the conditions in the body that allow you to survive. For instance, when blood sugar becomes too high, as occurs in **diabetes mellitus** (dye ah **BEE** teez **MELL** ih tus), the extra sugar is filtered from the blood and then removed from the body in the urine.

Each nephron consists of the **renal corpuscle** (**REE** nal **KOR** pus ehl) and the **renal tubule** (**REE** nal **TOOB** yool) (see Figure 10.5). The renal corpuscle is a double-walled

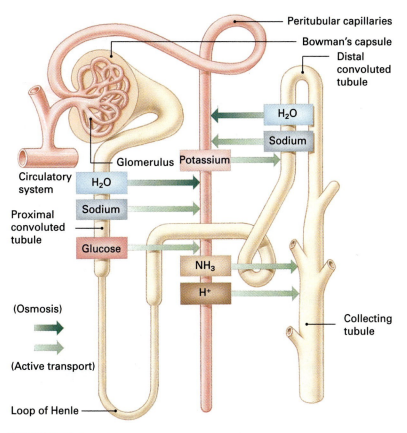

FIGURE 10.5 Mechanism of urine production.

cuplike structure called the **glomerular** (glom **AIR** yoo lar) or **Bowman's capsule** (Bow manz **CAP** sool), which is part of the blood-filtering portion of the nephron. This capsule contains a twisted group of capillary channels called the **glomerulus** (glom **AIR** yoo lus). An **afferent arteriole** (**AFF** er ent ar **TEE** ree ol) carries blood to the glomerulus, and the smaller **efferent arteriole** (**EF** er ent ar **TEE** ree ohl) carries blood away from the glomerulus.

MED TERM TIP

Afferent, meaning moving toward, and *efferent,* meaning moving away from, are terms used when discussing moving either toward or away from the central point in many systems. For example, there are afferent and efferent nerves in the nervous system.

The renal tubule is divided into four areas: (1) the **proximal convoluted tubule,** followed by the narrow (2) **loop of Henle,** then the (3) **distal convoluted tubule,** and finally, the (4) **collecting tubule.**

Blood flowing through the glomerulus forces material through the glomerular wall of the Bowman's capsule into the nephron. This fluid in the nephron is called **glomerular filtrate** (glom **AIR** yoo lar **FILL** trayt) and consists of water, **electrolytes** (ee **LEK** troh lites), nutrients, soluble wastes, and toxins. This waste must be eliminated from the body, but the rest of the materials (water, electrolytes, nutrients) must be returned to the blood. This process of reabsorption is called *tubular reabsorption.*

MECHANISMS OF URINE PRODUCTION

Waste products are removed from the blood in three stages: filtration, reabsorption, and secretion. Each of these steps is performed by a different section of the hardworking nephrons. Following are the three stages of urine production. (See Figure 10.6 for a CAT scan of the working kidneys.)

1. *Filtration.* The first stage is the sifting of particles, which occurs in the renal corpuscle. This process removes water, sugar, amino acids, electrolytes, and other materials from the blood by moving the fluid into the glomerulus and into Bowman's capsule. This fluid is called filtrate.

FIGURE 10.6 Enhanced color CAT scan of kidneys (in red). (CNRI/GJLP/ Phototake NYC)

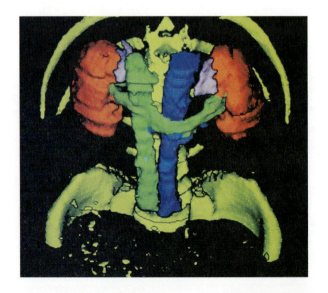

2. *Reabsorption.* After filtration, the filtrate passes through the four sections of the tubule. As the filtrate moves along its twisted journey, most of the water and some electrolytes and amino acids are absorbed by the peritubular capillaries. They can then reenter the circulating blood.

3. *Secretion.* The final stage of urine production occurs when the special cells of the collecting tubules secrete ammonia, uric acid, and other substances directly into the tubule. Urine formation is now finished; it is passed from the collecting tubules to the renal pelvis, which is the collecting basin of the kidney.

MED TERM TIP

The amount of water and other fluids processed by the kidneys each day is astonishing. Approximately 190 quarts of fluid is filtered out of the glomerular blood every day. Most of this fluid returns to the body through the reabsorption process. About 99 percent of the water that leaves the blood each day through the filtration process returns to the blood by proximal tubule reabsorption.

BLOOD SUPPLY TO THE KIDNEYS

aorta	hypertension
hemorrhage	hypotension

The blood supply to the kidney is rich and enters through the renal artery, which is a branch of the **aorta** (ay **OR** tah). The renal artery divides into smaller vessels as it meanders through kidney tissue. Eventually, the blood is brought into the Bowman's capsule and then circulated through the glomerulus within the capsule.

Blood pressure affects the speed of blood filtering through the kidneys. When systemic blood pressure drops, the filtration of the blood may slow down to the point at which the kidneys will stop functioning. This may occur in the condition called shock, which can result from **hemorrhage** (**HEM** eh rij). If the systemic pressure is too high, as in persistent high blood pressure, kidney damage may result.

Blood pressure regulation is an important kidney function. Salt, or sodium, in the body is processed by the kidney. Many patients with high blood pressure are encouraged to lower their intake of salt. This lessens the burden on the kidneys and helps to regulate blood pressure.

MED TERM TIP

The term **hypotension** (high poh **TEN** shun) refers to a lower-than-normal blood pressure, while **hypertension** (high per **TEN** shun) is the opposite, with an elevated blood pressure. Normal blood pressure in an adult is generally 120/80, with a range of normal between 100/60 and 140/90. Hypotensive and hypertensive drugs are used to treat these conditions.

REGULATION OF THE URINE COMPOSITION

antidiuretic	pH
atrial natriuretic hormone (ANH)	

Many processes regulate the composition and **pH** (acidity versus alkalinity) of the urine during its trip through the kidney. The pituitary hormone (antidiuretic hormone) (ADH) decreases the amount of urine by making the collecting cells more receptive to water. When the water is reabsorbed by the collecting tubules, less water is lost as urine.

The **adrenal cortex,** located in the adrenal glands, secretes the hormone aldosterone, which assists the tubules' reabsorption of salt.

This is in contrast to **atrial natriuretic hormone (AY** tree al nay tree yoo **RET** ik **HOR** mohn) **(ANH),** which is produced by the heart's atrial wall. This hormone stimulates the kidney tubules to secrete more sodium and in this way lose more water. Therefore, ANH is a water- and salt-losing hormone.

Antidiuretic hormone (ADH **ureters**) can be thought of as the water-retaining hormone, since it is **antidiuretic** (an tye dye yoo **RET** ik) against forming urine. Atrial natriuretic hormone (ANH) can be thought of as the water-losing hormone.

URETERS

cystitis   **peristaltic waves**

Once urine is formed in the collecting tubules, it then drains out of each kidney into the renal pelvis and down the ureter into the urinary bladder. Ureters are very narrow tubes measuring less than 1/4 inch wide and 10 to 12 inches long that extend from the renal pelvis to the urinary bladder. Mucous membrane lines the ureters just as it lines most internal passages. Figure 10.7 shows the kidneys and surrounding structures, including the ureters.

Mucous membranes will carry infections up the urinary tract from the urinary meatus and urethra into the bladder and eventually up the ureters and into the kidneys if not stopped. It is never wise to ignore a *simple bladder infection* or what is called **cystitis** (siss **TYE** tis).

FIGURE 10.7 Enhanced color three-dimensional model showing kidneys and surrounding structures. (Clinique Ste. Catherine/ CNRI/Science Photo Library/ Photo Researchers, Inc.)

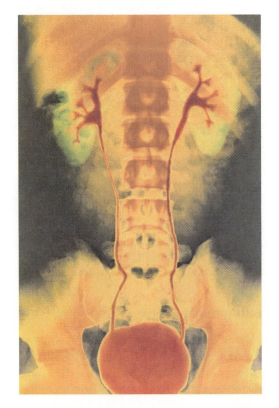

Urine goes into the bladder through the ureters every few seconds. It enters as spurts through the urethral openings into the bladder. This orifice opens and closes through a process of **peristaltic** (pair ih **STALL** tik) **waves.**

URINARY BLADDER

rugae   **sphincter**

The bladder is an elastic muscular sac that lies in the base of the pelvis just behind the pubic symphysis. It is composed of three layers of smooth muscle tissue lined with mucous membrane containing **rugae** (**ROO** gay) or wrinkles. The bladder receives the urine directly from the ureters through two openings, stores urine, and excretes it through the urethra.

Generally, the bladder will hold 250 mL of urine. This amount then creates an urge to void or empty the bladder.

Involuntary muscle action causes the bladder to contract and the internal muscle **sphincter** (**SFINGK** ter) to relax. The internal muscle sphincter protects us from having our bladder empty at the wrong time. Voluntary action controls the external muscle sphincter. The act of controlling the emptying of urine is developed sometime after a child is 2 years of age.

URETHRA

semen

The urethra is a tubular canal that carries the flow of urine from the bladder to the outside of the body. The external opening is called the urinary meatus. Mucous membrane also lines the urethra as it does the renal pelvis. This is one of the reasons that infection spreads up the urinary tract. The urethra is 1-1/2 inches long in the female and 8 inches long in the male. In a woman it functions only as the outlet for urine and is in the muscle of the front wall of the vagina. In the male, however, it has two functions: an outlet for urine and the passageway for the reproductive fluid **semen** (**SEE** men) to leave the body.

MED TERM TIP

The terms *ureter* and *urethra* are frequently confused. Remember that there are two ureters carrying urine from the kidneys into the bladder. There is only one urethra and it carries urine from the bladder to the outside of the body.

URINE CHARACTERISTICS

albumin   **hormones**

blood   **nitrogenous wastes**

glucose   **toxins**

Urine is normally straw colored to clear. Although it is 95 percent water, it also contains many dissolved substances, such as electrolytes, **toxins** (**TOKS** ins), **nitrogenous** (nigh **TROJ** eh nus) **wastes,** and **hormones** (**HOR** mohnz). At times the urine will also contain abnormal materials, such as **glucose** (**GLOO** kohs), **blood,** or **albumin** (al **BEW** min). Normally, during a 24-hour period the output of urine will be 1,000 to 2,000 mL, depending on the amount of fluid consumed and the general health of the person. Normal urine has an acid reaction, and the specific gravity varies from 1.001 to 1.030.

The color, odor, volume, and sugar content of urine have been examined for centuries. Color charts for urine were developed by 1140 A.D., and "taste testing" was common in the late seventeenth century. By the nineteenth century, urinalysis was a routine part of a physical examination.

See Table 10.1 for the normal values for urine testing and Table 10.2 for abnormal findings.

Table 10.1 Values for Urinalysis Testing	
Element	**Normal Findings**
Color	Straw colored, pale yellow, to deep gold
Odor	Aromatic
Appearance	Clear
Specific gravity	1.010–1.030
pH	5.0–8.0
Protein	Negative to trace
Glucose	None
Ketones	None
Blood	Negative

Table 10.2 Abnormal Urinalysis Findings	
Element	**Implications**
Color	Color varies depending on the patient's fluid intake and output or medication. Brown or black urine color indicates a serious disease process.
Odor	A fetid or foul odor may indicate infection. For instance, a fruity odor may be found in diabetes mellitus, dehydration, or starvation. Other odors may be due to medication or foods.
Appearance	Cloudiness may mean that an infection is present.
Specific gravity	Concentrated urine has a higher specific gravity. Dilute urine, such as can be found with diabetes insipidus, acute tubular necrosis, or salt-restricted diets, has a lower specific gravity.
pH	A pH value below 7.0 (acidic) is common in urinary tract infections, metabolic or respiratory acidosis, diets high in fruits or vegetables, or administration of some drugs. A pH higher than 7.0 (basic or alkaline) is common in metabolic or respiratory alkalosis, fever, high-protein diets, and taking ascorbic acid.
Protein	Protein may indicate glomerulonephritis or preeclampsia in a pregnant woman.
Glucose	Small amounts of glucose may be present as the result of eating a high-carbohydrate meal, stress, pregnancy, and taking some medications, such as aspirin or corticosteroids. Higher levels may indicate poorly controlled diabetes, Cushing's syndrome, or infection.
Ketones	The presence of ketones may indicate poorly controlled diabetes, dehydration, starvation, or ingestion of large amounts of aspirin.
Blood	Blood may indicate some anemias, taking some medications (such as blood thinners), arsenic poisoning, reactions to transfusion, trauma, burns, and convulsions.

Word Building Relating to the Urinary System

The following list contains examples of medical terms built directly from word parts. The definition for these terms can be determined by a straightforward translation of the word parts.

Combining Form	Prefix/ Suffix	Medical Term	Definition
cyst/o	-algia	cystalgia (sis **TAL** jee ah)	bladder pain
	-cele	cystocele (**SIS** toh seel)	bladder protrusion (through vaginal wall)
	-ectomy	cystectomy (sis **TEK** toh me)	excision of the bladder
	-itis	cystitis (siss **TYE** tis)	bladder inflammation
	-lith	cystolith (**SIS** toh lith)	bladder stone
	-ostomy	cystostomy (sis **TOSS** toh mee)	create a new opening into the bladder
	-otomy	cystotomy (sis **TOT** oh me)	incision into the bladder
	-plasty	cystoplasty (**SIS** toh plas tee)	surgical repair of the bladder
	-rrhagia	cystorrhagia (sis toh **RAH** jee ah)	rapid bleeding from bladder
	-scopy	cystoscopy (sis **TOSS** koh pee)	procedure to visually examine the bladder
glycos/o	-uria	glycosuria (glye kohs **YOO** ree ah)	condition of sugar in the urine
lith/o	-tripsy	lithotripsy (**LITH** oh trip see)	surgical crushing of a stone
nephr/o	-ectomy	nephrectomy (ne **FREK** toh mee)	excision of a kidney
	-graphy	nephrography (neh **FROG** rah fee)	process of recording (X-raying) the kidney
	-itis	nephritis (neh **FRYE** tis)	kidney inflammation
	-malacia	nephromalacia (nef roh mah **LAY** she ah)	softening of the kidney
	-megaly	nephromegaly (nef roh **MEG** ah lee)	enlarged kidney
	-oma	nephroma (neh **FROH** ma)	kidney tumor
	-optosis	nephroptosis (nef rop **TOH** sis)	drooping kidney
	-ostomy	nephrostomy (neh **FROS** toh mee)	create a new opening into the kidney
	-otomy	nephrotomy (neh **FROP** ah thee)	incision into a kidney
	-pathy	nephropathy (neh **FROP** ah thee)	kidney disease
	-pexy	nephropexy (**NEF** roh pek see)	surgical fixation of (floating) kidney
	-rrhaphy	nephrorrhaphy (nef **ROR** ah fee)	suturing a kidney
	-sclerosis	nephrosclerosis (nef roh skleh **ROH** sis)	hardening of the kidney
noct/i	-uria	nocturia (nok **TOO** ree ah)	condition of frequent night-time urination

(continued)

Combining Form	Prefix/ Suffix	Medical Term	Definition
olig/o	-uria	oliguria (ol ig **YOO** ree ah)	condition of scanty amount of urine
py/o	-uria	pyuria (pye **YOO** ree ah)	condition of pus in the urine
pyel/o	-gram	pyelogram (**PYE** eh loh gram)	X-ray record of the renal pelvis
	-itis	pyelitis (pye eh **LYE** tis)	renal pelvis inflammation
	-plasty	pyeloplasty (**PIE** ah loh plas tee)	surgical repair of the renal pelvis
ur/o	an-	anuria (an **YOO** ree ah)	condition of no urine (produced by kidney)
	dys-	dysuria (dis **YOO** ree ah)	condition of difficult or painful urination
	hemato-	hematuria (hee mah **TOO** ree ah)	condition of blood in the urine
	-logist	urologist (yoo **RALL** oh jist)	specialist in the urinary system
	-logy	urology (yoo **RALL** oh jee)	study of the urinary system
	poly-	polyuria (pol ee **YOO** ree ah)	condition of (too) much urine
ureter/o	-ectasis	ureterectasis (yoo ree ter **EK** tah sis)	ureter dilation
	-stenosis	ureterostenosis (yoo ree ter oh sten **OH** sis)	narrowing of a ureter
urethr/o	-algia	urethralgia (yoo ree **THRAL** jee ah)	urethra pain
	-itis	urethritis (yoo ree **THRIGH** tis)	urethra inflammation
	-rrhagia	urethrorrhagia (yoo ree throh **RAH** jee ah)	rapid bleeding from the urethra
	-scope	urethroscope (yoo **REE** throh scope)	instrument to visually examine the urethra
	-stenosis	urethrostenosis (yoo ree throh steh **NOH** sis)	narrowing of the urethra

Vocabulary Relating to the Urinary System

anuria (an **YOO** ree ah)	Complete suppression of urine formed by the kidneys and a complete lack of urine excretion.
calculus (**KAL** kew lus)	A stone formed within an organ by an accumulation of mineral salts. Found in the kidney, renal pelvis, ureters, bladder, or urethra. Plural is *calculi* (see Figure 10.8).
diuresis (dye yoo **REE** sis)	Abnormal secretion of large amounts of urine.

electrolyte **(ee LEK troh lite)**	Chemical compound that separates into charged particles, or ionizes, in a solution. Sodium chloride (NaCl) and potassium (K) are examples of electrolytes.
enuresis **(en yoo REE sis)**	Involuntary discharge of urine after the age by which bladder control should have been established. This usually occurs by the age of 5. Also called bed-wetting at night.
Escherichia coli **(E. coli)(esh er IK ee ah KOH lye)**	Normal bacteria found in the intestinal track; the most common cause of lower urinary track infections due to improper hygiene after bowel movements.
extracellular (eks trah SELL yoo lar) fluid	Water found outside the cells; also called *interstitial fluid*.
frequency	A greater-than-normal occurrence in the urge to urinate, without an increase in the total daily volume of urine. Frequency is an indication of inflammation of the bladder or urethra.
hematuria **(he muh TOO ree ah)**	Condition of blood in the urine.
hesitancy	A decrease in the force of the urine stream, often with difficulty initiating the flow. It is often a symptom of a blockage along the urethra, such as an enlarged prostate gland.
homeostasis **(hoh mee oh STAY sis)**	Steady state or state of balance within the body. The kidneys assist in maintaining this regulatory, steady state.
micturition **(mik too RIH shun)**	Another term for urination.
nocturia **(nok TOO ree ah)**	Excessive urination during the night. May or may not be abnormal.
osmosis (oz MOH sis)	Diffusion of water through a permeable membrane that allows the passage of the water (the solvent) but does not permit the solute to pass.
peritoneum **(pair ih toh NEE um)**	Membranous sac that lines the abdominal cavity and encases the abdominopelvic organs. The kidneys are an exception since they lay outside the peritoneum and alongside the vertebral column.
pyuria **(pye YOO ree ah)**	Presence of pus in the urine.
stricture (STRIK chur)	Narrowing of a passageway in the urinary system.
urgency (ER jen see)	Feeling the need to urinate immediately.
urinary incontinence **(YOO rih nair ee in CON tin ens)**	Involuntary release of urine. In some patients an indwelling catheter is inserted into the bladder for continuous urine drainage (see Figure 10.9).
urine (YOO rin)	The fluid that remains in the urinary system following the three stages of urine production: filtration, reabsorption, and secretion.
urologist **(yoo RALL oh jist)**	A physician specialized in treating conditions and diseases of the urinary system and male reproductive system.
urology **(yoo RALL oh jee)**	Study of the urinary system.

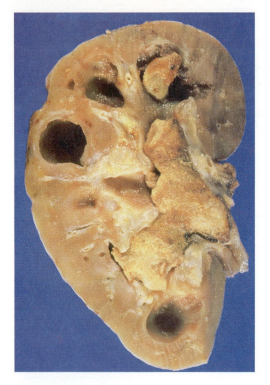

FIGURE 10.8 Sectioned kidney with calculi. (Dr. E. Walker/Science Photo Library/Photo Researchers, Inc.)

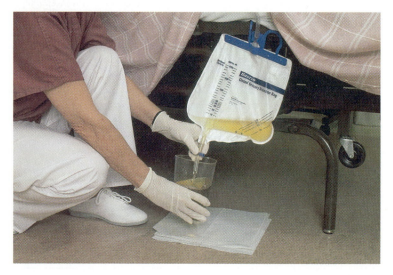

FIGURE 10.9 Closed urinary drainage system. Urine being measured after it leaves patient's body via catheter.

Pathology of the Urinary System

bladder neck obstruction	Blockage of the bladder outlet.
dysuria (dis YOO ree ah)	Painful or difficult urination. This is a symptom in many disorders, such as cystitis, urethritis, enlarged prostate in the male, and prolapsed uterus in the female.
glomerulonephritis (gloh mair yoo loh neh FRYE tis)	Inflammation of the kidney (primarily of the glomerulus). Since the glomerular membrane is inflamed, it becomes more permeable and will allow protein and blood cells to enter the filtrate. Results in protein in the urine (proteinuria) and hematuria.
hydronephrosis (high droh neh FROH sis)	Distention of the pelvis due to urine collecting in the kidney resulting from an obstruction.
hypospadias (high poh SPAY dee as)	Congenital opening of the male urethra on the undersurface of the penis.
interstitial cystitis (in ter STISH al sis TYE tis)	Disease of unknown cause in which there is inflammation and irritation of the bladder. Most commonly seen in middle-aged women.
nephrolithiasis (nef roh lith EYE ah sis)	The presence of calculi in the kidney.
phimosis (fih MOH sis)	Narrowing or stenosis of the opening of the foreskin over the glans of penis on males. May cause difficulty in urination and eventual infection. Treatment is circumcision, or removal of the foreskin.
pyelitis (pye eh LYE tis)	Inflammation of the renal pelvis.

pyelonephritis (pye eh loh neh FRYE tis)	Inflammation of the renal pelvis and the kidney. One of the most common types of kidney disease. It may be the result of a lower urinary tract infection that moved up to the kidney by way of the ureters. There may be large quantities of white blood cells and bacteria in the urine. Blood (hematuria) may even be present in the urine in this condition. Can occur with any untreated or persistent case of cystitis.
renal colic (REE nal KOL ik)	Pain caused by a kidney stone. Can be an excrutiating pain and generally requires medical treatment.
ureterolith (yoo REE ter oh lith)	A calculus in the ureter.
urinary retention (YOO rih nair ee ree TEN shun)	An inability to fully empty the bladder, often indicates a blockage in the urethra.
Wilm's tumor (VILMZ TOO mor)	Malignant kidney tumor found most often in children.

Diagnostic Procedures Relating to the Urinary System

blood urea nitrogen (BUN) (BLUD yoo REE ah NIGH troh jen)	Blood test to measure kidney function by the level of nitrogenous waste, urea, that is in the blood.
clean catch specimen (CC)	Urine sample obtained after cleaning off the urinary opening and catching or collecting a sample in midstream (halfway through the urination process) to minimize contamination from the genitalia.
cystography (sis TOG rah fee)	Process of instilling a contrast material or dye into the bladder by catheter to visualize the urinary bladder on X-ray.
cystoscopy (sis TOSS koh pee)	Visual examination of the urinary bladder using an instrument called a cystoscope.
excretory urography (EKS kreh tor ee yoo RIG rah fee)	Injecting dye into the bloodstream and then taking an X-ray to trace the action of the kidney as it excretes the dye.
intravenous pyelogram (IVP) (in trah VEE nus PYE eh loh gram)	Injecting a contrast medium into a vein and then taking an X-ray to visualize the renal pelvis.
retrograde pyelogram (RET roh grayd PYE eh loh gram)	A diagnostic X-ray in which dye is inserted through the urethra to outline the bladder, ureters, and renal pelvis.
serum electrolyte level (SEE rum ee LEK troh lite)	A laboratory test to measure the amount of sodium, potassium, and chloride ions in the blood.
sound	Metal rod curved at one end with a handle at the other end, used to treat a stricture or an obstruction in the urethra. A physician will pass the sound up the urethra.
urinalysis (U/A, UA) (yoo rih NAL ih sis)	Laboratory test that consists of the physical, chemical, and microscopic examination of urine.
urography (yoo ROG rah fee)	Use of a contrast medium to provide an X-ray of the urinary tract.

Treatment Procedures Relating to the Urinary System

catheterization **(kath eh ter ih ZAY shun)**	Insertion of a tube through the urethra and into the urinary bladder for the purpose of withdrawing urine or inserting dye.
extracorporeal shockwave lithotripsy (ESWL) **(eks trah cor POR ee al shockwave LITH oh trip see)**	Use of ultrasound waves to break up stones. Process does not require invasive surgery (see Figure 10.10).
hemodialysis (HD) **(hee moh dye AL ih sis)**	Use of an artificial kidney machine that filters the blood of a person to remove waste products. Use of this technique in patients who have defective kidneys is lifesaving (see Figure 10.11).
lithotomy **(lith OT oh mee)**	Surgical incision to remove kidney stones.
lithotripsy **(LITH oh trip see)**	Destroying or crushing kidney stones in the bladder or urethra with a device called a *lithotriptor*.
meatotomy **(mee ah TOT oh me)**	Surgical enlargement of the urinary opening (meatus).
peritoneal dialysis **(pair ih TOH nee al dye AL ih sis)**	Removal of toxic waste substances from the body by placing warm chemically balanced solutions into the peritoneal cavity. Used in treating renal failure and certain poisonings.
renal transplant (REE nal)	Surgical placement of a donor kidney.

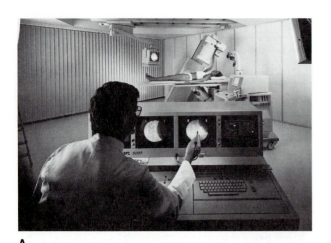

A

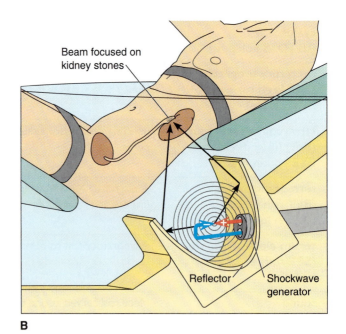

B

FIGURE 10.10 Extracorporeal shockwave lithotripsy. Acoustic shockwaves created by the shockwave generator travel through soft tissue to shatter the renal stone into fragments, which are then eliminated in the urine. (A) A shockwave generator that does not require water immersion. (B) An illustration of water immersion lithotripsy procedure.

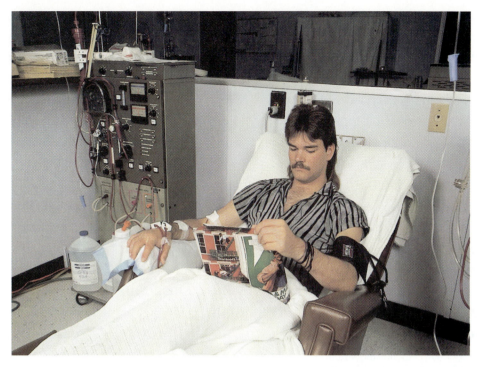

FIGURE 10.11 Patient undergoing hemodialysis in dialysis unit. (Southern Illinois University/ Photo Researchers, Inc.)

Professional Profile

Occupational Therapist

Occupational therapists specialize in rehabilitating patients/clients to perform activities that are essential for daily living. They develop a treatment plan and programs to restore personal care skills to persons with physical, mental, emotional, and/or developmental problems. Occupational therapists work in a wide variety of settings such as hospitals, mental health agencies, and rehabilitation centers. To become an occupational therapist, students must graduate from an accredited master's level occupational therapy program, complete six months of clinical experience, and pass a national certification examination given by the American Occupational Therapy Association. For more information on a career in occupational therapy, visit the American Occupational Therapy Association's web site at www.aota.org.

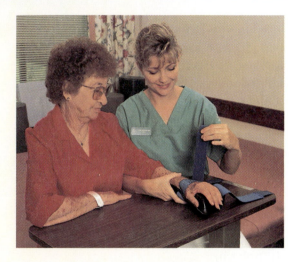

Occupational Therapist (OTR)

- **Provides occupational therapy as ordered by a physician**

- **Graduates from an approved four-year college or university occupational therapy program**
- **Completes six months of clinical experience**
- **Passes a national certification examination**

Abbreviations Relating to the Urinary System

ADH	antidiuretic hormone		**IPD**	intermittent peritoneal dialysis
ARF	acute renal failure		**IVP**	intravenous pyelogram
BUN	blood urea nitrogen		**IVU**	intravenous urogram
C & S	culture and sensitivity test		**K**	potassium
CAPD	continuous ambulatory peritoneal dialysis		**KUB**	kidney, ureter, bladder
CC	clean-catch urine specimen		**mL**	milliliter
Cl	chloride		**Na**	sodium
CRF	chronic renal failure		**pH**	acidity or alkalinity of urine
cysto	cystoscopic exam		**RP**	retrograde pyelogram
E. coli	*Escherichia coli*		**SG**	specific gravity
ESWL	extracorporeal shockwave lithotripsy		**TUR**	transurethral resection
GU	genitourinary		**U/A, UA**	urinalysis
HD	hemodialysis		**UC**	urine culture
H$_2$O	water		**UTI**	urinary tract infection
I & O	intake and output			

KEY TERMS

- adrenal correx
- afferent arteriole (**AFF** er ent ar **TEE** ree ohl)
- albumin (al **BEW** min)
- aldosterone (al **DOSS** ter ohn)
- antidiuretic (an tye dye yoo **RET** ik)
- antidiuretic hormone (ADH) (an tye dye yoo **RET** tik **HOR** mohn)
- anuria (an **YOO** ree ah)
- aorta (ay **OR** tah)
- atrial natriuretic hormone (ANH) (**AY** tree al nay tree yoo **RET** ik **HOR** mohn)
- bladder neck obstruction
- blood
- blood urea nitrogen (BUN) (**BLUD** yoo **REE** ah **NIGH** troh jen)
- Bowman's capsule (**BOW** manz **CAP** sool)
- calculus (**KAL** kew lus)
- calyx (**KAY** liks)
- catheterization (kath eh ter ih **ZAY** shun)
- clean catch specimen (CC)
- collecting tubule (**TOOB** yool)
- cortex (**KOR** teks)
- cystalgia (sis **TAL** jee ah)
- cystectomy (sis **TEK** toh mee)
- cystitis (siss **TYE** tis)
- cystocele (**SIS** toh seel)

- cystography (sis **TOG** rah fee)
- cystolith (**SIS** toh lith)
- cystoplasty (**SIS** toh plas tee)
- cystorrhagia (sis toh **RAH** jee ah)
- cystoscopy (sis **TOSS** koh pee)
- cystostomy (sis **TOSS** toh mee)
- cystotomy (sis **TOT** oh mee)
- diabetes mellitus (dye ah **BEE** teez **MELL** ih tus)
- distal convoluted tubule (**TOOB** yool)
- diuresis (dye yoo **REE** sis)
- dysuria (dis **YOO** ree ah)
- efferent arteriole (**EF** er ent ar **TEE** ree ohl)
- electrolyte (ee **LEK** troh lite)
- enuresis (en yoo **REE** sis)
- *Escherichia coli* (E. coli) (esh er **IK** ee ah **KOH** lye)
- excretory urography (**EKS** kreh tor ee yoo **ROG** rah fee)
- extracellular fluid (eks trah **SELL** yoo lar)
- extracorporeal shockwave lithotripsy (ESWL) (eks trah cor **POR** ee al shockwave **LITH** oh trip see)
- fascia (**FASH** ee ah)
- frequency
- genital tract (**JEN** ih tal)
- genitourinary (GU) (jen ih toh **YOO** rih nair ee)
- glomerular capsule (glom **AIR** yoo lar **CAP** sool)

- glomerular filtrate (glom **AIR** yoo lar **FILL** trayt)
- glomerulonephritis
  (gloh mair yoo loh neh **FRYE** tis)
- glomerulus (glom **AIR** yoo lus)
- glucose (**GLOO** kohs)
- glycosuria (glye kohs **YOO** ree ah)
- hematuria (hee mah **TOO** ree ah)
- hemodialysis (HD) (hee moh dye **AL** ih sis)
- hemorrhage (**HEM** eh rij)
- hesitancy
- hilum (**HIGH** lum)
- homeostasis (hoh mee oh **STAY** sis)
- hormones (**HOR** mohnz)
- hydronephrosis (high droh neh **FROH** sis)
- hypertension (high per **TEN** shun)
- hypospadias (high poh **SPAY** dee as)
- hypotension (high poh **TEN** shun)
- interstitial cystitis (in ter **STISH** al sis **TYE** tis)
- intravenous pyelogram (IVP)
  (in trah **VEE** nus **PYE** eh loh gram)
- kidneys
- lithotomy (lith **OT** oh mee)
- lithotripsy (**LITH** oh trip see)
- loop of Henle
- meatotomy (mee ah **TOT** oh mee)
- medulla (meh **DULL** ah)
- micturition (mik too **RIH** shun)
- nephrectomy (neh **FREK** toh mee)
- nephritis (neh **FRYE** tis)
- nephrography (neh **FROG** rah fee)
- nephrolithiasis (nef roh lith **EYE** ah sis)
- nephrologists (neh **FRALL** oh jist)
- nephrology (neh **FRALL** oh jee)
- nephroma (neh **FROH** mah)
- nephromalacia (nef roh mah **LAY** she ah)
- nephromegaly (nef roh **MEG** ah lee)
- nephrons (**NEF** ronz)
- nephropathy (neh **FROP** ah thee)
- nephropexy (**NEF** roh pek see)
- nephroptosis (nef rop **TOH** sis)
- nephrorrhaphy (nef **ROR** ah fee)
- nephrosclerosis (nef roh skleh **ROH** sis)
- nephrosis (neh **FROH** sis)
- nephrostomy (neh **FROS** toh mee)
- nephrotomy (neh **FROT** oh mee)
- nitrogenous wastes (nigh **TROJ** eh nus)
- nocturia (nok **TOO** ree ah)
- oliguria (ol ig **YOO** ree ah)
- osmosis (oz **MOH** sis)
- papilla (pah **PILL** ah)
- peristaltic waves (pair ih **STALL** tik)
- peritoneal dialysis
  (pair ih **TOH** nee al dye **AL** ih sis)

- peritoneum (pair ih toh **NEE** um)
- pH
- phimosis (fih **MOH** sis)
- polyuria (pol ee **YOO** ree ah)
- proximal convoluted tubule (**PROK** sim al con voh **LOOT** ed **TOOB** yool)
- pyelitis (pye eh **LYE** tis)
- pyelogram (**PYE** eh loh gram)
- pyelonephritis (pye eh loh neh **FRYE** tis)
- pyeloplasty (**PYE** ah loh plas tee)
- pyramids (**PEER** ah mids)
- pyuria (pye **YOO** ree ah)
- renal artery (**REE** nal **AR** teh ree)
- renal colic (**REE** nal **KOL** ik)
- renal corpuscle (**REE** nal **KOR** pus ehl)
- renal pelvis (**REE** nal **PELL** vis)
- renal transplant (**REE** nal)
- renal tubule (**REE** nal **TOOB** yool)
- renal vein (**REE** nal)
- retrograde pyelogram (RP)
  (**RET** roh grayd **PYE** eh loh gram)
- retroperitoneal (ret roh pair ih toh **NEE** al)
- rugae (**ROO** gay)
- semen (**SEE** men)
- serum electrolyte level (**SEE** rum ee **LEK** troh lite)
- sound
- sphincter (**SFINGK** ter)
- stricture (**STRIK** chur)
- toxins (**TOKS** ins)
- uremia (yoo **REE** mee ah)
- ureterectasis (yoo ree ter **EK** tah sis)
- ureterolith (yoo **REE** ter oh lith)
- ureterostenosis (yoo ree ter oh sten **OH** sis)
- ureters (yoo **REE** ters)
- urethra (yoo **REE** thrah)
- urethralgia (yoo ree **THRAL** jee ah)
- urethritis (yoo ree **THRIGH** tis)
- urethrorrhagia (yoo ree throh **RAH** jee ah)
- urethroscope (yoo **REE** throh scope)
- urethrostenosis (yoo ree throh steh **NOH** sis)
- urgency (**ER** jen see)
- urinalysis (U/A, UA) (yoo rih **NAL** ih sis)
- urinary bladder (**YOO** rih nair ee)
- urinary incontinence
  (**YOO** rih nair ee in **CON** tin ens)
- urinary meatus (**YOO** rih nair ee mee **AY** tus)
- urinary retention (**YOO** rih nair ee ree **TEN** shun)
- urine (**YOO** rin)
- urography (yoo **ROG** rah fee)
- urologist (yoo **RALL** oh jist)
- urology (yoo **RALL** oh jee)
- Wilm's tumor (**VILMZ TOO** mor)

Case Study

DISCHARGE SUMMARY

Admitting Diagnosis: Severe right side pain, visible blood in his urine.

Final Diagnosis: Pyelonephritis right kidney, complicated by chronic cystitis.

History of Present Illness: Patient has long history of frequent bladder infections, but denies any recent lower pelvic pain or dysuria. Earlier today he had rapid onset of severe right side pain, and is unable to stand fully erect. His temperature was 101°F and his skin was sweaty and flushed. He was admitted from the ER for further testing and diagnosis.

Summary of Hospital Course: Clean catch urinalysis revealed gross hematuria and pyuria, but no protenuria. A culture and sensitivity was ordered to identify the pathogen and a broad-spectrum IV antibiotic was started. An intravenous pyelogram indicated no calculi or obstructions in the ureters. Cystoscopy discovered evidence of chronic cystitis, bladder irritation, and a bladder neck obstruction. The obstruction appears to be congenital and the probable cause of the chronic cystitis. The patient was catheterized to insure complete emptying of the bladder and fluids were encouraged. Patient responded well to the antibiotic therapy and fluids, and his symptoms improved.

Discharge Plans: Patient was discharged home after three days in the hospital. He was switched to an oral antibiotic for the pyelonephritis and chronic cystitis. A repeat urinalysis is scheduled for next week. After all inflammation is corrected, will repeat cystoscopy to re-evaluate bladder neck obstruction. Will discuss if urethroplasty is indicated at that time.

CRITICAL THINKING QUESTIONS

1. This patient has a long history of frequent bladder infections. What did the physician discover that explained this?

2. Describe, in your own words, the patient's condition when he came to the emergency room.

3. This patient has gross hematuria. What do you think the term *gross* means in this context?

4. The following terms are not referred to in the Urinary System chapter. Define each in your own words, using your text as a dictionary.

   a. congenital

   b. chronic

   c. pathogen

   d. oral

5. Which of the following substances was not found in the patient's urine?

   a. protein

   b. pus

   c. blood

6. Compare and contrast pyelonephritis and glomerulonephritis.

Chart Note Transcription

Chart Note

The chart note below contains eleven phrases that can be reworded with a medical term that you learned in this chapter. Each phrase is identified with an underline. Determine the medical term and write your answers in the space provided.

Current Complaint: A 36-year-old male was seen by the specialist in the treatment of diseases of the urinary system[1] because of right flank pain and blood in the urine.[2]

Past History: Patient has a history of bladder infection;[3] denies experiencing any symptoms for two years.

Signs and Symptoms: A technique used to obtain an uncontaminated urine sample[4] obtained for laboratory analysis of the urine[5] revealed blood in the urine, but no pus in the urine.[6] A kidney X-ray made after inserting dye into the bladder[7] was normal on the left, but dye was seen filling the right tube between the kidney and bladder[8] only halfway to the kidney.

Diagnosis: Stone in the tube between the kidney and the bladder[9] on the right.

Treatment: Patient underwent the use of ultrasound waves to break up stones.[10] Pieces of dissolved kidney stones[11] were flushed out, after which symptoms resolved.

1 _____

2 _____

3 _____

4 _____

5 _____

6 _____

7 _____

8 _____

9 _____

10 _____

11 _____

Practice Exercises

A. STATE THE TERMS DESCRIBED USING THE COMBINING FORMS INDICATED.

The combining form ren/o refers to the kidney. Use it to write a term that means

1. Pertaining to the kidney _____
2. Acute pain in the kidney _____
3. Kidney stones _____

The combining form nephr/o also refers to the kidney. Use it to write a term that means

4. Removal of a kidney _____
5. Inflammation of the kidney _____
6. Kidney disease (general term) _____
7. Hardening of the kidney _____

The combining form cyst/o refers to the urinary bladder. Use it to write a term that means

8. Inflammation of the bladder _____
9. Suturing of the bladder _____
10. Surgical repair of the bladder _____
11. Herniation of the bladder _____

The combining form ur/o refers to urine and the urinary tract. Use it to write a term that means

12. X-ray study of the urinary tract _____
13. A urinary stone _____
14. Absence of urine _____
15. Painful urination _____

The combining form ureter/o refers to one or both of the ureters. Use it to write a term that means

16. A ureteral stone _____
17. Surgical repair of a ureter _____
18. Surgical removal of a ureter _____

The combining form urethr/o refers to the urethra. Use it to write a term that means

19. Surgical repair of the urethra _____
20. Surgical creation of an opening _____

B. DEFINE THE FOLLOWING TERMS.

1. dysuria _____
2. diuretic _____
3. nocturia _____
4. pyuria _____
5. pyelitis _____
6. nephropyelitis _____

7. lithotomy _____

8. enuresis _____

9. meatotomy _____

10. polyuria _____

11. oliguria _____

12. cystocele _____

C. WRITE THE MEDICAL TERM THAT MEANS

1. absence of urine _____

2. blood in the urine _____

3. kidney stone _____

4. crushing a kidney stone _____

5. inflammation of the urethra _____

6. pus in the urine _____

7. inflammation of the renal pelvis _____

8. painful urination _____

9. presence of blood in urine _____

10. presence of serum albumin in urine _____

11. excessive amount of urine _____

D. WRITE THE ABBREVIATION FOR THE FOLLOWING TERMS.

1. potassium _____

2. sodium _____

3. urinalysis _____

4. blood urea nitrogen _____

5. specific gravity _____

6. intravenous pyelogram _____

7. transurethral resection _____

E. IDENTIFY THE FOLLOWING ABBREVIATIONS.

1. KUB _____

2. ADH _____

3. cysto _____

4. GU _____

5. ESWL _____

6. UTI _____

7. UC _____

8. RP _____

9. ARF _____

10. CC _____

11. CRF _____

12. H_2O _____

F. Match the terms in column A with the definitions in column B.

A		B
1. _____	Wilm's tumor	a. kidney stones
2. _____	dysuria	b. involuntary urinating at night
3. _____	polyuria	c. childhood malignant kidney tumor
4. _____	pyuria	d. frequent voiding during the night
5. _____	oliguria	e. albumin in the urine
6. _____	albuminuria	f. reduced urine
7. _____	nocturia	g. painful urination
8. _____	enuresis	h. excessive urine
9. _____	nephrolithiasis	i. pus in the urine
10. _____	polycystic kidneys	j. multiple cysts in the kidneys

G. Use the following terms in the sentences that follow.

cystoscopy	cystostomy
intravenous pyelogram (IVP)	renal biopsy
nephropexy	ureterectomy
urinary tract infection	pyelolithectomy
renal transplant	

1. Juan suffered from chronic renal failure. His sister, Maria, donated one of her normal kidneys to him and he had a(n) _____ .

2. Anesha's floating kidney needed surgical fixation. Her physician performed a surgical procedure known as _____ .

3. Kenya's physician stated that she had a general infection that he referred to as a UTI. The full name for this infection is _____ .

4. The surgeons operated on Robert to remove calculus from his renal pelvis. The name of this surgery is _____ .

5. Charles had to have a small piece of his kidney tissue removed so that the physician could perform a microscopic evaluation. This procedure is called a(n) _____ .

6. Naomi had to have one of her ureters removed due to a stricture. This procedure is called _____ .

7. The physician had to create a temporary opening into Eric's bladder. This procedure is called _____ .

8. Sally's bladder and ureters were examined using a special instrument. This procedure is called a(n) _____ .

9. The doctors believe that Jacob has a tumor of the right kidney. They are going to do a test called a(n) _____ that requires them to inject a radiopaque contrast medium intravenously so that they can see the kidney on X-ray.

Getting Connected

Multimedia Extension Activities

CD-ROM
Use the CD-ROM enclosed with your textbook to gain additional reinforcement through interactive word building exercises, spelling games, labeling activities, and additional quizzes.

www.prenhall.com/fremgen
Use the above address to access the free, interactive Companion Website created for this textbook. Get hints, instant feedback, and textbook references to chapter-related multiple choice questions, and labeling and matching exercises. In addition, you will find an audio glossary, case studies, Internet exploration exercises, flashcards, and a comprehensive exam.

Answers

CASE STUDY (CRITICAL THINKING QUESTIONS)

1. Bladder neck obstruction   2. Severe right side pain, unable to stand fully erect, 101°F temperature, sweaty and flushed skin   3. Large enough to be visible with the naked eye   4. Present from birth, of long duration, disease-causing, by mouth   5. a—protein   6. Compare: both are infections of kidney tissue   Contrast: glomerulonephritis—infection is in the glomerulus and it allows protein to leak into the urine   Pyelonephritis—infection is in the renal pelvis portion of the kidney, more common, often caused by bladder infection moving up the ureters to the kidney.

CHART NOTE

1. urologist—specialist in the treatment of diseases of the urinary system   2. hematuria—blood in the urine
3. cystitis—bladder infection   4. clean catch specimen—technique used to obtain an uncontaminated urine sample
5. urinalysis (U/A, UA)—laboratory analysis of the urine   6. pyuria—pus in the urine   7. retrograde pyelogram—
a kidney X-ray made after inserting dye into the bladder   8. ureter—tube between the kidney and bladder
9. ureterolith—stone in the tube between the kidney and the bladder   10. extracorporeal shockwave lithotripsy
(ESWL)—use of ultrasound waves to break up stones   11. calculi—kidney stones

PRACTICE EXERCISES

A. 1. renal   2. renal colic   3. renal calculi   4. nephrectomy   5. nephritis   6. nephropathy   7. nephrosclerosis
8. cystitis   9. cystorrhaphy   10. cystoplasty   11. cystocele   12. urogram   13. urolith   14. anuria   15. dysuria
16. ureterolith   17. ureteroplasty   18. ureterectomy   19. urethroplasty   20. urethrostomy
B. 1. painful urination   2. increases urine production   3. urination at night   4. pus in urine   5. inflammation of renal
pelvis   6. inflammation of kidney and renal pelvis   7. incision to remove stone   8. bed-wetting   9. enlargement of
urinary opening   10. excessive urination   11. reduced urination   12. herniation of bladder
C. 1. anuria   2. hematuria   3. calculus/nephrolith   4. lithotripsy   5. urethritis   6. pyuria   7. pyelitis   8. dysuria
9. hematuria   10. albuminuria   11. polyuria
D. 1. K   2. Na   3. UA   4. BUN   5. SG   6. IVP   7. TUR
E. 1. kidneys, ureters, bladder   2. antidiuretic hormone   3. cystoscopy   4. genitourinary   5. extracorporeal
shock-wave lithotripsy   6. urinary tract infection   7. urine culture   8. retrograde pyelogram   9. acute renal failure
10. clean-catch urine specimen   11. chronic renal failure   12. water
F. 1. c   2. g   3. h   4. i   5. f   6. e   7. d   8. b   9. a   10. j
G. 1. renal transplant   2. nephropexy   3. urinary tract infection   4. pyelolithectomy   5. renal biopsy
6. ureterectomy   7. cystostomy   8. cystoscopy   9. IVP

Chapter 11

REPRODUCTIVE SYSTEM

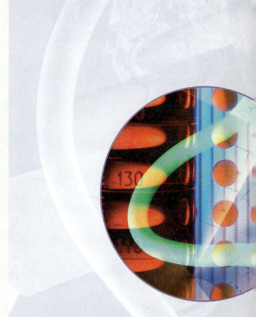

LEARNING OBJECTIVES

Upon completion of this chapter, you will be able to:

- Recognize the combining forms and suffixes introduced in this chapter.

- Gain the ability to pronounce medical terms and major anatomical structures.

- List the major organs of the male and female reproductive systems and their functions.

- Use medical terms to describe circumstances relating to pregnancy.

- Identify the symptoms and origin of sexually transmitted diseases.

- Describe genetic disorders.

- Build male and female reproductive system medical terms from word parts.

- Define vocabulary, pathology, diagnostic, and therapeutic medical terms relating to the male and female reproductive systems.

- Interpret abbreviations associated with the male and female reproductive systems.

Overview

fertilization	**impregnation**	**sperm**
genitalia	**ova**	

The reproductive organs are not necessary to sustain the life of the individual, but they are necessary for a continuation of the human race. The actual reproductive process consists of the male cells called **sperm** joining the female cells called **ova** (**OH** vah) or eggs. This process is called **fertilization** (fer til ih **ZAY** shun) or **impregnation** (im preg **NAY** shun). The term **genitalia** (jen ih **TAY** lee ah) is a general term used to refer to both male and female reproductive organs.

PART I: *Female Reproductive System*

ORGANS OF THE FEMALE REPRODUCTIVE SYSTEM

fallopian tubes (2)	**uterus**	**vulva**
ovaries (2)	**vagina**	

COMBINING FORMS RELATING TO THE FEMALE REPRODUCTIVE SYSTEM

amni/o	amnion	**mast/o**	breast
amnion/o	amnion	**men/o**	menses, menstruation
cervic/o	neck, cervix	**metr/o**	uterus
cervis/o	cervix, neck	**nat/i, nat/o**	birth
chori/o	chorion	**o/o**	egg
colp/o	vagina	**omphal/o**	navel, umbilicus
culd/o	cul-de-sac	**oophor/o**	ovary
embry/o	embryo	**ov/i, ov/o**	egg
episi/o	vulva, episiotomy	**ovari/o**	ovary
fet/i, fet/o	fetus	**ovul/o**	ovary
galact/o	milk	**par/o, part/o**	labor, childbirth
gravid/o	pregnancy	**perine/o**	perineum
gynec/o	woman, female	**salping/o**	fallopian tubes, uterine tubes
hymen/o	hymen	**umbilic/o**	umbilical
hyster/o	uterus, womb	**uter/o**	uterus
labi/o	lip	**vagin/o**	vagina
lact/o	milk	**vulv/o**	vulva
mamm/o	breast		

Suffix	Meaning	Example
-arche	beginning	menarche
-cyesis	state of pregnancy	pseudocyesis
-gravida	pregnancy	multigravida
-para	to bear	nullipara
-rrhea	discharge; flow	lactorrhea
-salpinx	fallopian tube	pyosalpinx
-tocia	labor, childbirth	dystocia
-version	turning of	anteversion

ANATOMY AND PHYSIOLOGY OF THE FEMALE REPRODUCTIVE SYSTEM

Bartholin's glands	**labia minora**	**vagina**
clitoris	**ovaries**	**vaginal orifice**
fallopian tubes	**perineum**	**vulva**
hymen	**urinary meatus**	
labia majora	**uterus**	

The female reproductive system consists of both internal and external organs. The internal organs of reproduction are located in the pelvic cavity and consist of one **uterus** (**YOO** ter us), two **ovaries** (**OH** vah reez), two **fallopian tubes** (fah **LOH** pee an **TOOBS**), and the **vagina** (vah **JIGH** nah), which extends to the external part of the body (see Figure 11.1).

The external genitalia are also referred to as the **vulva** (**VULL** vah) and contain the **labia majora** (**LAY** bee ah mah **JOR** ah), **labia minora** (**LAY** bee ah mih **NOR** ah), **urinary meatus** (**YOO** rih nair ee mee **AY** tus), **clitoris** (**KLIT** oh ris), **hymen** (**HIGH** men), **vaginal orifice** (**VAJ** ih nal **OR** ih fis), and **Bartholin's** (**BAR** toh linz) **glands**. The region between the vaginal opening and the anus is referred to as the **perineum** (pair ih **NEE** um).

INTERNAL ORGANS OF REPRODUCTION

Uterus

anteflexion	**endometrium**	**menstruation**
anteversion	**fetus**	**ovum**
cervix (Cx)	**fundus**	**retroflexion**
corpus	**ligaments**	**retroversion**

The uterus is a hollow, pear-shaped organ that contains a thick muscular wall, a mucous membrane lining, and a rich supply of blood. It lies in the center of the pelvic cavity. The

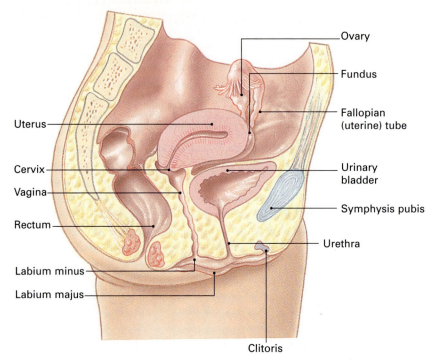

Labium minus (singular), Labia minora (plural)
Labium majus (singular), Labia majora (plural)

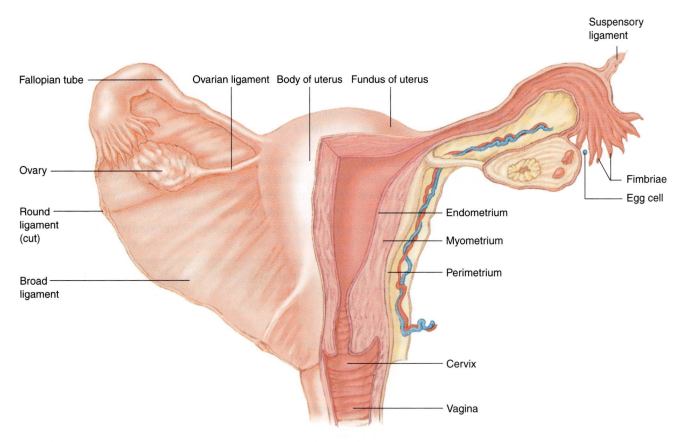

FIGURE 11.1 Female organs of reproduction.

position of the uterus is between the bladder and the rectum. It is normally bent slightly forward, which is called **anteflexion** (an tee **FLEK** shun) and contains three parts: (1) **fundus** (**FUN** dus) or upper portion, with a rounded edge; (2) **corpus** (**KOR** pus) or body, which is the central portion; and (3) **cervix** (**SER** viks) **(Cx)**, or lower portion, which is also called the neck of the uterus and opens into the vagina.

The uterus is the organ that receives the fertilized egg or **ovum** (**OH** vum). The fertilized egg becomes implanted in the uterus, which provides nourishment and protection for the developing **fetus** (**FEE** tus) until birth. The thick muscular walls of the uterus assist in propelling the fetus through the birth canal at delivery.

The inner layer, or **endometrium** (en doh **MEE** tre um), of the uterine wall contains a rich blood supply. The endometrium reacts to hormonal changes every month, which results in **menstruation** (men stroo **AY** shun). During a pregnancy, the lining of the uterus does not leave the body but remains to nourish the unborn child.

The cervix is the area from which a **PAP (Papanicolaou) smear** is taken by the physician. This test, named for George Papanicolaou (pap ah **NIK** oh low), a Greek physician, is a life-saving test to detect early cancer. The physician removes scrapings of cervical cells, which are then examined to detect the presence of cellular changes or cancer.

The position of the uterus is important to note since an incorrect position, or malposition, can result in the inability to either conceive a child or to carry a fetus to full-term delivery. The terminology for abnormal positions of the uterus is as follows:

anteflexion (an tee **FLEK** shun): While the uterus is normally in this position, an exaggeration of the forward bend of the uterus is abnormal. The forward bend is near the neck of the uterus. The position of the cervix, or opening of the uterus, remains normal.

retroflexion (ret roh **FLEK** shun): In this position the uterus is bent back (retro-) upon itself. However, the cervix remains in its normal position.

anteversion (an tee **VER** zhun): In this position the uterus is actually tipped forward without bending, so that the cervix becomes tipped toward the sacrum and the fundus is tipped toward the pubis.

retroversion (ret roh **VER** zhun): The uterus is turned backward with the cervix in an exaggerated direction of the pubis.

These conditions can be caused by a variety of conditions, such as pregnancies or injury, that weaken the fibrous **ligaments** (**LIG** ah ments) that support the uterus. In some cases surgery is necessary to correct the condition.

It is important to know the various parts of the uterus since they are used in descriptions of medical examinations and surgical procedures. For instance, during pregnancy, the height of the fundus is an important measurement for estimating the stage of pregnancy and the size of the fetus. Following birth, massaging the fundus with pressure applied in a circular pattern stimulates the uterine muscle to contract to help stop bleeding. Patients may be more familiar with a common term for uterus: *womb*. However, the correct medical term is uterus.

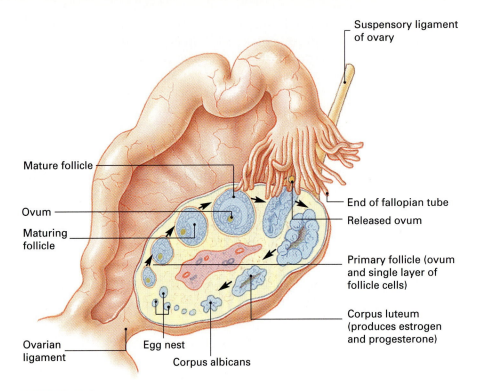

Suspensory ligament
of ovary

Mature follicle

Ovum

Maturing
follicle

End of fallopian tube

Released ovum

Primary follicle (ovum
and single layer of
follicle cells)

Corpus luteum
(produces estrogen
and progesterone)

Ovarian
ligament

Egg nest

Corpus albicans

FIGURE 11.2 The ovary.

Ovaries

estrogen	**ovulation**	**progesterone**
menopause	**parasites**	

There are two ovaries located on each side within the pelvic cavity (see Figure 11.2). These are small almond-shaped glands that produce the ovum, or egg, and hormones.

The singular for egg is *ovum*. The plural term for many eggs is *ova*. The term ova is not used exclusively when discussing the human reproductive system. For instance, testing the stool for ova and **parasites** (**PAR** ah sites) is used to detect the presence of parasites or their ova in the digestive tract, a common cause for severe diarrhea.

The ovaries produce important hormones that are also discussed in the endocrine system. **Estrogen** (**ESS** troh jen) and **progesterone** (proh **JES** ter ohn) are critical during the process of menstruation and **menopause** (**MEN** oh pawz). After **ovulation** (ov yoo **LAY** shun), which is the release of an ovum from the ovary during the menstrual cycle, the ovum is captured by the fingerlike projections of the fallopian tubes (see Figure 11.3)

Fallopian (or Uterine) Tubes

ectopic pregnancy

fimbriae

The fallopian tubes are approximately 5-½ inches long and project from either side of the upper area of the uterus. These two tubes end with fingerlike projections, **fimbriae**

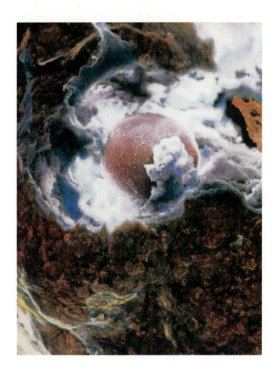

FIGURE 11.3 Enhanced color scanning electron micrography of the ovulation process. The egg (pink in center) has ruptured. The external surface of the ovary is brown in this photo. (P. M. Motta and J. Van Blekrom/Science Photo Library/Photo Researchers, Inc.)

(**FIM** bree ay), near the ovaries. The primary purpose of the fallopian tubes is to propel the ovum from the ovary to the uterus so that it can implant. The meeting of the egg and sperm, called fertilization, may actually take place within the upper one-half of the fallopian tubes. When the fertilized egg adheres or implants to the fallopian tube instead of moving into the uterus, a condition called **ectopic** (ek **TOP** ik) **pregnancy** exists, which will require surgical intervention. Implantation of the fertilized egg occurring in any area of the abdomen other than the uterus is abnormal.

Vagina

hymen	**vaginal orifice**
semen	

The vagina is a muscular tube, lined with mucous membranes, that extends from the cervix of the uterus to the outside of the body. The vagina allows for the passage of the monthly menstrual flow of blood and tissue. In addition, it is the receptacle for the male sex cells, or **semen** (**SEE** men), which is the fluid containing sperm, during sexual intercourse. The vagina also serves as the birth canal through which the baby passes during a normal vaginal birth.

The **hymen** is a thin membraneous tissue that covers the external vaginal opening or **vaginal orifice.** This membrane is broken during the first sexual encounter of the female and can also be broken prematurely by the use of tampons and during physical activity.

EXTERNAL ORGANS OF REPRODUCTION

Bartholin's glands	**labia majora**
clitoris	**labia minora**
erectile tissue	

The vulva is a general term meaning the external female genitalia. **Bartholin's glands,** which secrete mucus for lubrication, are located on each outer side of the vaginal opening.

The **labia majora** and **labia minora** are folds of skin that serve as protection for the genitalia and, in particular, the urinary meatus. Since the urinary tract and the reproductive organs are located in close proximity to one another and each contains mucous membranes that can transport infection, there is a danger of infection entering the urinary tract. The **clitoris** is a small organ containing **erectile** (ee **REK** tile) **tissue** that is covered by the labia minora. The clitoris contains sensitive tissue that is aroused during sexual stimulation and corresponds to the penis in the male.

PREGNANCY

abortion	dilation stage	placental stage
amnion	effacement	pregnancy
amniotic fluid	embryo	premature
breech presentation	fetus	spontaneous abortion
chorion	gestational period	umbilical cord
congenital anomalies	labor	viable
contractions	miscarriage	
crowning	placenta	

Pregnancy (**PREG** nan see) refers to the period of time during which a baby grows and develops in its mother's uterus (see Figure 11.4). The normal length of time for a pregnancy, its **gestational** (jess **TAY** shun al) **period,** is 40 weeks. If a baby is born before completing at least 37 weeks of gestation, it is considered **premature.**

FIGURE 11.4 Anatomy of pregnancy.

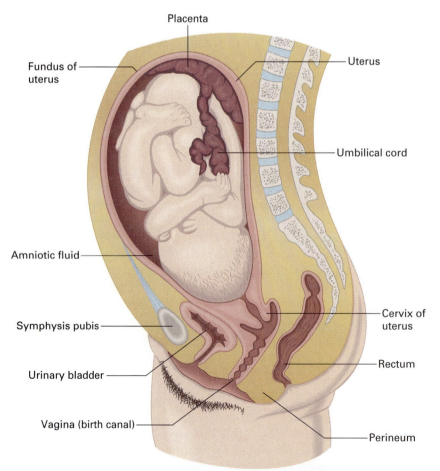

The term **abortion** (ah **BOR** shun) has different meanings for medical professionals and the general population. The medical term for the termination of a pregnancy before a fetus becomes **viable** (**VYE** ah bull), meaning that it can live on its own, is *abortion*. However, the general population equates the term *abortion* with an induced termination of pregnancy. The term **miscarriage,** although not the accepted medical term, can be used when discussing an unplanned loss of the fetus with the parents. The correct medical term for a miscarriage is **spontaneous abortion.**

During pregnancy the female body undergoes many changes. In fact, all of the body systems become involved in the development of a healthy infant (see Figures 11.5 to 11.7). The actual process, and relevant terminology, will be discussed briefly. From the time the fertilized egg implants in the uterus until approximately the end of the eighth week, the infant is referred to as an **embryo** (**EM** bree oh). This is a period of rapid growth and formation of the major organ systems. Following the embryo stage until birth, the infant is a **fetus** (**FEE** tus).

During the embryo stage of gestation, the organs and organ systems of the body are formed. Therefore, this is a very common time for **congenital anomalies** (con **JEN** ih tal ah **NOM** ah lees), or birth defects, to occur. This may happen before the woman is even aware of being pregnant.

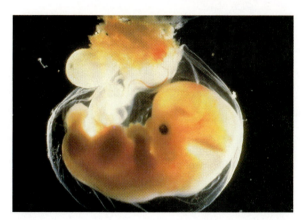

FIGURE 11.5   Fetus at five to six weeks in utero. (Petit Format/Nestle/Photo Researchers, Inc.)

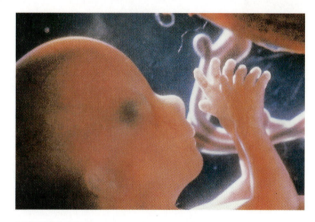

FIGURE 11.6   Fetus at four months in utero. (Petit Format/Nestle/Photo Researchers, Inc.)

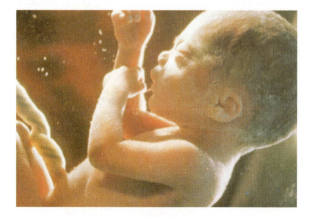

FIGURE 11.7   Fetus at eight to nine months (almost full term) in utero. (Petit Format/Nestle/Science Source/Photo Researchers, Inc.)

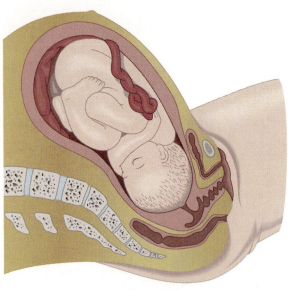

FIRST STAGE:
First uterine contraction to dilation of cervix

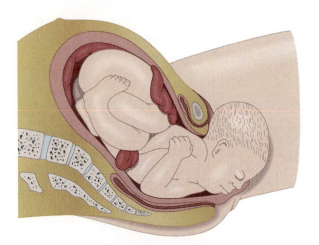

SECOND STAGE:
Birth of baby or expulsion

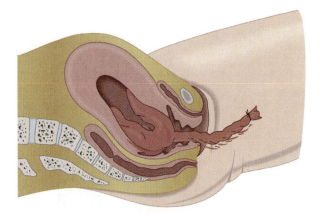

THIRD STAGE:
Delivery of placenta

FIGURE 11.8 Three stages of labor.

One of the most important developments is the **placenta** (plah **SEN** tah), which is the spongy structure through which the fetus is nourished. The fetus is attached to the placenta by way of the **umbilical cord** (um **BILL** ih kal **KORD**).

The fetus is surrounded by two membranous sacs, the **amnion** (**AM** nee on) and the **chorion** (**KOR** ree on). The amnion is the innermost sac and it holds the **amniotic** (am nee **OT** ik) **fluid** in which the fetus floats. The chorion is an outer, protective sac and also forms part of the placenta.

Labor (**LAY** bor) is the actual process of expelling the fetus from the uterus and through the vagina (see Figure 11.8). The first stage is referred to as the **dilation** (dye **LAY** shun) **stage,** in which the uterine muscles contract in an attempt to expel the fetus. During this process the fetus presses on the cervix and causes it to dilate or expand. When the cervix is completely dilated at 10 centimeters, the second stage of labor begins. The thinning of the cervix is referred to as **effacement** (eh **FACE** ment). This stage ends with the birth of the baby (Figure 11.9). Generally, the head of the baby appears first, which is referred to as **crowning** (see Figures 11.10 and 11.11). In some cases the baby's buttocks will appear first, and this is referred to as a **breech presentation** (see Figure 11.12).

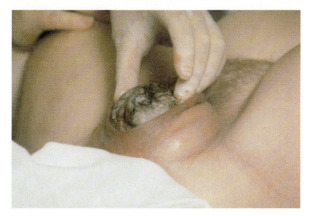

FIGURE 11.9 Baby's head at vaginal opening. (D. Van Rossum/Petit Format/Photo Researchers, Inc.)

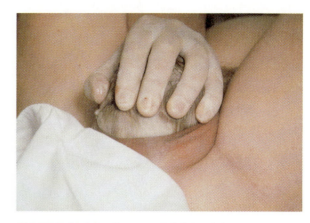

FIGURE 11.10 Crowning. Baby's head almost completely out of birth canal. (D. Van Rossum/Petit Format/Photo Researchers, Inc.)

FIGURE 11.11 Head completely out of birth canal. (D. Van Rossum/ Petit Format/Photo Researchers, Inc.)

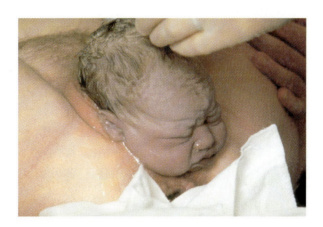

FIGURE 11.12 Breech presentation.

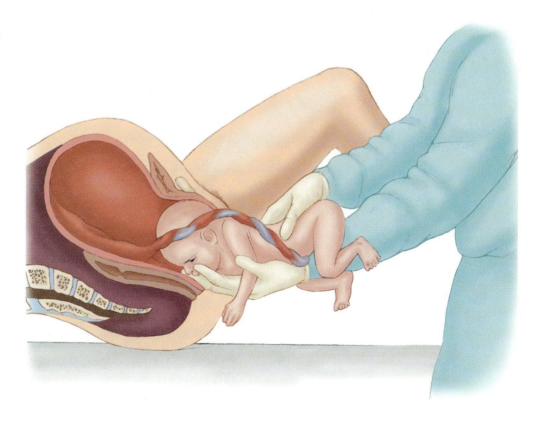

FIGURE 11.13 Neonate
(newborn).

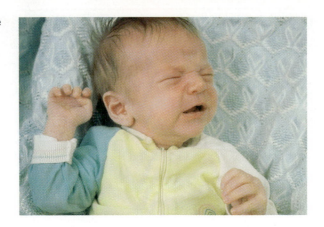

The last stage of labor is the **placental** (plah **SEN** tal) **stage,** during which the *placenta* or *afterbirth* is delivered (see also Figure 11.8). Immediately after childbirth, the uterus again begins **contractions,** causing the placenta to be expelled through the vagina. See Figure 11.13 for illustration of neonate.

MAMMARY GLAND (BREAST)

areola	**lactation**	**nurse**
breasts	**mammary glands**	

The **mammary** (**MAM** ah ree) **glands,** or **breasts** (see Figure 11.14), play a vital role in the reproductive process since they nourish the newborn. The size of the breasts, which vary greatly from woman to woman, has no bearing on the ability to **nurse** or feed a baby. **Lactation** (lak **TAY** shun), or milk production, causes an enlargement of the breasts to the point of becoming uncomfortable. A nursing child relieves this discomfort.

The **areola** (ah **REE** oh la) is the area around the nipple of the breast, which changes during pregnancy from pink to a brownish color. The areola portion of the breast contains glands that secrete milk after the birth of a child. As long as the breast is stimulated by the nursing infant, the breast will continue to secrete milk.

FIGURE 11.14 Mammary gland.

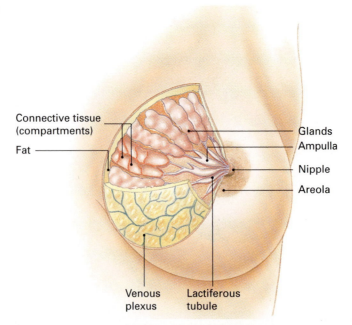

Word Building Relating to the Female Reproductive System

The following list contains examples of medical terms built directly from word parts. The definition for these terms can be determined by a straightforward translation of the word parts.

Combining Form	Combined With	Medical Term	Definition
amni/o	-centesis	amniocentesis (am nee oh sen **TEE** sis)	puncture to withdraw amniotic fluid
	-otomy	amniotomy (am nee **OT** oh mee)	incision into amnion
	-rrhea	amniorrhea (am nee oh **REE** ah)	flow of fluid from amnion
	-scopy	amnioscopy (am nee **OSS** koh pee)	process of viewing amnion
cervic/o	-ectomy	cervicectomy (ser vih **SEK** toh mee)	excision of cervix
	endo- -itis	endocervicitis (en doh ser vih **SIGH** tis)	inflammation within cervix
colp/o	-scope	colposcope (**KOL** poh scope)	instrument to view inside vagina
	-scopy	colposcopy (kol **POSS** koh pee)	process of viewing vagina
episi/o	-otomy	episiotomy (eh peez ee **OT** oh mee)	incision into vulva
	-rrhaphy	episiorrhaphy (eh peez ee **OR** ah fee)	suture of vulva
gynec/o	-ologist	gynecologist (gigh neh **KOL** oh jist)	specialist in female (reproductive system)
	-ology	gynecology (gigh ne **KOL** oh jee)	study of female (reproductive system)
hyster/o	-ectomy	hysterectomy (hiss ter **EK** toh mee)	excision of the uterus
	-pexy	hysteropexy (**HISS** ter oh pek see)	surgical fixation of the uterus
	-rrhexis	hysterorrhexis (hiss ter oh **REK** sis)	ruptured uterus
lact/o	-ic	lactic (**LAK** tik)	pertaining to milk
	-rrhea	lactorrhea (lak toh **REE** ah)	milk discharge
mamm/o	-algia	mastalgia (mas **TAL** jee ah)	breast pain
	-gram	mammogram (**MAM** moh gram)	record of the breast
	-graphy	mammography (mam **OG** rah fee)	process of recording the breast
	-plasty	mammoplasty (**MAM** moh plas tee)	surgical repair of breast
mast/o	-ectomy	mastectomy (mass **TEK** toh mee)	excision of the breast
men/o	a- -rrhea	amenorrhea (ah men oh **REE** ah)	no menstrual flow
	dys- -rrhea	dysmenorrhea (dis men oh **REE** ah)	difficult menstrual flow
	oligo- -rrhea	oligomenorrhea (ol lih goh men oh **REE** ah)	scanty menstrual flow
	-rrhagia	menorrhagia (men oh **RAY** jee ah)	abnormal, rapid menstrual flow
metr/o	endo- -itis	endometritis (en doh meh **TRY** tis)	inflammation within the uterus
	peri- -itis	perimetritis (pair ih meh **TRY** tis)	inflammation around the uterus
	-rrhea	metrorrhea (meh troh **REE** ah)	flow from uterus
nat/o	neo-	neonate (**NEE** oh nayt)	newborn
	neo- -ology	neonatology (nee oh nay **TALL** oh jee)	study of the newborn
oophor/o	-ectomy	oophorectomy (oh off oh **REK** toh mee)	excision of the ovary
	-itis	oophoritis (oh off oh **RIGH** tis)	inflammation of the ovary
part/o	ante- -um	antepartum (an tee **PAR** tum)	before birth
	post- -um	postpartum (post **PAR** tum)	after birth
salping/o	-cyesis	salpingocyesis (sal ping goh sigh **EE** sis)	tubal pregnancy
	-ostomy	salpingostomy (sal ping **GOS** toh mee)	create an opening in the fallopian tube

(continued)

Prefix	Suffix	Medical Term	Definition
pseudo-	-cyesis	pseudocyesis (soo doh sigh **EE** sis)	false pregnancy
nulli-	-gravida	nulligravida (null ih **GRAV** ih dah)	no pregnancies
primi-		primigravida (**PREM** i grav i da)	first pregnancy
nulli-	-para	nullipara (null **IP** ah rah)	no births
primi-		primipara (prem **IP** ah rah)	first birth
hemato-	-salpinx	hematosalpinx (hee mah toh **SAL** pinks)	blood in fallopian tube
hydro-		hydrosalpinx (high droh **SAL** pinks)	water in fallopian tube
pyo-		pyosalpinx (pie oh **SAL** pinks)	pus in fallopian tube

Vocabulary Relating to the Female Reproductive System

breech presentation	Placement of the fetus in which the buttocks or feet are presented first for delivery rather than the head.
congenital anomaly (con JEN ih tal ah NOM ah lee)	Any abnormality present at birth. A *birth defect.*
contraception (kon trah SEP shun)	Prevention of a pregnancy using artificial means such as an intrauterine device (IUD) or medication (birth control pills).
crowning	When the head of the baby is visible through the vaginal opening. A sign that birth is imminent.
dystocia (dis TOH she ah)	Abnormal or difficult labor and childbirth.
emergency childbirth	Childbirth that happens quickly before the mother and assistants are prepared. The signs and symptoms of an impending delivery are • A bloody show of mucus • Strong uterine contractions that become close together • A feeling and desire of the mother to bear down or push with the contractions • The visible bulging of the baby's head against the bag of waters (if it has not broken) • The baby's head *crowning* or appearing at the vaginal opening
estimated date of confinement (EDC)	Estimation date when the baby will be born based on a calculation from the last menstrual period of the mother.
fetal (FEE tal) heart rate (FHR)	The heart rate of the fetus can be monitored with an electronic device during labor to detect signs of fetal distress. The normal heart rate of the fetus is rapid, at ranges from 120 to 160 beats per minute.
fetal (FEE tal) heart tone (FHT)	Listening for the fetal heart sound to determine strength and general condition of the fetus. This is also done during the labor process.
gestation (jess TAY shun)	Length of time from conception to birth, generally nine months. Calculated from the first day of the last menstrual period, with a range of from 259 days to 280 days.
gravida (GRAV ih dah)	A pregnant woman.
gynecologist (gigh neh KOL oh jist)	A physician specializing in treating conditions and diseases of the female reproductive system.

gynecology (GYN, gyn) (gigh neh KOL oh jee)	Study of the diseases of the female reproductive system, including the breasts.
intrauterine (in trah YOO ter in) **device (IUD)**	Device that is inserted into the uterus by a physician for the purpose of contraception.
lactation (lak TAY shun)	The function of secreting milk after childbirth from the breasts or mammary glands.
last menstrual period (LMP)	Date when the last menstrual period started.
low birth weight (LBW)	Abnormally low weight in a newborn. It is usually considered to be less than 5.5 pounds.
menarche (men AR kee)	The first menstrual period.
menopause (MEN oh pawz)	Cessation or ending of menstrual activity. This is generally between the ages of 40 and 55.
multigravida (mul ti GRAV ih da)	Woman who has had more than one pregnancy.
multipara (mull TIP ah rah)	Woman who has given birth to more than one child.
neonate (NEE oh nayt)	Term used to describe the newborn infant during the first four weeks of life.
newborn (NB)	Interchangeable with the term *neonate,* meaning infants less than one month old.
nulligravida (null ih GRAV ih dah)	Woman who has never been pregnant.
nullipara (null IP ah rah)	Woman who has never produced a viable baby.
obstetrician (ob steh TRISH an)	A physician specializing in providing care for pregnant women and delivering infants.
obstetrics (OB) (ob STET riks)	Branch of medicine that treats women during pregnancy and childbirth, and immediately after childbirth.
postpartum (post PAR tum)	Period immediately after delivery or childbirth.
premature birth	Delivery in which the infant (neonate) is born before the thirty-seventh week of gestation (pregnancy).
premenstrual syndrome (PMS) (pre MEN stroo al SIN drohm)	Symptoms that develop just prior to the onset of a menstrual period, which can include irritability, headache, tender breasts, and anxiety.
prenatal visits (pre NAY tl)	Appointments with a physician or nurse practitioner for the purpose of monitoring the mother's pregnancy.
puberty (PEW ber tee)	Beginning of menstruation and the ability to reproduce.
puerperium (pew er PEER ee um)	Term used when discussing the mother's first three to six weeks after childbirth.

Pathology of the Female Reproductive System

abruptio placenta (ah BRUP she oh plah SEN tah)	Emergency condition in which the placenta tears away from the uterine wall before the twentieth week of pregnancy. Requires immediate delivery of the baby.
amenorrhea (ah men oh REE ah)	Absence of menstruation, which can be the result of many factors, including pregnancy, menopause, and dieting.
cervical cancer (SER vih kal CAN ser)	Malignant growth in the cervix. An especially difficult type of cancer to treat that causes 5 percent of the cancer deaths in women. PAP tests have helped to detect early cervical cancer.
cervical polyps (SER vih kal PALL ips)	Fibrous or mucous tumor or growth found in the cervix. These are removed surgically if there is a danger that they will become malignant.
cervicitis (ser vih SIGH tis)	Inflammation of the cervix.
choriocarcinoma (kor ee oh kar sih NOH mah)	Rare type of cancer of the uterus. May occur following a normal pregnancy or abortion.
condyloma (kon dih LOH ma)	Wartlike growth on the external genitalia.
cystocele (SIS toh seel)	Hernia or outpouching of the bladder that protrudes into the vagina. This may cause urinary frequency and urgency.
dysmenorrhea (dis men oh REE ah)	Painful cramping that is associated with menstruation.
eclampsia (eh KLAMP see ah)	Convulsive seizures and coma occurring in the woman between the twentieth week of pregnancy and the first week of postpartum. Often associated with hypertension.
ectopic (ek TOP ik) pregnancy	Fetus that becomes abnormally implanted outside the uterine cavity. This is a condition requiring immediate surgery.
endometrial (en doh MEE tree al) cancer	Cancer of the endometrial lining of the uterus.
endometriosis (en doh mee tree OH sis)	Abnormal condition of endometrium tissue appearing throughout the pelvis or on the abdominal wall. This tissue is usually found within the uterus.
erythroblastosis fetalis (eh rith roh blass TOH sis fee TAL iss)	Condition developing in the baby when the mother's blood type is Rh-negative and the father's is Rh-positive. The baby's red blood cells can be destroyed as a result of this condition. Treatment is early diagnosis and blood transfusion.
fibroid tumor (FIGH broyd TOO mor)	Benign tumor or growth that contains fiberlike tissue. Uterine fibroid tumors are the most common tumors in women.
mastitis (mas TYE tis)	Inflammation of the breast, which is common during lactation but can occur at any age.
menorrhagia (men oh RAY jee ah)	Excessive bleeding during the menstrual period. Can be measured either in the total number of days or the amount of blood or both.
ovarian carcinoma (oh VAY ree an kar sih NOH mah)	Cancer of the ovary.

ovarian cyst (oh VAY ree an SIST)	Sac that develops within the ovary.
pelvic inflammatory disease (PID) (PELL vik in FLAM mah toh ree dih ZEEZ)	Any inflammation of the female reproductive organs, generally bacterial in nature.
placenta previa (plah SEN tah PREE vee ah)	When the placenta has become placed in the lower portion of the uterus and, in turn, blocks the birth canal (see Figure 11.15).
preeclampsia (pre eh KLAMP see ah)	Toxemia of pregnancy that, if untreated, can result in true eclampsia. Symptoms include hypertension, headaches, albumin in the urine, and edema.
prolapsed umbilical cord (pro LAPS'D um BILL ih kal)	When the umbilical cord of the baby is expelled first during delivery and is squeezed between the baby's head and the vaginal wall. This presents an emergency situation since the baby's circulation is compromised.
prolapsed uterus (pro LAPS'D YOO ter us)	Fallen uterus that can cause the cervix to protrude through the vaginal opening. Generally caused by weakened muscles from vaginal delivery or as the result of pelvic tumors pressing down.
salpingitis (sal pin JIGH tis)	Inflammation of the fallopian tube or tubes.
spontaneous abortion	Loss of a fetus without any artificial aid. Also called a *miscarriage*.
stillbirth	Birth in which a viable-aged fetus dies before or at the time of delivery.
toxic shock syndrome (TSS)	Rare and sometimes fatal staphylococcus infection that generally occurs in menstruating women.
tubal pregnancy (TOO bal PREG nan see)	Implantation of a fetus within the fallopian tube instead of the uterus. Requires immediate surgery.
vaginitis (vaj in EYE tis)	Inflammation of the vagina, generally caused by a microorganism.

FIGURE 11.15 Placenta previa.

PLACENTA PREVIA

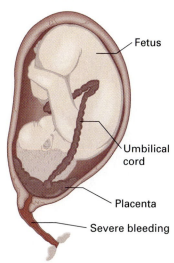

Fetus

Umbilical cord

Placenta

Severe bleeding

Diagnostic Procedures Relating to the Female Reproductive System

amniocentesis (am nee oh sen TEE sis)	Puncturing of the amniotic sac using a needle and syringe for the purpose of withdrawing amniotic fluid for testing. Can assist in determining fetal maturity, development, and genetic disorders.
cervical biopsy (SER vih kal BYE op see)	Taking a sample of tissue from the cervix to test for the presence of cancer cells.
Doppler ultrasound (DOP ler ULL trah sound)	Using an instrument placed externally over the uterus to examine the fetal heart. Named after Christian Doppler, an Austrian physicist.
endometrial biopsy (en doh MEE tre al BYE op see)	Taking a sample of tissue from the lining of the uterus to test for abnormalities.
fetal (FEE tal) monitoring	Using electronic equipment placed on the mother's abdomen to check the baby's heart rate and strength during labor.
hysterosalpingography (HSG) (hiss ter oh sal pin GOG rah fee)	Taking an X-ray after injecting radiopaque material into the uterus and oviducts.
hysteroscopy (hiss ter OS koh pee)	Inspection of the uterus using a special endoscope instrument.
laparotomy (lap ah ROT oh mee)	Surgical opening of the abdomen; an abdominal operation.
PAP (Papanicolaou) (pap ah NIK oh low) smear	Test for the early detection of cancer of the cervix named after the developer of the test, George Papanicolaou, a Greek physician. A scraping of cells is removed from the cervix for examination under a microscope.
pelvic examination	Physical examination of the vagina and adjacent organs performed by a physician placing the fingers of one hand into the vagina. A visual examination is performed using a speculum (see Figure 11.16).
pelvic ultrasonography (PELL vik ull trah son OG rah fee)	Use of ultrasound waves to produce an image or photograph of an organ, such as the uterus, ovaries, or fetus.
pelvimetry (pell VIM eh tree)	Measurement of the pelvic area that helps in determining if the fetus can be delivered vaginally.
pregnancy (PREG nan see) test	Chemical test that can determine a pregnancy during the first few weeks. Can be performed in a physician's office or with a home-testing kit.

FIGURE 11.16 Vaginal speculum. (Simon Fraser/ Science Photo Library/Photo Researchers, Inc.)

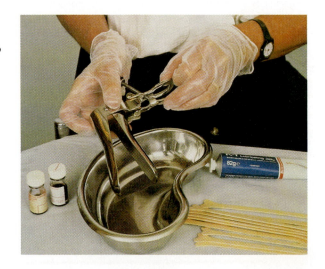

Treatment Procedures Relating to the Female Reproductive System

abortion (AB) (ah BOR shun)	Termination of a pregnancy before the fetus reaches a viable point in development.
cauterization (kaw ter ih ZAY shun)	Destruction of tissue using an electric current, a caustic product, a hot iron, or by freezing.
cesarean section (see SAYR ee an) (CS, C-section)	Surgical delivery of a baby through an incision into the abdominal and uterine walls. Legend has it that the Roman emperor, Julius Caesar, was the first person born by this method.
colposcopy (kol POSS koh pee)	Visual examination of the cervix and vagina using a colposcope or instrument with a magnifying lens.
conization (kon ih ZAY shun	Surgical removal of a core of cervical tissue. Also refers to partial removal of the cervix.
cryosurgery (cry oh SER jer ee)	Exposing tissues to extreme cold to destroy tissues. Used in treating malignant tumors, and to control pain and bleeding.
culdoscopy (kul DOS koh pee)	Examination of the female pelvic cavity by introducing an endoscope through the wall of the vagina.
dilation and curettage (D & C) (dye LAY shun and koo reh TAHZ)	Surgical procedure in which the opening of the cervix is dilated and the uterus is scraped or suctioned of its lining or tissue. Often performed after a spontaneous abortion and to stop excessive bleeding from other causes.
episiotomy (eh peez ee OT oh mee)	Surgical incision of the perineum to facilitate the delivery process. Can prevent an irregular tearing of tissue during birth.
hymenectomy (high men EK toh mee)	Surgical removal of the hymen. Performed when the hymen tissue is particularly tough.
hysterectomy (hiss ter EK toh mee)	Removal of the uterus.
Kegel exercises (KAY gull)	Exercises named after A. H. Kegel, an American gynecologist, who developed them to strengthen female pubic muscles. The exercises are useful in treating incontinence and as an aid in the childbirth process.
laparoscopy (lap ar OS koh pee)	Examination of the peritoneal cavity using an instrument called a laparoscope. The instrument is passed through a small incision made by the surgeon into the abdominopelvic cavity (see Figure 11.17).
oophorectomy (oh off oh REK to mee)	Surgical removal of an ovary.
panhysterectomy (pan hiss ter EK toh mee)	Excision of the entire uterus, including the cervix.
panhysterosalpingo-oophorectomy (pan hiss ter oh sal ping goh oh off oh REK toh mee)	Removal of the entire uterus, cervix, ovaries, and fallopian tubes. A total hysterectomy.
polypectomy (pall ih PEK toh mee)	Surgical removal of a polyp.
salpingo-oophorectomy (sal ping goh off oh REK toh mee)	Removal of a fallopian tube and ovary.
tubal ligation (TOO bal lye GAY shun)	Surgical tying off of the fallopian tubes to prevent conception from taking place. Results in sterilization of the female.

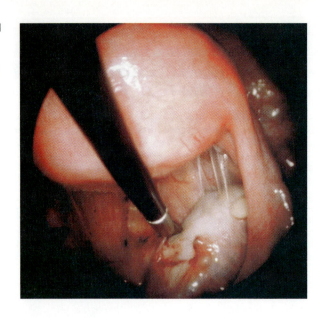

Abbreviations Relating to the Female Reproductive System

AH	abdominal hysterectomy	**IUD**	intrauterine device
Cx	cervix	**LMP**	last menstrual period
D&C	dilation and curettage	**MH**	marital history
DUB	dysfunctional uterine bleeding	**NGU**	nongonococcal urethritis
ECC	endocervical curettage	**PAP**	Papanicolaou test
ERT	estrogen replacement therapy	**PID**	pelvic inflammatory disease
FSH	follicle-stimulating hormone	**PMP**	previous menstrual period
GYN, gyn	gynecology	**PMS**	premenstrual syndrome
HRT	hormone replacement therapy	**TAH**	total abdominal hysterectomy
HSG	hysterosalpingography	**TSS**	toxic shock syndrome
HSO	hysterosalpingoophrectomy		

Obstetrical Abbreviations

AB	abortion	**GI, grav I**	first pregnancy
CPD	cephalopelvic disproportion	**HCG**	human chorionic gonadotropin
CS, CS-section	cesarean section	**HSG**	hysterosalpingography
CWP	childbirth without pain	**LBW**	low birth weight
DOB	date of birth	**NB**	newborn
EDC	estimated date of confinement	**OB**	obstetrics
FEKG	fetal electrocardiogram	**PI, para I**	first delivery
FHR	fetal heart rate	**PKU**	phenylketonuria
FHT	fetal heart tone	**RML**	right mediolateral (episiotomy)
FTND	full-term normal delivery	**UC**	uterine contractions

- abortion (AB) (ah **BOR** shun)
- abruptio placenta (ah **BRUP** she oh plah **SEN** tah)
- amenorrhea (ah men oh **REE** ah)
- amniocentesis (am nee oh sen **TEE** sis)
- amnion (**AM** nee on)
- amniotic fluid (am nee **OT** ik)
- amniorrhea (am nee oh **REE** ah)
- amnioscopy (am nee **OSS** koh pee)
- amniotomy (am nee **OT** oh mee)
- anteflexion (an tee **FLEK** shun)
- antepartum (an tee **PAR** tum)
- anteversion (an tee **VER** zhun)
- areola (ah **REE** oh la)
- Bartholin's glands (**BAR** toh linz)
- breasts
- breech presentation
- cauterization (kaw ter ih **ZAY** shun)
- cervical biopsy (**SER** vih kal **BYE** op see)
- cervical cancer (**SER** vih kal **CAN** ser)
- cervical polyps (**SER** vih kal **PALL** ips)
- cervicectomy (ser vih **SEK** toh mee)
- cervicitis (ser vih **SIGH** tis)
- cervix (Cx) (**SER** viks)
- cesarean section (CS, C-section) (see **SAYR** ee an)
- choriocarcinoma (kor ee oh kar sih **NOH** mah)
- chorion (**KOR** ree on)
- clitoris (**KLIT** oh ris)
- colposcope (**KOL** poh scope)
- colposcopy (kol **POSS** koh pee)
- condyloma (kon dih **LOH** mah)
- congenital anomalies (con **JEN** ih tal ah **NOM** ah lees)
- conization (kon ih **ZAY** shun)
- contraception (kon trah **SEP** shun)
- contractions
- corpus (**KOR** pus)
- crowning
- cryosurgery (cry oh **SER** jer ee)
- culdoscopy (kul **DOS** koh pee)
- cystocele (**SIS** toh seel)
- dilation and curettage (D & C) (dye **LAY** shun and koo reh **TAHZ**)
- dilation stage (dye **LAY** shun)
- Doppler ultrasound (**DOP** ler **ULL** trah sound)
- dysmenorrhea (dis men oh **REE** ah)
- dystocia (dis **TOH** she ah)
- eclampsia (eh **KLAMP** see ah)
- ectopic pregnancy (ek **TOP** ik)
- effacement (eh **FACE** ment)
- embryo (**EM** bree oh)

- emergency childbirth
- endocervicitis (en doh ser vih **SIGH** tis)
- endometrial biopsy (en doh **MEE** tree al **BYE** op see)
- endometrial cancer (en doh **MEE** tree al **CAN** ser)
- endometriosis (en doh mee tree **OH** sis)
- endometritis (en doh meh **TRY** tis)
- endometrium (en doh **MEE** tree um)
- episiorrhaphy (eh peez ee **OR** ah fee)
- episiotomy (eh peez ee **OT** oh mee)
- erectile tissue (ee **REK** tile)
- erythroblastosis fetalis (eh rith roh blas **TOH** sis fee **TAL** iss)
- estimated date of confinement (EDC)
- estrogen (**ESS** troh jen)
- fallopian tubes (fah **LOH** pee an **TOOBS**)
- fertilization (fer til ih **ZAY** shun)
- fetal heart rate (FHR) (**FEE** tal)
- fetal heart tone (FHT) (**FEE** tal)
- fetal monitoring (**FEE** tal)
- fetus (**FEE** tus)
- fibroid tumor (**FIGH** broyd **TOO** mor)
- fimbriae (**FIM** bree ay)
- fundus (**FUN** dus)
- genitalia (jen ih **TAY** lee ah)
- gestation (jess **TAY** shun)
- gestational period (jess **TAY** shun al)
- gravida (**GRAV** ih dah)
- gynecologist (gigh neh **KOL** oh jist)
- gynecology (GYN, gyn) (gigh neh **KOL** oh jee)
- hematosalpinx (hee mah toh **SAL** pinks)
- hydrocephalus (high droh **SEFF** ah lus)
- hydrosalpinx (high droh **SAL** pinks)
- hymen (**HIGH** men)
- hymenectomy (high men **EK** toh mee)
- hysterectomy (hiss ter **EK** toh mee)
- hysteropexy (**HISS** ter oh pek see)
- hysterorrhexis (hiss ter oh **REK** sis)
- hysterosalpingography (HSG) (hiss ter oh sal pin **GOG** rah fee)
- hysteroscopy (hiss ter **OS** koh pee)
- impregnation (im preg **NAY** shun)
- intrauterine device (IUD) (in trah **YOO** ter in)
- Kegel exercises (**KAY** gull)
- labia majora (**LAY** bee ah mah **JOR** ah)
- labia minora (**LAY** bee ah mih **NOR** ah)
- labor (**LAY** bor)
- lactation (lak **TAY** shun)
- lactic (**LAK** tik)
- lactorrhea (lak toh **REE** ah)

- laparoscopy (lap ar **OS** koh pee)
- laparotomy (lap ah **ROT** oh mee)
- last menstrual period (LMP)
- ligaments (**LIG** ah ments)
- low birth weight (LBW)
- mammary glands (**MAM** ah ree)
- mammogram (**MAM** moh gram)
- mammography (mam **OG** rah fee)
- mammoplasty (**MAM** moh plas tee)
- mastalgia (mas **TAL** jee ah)
- mastectomy (mass **TEK** toh mee)
- mastitis (mas **TYE** tis)
- menarche (men **AR** kee)
- menopause (**MEN** oh pawz)
- menorrhagia (men oh **RAY** jee ah)
- menstruation (men stroo **AY** shun)
- metrorrhea (meh troh **REE** ah)
- miscarriage
- multigravida (mull tih **GRAV** ih da)
- multipara (mull **TIP** ah rah)
- neonate (**NEE** oh nayt)
- neonatology (nee oh nay **TALL** oh jee)
- newborn (NB)
- nulligravida (null ih **GRAV** ih dah)
- nullipara (null **IP** ah rah)
- nurse
- obstetrician (ob steh **TRISH** an)
- obstetrics (OB) (ob **STET** riks)
- oligomenorrhea (ol ih goh men oh **REE** ah)
- oophorectomy (oh off oh **REK** toh mee)
- oophoritis (oh off oh **RIGH** tis)
- ova (**OH** vah)
- ovarian carcinoma
  (oh **VAY** ree an kar sih **NOH** mah)
- ovarian cyst (oh **VAY** ree an **SIST**)
- ovaries (**OH** vah reez)
- ovulation (ov yoo **LAY** shun)
- ovum (**OH** vum)
- panhysterectomy (pan hiss ter **EK** toh mee)
- panhysterosalpingo-oophorectomy (pan hiss ter
  oh sal ping goh oh off oh **REK** toh mee)
- PAP smear (Papanicolaou) (pap ah **NIK** oh low)
- parasites (**PAR** ah sites)
- pelvic examination (**PELL** vik)
- pelvic inflammatory disease (PID) (**PELL** vik in
  FLAM mah toh ree dih **ZEEZ**)
- pelvic ultrasonography
  (**PELL** vik ull trah son **OG** rah fee)

- pelvimetry (pell **VIM** eh tree)
- perimetritis (pair ih meh **TRY** tis)
- perineum (pair ih **NEE** um)
- placenta (plah **SEN** tah)
- placenta previa (plah **SEN** tah **PRE** vee ah)
- placental stage (plah **SEN** tal)
- polypectomy (pall ih **PEK** toh mee)
- postpartum (post **PAR** tum)
- preeclampsia (pre eh **KLAMP** see ah)
- pregnancy (**PREG** nan see)
- pregnancy test (**PREG** nan see)
- premature
- premature birth
- premenstrual syndrome (PMS)
  (pre **MEN** stroo al **SIN** drohm)
- prenatal visits (pre **NAY** tl)
- primigravida (pri mih **GRAV** ih dah)
- primipara (prem **IP** ah rah)
- progesterone (proh **JES** ter ohn)
- prolapsed umbilical cord
  (pro **LAPS'D** um **BILL** ih kal)
- prolapsed uterus (pro **LAPS'D YOO** ter us)
- pseudocyesis (soo doh sigh **EE** sis)
- puberty (**PEW** ber tee)
- puerperium (pew er **PEER** ee um)
- pyosalpinx (pie oh **SAL** pinks)
- retroflexion (ret roh **FLEK** shun)
- retroversion (ret roh **VER** zhun)
- salpingitis (sal pin **JIGH** tis)
- salpingocyesis (sal ping goh sigh **EE** sis)
- salpingo-oophorectomy
  (sal ping goh oh off oh **REK** toh mee)
- salpingostomy (sal ping **GOS** toh mee)
- semen (**SEE** men)
- sperm
- spontaneous abortion
- stillbirth
- toxic shock syndrome (TSS)
- tubal ligation (**TOO** bal lye **GAY** shun)
- tubal pregnancy (**TOO** bal **PREG** nan see)
- umbilical cord (um **BILL** ih kal **KORD**)
- urinary meatus (**YOO** rih nair ee mee **AY** tus)
- uterus (**YOO** ter us)
- vagina (vah **JIGH** nah)
- vaginal orifice (**VAJ** ih nal **OR** ih fis)
- vaginitis (vaj in **EYE** tis)
- viable (**VYE** ah b'l)
- vulva (**VULL** vah)

Case Study I

HIGH-RISK OBSTETRICS CONSULTATION REPORT

Reason for Consultation: High-risk pregnancy with late-term bleeding.

History of Present Illness: Patient is 23-years-old. She is currently estimated to be at 240 days of gestation. She has had a 23# weight gain with this pregnancy. Amniocentesis at 20 weeks indicated male fetus with no evidence of genetic or developmental disorders. She noticed moderate degree of vaginal bleeding this morning but denies any cramping or pelvic pain. She immediately saw her obstetrician who referred her for high-risk evaluation.

Past Medical History: This patient is multigravida but nullipara with 3 early miscarriages without obvious cause. She was diagnosed with cancer of the left ovary 4 years ago. It was treated with a left oophorectomy and chemotherapy. She continues to undergo full-body CT-scan every six months, and there has been no evidence of metastasis since that time. Menarche was at age 13 and her menstrual history is significant for menorrhagia resulting in chronic anemia.

Results of Physical Examination: Patient appears well nourished and abdominal girth appears consistent with length of gestation. She is understandably quite anxious regarding the sudden spotting. Pelvic ultrasound indicates placenta previa with placenta almost completely overlying cervix. However, there is no evidence of abruptio placentae at this time. Fetal size estimate is consistent with 25 weeks of gestation. The fetus is turned head down and the umbilical cord is not around the neck. The fetal heart tones are strong with a rate of 90 beats/minute. There is no evidence of cervical effacement or dilation at this time.

Recommendations: Fetus appears to be developing well and in no distress at this time. The placenta appears to be well-attached on ultrasound, but the bleeding is cause for concern. With the extremely low position of the placenta, this patient is at very high risk for abruptio placentae when cervix begins effacement and dilation. She may require early delivery by cesarean section at that time. She will definitely require c-section at onset of labor. At this time, recommend bed rest with bathroom privileges. She is to return every other day for two weeks and every day after that for evaluation of cervix and fetal condition. She is to call immediately if she notes any further bleeding or change in activity level of the fetus.

CRITICAL THINKING QUESTIONS

1. Describe in your own words the treatment this patient received for her ovarian cancer. What procedure does she continue to have every six months?

2. Describe in your own words this patient's menstrual history.

3. Which of the following choices describes this patient?

    a. She has never been pregnant.

    b. She has several live children.

    c. She has no live children.

    d. She has been pregnant several times.

4. This patient has placenta previa. What procedure discovered this condition? However, the physician is much more concerned about abruptio placentae. Explain why?

5. Describe the condition of the fetus.

6. The following two phrases are not specifically defined by your text. Explain what you believe them to mean based on the context of this consultation report.

    a. high-risk pregnancy

    b. abdominal girth appears consistent with length of gestation

Chart Note Transcription I

Chart Note

The chart note below contains eleven phrases that can be reworded with a medical term that you learned in this chapter. Each phrase is identified with an underline. Determine the medical term and write your answers in the space provided.

Current Complaint: Patient is a 45-year-old female is seen by her <u>physician who specializes in treating diseases of the female reproductive tract's</u>[1] office with complaints of increasingly severe <u>painful cramping with menstruation.</u>[2]

Past History: Patient has <u>given birth to more than one child</u>[3] and had a <u>tying off of the tubes between ovaries and uterus</u>[4] six months after the birth of her youngest child.

Signs and Symptoms: No abnormalities were identified with an <u>image of the pelvic cavity produced by ultrasound waves.</u>[5] However, results of an <u>X-ray taken after injecting dye into the uterus and tubes</u>[6] indicated <u>blocked bilateral tubes between the ovaries and uterus.</u>[7] <u>Examination of the abdominopelvic cavity using a laparoscope</u>[8] found scarring around bilateral tubes between the ovaries and uterus. Biopsies found evidence of <u>inner layer of the uterus</u>[9] in all scarred areas.

Diagnosis: <u>Abnormal condition of inner uterine layer appearing in the pelvis.</u>[10]

Treatment: Surgical <u>removal of entire uterus, ovaries, and fallopian tubes.</u>[11]

1 _____

2 _____

3 _____

4 _____

5 _____

6 _____

7 _____

8 _____

9 _____

10 _____

11 _____

Practice Exercises I

A. COMPLETE THE FOLLOWING STATEMENTS.

1. The study of the female reproductive system is the medical specialty of _____ .
2. A physician who specializes in the treatment of women is called a(n) _____ .
3. A general term that refers to both the male and female reproductive organs is _____ .
4. The time required for the development of a fetus is called the _____ period.
5. The absence of menstruation is called _____ .
6. The female sex cell is a(n) _____ .
7. The inner lining of the uterus is called the _____ .
8. The organ in which the developing fetus resides is called the _____ .
9. The tubes that extend from the outer edges of the uterus and assist in transporting the ova and sperm are called _____ .
10. One of the longest terms used in medical terminology refers to the removal of the uterus, cervix, ovaries, and fallopian tubes. This term is _____ .

B. STATE THE TERMS DESCRIBED USING THE COMBINING FORMS PROVIDED.

The combining form vagin/o refers to the vagina. Use it to write a term that means

1. relating to the vagina _____
2. inflammation of the vagina _____
3. vaginal hernia _____
4. related to the vagina and labia _____
5. fungus infection (mycosis) of the vagina _____
6. relating to the vagina and the perineum _____

The combining form colp/o also refers to the vagina. Use it to write a term that means

7. visual examination of the vagina using an instrument _____
8. instrument used to examine the vagina and cervix _____
9. suture of the vagina _____

The combining form cervic/o refers to the cervix. Use it to write a term that means

10. inflammation of the cervix _____
11. pertaining to the cervix _____

The combining form uter/o refers to the uterus. Use it to write a term that means

12. relating to the uterus and the cervix _____
13. pertaining to the uterus and the rectum _____

The combining form hyster/o also refers to the uterus. Use it to write a term that means

14. uterine disease _____
15. surgical fixation of the uterus _____
16. uterine spasm _____
17. removal of the uterus _____
18. hernia of the uterus _____
19. rupture of the uterus _____
20. suture of the uterus _____

The combining form metr/o also refers to the uterus. Use it to write a term that means

21. any uterine disease _____

22. inflammation of the uterus and peritoneum _____

23. uterine hemorrhage _____

The combining form gyne/o refers to the female. Use it to write a term that means

24. study of the diseases of the female _____

25. physician who specializes in diseases of women _____

The combining form oophor/o refers to the ovaries. Use it to write a term that means

26. inflammation of an ovary and a fallopian tube _____

27. inflammation of an ovary _____

The combining form salping/o refers to the fallopian tubes. Use it to write a term that means

28. inflammation of the fallopian tube _____

29. inflammation of a fallopian tube and ovary _____

30. removal of the uterus, fallopian tubes, and ovaries _____

C. CHANGE THE FOLLOWING SINGULAR TERMS TO PLURAL TERMS.

1. ovum _____

2. labium _____

D. USE THE SUPPLIED SUFFIXES TO CREATE A MEDICAL TERM FOR EACH DEFINITION RELATING TO THE FEMALE REPRODUCTIVE SYSTEM.

1. -arche for a word that means beginning of menses _____

2. -gravida for a word that means many pregnancies _____

3. -para for a word that means having had no births _____

E. IDENTIFY THE FOLLOWING ABBREVIATIONS.

1. Cx	_____	9. FHT	_____
2. LMP	_____	10. CS	_____
3. TAH	_____	11. NB	_____
4. OB	_____	12. PMS	_____
5. PAP	_____	13. TSS	_____
6. MH	_____	14. LBW	_____
7. PID	_____	15. ERT	_____
8. DOB	_____		

F. WRITE THE ABBREVIATIONS FOR THE FOLLOWING TERMS.

1. phenylketonuria	_____	6. dilation and curettage	_____
2. right mediolateral	_____	7. dysfunctional uterine bleeding	_____
3. uterine contractions	_____	8. gynecology	_____
4. full-term normal delivery	_____	9. abortion	_____
5. childbirth without pain	_____		

G. DEFINE THE FOLLOWING COMBINING TERMS.

1. metr/o _____
2. hyster/o _____
3. gynec/o _____
4. episi/o _____
5. oophor/o _____
6. ovar/o _____
7. salping/o _____
8. gravid/o _____
9. vagin/o _____
10. mamm/o _____

H. MATCH THE TERMS IN COLUMN A WITH THE DEFINITIONS IN COLUMN B.

A	B
1. _____ uterus	a. thin membrane
2. _____ ovary	b. secrete oil
3. _____ vagina	c. outer lip
4. _____ labia majora	d. erectile tissue, similar to penis in male
5. _____ labia minora	e. normal position of uterus
6. _____ endometrium	f. uterus abnormally tipped
7. _____ clitoris	g. pear-shaped organ
8. _____ hymen	h. birth canal
9. _____ Bartholin's gland	i. inner lip
10. _____ anteversion	j. top of uterus
11. _____ anteflexion	k. produces eggs
12. _____ fundus	l. uterine lining

I. MATCH THE TERMS IN COLUMN A WITH THE DEFINITIONS IN COLUMN B.

A	B
1. _____ dysmenorrhea	a. after birth
2. _____ menarche	b. nursing
3. _____ menopause	c. newborn
4. _____ neonate	d. abort
5. _____ gravida	e. painful menstruation
6. _____ lactation	f. cessation of menstruation
7. _____ prenatal	g. beginning of menstruation
8. _____ postpartum	h. before birth
9. _____ miscarry	i. a pregnant woman

J. USE THE FOLLOWING TERMS IN THE SENTENCES THAT FOLLOW.

premenstrual syndrome   puberty   eclampsia
gestational   Rh-factor   D&C
fibroid tumor   conization   cesarean section
stillbirth   endometriosis   laparoscopy

1. Roberta has a negative blood factor and her husband's is positive. What condition will the physician test for in her baby? _____

2. Kesha had a core of tissue from her cervix removed for testing. This is called _____ .

3. Joan delivered a baby that had died while still in the uterus. She had a(n) _____ .

4. Emily's doctor asked her when her last menstrual period was in order to calculate the date of arrival for her baby. The time period for the baby's development is called the _____ period.

5. Ashley has just started her first menstrual cycle. She is said to have entered _____ .

6. Kimberly is experiencing tender breasts, headaches, and some irritability just prior to her monthly menstrual cycle. This may be _____ .

7. Ana has been scheduled for an examination in which her physician will use an instrument to observe her abdominal cavity to rule out the diagnosis of severe endometriosis. The physician will insert the instrument through a small incision. This procedure is called a(n) _____ .

8. Lenora is scheduled to have a hysterectomy as a result of a long history of large benign growths in her uterus that have caused pain and bleeding. Lenora has a(n) _____ .

9. Tiffany's physician has recommended that she have a uterine scraping to stop excessive bleeding after a miscarriage. She will be scheduled for a _____ .

10. Stacey is having frequent prenatal checkups to prevent the serious condition of pregnancy called _____ .

11. Marion has experienced painful menstrual periods as a result of the lining of her uterus being displaced into her pelvic cavity. This is called _____ .

12. The results of Shataundra's pelvimetry indicate that she will probably require a(n) _____ for her baby's delivery.

Getting Connected

Multimedia Extension Activities

CD-ROM

Use the CD-ROM enclosed with your textbook to gain additional reinforcement through interactive word building exercises, spelling games, labeling activities, and additional quizzes.

www.prenhall.com/fremgen

Use the above address to access the free, interactive Companion Website created for this textbook. Get hints, instant feedback, and textbook references to chapter-related multiple choice questions, and labeling and matching exercises. In addition, you will find an audio glossary, case studies, Internet exploration exercises, flashcards, and a comprehensive exam.

Overview

PART II: *Male Reproductive System*

ORGANS OF THE MALE REPRODUCTIVE SYSTEM

bulbourethral gland	**prostate gland**	**testes (2)**
epididymis	**scrotum**	**vas deferens**
penis	**seminal vesicle (2)**	

COMBINING FORMS RELATING TO THE MALE REPRODUCTIVE SYSTEM

andr/o	male	**prostat/o**	prostate
balan/o	glans penis	**semin/o**	semen
crypt/o	hidden	**sperm/o**	sperm, spermatozoa, aspermia
epididym/o	epididymis	**spermat/o**	sperm
gon/o	seed	**test/o**	testes
hydr/o	water, fluid	**varic/o**	varicose veins
orch/o	testes	**vas/o**	vas deferens
orchi/o	testes	**vesicul/o**	seminal vesicle
orchid/o	testes		

ANATOMY AND PHYSIOLOGY OF THE MALE REPRODUCTIVE SYSTEM

bulbourethral gland	**prostate gland**	**testes**
Cowper's gland	**scrotum**	**urethra**
epididymis	**semen**	**vas deferens**
penis	**seminal vesicles**	

The male reproductive system is a combination of reproduction and urinary systems. In the male, the major organs of reproduction are located outside the body in the **scrotum** (**SKROH** tum) and **penis** (**PEE** nis). The scrotum contains the two **testes** (**TESS** teez) and the **epididymis** (ep ih **DID** ih mis). The penis contains the **urethra** (yoo **REE** thrah), which carries both urine and **semen** (**SEE** men) to the outside of the body (see Figure 11.18).

The internal organs of reproduction are the **seminal vesicles** (**SEM** ih nal **VESS** ih kls), **vas deferens** (**VAS DEF** er enz), the **prostate** (**PROSS** tayt) **gland,** and **bulbourethral** (buhl boh yoo **REE** thral) or **Cowper's** (**KOW** perz) **gland.**

EXTERNAL ORGANS OF REPRODUCTION

Scrotum

perineum

The scrotum is actually a sac that serves as a container for the testes or testicles. This sac, which is divided by a septum, supports the testicles and lies between the legs and behind

Reproductive System • **361**

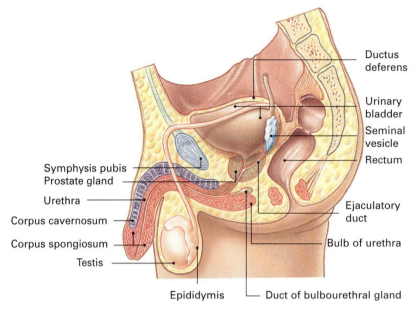

FIGURE 11.18　Male reproductive organs.

the penis. During early childhood, the testes will frequently retract up into the pelvic cavity. However, as the young boy reaches one year in age, the testes will remain permanently in the scrotum.

The **perineum** (pair ih **NEE** um) of the male is similar to that in the female. It is the area between the anus, or rectal opening, and the scrotum.

Testes

seminiferous tubules	**spermatozoon**
sperm	**testicles**
spermatozoa	**testosterone**

The testes are oval in shape and are responsible for the development of **sperm** (see Figure 11.19) within the **seminiferous tubules** (sem ih **NIF** er us **TOO** byoo ls). The testes must be maintained at the proper temperature for the sperm to survive. This lower temperature level is controlled by the placement of the scrotum outside the body. The hormone **testosterone** (tess **TOSS** ter ohn), which is responsible for the growth and development of the male reproductive organs, is also produced by the testes. The testes are also referred to as the **testicles** (**TESS** tih kls). The singular for *testes* is *testis*.

Spermatozoon (sper mat oh **ZOH** on) and its plural form, **spermatozoa** (sper mat oh **ZOH** ah), are other terms that mean *sperm*. You have no doubt realized that there can be several terms with the same meaning in medical terminology. You must continue to remain flexible when working with these terms in your career. In some cases, one term will be more commonly used, depending on the type of medical specialty or even what part of the country you are in.

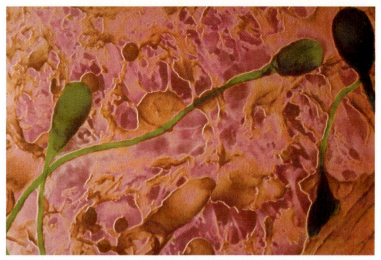

FIGURE 11.19 Enhanced color photo of sperm through electron microscope. (Dennis Kunkel/CNRI/Phototake NYC)

Penis

circumcision   erectile tissue   glans penis

ejaculation   foreskin   prepuce

The penis is the male sex organ containing **erectile** (ee **REK** tile) **tissue** that is encased in skin. This organ transports the semen into the female vagina. The soft tip of the penis is referred to as the **glans penis** (**GLANS PEE** nis). It is protected by a covering called the **prepuce** (**PREE** pyoos) or **foreskin** (**FOR** skin). It is this covering of skin that is removed during the procedure known as **circumcision** (ser kum **SIH** zhun). The penis becomes erect during sexual stimulation, which allows it to be placed within the female for the **ejaculation** (ee jak yoo **LAY** shun) of semen.

Epididymis

ductus deferens

The epididymis is a coiled tubule that lies on top of the testes within the scrotum. This tube is placed partially inside and partially outside the body since it runs down the testicles and then turns back up to become the vas deferens as it enters the abdominal cavity. The vas deferens is also known as the **ductus deferens** (**DUCK** tus **DEF** er enz).

INTERNAL ORGANS OF REPRODUCTION

Vas Deferens or Ductus Deferens

spermatic cord

vasectomy

The vas deferens carries sperm from the epididymis up into the pelvic cavity of the male and becomes contained within the **spermatic cord** (sper **MAT** ik **KORD**). This cord contains nerves, arteries, veins, and lymphatic tissue. It continues around the bladder and empties into the urethra.

Seminal Vesicles

semen

The two seminal vesicles are small glands located at the base of the urinary bladder. These vesicles join the vas deferens at the point the vas deferens empties into the urethra. The seminal vesicles secrete a fluid that nourishes the sperm. This liquid, along with the sperm, constitutes **semen,** which is the fluid that is eventually ejaculated during sexual intercourse.

Prostate Gland

The prostate gland is located just below the urinary bladder. It surrounds the urethra and when enlarged can cause difficulty in urination. The prostate is important for the reproductive process since it secretes an alkaline fluid that assists in keeping the sperm alive.

Bulbourethral or Cowper's Glands

The bulbourethral glands or Cowper's glands, are small glands located on either side of the urethra just below the prostate. They also produce a fluid that joins with semen to become a part of the ejaculate during sexual intercourse. The alkaline fluid from this gland neutralizes the acidity in the urethra.

Urethra

coitus	sexual intercourse
copulation	sphincter

The male urethra extends from the urinary bladder to the external opening in the penis. It serves a dual function: the elimination of urine and the ejaculation of semen containing sperm. During the ejaculation process, a **sphincter** (**SFINGK** ter), which is a contracting muscle at the base of the bladder, closes to keep urine from escaping.

Word Building Relating to the Male Reproductive System

The following list contains examples of medical terms built directly from word parts. The definition for these terms can be determined by a straightforward translation of the word parts.

Combining Form	Combined With	Medical Term	Definition
balan/o	-itis	balanitis (bal ah **NYE** tis)	inflammation of glans penis
	-plasty	balanoplasty (**BAL** ah noh plas tee)	surgical repair of glans penis
	-rrhea	balanorrhea (bah lah noh **REE** ah)	discharge from glans penis
epididym/o	-ectomy	epididymectomy (ep ih did ih **MEK** toh mee)	excision of epididymis
	-itis	epididymitis (ep ih did ih **MYE** tis)	inflammation of the epididymis
orch/o	an- -ism	anorchism (an **OR** kizm)	condition of no testes
orchi/o	-ectomy	orchiectomy (or kee **EK** toh mee)	excision of testes
	-otomy	orchiotomy (or kee **OT** oh mee)	incision into testes
	-plasty	orchioplasty (**OR** kee oh plas tee)	surgical repair of testes
orchid/o	crypto- -ism	cryptorchidism (kript **OR** kid izm)	condition of hidden testes
	-ectomy	orchidectomy (or kid **EK** toh mee)	excision of the testes
	-pexy	orchidopexy (**OR** kid oh peck see)	surgical fixation of testes
prostat/o	cyst/o -itis	prostatocystitis (pross tah toh sis **TYE** tis)	prostate and bladder inflammation
	-ectomy	prostatectomy (pross tah **TEK** toh mee)	excision of prostate
	-lith	prostatolith (pross **TAT** oh lith)	stone in prostate
	lith/o -otomy	prostatolithotomy (pross tah toh lih **THOT** oh mee)	prostate stone incision
	-rrhea	prostatorrhea (pross tah toh **REE** ah)	discharge from prostate
sperm/o	a- -ia	aspermia (ah **SPER** mee ah)	state of no sperm
	oligo- -ia	oligospermia (ol ih goh **SPER** mee ah)	state of scanty (few) sperm
spermat/o	-genesis	spermatogenesis (sper mat oh **JEN** eh sis)	sperm forming
	-lysis	spermatolysis (sper mah **TOL** ih sis)	sperm destruction
vas/o	-ectomy	vasectomy (vas **EK** toh mee)	excision of vas deferens
	vas/o -ostomy	vasovasostomy (vas oh vay **ZOS** toh mee)	create an opening between the one severed end of the vas deferens and the other severed end of the vas deferens (reversal of vasectomy)

Vocabulary Relating to the Male Reproductive System

aspermia (ah SPER mee ah)	Lack of, or failure to ejaculate, sperm.
azoospermia (ah zoh oh SPER mee ah)	Absence of sperm in the semen.
ejaculation (ee jak yoo LAY shun)	The impulse of forcing seminal fluid from the male urethra.
impotent (IM poh tent)	Inability to copulate due to inability to maintain an erection.
perineum (pair ih NEE um)	In the male, the external region between the scrotum and anus.
sexual intercourse	Process of sexual relations or coitus.
spermatogenesis (sper mat oh JEN eh sis)	Formation of mature sperm.
spermatolytic (sper mah toh LIT ik)	Destruction of spermatozoa.

Pathology of the Male Reproductive System

anorchism (an OR kizm)	Congenital absence of one or both testes.
balanitis (bal ah NYE tis)	Inflammation of the skin covering the glans penis.
benign prostatic hypertrophy (BPH) (bee NINE pross TAT ik high PER troh fee)	Enlargement of the prostate gland commonly seen in males over 50.
carcinoma (kar sih NOH mah) **of the testes**	Cancer of one or both testicles.
cryptorchidism (kript OR kid izm)	Failure of the testes to descend into the scrotal sac before birth. Generally, the testes will descend before the boy is one year old. A surgical procedure called **orchidopexy** (OR kid oh peck see) may be required to bring the testes down into the scrotum permanently. Failure of the testes to descend could result in sterility in the male.
epididymitis (ep ih did ih MYE tis)	Inflammation of the epididymis that causes pain and swelling in the inguinal area.

epispadias (ep ih **SPAY** dee as)	Congenital opening of the urethra on the dorsal surface of the penis.
hydrocele (**HIGH** droh seel)	Accumulation of fluid within the testes.
hypospadias (high poh **SPAY** dee as)	Congenital opening of the male urethra on the underside of the penis.
phimosis (fih **MOH** sis)	Narrowing of the foreskin over the glans penis that results in difficulty with hygiene. This condition can lead to infection or difficulty with urination. The condition is treated with circumcision, the surgical removal of the foreskin.
prostate cancer (**PROSS** tayt **CAN** ser)	Slow-growing cancer that affects a large number of males after 50. The PSA (prostate-specific antigen) test is used to assist in early detection of this disease.
prostatic hyperplasia (pross **TAT** ik high per **PLAY** zee ah)	Abnormal cell growth within the prostate.
prostatitis (pross tah **TYE** tis)	Inflamed condition of the prostate gland that may be a result of an infection.
varicocele (**VAIR** ih koh seel)	Enlargement of the veins of the spermatic cord that commonly occurs on the left side of adolescent males. Seldom needs treatment.

Diagnostic Procedures Relating to the Male Reproductive System

digital rectal exam (**DIJ** ih tal **REK** tal) (**DRE**)	Manual examination for an enlarged prostate gland performed by palpating (feeling) the prostate gland through the wall of the rectum.
prostate-specific antigen (PSA) (**PROSS** tayt-specific **AN** tih jen)	A blood test to screen for prostate cancer. Elevated blood levels of PSA are associated with prostate cancer.
semen analysis (**SEE** men ah **NAL** ih sis)	This procedure is used when performing a fertility workup to determine if the male is able to produce sperm. Semen is collected by the patient after abstaining from sexual intercourse for a period of three to five days. The sperm in the semen are analyzed for number, swimming strength, and shape. Also used to determine if a vasectomy has been successful. After a period of six weeks, no further sperm should be present in a sample from the patient.

Treatment Procedures Relating to the Male Reproductive System

castration (kass TRAY shun)	Excision of the testicles in the male or the ovaries in the female.
cauterization (kaw ter ih ZAY shun)	Destruction of tissue with an electric current, caustic agent, hot iron, by freezing.
circumcision (ser kum SIH zhun)	Surgical removal of the end of the prepuce or foreskin of the penis. Generally performed on the newborn male at the request of the parents. The primary reason is for ease of hygiene. Circumcision is also a ritual practice in some religions.
epididymectomy (ep ih did ih MEK toh mee)	Surgical excision of the epididymis.
orchidopexy (OR kid oh peck see)	Surgical fixation to move undescended testes into the scrotum, and to attach them to prevent retraction.
orchiectomy (or ke EK toh mee)	Surgical removal of the testes.
prostatectomy (pross tah TEK toh mee)	Surgical removal of the prostate gland.
sterilization (ster ih lih ZAY shun)	Process of rendering a male or female sterile or unable to conceive children.
transurethral resection of the prostate (TUR) (trans yoo REE thral REE sek shun of the PROSS tayt)	Surgical removal of the prostate gland by inserting a device through the urethra and removing prostate tissue.
vasectomy (vas EK toh mee)	Removal of a segment or all of the vas deferens to prevent sperm from leaving the male body. Used for contraception purposes.

Abbreviations Relating to the Male Reproductive System

AIH	artificial insemination homologous		**NCU**	nongonococcal urethritis
BPH	benign prostatic hypertrophy		**PSA**	prostate-specific antigen
DRE	digital rectal exam		**SPP**	suprapubic prostatectomy
GU	genitourinary		**TUR**	transurethral resection

- anorchism (an **OR** kizm)
- aspermia (ah **SPER** mee ah)
- azoospermia (ah zoh oh **SPER** mee ah)
- balanitis (bal ah **NYE** tis)
- balanoplasty (**BAL** ah noh plas tee)
- balanorrhea (bah lah noh **REE** ah)
- benign prostatic hypertrophy (BPH)
  (bee **NINE** pross **TAT** ik high **PER** troh fee)
- bulbourethral gland (buhl boh yoo **REE** thral)
- carcinoma of the testes (kar sih **NOH** mah)
- castration (kass **TRAY** shun)
- cauterization (kaw ter ih **ZAY** shun)
- circumcision (ser kum **SIH** zhun)
- coitus (**KOH** ih tus)
- copulation (kop yoo **LAY** shun)
- Cowper's glands (**KOW** perz)
- cryptorchidism (kript **OR** kid izm)
- digital rectal exam (DRE) (**DIJ** ih tal **REK** tal)
- ductus deferens (**DUCK** tus **DEF** er enz)
- ejaculation (ee jak yoo **LAY** shun)
- epididymectomy (ep ih did ih **MEK** toh mee)
- epididymis (ep ih **DID** ih mis)
- epididymitis (ep ih did ih **MYE** tis)
- epispadias (ep ih **SPAY** dee as)
- erectile tissue (ee **REK** tile)
- foreskin (**FOR** skin)
- glans penis (**GLANS PEE** nis)
- hydrocele (**HIGH** droh seel)
- hypospadias (high poh **SPAY** dee as)
- impotent (**IM** poh tent)
- oligospermia (ol ih goh **SPER** mee ah)
- orchidectomy (or kid **EK** toh mee)
- orchidopexy (**OR** kid oh peck see)
- orchiectomy (or kee **EK** toh mee)
- orchioplasty (**OR** kee oh plas tee)
- orchiotomy (or kee **OT** oh mee)
- penis (**PEE** nis)
- perineum (pair ih **NEE** um)
- phimosis (fih **MOH** sis)
- prepuce (**PREE** pyoos)

- prostate cancer (**PROSS** tayt **CAN** ser)
- prostate gland (**PROSS** tayt)
- prostate-specific antigen (PSA)
  (**PROSS** tayt-specific **AN** tih jen)
- prostatectomy (pross tah **TEK** toh mee)
- prostatic hyperplasia
  (pross **TAT** ik high per **PLAY** zee ah)
- prostatitis (pross tah **TYE** tis)
- prostatocystitis (pross tah toh sis **TYE** tis)
- prostatolith (pross **TAT** oh lith)
- prostatolithotomy (pross tah toh lih **THOT** oh mee)
- prostatorrhea (pross tah toh **REE** ah)
- scrotum (**SKROH** tum)
- semen (**SEE** men)
- semen analysis (**SEE** men ah **NAL** ih sis)
- seminal vesicles (**SEM** ih nal **VESS** ih kls)
- seminiferous tubules
  (sem ih **NIF** er us **TOO** byools)
- sexual intercourse
- sperm
- spermatic cord (sper **MAT** ik **KORD**)
- spermatogenesis (sper mat oh **JEN** eh sis)
- spermatolysis (sper mah **TOL** ih sis)
- spermatolytic (sper mah toh **LIT** ik)
- spermatozoa (sper mat oh **ZOH** ah)
- spermatozoon (sper mat oh **ZOH** on)
- sphincter (**SFINGK** ter)
- sterilization (ster ih lih **ZAY** shun)
- testes (**TESS** teez)
- testicles (**TESS** tih kls)
- testosterone (tess **TOSS** ter ohn)
- transurethral resection of the prostate (TUR)
  (trans yoo **REE** thrall **REE** sek shun
  of the **PROSS** tayt)
- urethra (yoo **REE** thrah)
- varicocele (**VAIR** ih koh seel)
- vas deferens (**VAS DEF** er enz)
- vasectomy (vas **EK** toh mee)
- vasovasostomy (vas oh vay **ZOS** toh mee)

Case Study II

DISCHARGE REPORT

Admitting Diagnosis: Right testicular carcinoma.

Final Diagnosis: Right testicular carcinoma with orchidectomy.

History of Present Illness: Patient is a 32-year-old male who first noted a lump along the anterior surface of his right testicle during a self-examination. Outpatient needle biopsy confirmed testicular carcinoma. He is admitted at this time for orchidectomy. He reports feeling well and denies any pain. Past medical history is significant for cryptorchidism noted at 2 months of age, which was promptly corrected with an orchidopexy at 6 months of age. Patient has recently married and does not have any children. After discussing alternatives, such as adoption, with his wife, he chose to have semen collected and stored at a sperm bank. Although no difficulties with impotence are anticipated, post-surgical cancer treatment will result in sterility, necessitating artificial insemination for conception.

Summary of Hospital Course: Patient underwent right orchidectomy. Pathological report confirmed well-encapsulated testicular cancer without any evidence of metastasis. Full body CT-scan also failed to show any evidence of metastasis. Patient recovered from the surgery without incident and was discharged on the third post-op day.

Discharge Plans: Patient was referred for oncology consultation to evaluate treatment options and choose a chemotherapy or radiation therapy protocol. He is to refrain from sexual intercourse and vigorous activity for two weeks. He is to return to the office for post-op follow-up in two weeks and may return to full activity after that time.

CRITICAL THINKING QUESTIONS

1. It is not anticipated that this patient's treatment will result in problems with impotence, but will result in sterility. In your own words, explain the difference between these terms.

2. How was this patient's cancer first discovered? How was the diagnosis confirmed?

3. The term *artificial insemination* is not referred to in your text. Explain what you think it means based on the context of this discharge report.

4. What pathology did this patient have as a baby? How was it corrected? Describe in your own words.

5. Which of the following is NOT true regarding this patient?

   a. The tumor was enclosed in a sheath.

   b. The tumor was benign.

   c. He has an appointment with a cancer specialist.

   d. The cancer does not appear to have spread.

Chart Note Transcription II

Chart Note

The chart note below contains ten phrases that can be reworded with a medical term that you learned in this chapter. Each phrase is identified with an underline. Determine the medical term and write your answers in the space provided.

Current Complaint: Patient is a 77-year-old male seen by the urologist with complaints of nocturia and difficulty with the release of semen from the urethra.[1]

Past History: Medical history revealed that the patient had failure of the testes to descend into the scrotum[2] at birth, which was repaired by surgical fixation of the testes.[3] He had also undergone elective sterilization by removal of a segment of the vas deferens[4] at the age of 41.

Signs and Symptoms: Patient states he first noted these symptoms about 5 years ago. They have become increasingly severe and now he is not able to sleep without waking up to urinate up to 20 times a night and has difficulty completing the process of sexual relations.[5] Palpation of the prostate gland through the rectum[6] revealed multiple round firm nodules in prostate gland. A needle biopsy was negative for slow-growing cancer that frequently affects males over 50[7] and a blood test for prostate cancer[8] was normal.

Diagnosis: Non-cancerous enlargement of the prostate gland.[9]

Treatment: Patient was scheduled for a surgical removal of prostate tissue through the urethra.[10]

1 _____

2 _____

3 _____

4 _____

5 _____

6 _____

7 _____

8 _____

9 _____

10 _____

Practice Exercises II

A. COMPLETE THE FOLLOWING STATEMENTS.

1. The male reproductive system is a combination of the _____ and _____ systems.
2. The male's external organs of reproduction consist of the _____ and the _____ .
3. Another term for the prepuce is the _____ .
4. The organs responsible for developing the sperm cells are the _____ .
5. The glands of lubrication and fluid production at each side of the male urethra are the _____ .
6. The male sex hormone is _____ .
7. The area between the scrotum and the anus is called the _____ .

B. STATE THE TERMS DESCRIBED USING THE COMBINING FORMS PROVIDED.

The combining form prostat/o refers to the prostate gland. Use this word root to write a term that means

1. removal of prostate
2. pertaining to the prostate gland
3. inflammation of the prostate
4. flow from the prostate

The combining forms orchid/o, orchi/o and orch/o refer to the testes. Use these word roots to write a term that means

5. pertaining to the testes
6. inflammation of the testes
7. inflammation of the testes and epididymis
8. disease of the testes
9. testicular pain

The combining form vesicul/o refers to the seminal vesicle. Use this word root to write a term that means

10. disease of the seminal vesicle
11. inflammation of the seminal vesicle

C. IDENTIFY THE FOLLOWING ABBREVIATIONS.

1. SPP _____
2. TUR _____
3. GU _____
4. BPH _____
5. AIH _____
6. PSA _____

D. DEFINE THE FOLLOWING TERMS.

1. spermatogenesis _____
2. hydrocele _____
3. transurethral resection of the prostate (TUR) _____
4. aspermia _____
5. orchiectomy _____
6. vasectomy _____
7. cauterization _____

SEXUALLY TRANSMITTED DISEASES (STD)

acquired immunodeficiency syndrome (AIDS) (acquired im yoo noh dee FIH shen see SIN drohm) The final stage of infection from the human immunodeficiency virus (HIV). At present there is no cure.

candidiasis (kan dih DYE ah sis) Yeastlike infection of the skin and mucous membranes that can result in white plaques on the tongue and vagina.

chancroid (SHANG kroyd) Highly infectious nonsyphilitic venereal ulcer.

chlamydial (klah MID ee al) infection Parasitic microorganism causing genital infections in males and females. Can lead to pelvic inflammatory disease in females and eventual infertility.

genital herpes (JEN ih tal HER peez) Creeping skin disease that can appear like a blister or vesicle, caused by a sexually transmitted virus.

genital (JEN ih tal) warts Growths and elevations of warts on the genitalia of both males and females that can lead to cancer of the cervix in females.

gonorrhea (gon oh REE ah) Sexually transmitted inflammation of the mucous membranes of either sex. Can be passed on to an infant during the birth process.

hepatitis (hep ah TYE tis) Infectious, inflammatory disease of the liver. Hepatitis B and C types are spread by contact with blood and bodily fluids of an infected person.

syphilis (SIF ih lis) Infectious, chronic, venereal disease that can involve any organ. May exist for years without symptoms. Treated with the antibiotic penicillin.

trichomoniasis (trik oh moh NYE ah sis) Genitourinary infection that is usually without symptoms (asymptomatic) in both males and females. In women the disease can produce itching and/or burning, a foul-smelling discharge, and result in vaginitis.

venereal disease (VD) (veh NEER ee al dih ZEEZ) Disease usually acquired as the result of heterosexual or homosexual intercourse.

GENETICS

chromosomes	genes	recessive
dominant	genetics	
Down syndrome	hemophilia	

Each sex cell, ova in the female and sperm in the male, carries the genetic material, or **chromosomes (KROH** moh sohmz), necessary for reproduction. Each chromosome is an extremely large molecule containing hundreds or thousands of **genes.** Each individual gene is responsible for producing one of the new baby's **traits,** such as eye color or height. At the union of the male and female sex cells in sexual intercourse, the fetus, or developing child, receives one-half of its genetic material (chromosomes) from the male parent and one-half from the female parent. If any of the genetic material is missing or damaged, a genetic defect, such as **Down syndrome (DOWN SIN** drohm), can result.

For a complete understanding of how genetic defects can occur, it is necessary to learn about **genetics** (jen **ET** iks), the study of heredity and how genes result in the expression of traits. Genes can be either **dominant** or **recessive.** A dominant gene is able to mask a recessive gene, meaning that only the dominant gene's trait will be visible.

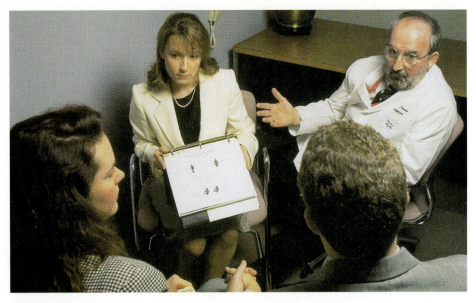

FIGURE 11.20 Genetic counseling with parents. (Will and Demi McIntyre/Photo Researchers, Inc.)

Therefore, each time a fetus receives at least one dominant gene from a parent, the dominant trait will result. The only way for a recessive trait to appear is for the fetus to receive a recessive gene from each parent. An example is eye color. The gene for brown eyes is dominant and the gene for blue eyes is recessive. Therefore, any person with brown eyes has to have only one brown eye color gene. It does not matter if the second gene is for blue or brown eyes. However, a person with blue eye color must have two blue eye color genes. A recessive gene is responsible for disorders such as **hemophilia** (hee moh **FILL** ee ah).

Genetic counseling provides advice to parents or potential parents regarding the possibility that their offspring may or may not have genetic abnormalities. This is an especially important service for those who have a history of genetic diseases in their families. The counseling is provided by medical professionals trained in this field (see Figure 11.20).

COMMON GENETIC DISORDERS

Cooley's anemia (KOO leez an NEE mee ah) Condition named after Thomas Cooley, an American pediatrician, in which a rare form of anemia or a reduction of red blood cells is found in some people of Mediterranean origin.

cystic fibrosis (SIS tik fye BROH sis) Disorder of the exocrine glands that causes those glands to produce abnormally thick secretions of mucus. The disease affects many organs, including the pancreas and the respiratory system. One reliable diagnostic test in children is the sweat test, which will show elevated sodium and potassium levels. There is presently no known cure for the disease, which can shorten the life span.

Down syndrome (DOWN SIN drohm) Disorder named after J. H. L. Down, a British physician, that produces moderate-to-severe mental retardation and multiple defects. The physical characteristics of a child with this disorder are a sloping forehead, flat nose or absent bridge to the nose, low-set eyes, and a generally dwarfed physical growth. The disorder occurs more commonly when the mother is over forty (see Figure 11.21).

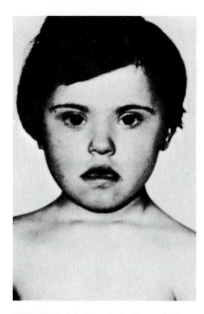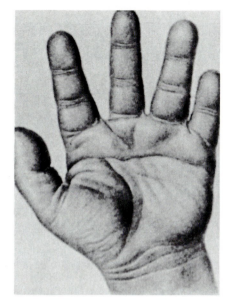

FIGURE 11.21   Left: Face of a five-year-old girl with Down syndrome. Note widely set eyes, underdeveloped bridge of the nose, partially open mouth, and protruding tongue. Right: Short, broad hand of a nine-year-old Down syndrome patient, showing shortened fifth finger and transverse crease across palm.

Duchenne muscular dystrophy (doo SHEN MUSS kew ler DIS troh fee)   Muscular disorder named after G. B. A. Duchenne, a French neurologist, in which there is progressive wasting away of various muscles, including leg, pelvic, and shoulder muscles. Children with this disorder have difficulty climbing stairs and running, and may eventually be confined to a wheelchair. Other complications relating to the heart and respiratory system can be present. Caused by a recessive gene and is more common in males. Often results in a shortened life-span.

hemophilia (hee moh FILL ee ah)   Bleeding disorder in which there is a deficiency in one of the factors necessary for blood to clot. There is an abnormal tendency to bleed, and victims of this disorder may require frequent blood transfusions. The female (mother) carries this recessive gene and it is passed on to males. Therefore, it is found almost exclusively in boys.

Huntington's chorea (HUNT ing tonz koh REE ah)   Rare condition, named after George Huntington, an American physician, characterized by bizarre involuntary movements called chorea. The patient may have progressive mental and physical disturbances, which generally begin around forty.

male pattern baldness   Genetically determined pattern of progressive hair loss. It begins with a receding hairline at the forehead and eventually leads to loss of hair on the top of the head.

retinitis pigmentosa (ret ih NIGH tis pig men TOH sah)   Chronic progressive disease that begins in early childhood and is characterized by degeneration of the retina. This can lead to blindness by middle age.

sickle cell anemia (SIKL SELL an NEE mee ah)   Severe, chronic, incurable disorder that results in anemia and causes joint pain, chronic weakness, and infections. Occurs more commonly in people of Mediterranean and African heritage. The actual blood cell is crescent-shaped.

Tay–Sachs (TAY-SACKS) disease   Disorder named after Warren Tay, a British physician, and Bernard Sachs, an American urologist. Caused by a deficiency of an enzyme, it can result in mental and physical retardation and blindness. It is transferred by a recessive trait and is most commonly found in families of Eastern European Jewish decent. Death generally occurs before the age of four.

Abbreviations Relating to Sexually Transmitted Diseases

AIDS	acquired immunodeficiency syndrome	**STD**	sexually transmitted disease
ARC	AIDS-related complex	**VD**	venereal disease
HIV	human immunodeficiency virus	**VDRL**	Venereal Disease Research Laboratory
HSV	herpes simplex virus		

KEY TERMS

- acquired immunodeficiency syndrome (AIDS) (acquired im yoo noh dee **FIH** shen see **SIN** drohm)
- candidiasis (kan dih **DYE** ah sis)
- chancroid (**SHANG** kroyd)
- chlamydial infection (klah **MID** ee al)
- chromosomes (**KROH** moh sohmz)
- Cooley's anemia (**KOO** leez an **NEE** mee ah)
- cystic fibrosis (**SIS** tik fye **BROH** sis)
- dominant
- Down syndrome (**DOWN SIN** drohm)
- Duchenne muscular dystrophy (doo **SHEN MUSS** kew ler **DIS** troh fee)
- genes
- genetics (jen **ET** iks)
- genital herpes (**JEN** ih tal **HER** peez)
- genital warts (**JEN** ih tal)
- gonorrhea (gon oh **REE** ah)
- hemophilia (hee moh **FILL** ee ah)
- hepatitis (hep ah **TYE** tis)
- Huntington's chorea (**HUNT** ing tonz koh **REE** ah)
- male pattern baldness
- recessive
- retinitis pigmentosa (ret ih **NIGH** tis pig men **TOH** sah)
- sickle cell anemia (**SIKL SELL** an **NEE** mee ah)
- syphilis (**SIF** ih lis)
- Tay–Sachs disease (**TAY-SACKS**)
- traits
- trichomoniasis (trik oh moh **NYE** ah sis)
- venereal disease (VD) (veh **NEER** ee al)

Professional Profile

Nursing Assistant

A certified nurse's assistant (CNA) is responsible for providing basic patient/client care, such as bathing and feeding, to those who are physically ill or disabled. They may also take and record a patient/client's vital signs. CNA's have many career options. They can work under the supervision of an RN or LPN in a wide variety of settings such as acute and long-term care facilities, home health agencies, and clinics. To become a certified nurse's aide, an approved on-the-job certification program must be completed.

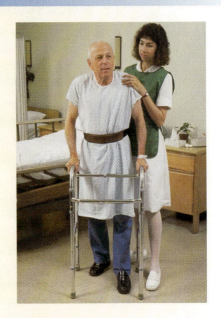

Practice Exercises III

A. MATCH THE TERMS IN COLUMN A WITH THE DEFINITIONS IN COLUMN B.

A	B
1. _____ hepatitis	a. final stage of HIV virus
2. _____ herpes	b. caused by parasitic microorganism
3. _____ candidiasis	c. treated with penicillin
4. _____ syphilis	d. elevated growths
5. _____ AIDS	e. disease of the liver
6. _____ genital warts	f. genitourinary infection
7. _____ chancroid	g. venereal ulcer
8. _____ chlamydial infection	h. yeastlike infection
9. _____ trichomoniasis	i. skin disease with vesicles

B. MATCH THE TERMS IN COLUMN A WITH THE DEFINITIONS IN COLUMN B.

A	B
1. _____ cystic fibrosis	a. crescent-shaped blood cell
2. _____ Huntington's chorea	b. bleeding disorder predominately in males
3. _____ Down syndrome	c. atrophying of muscles
4. _____ sickle cell anemia	d. exocrine gland disorder
5. _____ hemophilia	e. rare anemia in Mediterranean people
6. _____ muscular dystrophy	f. enzyme-deficiency disease
7. _____ Tay–Sachs disease	g. involuntary movements
8. _____ Cooley's anemia	h. more common with older mothers

C. IDENTIFY THE FOLLOWING ABBREVIATIONS.

1. VD   _____
2. AIDS   _____
3. HIV   _____

4. STD   _____
5. HSV   _____

Getting Connected

Multimedia Extension Activities

CD-ROM

Use the CD-ROM enclosed with your textbook to gain additional reinforcement through interactive word building exercises, spelling games, labeling activities, and additional quizzes.

www.prenhall.com/fremgen

Use the above address to access the free, interactive Companion Website created for this textbook. Get hints, instant feedback, and textbook references to chapter-related multiple choice questions, and labeling and matching exercises. In addition, you will find an audio glossary, case studies, Internet exploration exercises, flashcards, and a comprehensive exam.

Answers

Case Study I (Critical Thinking Questions)

1. oophorectomy and chemotherapy; full body CT-scan   2. menarche at 13, menorrhagia with chronic anemia
3. c—nullipara and d—multigravida   4. pelvic ultrasound; because the placenta overlies the cervix, it will detach before the baby can physically be born   5. size consistent with 25-weeks gestation, turned head down, umbilical cord is not around the neck, fetal heart tones are strong, male, no evidence of developmental or genetic disorders
6. a. a greater than normal level of risk of problems developing or fetal death with this pregnancy; b. she looks like she is 8-months pregnant (her abdomen is not too small or too large)

Chart Note I

1. gynecologist—physician specialized in treating diseases of the female reproductive tract   2. dysmenorrhea—painful cramping with menstruation   3. multipara—given birth to more than one child   4. tubal ligation—tying off of the tubes between the ovaries and uterus   5. pelvic ultrasonography—image of the pelvic cavity produced by ultrasound waves
6. hysterosalpingography—X-ray taken after injecting dye into the uterus and tubes   7. fallopian tubes—tubes between the ovaries and uterus   8. laparoscopy—examination of the abdominopelvic cavity using a laparoscope
9. endometrium—inner layer of the uterus   10. endometriosis—abnormal condition of inner uterine layer appearing in the pelvis.   11. pan hysterosalpingo-oophorectomy—removal of entire uterus, ovaries, and fallopian tubes

Practice Exercises I

A. 1. gynecology   2. gynecologist   3. genitalia   4. gestational   5. amenorrhea   6. ovum   7. endometrium
8. uterus   9. fallopian tubes   10. panhysterosalpingo-oophorectomy
B. 1. vaginal   2. vaginitis   3. vaginocele   4. vaginolabial   5. vaginomycosis   6. vaginoperineal   7. colposcopy
8. colposcope   9. colporrhaphy   10. cervicitis   11. cervical   12. uterocervical   13. uterorectal   14. hysteropathy
15. hysteropexy   16. hysterospasms   17. hysterectomy   18. hysterocele   19. hysterorrhexis   20. hysterorrhaphy
21. metropathy   22. metroperitonitis   23. metrorrhagia   24. gynecology   25. gynecologist   26. oophorosalpingitis
27. oophoritis   28. salpingitis   29. salpingo-oophoritis   30. hysterosalpingo-oophorectomy
C. 1. ova   2. labia
D. 1. menarche   2. multigravida   3. nullipara
E. 1. cervix   2. last menstrual period   3. total abdominal hysterectomy   4. obstetrics   5. Papanicolaou test   6. marital history   7. pelvic inflammatory disease   8. date of birth   9. fetal heart tone   10. cesarean section   11. newborn
12. premenstrual syndrome   13. toxic shock syndrome   14. low birth weight   15. estrogen replacement therapy
F. 1. PKU   2. RML   3. UC   4. FTND   5. CWP   6. D&C   7. DUB   8. gyne   9. AB
G. 1. uterus   2. uterus   3. female   4. vulva   5. ovary   6. ovary   7. fallopian tube   8. pregnancy   9. vagina
10. breast
H. 1. g   2. k   3. h   4. c   5. i   6. l   7. d   8. a   9. b   10. f   11. e   12. j
I. 1. e   2. g   3. f   4. c   5. i   6. b   7. h   8. a   9. d
J. 1. Rh-factor   2. conization   3. stillbirth   4. gestational   5. puberty   6. premenstrual syndrome   7. laparoscopy
8. fibroid tumor   9. D&C   10. eclampsia   11. endometriosis   12. cesarean section

Case Study II (Critical Thinking Questions)

1. impotence—unable to achieve or maintain an erection; sterility—lack of sperm in the semen (aspermia)   2. he felt it on a self-examination; needle biopsy   3. sperm are artificially introduced into the wife's vagina, not during intercourse   4. cryptorchidism, orchidopexy   5. b—the tumor was benign

CHART NOTE II

1. ejaculation—release of semen from the urethra   2. cryptorchidism—failure of the testes to descend into the scrotum   3. orchidopexy—surgical fixation of the testes   4. vasectomy—removal of a segment of the vas deferens   5. sexual intercourse—the process of sexual relations   6. digital rectal exam (DRE)—palpation of the prostate gland through the rectum   7. prostate cancer—slow-growing cancer that frequently affects males over 50   8. prostate-specific antigen (PSA)—blood test for prostate cancer   9. benign prostatic hypertrophy (BPH)—non-cancerous enlargement of prostate gland   10. transurethral resection (TUR)—surgical removal of prostate tissue through the urethra

PRACTICE EXERCISES II

A. 1. urinary, reproductive   2. scrotum, penis   3. foreskin   4. testes   5. Cowper's glands   6. testosterone   7. perineum

B. 1. prostatectomy   2. prostatic   3. prostatitis   4. prostatorrhea   5. orchidic   6. orchitis   7. orchiepididymitis   8. orchiopathy   9. orchialgia   10. vesiculopathy   11. vesiculitis

C. 1. suprapubic prostatectomy   2. transurethral resection   3. genitourinary   4. benign prostatic hypertrophy   5. artificial insemination homologous   6. prostate-specific antigen

D. 1. The formation of mature sperm.   2. Accumulation of fluid within the testes.   3. Surgical removal of the prostate gland by inserting a device through the urethra and removing prostate tissue.   4. Failure to ejaculate sperm.   5. Surgical removal of the testes.   6. Surgical removal of part or all of the vas deferens.   7. Destruction of tissue with an electric current, caustic agent, hot iron, or by freezing.

PRACTICE EXERCISES III

A. 1. e   2. i   3. h   4. c   5. a   6. d   7. g   8. b   9. f

B. 1. d   2. g   3. h   4. a   5. b   6. c   7. f   8. e

C. 1. venereal disease   2. acquired immune deficiency syndrome   3. human immunodeficiency virus   4. sexually transmitted disease   5. herpes simplex virus

Chapter 12

NERVOUS SYSTEM

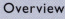
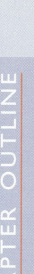

LEARNING OBJECTIVES

Upon completion of this chapter, you will be able to:

- Recognize the combining forms, prefixes, and suffixes introduced in this chapter.

- Gain the ability to pronounce medical terms and major anatomical structures.

- List the major organs of the nervous system and their functions.

- Describe the components of a nerve.

- Distinguish between the central nervous system, peripheral nervous system, and autonomic nervous system.

- Build nervous system medical terms from word parts.

- Define vocabulary, pathology, diagnostic, and therapeutic medical terms relating to the nervous system.

- Interpret abbreviations associated with the nervous system.

Overview

ORGANS OF THE NERVOUS SYSTEM

brain

nerves

spinal cord

COMBINING FORMS RELATING TO THE NERVOUS SYSTEM

cephal/o	head	**mening/o**	meninges
cerebell/o	cerebellum	**meningi/o**	meninges
cerebr/o	brain	**ment/o**	mind
comat/o	deep sleep (coma)	**myel/o**	spinal cord
crani/o	head, skull	**neur/o**	nerve
dur/o	hard	**phas/o**	speech
encephal/o	brain	**poli/o**	gray matter
gangli/o	ganglion	**radicul/o**	nerve root
ganglion/o	ganglion	**spondyl/o**	vertebra
gli/o	glue	**vag/o**	vagus nerve
medull/o	medulla		

PREFIXES RELATING TO THE NERVOUS SYSTEM

Prefix	Meaning	Example
cryo-	cold	cryosurgery
hydro-	water	hydrocephalus

SUFFIXES RELATING TO THE NERVOUS SYSTEM

Suffix	Meaning	Example
-algesia	pain, sensitivity	analgesia
-algia	pain	cephalgia
-esthesia	feeling, sensation	anesthesia
-kinesia	movement	bradykinesia
-lepsy	seizure	narcolepsy
-paresis	weakness	hemiparesis
-plegia	paralysis	paraplegia
-sthenia	strength	myasthenia
-taxia	muscular coordination	ataxia

ANATOMY AND PHYSIOLOGY OF THE NERVOUS SYSTEM

DIVISIONS OF THE NERVOUS SYSTEM

autonomic nervous system (ANS)

brain

central nervous system (CNS)

cranial nerves

peripheral nervous system (PNS)

spinal cord

spinal nerves

The nervous system is composed of three parts: the **central nervous system (CNS),** the **peripheral** (per **IF** er al) **nervous system (PNS),** and the **autonomic nervous system (ANS)** (aw toh **NOM** ik **NER** vus **SIS** tem) (see Figure 12.1).

FIGURE 12.1 The nervous system.

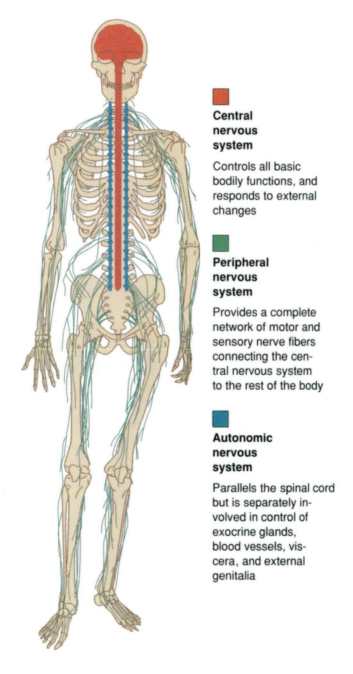

Central nervous system

Controls all basic bodily functions, and responds to external changes

Peripheral nervous system

Provides a complete network of motor and sensory nerve fibers connecting the central nervous system to the rest of the body

Autonomic nervous system

Parallels the spinal cord but is separately involved in control of exocrine glands, blood vessels, viscera, and external genitalia

The central nervous system consists of the **brain** and **spinal cord.** The peripheral nervous system contains the **cranial** (**KRAY** nee al) **nerves** and **spinal nerves.** These two systems regulate functions that are mainly voluntary, or within our control, such as muscle movement, smell, taste, sight, and hearing. The autonomic nervous system consists of nerves to the internal organs that function involuntarily or without our conscious control.

NERVES

afferent neurons	**dendrites**	**impulse**
axon	**efferent neurons**	**neuron**
cell body	**ganglion**	**stimulus**

A nerve is a group or bundle of fibers located outside the central nervous system that connects the brain and spinal cord with various parts of the body (see Figure 12.2 for a nerve cell). Terminology relating to the nerves is as follows:

afferent (AFF er ent) neurons Carry impulses to the brain and spinal cord from the skin and sense organs. Also called *sensory neurons.*

axon (AK son) Single projection of neuron that conducts impulse away from cell body.

cell body Part of the neuron that contains the nucleus.

dendrites (DEN drights) Branched process of a neuron that receives impulses and carries them to the cell body.

efferent (EFF er ent) neurons Carry impulses away from the brain and spinal cord to the muscles and glands. Also called *motor neurons.*

ganglion (GANG lee on) Knotlike mass of nerve tissue located outside the brain and spinal cord.

impulse Wave of sudden excitement.

neuron (NOO ron) Basic, individual, microscopic nerve cell (see Figure 12.3).

stimulus (STIM yoo lus) Something that activates or excites the nerve and results in an impulse.

FIGURE 12.2 Enhanced color scanning electron micrograph of neuron. (CNRI/Science Photo Library/Photo Researchers, Inc.)

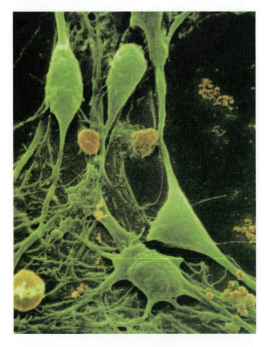

FIGURE 12.3   Neuron.

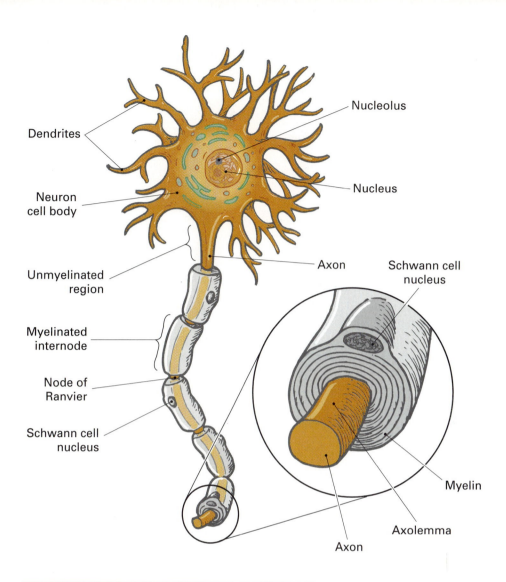

Labels: Dendrites, Nucleolus, Neuron cell body, Nucleus, Unmyelinated region, Axon, Schwann cell nucleus, Myelinated internode, Node of Ranvier, Schwann cell nucleus, Myelin, Axolemma, Axon

CENTRAL NERVOUS SYSTEM

gray matter	**myelin**	**tract**
meninges	**myelinated**	**white matter**
multiple sclerosis (MS)	**poliomyelitis**	

Since this system is a combination of the brain and spinal cord, it is able to receive impulses from all over the body, process this information, and then respond with an action. This system consists of both gray and white matter. **Gray matter** is unsheathed or uncovered cell bodies and dendrites. **White matter** is **myelinated** (**MY** eh lih nayt ed) nerve fibers (see Figure 12.4). Bundles of nerve fibers interconnecting different parts of the central nervous system (CNS) are called **tracts.** The central nervous system (CNS) is encased and protected by three membranes known as the **meninges** (men **IN** jeez).

MED TERM TIP

There are disease processes that attack the gray matter and the white matter of the central nervous system. For instance, **poliomyelitis** (poh lee oh my ell **EYE** tis) is a viral infection of the gray matter of the spinal cord. The combining term *polio* means gray matter. This disease has almost been conquered, due to the polio vaccine. The inflammatory disease **multiple sclerosis** (**MULL** tih pl skleh **ROH** sis) (**MS**) attacks the protective **myelin** (**MY** eh lin) sheath of nerves.

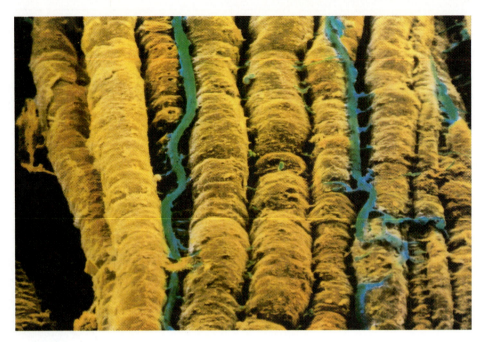

FIGURE 12.4 Enhanced color nerve fibers. (Prof. P. Motta/Photo Researchers, Inc.)

The Brain

brain stem	frontal lobe	parietal lobe
cerebellum	gyri	pons
cerebral cortex	hemisphere	spinal puncture
cerebrospinal fluid (CSF)	hypothalamus	sulci
cerebrovascular accident (CVA)	lumbar puncture (LP)	temporal lobe
cerebrum	medulla oblongata	thalamus
diencephalon	midbrain	ventricles
fissures	occipital lobe	

The brain is one of the largest organs in the body and coordinates most body activities. It is the center for all thought, memory, judgment, and emotion. Each part of the brain is responsible for controlling different body functions, such as temperature regulation and breathing.

There are four sections to the brain: **cerebrum** (**SER** eh brum), **cerebellum** (ser eh **BELL** um), **diencephalon** (dye en **SEFF** ah lon), and **brain stem** (see Figure 12.5). The largest section of the brain is the cerebrum. It is located in the upper portion of the brain and is the area that processes thoughts, judgment, memory, association skills, and the ability to discriminate between items. The outer layer of the cerebrum is the **cerebral cortex** (seh **REE** bral **KOR** teks), which is composed of folds of gray matter. The elevated portions of the cerebrum, or convolutions, are called **gyri** (**JYE** rye) and are separated by **fissures** (**FISH** ers) or **sulci** (**SULL** kye).

The cerebrum has both a left and a right division or **hemisphere** (**HEM** is feer). Each hemisphere has four lobes. The areas controlled by the lobes are as follows (see Figure 12.6):

1. **Frontal lobe:** Controls motor function.
2. **Parietal** (pah **RYE** eh tal) **lobe:** Receives and interprets nerve impulses from sensory receptors.
3. **Occipital** (ock **SIP** ih tal) **lobe:** Controls eyesight.
4. **Temporal** (**TEM** por al) **lobe:** Controls hearing and smell.

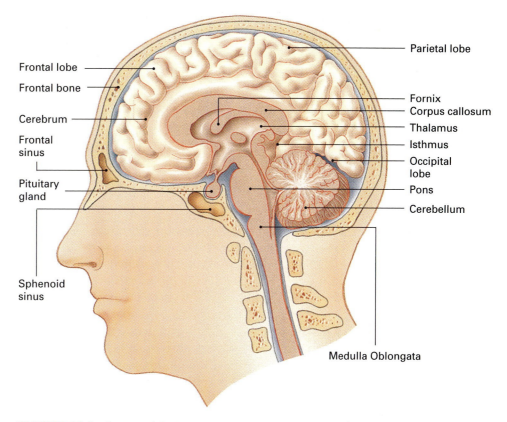

FIGURE 12.5 Section of the brain.

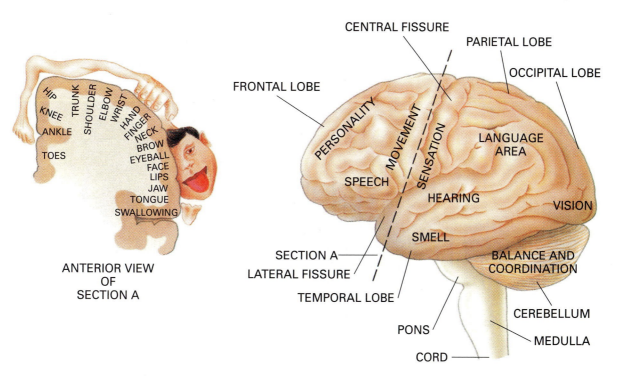

**ANTERIOR VIEW
OF
SECTION A**

FIGURE 12.6 The brain: lateral view.

Within the middle portion of the cerebrum are spaces or cavities called **ventricles** (**VEN** trik lz). These contain **cerebrospinal fluid** (ser eh broh **SPY** nal **FLOO** id) **(CSF),** which is the watery, clear fluid that provides protection from shock or sudden motion to the brain.

MED TERM *TIP*

The term for withdrawing cerebrospinal fluid is **spinal puncture** (**PUNK** chur) or **lumbar puncture** (**LUM** bar **PUNK** chur) **(LP)** (see Figure 12.7). This spinal fluid is withdrawn by syringe to relieve pressure on the brain or for testing purposes.

The diencephalon, located below the cerebrum, contains two of the most critical areas of the brain, the **thalamus** (**THAL** ah mus) and the **hypothalamus** (high poh **THAL** ah mus). The thalamus is composed of gray matter and acts as a center for relaying impulses from the eyes, ears, and skin to the cerebrum. Our pain perception is controlled by the thalamus. The hypothalamus, lying just below the thalamus, controls body temperature, appetite, sleep, sexual desire, and emotions such as fear. The hypothalamus is actually responsible for controlling the autonomic nervous system, cardiovascular system, and the gastrointestinal system. It also regulates the parasympathetic and sympathetic nervous systems, and the release of hormones from the pituitary gland.

The cerebellum, the second largest portion of the brain, is located beneath the posterior part of the cerebrum. This part of the brain aids in coordinating voluntary body movements and maintaining balance and equilibrium. It is attached to the brain stem by the **pons** (**PONZ**) or bridge. The cerebellum refines the muscular movement that is initiated in the cerebrum.

The final portion of the brain is the brain stem. This area has three components: **medulla oblongata** (meh **DULL** ah ob long **GAH** tah), pons, and **midbrain.** The medulla oblongata connects the spinal cord with the brain. This is the area where the nerve cells cross from one side of the brain to control functions and movement on the other side of the brain.

FIGURE 12.7 Site for lumbar puncture.

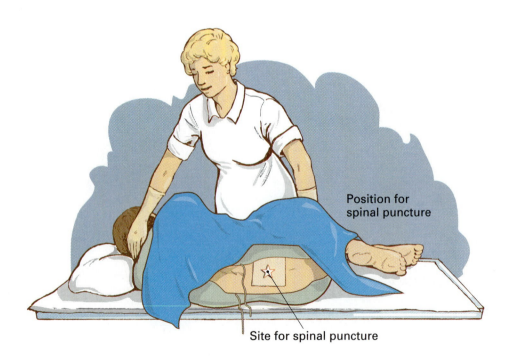

Position for spinal puncture

Site for spinal puncture

An injury or damage to one side of the brain causes paralysis on the opposite side of the body. Since nerve cells that control the movement of the right side of the body are located in the left side of the medulla oblongata, a **cerebrovascular accident** (ser eh broh **VASS** kyoo lar **AK** sih dent) **(CVA),** or stroke, paralyzing the right side of the body would actually have occurred in the left side of the brain.

The general function of the brain stem is to act as a pathway for impulses to be conducted between the brain and the spinal cord. In addition, the twelve pairs of cranial nerves begin in the brain stem. This vital area of the brain is the center that controls respiration, heart rate, and blood pressure.

A brain stem injury, such as occurs in a sports injury or auto accident, is especially serious because the functions of respiration, heart rate, and blood pressure are disturbed.

Spinal Cord

myelogram	**vertebral canal**
spinal canal	**vertebral column**
vertebra	

The function of the spinal cord is to provide a pathway for impulses traveling to and from the brain in addition to carrying the nerves for the lower part of the body. The spinal cord is actually a column of nervous tissue that extends from the medulla oblongata of the brain down to the second lumbar **vertebra** (**VER** teh brah) within the **vertebral** (**VER** teh bral) **column.** The vertebral column consists of the thirty-three vertebrae of the back bone. They line up to form a continuous canal for the spinal cord called the **spinal** or **vertebral** (**VER** teh bral) **canal** (see Figures 12.8 and 12.9).

The combining form *myel/o* means spinal cord. A **myelogram** (**MY** eh loh gram) is an X-ray reading of the spinal column after the injection of dye. Patients must remain flat for a period of time after this exam to prevent the dye from moving into the brain and causing a severe headache.

The spinal cord is also protected by cerebrospinal fluid just as in the brain. The inner core of the spinal cord contains gray matter that is not protected by a myelin sheath or covering. This inner core consists of cell bodies and dendrites of peripheral nerves. The outer portion of the spinal cord is myelinated white matter.

FIGURE 12.8 Divisions of
the spinal cord.

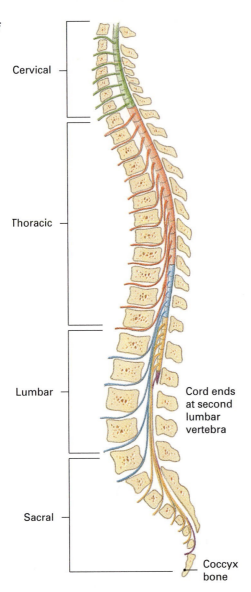

Cervical

Thoracic

Lumbar

Cord ends
at second
lumbar
vertebra

Sacral

Coccyx
bone

FIGURE 12.9 Enhanced-
color spinal cord. (Video
Surgery/Photo Researchers,
Inc.)

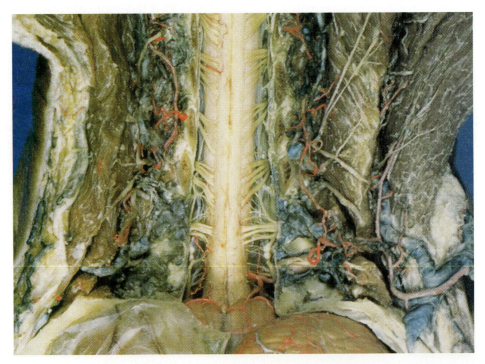

MENINGES

arachnoid layer	**subarachnoid space**
dura mater	**subdural hematoma**
meningitis	**subdural space**
pia mater	

The meninges are three layers of connective tissue membranes that surround the brain and spinal cord (see Figure 12.10). An inflammation of these due to infection, such as in **meningitis** (men in **JYE** tis), can cause serious complications since brain function is diminished.

Moving from external to internal, the meninges are

1. **Dura mater** (**DOO** rah **MATE** er): The name means *tough mother*; it is a tough, fibrous layer.

2. **Subdural** (sub **DOO** ral) **space:** The actual space between the dura mater and arachnoid layers.

3. **Arachnoid** (ah **RAK** noyd) **layer:** The name means *spider-like*; it is a thin, delicate layer attached to the pia mater by web-like filaments.

4. **Subarachnoid** (sub ah **RAK** noyd) **space:** The space between the arachnoid layer and the pia mater; it contains cerebrospinal fluid.

5. **Pia mater** (**PEE** ah **MATE** er): The name means *soft mother;* it is the innermost membrane layer and is applied directly to the surface of the brain.

MED TERM *TIP*

If the meninges are torn by trauma to the head, blood may collect in the subdural space. This is a **subdural hematoma** (sub **DOO** ral hee mah **TOH** mah) and can exert fatal pressure on the brain if the hematoma is not drained by surgery.

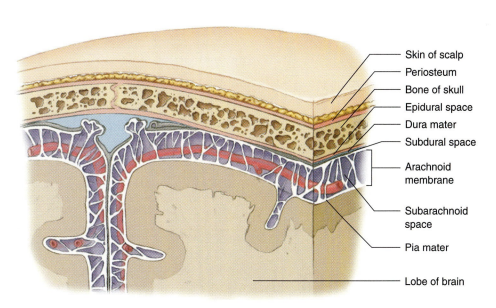

- Skin of scalp
- Periosteum
- Bone of skull
- Epidural space
- Dura mater
- Subdural space
- Arachnoid membrane
- Subarachnoid space
- Pia mater
- Lobe of brain

FIGURE 12.10 The meninges of the brain.

PERIPHERAL NERVOUS SYSTEM

The peripheral nervous system includes both the twelve pairs of cranial nerves and the thirty-one pairs of spinal nerves. This system carries both sensory information from the body to the central nervous system and motor instructions from the central nervous system to the muscles, organs, and glands of the body.

The cranial nerves originate within the brain. They are generally named for either the function they serve or their location. They are also identified using Roman numerals. The entire list of cranial nerves is found in Table 12.1.

Spinal nerves split off from the spinal cord, one pair between each pair of vertebrae. They are generally named for the area of body they serve or a major blood vessel with which they are associated. Figure 12.11 illustrates some of the major spinal nerves in the human body.

AUTONOMIC NERVOUS SYSTEM

adrenal medulla   **salivary glands**

gastric glands   **sweat glands**

parasympathetic   **sympathetic**

Table 12.1	*Cranial Nerves*	
Number	**Name**	**Function**
I	Olfactory	Transports impulses for sense of smell
II	Optic	Carries impulses for sense of sight
III	Oculomotor	Motor impulses for eye muscle movement and the pupil of eye
IV	Trochlear	Controls oblique muscle of eye on each side
V	Trigeminal	Carries sensory facial impulses and controls muscles for chewing; branches into eyes, forehead, upper and lower jaw
VI	Abducens	Controls an eyeball muscle to turn eye to side
VII	Facial	Controls facial motor muscles for expression, salivation, and taste on two-thirds of tongue (anterior)
VIII	Acoustic/auditory	Responsible for impulses of equilibrium and hearing; also called auditory nerve
IX	Glossopharyngeal	Carries sensory impulses from pharynx (swallowing) and taste on one-third of tongue
X	Vagus	Supplies most organs in abdominal and thoracic cavities
XI	Spinal accessory	Controls the neck and shoulder muscles
XII	Hypoglossal	Controls tongue muscles

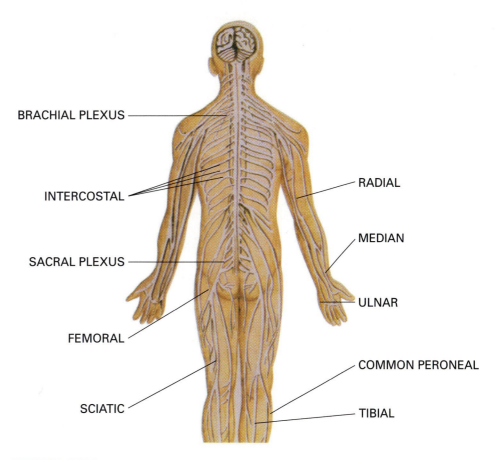

BRACHIAL PLEXUS

INTERCOSTAL

SACRAL PLEXUS

FEMORAL

SCIATIC

RADIAL

MEDIAN

ULNAR

COMMON PERONEAL

TIBIAL

FIGURE 12.11 Some of the major spinal nerves found in the human body.

The autonomic nervous system is concerned with the control of involuntary bodily functions. It serves to regulate the functions of the glands, especially the **salivary** (**SAL** ih vair ee), **gastric** (**GAS** trik), and **sweat glands.** The **adrenal medulla** (ad **REE** nal meh **DULL** ah), heart, and smooth muscle tissue are also controlled by the autonomic nervous system. The autonomic nervous system acts on these tissues either to initiate their function or to slow the function down.

This system is divided into two parts: **sympathetic** (sim pah **THET** ik) and **parasympathetic** (pair ah sim pah **THET** ik). The sympathetic nerves stimulate the body in times of stress and crisis. These nerves would increase the heart rate, dilate airways to allow for more oxygen, cause an increase in blood pressure, inhibit digestion, and stimulate the production of adrenalin during a crisis. The other group of nerves within this system are the parasympathetic nerves. This group of nerves serves as a counterbalance for the sympathetic nerves. Therefore, they would cause the heart rate to slow down, lower the blood pressure, constrict eye pupils, and increase digestion and the production of saliva.

Word Building Relating to the Nervous System

The following list contains examples of medical terms built directly from word parts. The definition for these terms can be determined by a straightforward translation of the word parts.

Combining Form	Combined With	Medical Term	Definition
cephal/o	-algia	cephalgia (seff **AL** jee ah)	head pain
cerebell/o	-ar	cerebellar (ser eh **BELL** ar)	pertaining to the cerebellum
	-itis	cerebellitis (ser eh bell **EYE** tis)	cerebellum inflammation
cerebr/o	-al	cerebral (seh **REE** bral)	pertaining to the cerebrum
	spin/o -al	cerebrospinal (ser eh broh **SPY** nal)	pertaining to the cerebrum and spine
dur/o	sub- -al	subdural (sub **DOO** ral)	pertaining to under the dura mater
encephal/o	electr/o -gram	electroencephalogram (ee lek troh en **SEFF** ah loh gram)	record of brain's electricity
	electr/o -graph	electroencephalograph (ee lek troh en **SEFF** ah loh graf)	instrument to record brain's electricity
	electr/o -graphy	electroencephalography (ee lek troh en seff ah **LOG** rah fee)	process of recording brain's electricity
	-itis	encephalitis (en seff ah **LYE** tis)	brain inflammation
	-malacia	encephalomalacia (en seff ah loh mah **LAY** she ah)	brain softening
	-sclerosis	encephalosclerosis (en seff ah loh skleh **ROH** sis)	brain hardening
mening/o	-cele	meningocele (men **IN** goh seel)	meninges hernia
	-itis	meningitis (men in **JYE** tis)	meninges inflammation
	myel/o -cele	myelomeningocele (my eh loh meh **NIN** goh seel)	meninges and spinal cord hernia
my/o	a- -sthenia	myasthenia (my ass **THEE** nee ah)	lack of muscle strength
myel/o	-gram	myelogram (**MY** eh loh gram)	record of spinal cord
	-malacia	myelomalacia (my eh loh mah **LAY** she ah)	spinal cord softening
	poli/o -itis	poliomyelitis (poh lee oh my ell **EYE** tis)	gray matter of spinal cord inflammation
neur/o	a- -sthenia	neurasthenia (noor ass **THEE** nee ah)	lack of nerve strength
	-algia	neuralgia (noo **RAL** jee ah)	nerve pain
	-ectomy	neurectomy (noo **REK** toh mee)	excision of nerve
	-lysis	neurolysis (noo **ROL** ih sis)	nerve destruction
	-ologist	neurologist (noo **RAL** oh jist)	specialist in nerves
	-ology	neurology (noo **RAL** oh jee)	study of nerves
	-oma	neuroma (noo **ROH** mah)	nerve tumor
	-otomy	neurotomy (noo **ROT** oh mee)	incision into a nerve

Prefix	Suffix	Medical Term	Definition
	-plasty	neuroplasty (**NOOR** oh plas tee)	surgical repair of nerves
	poly- -itis	polyneuritis (pol ee noo **RYE** tis)	inflammation of many nerves
	-rrhaphy	neurorrhaphy (noo **ROR** ah fee)	suture of nerve
radicul/o	-itis	radiculitis (rah dick yoo **LYE** tis)	nerve root inflammation
Prefix	**Suffix**	**Medical Term**	**Definition**
an-	-esthesia	anesthesia (an ess **THEE** zee ah)	lack of sensations
hyper-		hyperesthesia (high per ess **THEE** zee ah)	excessive sensations
hemi-	-paresis	hemiparesis (hem ee par **EE** sis)	weakness of half
mono-		monoparesis (mon oh pah **REE** sis)	weakness of one
a-	-phasia	aphasia (ah **FAY** zee ah)	lack of speech
dys-		dysphasia (dis **FAY** zee ah)	difficult speech
hemi-	-plegia	hemiplegia (hem ee **PLEE** jee ah)	paralysis of half
mono-		monoplegia (mon oh **PLEE** jee ah)	paralysis of one
pan-		panplegia (pan **PLEE** jee ah)	paralysis of all
quadri-		quadriplegia (kwod rih **PLEE** jee ah)	paralysis of four
tetra-		tetraplegia (tet rah **PLEE** jee ah)	paralysis of four

Vocabulary Relating to the Nervous System

analgesia (an al JEE zee ah)	A reduction in the perception of pain or sensation due to a neurological condition or medication.
anesthesia (an ess THEE zee ah)	Partial or complete loss of sensation with or without a loss of consciousness as a result of a drug, disease, or injury.
aphasia (ah FAY zee ah)	Loss of the ability to speak.
asthenia (as THEE nee ah)	Lack or loss of strength, causing extreme weakness.
astrocyte (ASS troh sight)	Star-shaped cells found in the nervous system that surround and support the neurons. They perform important metabolic functions, but do not participate in conducting electrical impulses.
ataxia (ah TAK see ah)	Having a lack of muscle coordination as a result of a disorder or disease.
bradykinesia (brad ee kin NEE see ah)	Slow movement, commonly seen with the rigidity of Parkinson's disease.
chorea (koh REE ah)	Involuntary nervous disorder that results in muscular twitching of the limbs or facial muscles.
coma (COH mah)	Abnormal deep sleep or stupor resulting from an illness or injury.
conscious (KON shus)	Condition of being awake and aware of surroundings.

(continued)

convulsion (kon VULL shun)	Severe involuntary muscle contractions and relaxations. These have a variety of causes, such as epilepsy, fever, and toxic conditions.
dementia (dee MEN she ah)	Progressive impairment of intellectual function that interferes with performing the activities of daily living. Patients have little awareness of their condition. Found in disorders such as Alzheimer's.
dysphasia (dis FAY zee ah)	Impairment of speech as a result of a brain lesion.
embolism (EM boh lizm)	Obstruction of a blood vessel by a blood clot or foreign substance, such as air and fat.
grand mal (GRAND MALL)	A type of severe epilepsy seizure characterized by a loss of consciousness and convulsions. It is also called a tonic-clonic seizure, indicating that the seizure alternates between strong continuous muscle spasms (tonic) and rhythmic muscle contraction and relaxation (clonic).
hemiparesis (hem ee par EE sis)	Weakness or loss of motion on one side of the body.
hemiplegia (hem ee PLEE jee ah)	Paralysis on only one side of the body.
idiopathic (id ee oh PATH ik)	When something occurs without a known cause.
lethargy (LETH ar jee)	Condition of sluggishness or stupor.
neurologist (noo RAL oh jist)	Physician who specializes in disorders of the nervous system.
neurology (noo RAL oh jee)	Specialty of medicine that deals with disorders of the nervous system.
neurosurgeon (noo roh SIR jen)	A physician specialized in treating conditions and diseases of the nervous systems by surgical means.
palsy (PAWL zee)	Temporary or permanent loss of the ability to control movement.
paralysis (pah RAL ih sis)	Temporary or permanent loss of function or voluntary movement.
paraplegia (pair ah PLEE jee ah)	Paralysis of the lower portion of the body and both legs.
petit mal (pet EE MALL)	A type of epilepsy seizure that lasts only a few seconds to half a minute, characterized by a loss of awareness and an absence of activity. It is also called an absence seizure.
quadriplegia (kwod rih PLEE jee ah)	Paralysis of all four limbs. Same as *tetraplegia*.
seizure (SEE zyoor)	Sudden attack of severe muscular contractions associated with a loss of consciousness. This is seen in grand mal epilepsy.
sleep disorder	Any condition that interferes with sleep other than environmental noises. Can include difficulty sleeping (insomnia), nightmares, night terrors, sleepwalking, and apnea.
syncope (SIN koh pee)	Fainting.
tetraplegia (tet rah PLEE jee ah)	Paralysis of all four limbs. Same as *quadriplegia*.
tic (TIK)	Spasmodic, involuntary muscular contraction involving the head, face, mouth, eyes, neck, and shoulders.
tremor (TREM or)	Involuntary quivering movement of a part of the body.
unconscious (un KON shus)	Condition or state of being unaware of surroundings, with the inability to respond to stimuli.

Pathology of the Nervous System

Alzheimer's (ALTS high merz) disease	Chronic, organic mental disorder consisting of dementia, which is more prevalent in adults between 40 and 60. Involves progressive disorientation, apathy, speech and gait disturbances, and loss of memory. Named for Alois Alzheimer, a German neurologist.
amyotrophic lateral sclerosis (ALS) (ah my oh TROFF ik LAT er al skleh ROH sis)	Disease with muscular weakness and atrophy due to degeneration of motor neurons of the spinal cord. Also called *Lou Gehrig's disease,* after the New York Yankees' baseball player who died from the disease.
aneurysm (AN yoo rizm)	Localized abnormal dilatation of a blood vessel, usually an artery; the result of a congenital defect or weakness in the wall of the vessel (see Figures 12.12 and 12.13).
astrocytoma (ass troh sigh TOH mah)	Tumor of the brain or spinal cord that is composed of astrocytes.
Bell's palsy (BELLZ PAWL zee)	One-sided facial paralysis with an unknown cause. The person cannot control salivation, tearing of the eyes, or expression. The patient will eventually recover. Named for Sir Charles Bell, a Scottish surgeon.
brain tumor	Intracranial mass, either benign or malignant. A benign tumor of the brain can be fatal since it will grow and cause pressure on normal brain tissue. The most malignant brain tumors in children are gliomas (see Figure 12.14).
cephalgia (seff AL jee ah)	A headache.
cerebral palsy (CP) (seh REE bral PAWL zee)	Nonprogressive paralysis resulting from a defect or trauma at the time of birth.
cerebrovascular accident (CVA) (ser eh broh VASS kyoo lar AK sih dent)	Also called a stroke. The development of an infarct due to loss in the blood supply to an area of the brain. Blood flow can be interrupted by a ruptured blood vessel (hemorrhage), a floating clot (embolus), a stationary clot (thrombosis), or compression (see Figure 12.15). The extent of damage depends on the size and location of the infarct and often includes speech problems and muscle paralysis.
concussion (kon KUSH un)	Injury to the brain that results from a blow or impact from an object. Can result in unconsciousness, dizziness, vomiting, unequal pupil size, and shock.
craniocele (KRAY nee oh seel)	Protrusion of the brain from within the skull.
encephalitis (en seff ah LYE tis)	Inflammation of the brain due to disease factors such as rabies, influenza, measles, or smallpox.
encephalocele (en SEFF ah loh seel)	Protrusion of the brain through the cranial cavity.
encephalosclerosis (en seff ah loh skleh ROH sis)	Condition of hardening of the brain.
epidural hematoma (ep ih DOO ral hee mah TOH mah)	Mass of blood in the space outside the dura mater of the brain and spinal cord.
epilepsy (EP ih lep see)	Recurrent disorder of the brain in which convulsive seizures and loss of consciousness occur.
glioma (glee OH mah)	Sarcoma of neurological origin.
hematoma (hee mah TOH mah)	Swelling or mass of blood confined in a specific area such as the brain.

(continued)

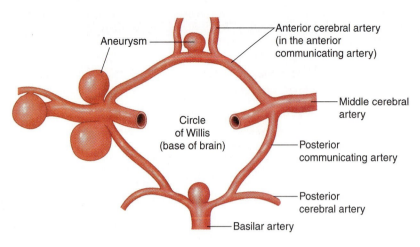

FIGURE 12.12 Aneurysms.

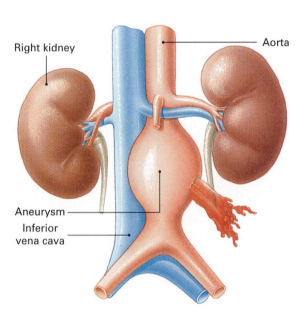

FIGURE 12.13 Abdominal aortic aneurysm.

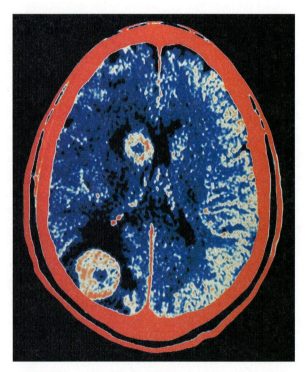

FIGURE 12.14 Enhanced-color malignant tumor of the brain. (Scott Camazine/Photo Researchers, Inc.)

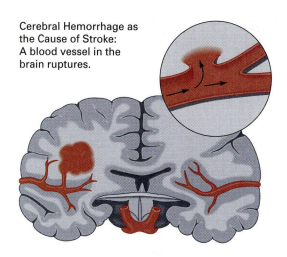

Cerebral Hemorrhage as the Cause of Stroke: A blood vessel in the brain ruptures.

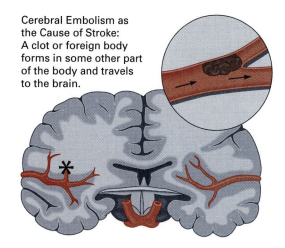

Cerebral Embolism as the Cause of Stroke: A clot or foreign body forms in some other part of the body and travels to the brain.

STROKE

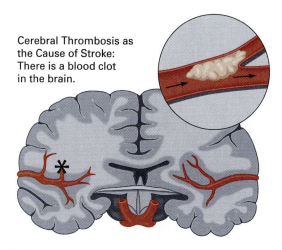

Cerebral Thrombosis as the Cause of Stroke: There is a blood clot in the brain.

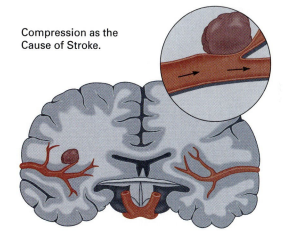

Compression as the Cause of Stroke.

FIGURE 12.15 Causes of stroke.

herniated nucleus pulposus (HNP) (HER nee ay ted NOO klee us pul POH sus)	Protrusion of the nucleus pulposus of the intervertebral disk into the spinal canal. Also called a *herniated disk,* or a *slipped disk.*
Huntington's chorea (HUNT ing tonz koh REE ah)	Disease of the central nervous system that results in progressive dementia with bizarre involuntary movements of parts of the body. Named for George Huntington, an American physician.
hydrocephalus (high droh SEFF ah lus)	Accumulation of cerebrospinal fluid within the ventricles of the brain, causing the head to be enlarged. It is treated by creating an artificial shunt for the fluid to leave the brain.
meningioma (meh nin jee OH mah)	Slow-growing tumor in the meninges of the brain.
meningitis (men in JYE tis)	Inflammation of the membranes of the spinal cord and brain that is caused by a microorganism.
meningocele (men IN goh seel)	Congenital hernia in which the meninges, or membranes, protrude through an opening in the spinal column or brain.
multiple sclerosis (MS) (MULL tih pl skleh ROH sis)	Inflammatory disease of the central nervous system in which there is extreme weakness and numbness.
myasthenia gravis (my ass THEE nee ah GRAV iss)	Disease with severe muscular weakness and fatigue.
narcolepsy (NAR koh lep see)	Chronic disorder in which there is an extreme uncontrollable desire to sleep.
neuritis (noo RYE tis)	Inflammation of a nerve or nerves, causing pain.
neuroblastoma (noo roh blass TOH mah)	Malignant hemorrhagic tumor that begins in the brain, especially in the adrenal medulla. Occurs mainly in infants and children.
Parkinson's disease (PARK in sons dih ZEEZ)	Chronic disorder of the nervous system with fine tremors, muscular weakness, rigidity, and a shuffling gait. Named for Sir James Parkinson, a British physician.
pica (PYE kah)	Eating disorder in which there is a craving for material that is not food, such as clay, grass, wood, paper, soap, and plaster.
Reye's syndrome (RISE SIN drohm)	Combination of symptoms first recognized by R.D.K. Reye, an Australian pathologist, in which there is acute encephalopathy and various organ damage. This occurs in children under 15 years of age who have had a viral infection.
shingles (SHING lz)	Eruption of vesicles on the trunk of the body along a nerve path. Can be painful and generally occurs on only one side of the body. Thought to be caused by a virus (see Figures 12.16 and 12.17).
spina bifida (SPY nah BIFF ih dah)	Congenital defect in the walls of the spinal canal in which the laminae of the vertebra do not meet or close. Results in membranes of the spinal cord being pushed through the opening. Can also result in other defects, such as hydrocephalus (see Figures 12.18 and 12.19).
subdural hematoma (sub DOO ral hee mah TOH mah)	Mass of blood forming beneath the dura mater of the brain (see Figure 12.20).
tic douloureux (TIK doo loo ROO)	Painful condition in which the trigeminal nerve is affected by pressure or degeneration. The pain is of a severe stabbing nature and radiates from the jaw and along the face.
transient ischemic (TRAN shent iss KEM ik) attack (TIA)	Temporary interference with blood supply to the brain, causing neurological symptoms such as dizziness, numbness, and hemiparesis. May eventually lead to a full-blown stroke (CVA).

FIGURE 12.16 Shingles.

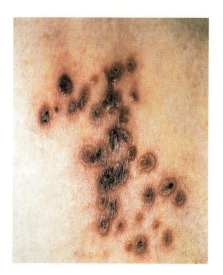

FIGURE 12.17 Shingles.

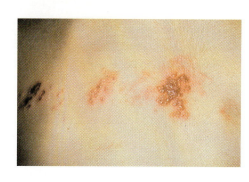

FIGURE 12.18 Forms of spina bifida.

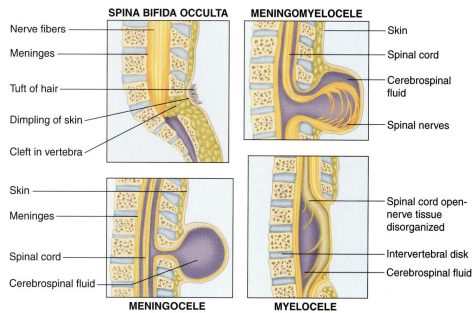

SPINA BIFIDA OCCULTA

- Nerve fibers
- Meninges
- Tuft of hair
- Dimpling of skin
- Cleft in vertebra

MENINGOMYELOCELE

- Skin
- Spinal cord
- Cerebrospinal fluid
- Spinal nerves

MENINGOCELE

- Skin
- Meninges
- Spinal cord
- Cerebrospinal fluid

MYELOCELE

- Spinal cord open-nerve tissue disorganized
- Intervertebral disk
- Cerebrospinal fluid

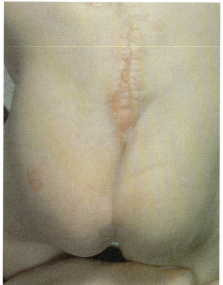

FIGURE 12.19 Child with spina bifida after surgical repair. (BioPhoto Associates/ Science Source/Photo Researchers, Inc.)

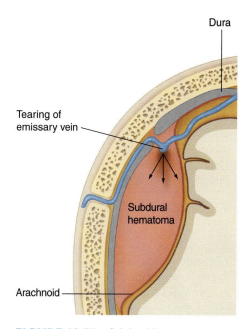

- Dura
- Tearing of emissary vein
- Subdural hematoma
- Arachnoid

FIGURE 12.20 Subdural hematoma.

Babinski's (bah BIN skeez) reflex	Reflex test developed by Joseph Babinski, a French neurologist, to determine lesions and abnormalities in the nervous system. The Babinski reflex is present if the great toe extends instead of flexes when the lateral sole of the foot is stroked. The normal response to this stimulation would be a flexion, or upward movement, of the toe.
brain scan	Injection of radioactive isotopes into the circulation to determine the function and abnormality of the brain.
cerebral angiography (seh REE bral an jee OG rah fee)	X-ray of the blood vessels of the brain after the injection of a radiopaque dye.
cerebrospinal fluid (CSF) analysis (ser eh broh SPY nal FLOO id an NAL ih sis)	Laboratory examination of the clear, watery, colorless fluid from within the brain and spinal cord. Infections and the abnormal presence of blood can be detected in this test.
computerized axial tomography (AK see al toh MOG rah fee) (CAT or CT)	Use of X-rays to examine a cross-section of the brain after dye has been injected. The outlines of tumors, blood clots, and hemorrhages can be seen.
echoencephalogram (ek oh en SEFF ah loh gram)	Recording of the ultrasonic echos of the brain. Useful in determining abnormal patterns of shifting in the brain.
electroencephalography (EEG) (ee lek troh en SEFF ah LOG rah fee)	Recording the electrical activity of the brain by placing electrodes at various positions on the scalp (see Figure 12.21). Also used in sleep studies to determine if there is a normal pattern of activity during sleep.
electromyogram (EMG) (ee lek troh MY oh gram)	Written recording of the contraction of muscles as a result of receiving electrical stimulation.
lumbar puncture (LP) (LUM bar PUNK chur)	Puncture with a needle into the lumbar area (usually the fourth intervertebral space) to withdraw fluid for examination and for the injection of anesthesia (see Figure 12.22). Also called spinal puncture or spinal tap.
magnetic resonance (mag NEH tik REHZ oh nance) imaging (MRI)	Use of electromagnetic energy to produce an image of the heart, blood vessels, brain, and soft tissues. Does not involve the use of radiation or an invasive procedure.
myelography (my eh LOG rah fee)	Injection of a radiopaque dye into the spinal canal. An X-ray is then taken to examine the normal and abnormal outlines made by the dye.
pneumoencephalography (PEG) (noo moh en seff ah LOG rah fee)	X-ray examination of the brain following withdrawal of cerebrospinal fluid and injection of air or gas via spinal puncture.
positron emission tomography (PET) (PAHZ ih tron ee MISH un toh MOG rah fee)	Use of positive radionuclides to reconstruct brain sections. Measurement can be taken of oxygen and glucose uptake, cerebral blood flow, and blood volume.
Romberg's (ROM bergs) test	Test developed by Moritz Romberg, a German physician, used to establish neurological function in which the person is asked to close his or her eyes and place the feet together. This test for body balance is positive if the patient sways when the eyes are closed.
transcutaneous electrical nerve stimulation (TENS) (tranz kyoo TAY nee us ee LEK trih kl nerve stim yoo LAY shun)	Application of a mild electrical stimulation to skin electrodes placed over a painful area, causing interference with the transmission of the painful stimuli. Can be used in pain management to interfere with the normal pain mechanism.

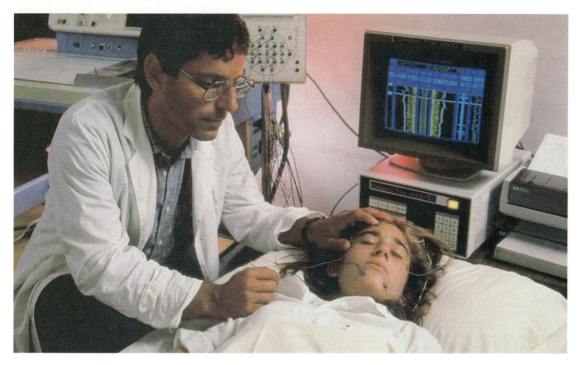

FIGURE 12.21   EEG in progress with computer display of brain waves in background. (Larry Mulvehill/Science Source/Photo Researchers, Inc.)

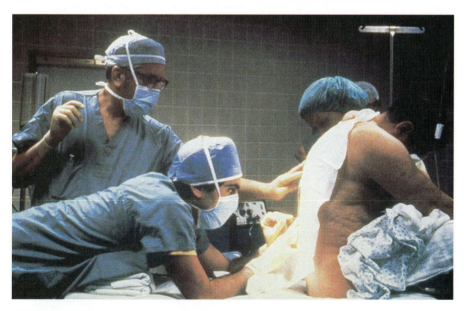

FIGURE 12.22   Spinal tap. (Mike Peres/Custom Medical Stock Photo, Inc.)

carotid endarterectomy (kah ROT id end ar ter EK toh mee)	Surgical procedure for removing an obstruction within the carotid artery, a major artery in the neck that carries oxygenated blood to the brain. Developed to prevent strokes, but is found to be useful only in severe stenosis with TIA.
cerebrospinal fluid (ser eh broh SPY nal FLOO id) shunts	A surgical procedure in which a bypass is created to drain cerebrospinal fluid. It is used to treat hydrocephalus by draining the excess cerebrospinal fluid from the brain and diverting it to the abdominal cavity.
cordectomy (kor DEK toh me)	Removal of part of the spinal cord.
craniotomy (kray nee OTT oh mee)	Surgical incision into the brain through the cranium.
cryosurgery (cry oh SER jer ee)	Use of extreme cold to destroy brain tissue. Used to control bleeding and treat brain tumors.
laminectomy (lam ih NEK toh mee)	Removal of a portion of a vertebra in order to relieve pressure on the spinal nerve.
nerve block	Method of regional anesthetic to stop the passage of sensory stimulation along a nerve path.
sympathectomy (sim pah THEK toh mee)	Excision of a portion of the sympathetic nervous system. Could include a nerve or a ganglion.
trephination (treff ih NAY shun)	Process of cutting out a piece of bone in the skull to gain entry into the brain or relieve pressure.
vagotomy (vah GOT oh mee)	An incision into the vagus nerve in order to cut away certain of its branches. One function of the vagus nerve is to stimulate the release of stomach acids. This procedure is performed to reduce the amount of stomach acid and therefore treat severe gastric ulcers.

Professional Profile

Psychiatrists

Psychiatrists promote their patient/client's mental health. They address issues that are disturbing to the client and outline various strategies and interventions in order to provide a treatment plan for the client/patient to work through these issues. Psychiatrists personally address issues such as adequacy, security and self-esteem. Psychiatrists may also counsel people who have been involved in traumatic situations, from car accident victims to victims of crime. Psychiatrists work in hospitals, rehabilitation facilities, and often have their own psychiatric practice. Psychiatrists who work in the field must graduate from medical school and obtain a license to practice medicine in the state where their

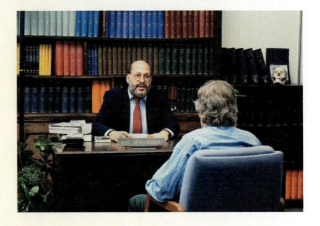

practice is based. For more information about a career as a Psychiatrist, visit the American Psychiatric Association's web site at www.psych.org.

Abbreviations Relating to the Nervous System

ALS	amyotrophic lateral sclerosis	**HNP**	herniated nucleus pulposus (herniated disk)
ANS	autonomic nervous system	**LP**	lumbar puncture
CAT, CT	computerized axial tomography	**MRI**	magnetic resonance imaging
CNS	central nervous system	**MS**	multiple sclerosis
CP	cerebral palsy	**PEG**	pneumoencephalogram
CSF	cerebrospinal fluid	**PET**	positron emission tomography
CVA	cerebrovascular accident	**PNS**	peripheral nervous system
EEG	electroencephalogram, electroencephalography	**TENS**	transcutaneous electrical nerve stimulation
EMG	electromyogram	**TIA**	transient ischemic attack
EST	electric shock therapy		

KEY TERMS

- adrenal medulla (ad **REE** nal meh **DULL** ah)
- afferent neurons (**AFF** er ent **NOO** rons)
- Alzheimer's disease (**ALTS** high merz)
- amyotrophic lateral sclerosis (ALS) (ah my oh **TROFF** ik **LAT** er al skleh **ROH** sis)
- analgesia (an al **JEE** zee ah)
- anesthesia (an ess **THEE** zee ah)
- aneurysm (**AN** yoo rizm)
- aphasia (ah **FAY** zee ah)
- arachnoid layer (ah **RAK** noyd)
- asthenia (as **THEE** nee ah)
- astrocyte (**ASS** troh sight)
- astrocytoma (ass troh sigh **TOH** mah)
- ataxia (ah **TAK** see ah)
- autonomic nervous system (ANS) (aw toh **NOM** ik **NER** vus **SIS** tem)
- axon (**AK** son)
- Babinski's sign (bah **BIN** skeez)
- Bell's palsy (**BELLZ PAWL** zee)
- bradykinesia (brad ee kin **NEE** see ah)
- brain
- brain scan
- brain stem
- brain tumor
- carotid endarterectomy (kah **ROT** id end ar ter **EK** toh mee)
- cell body
- central nervous system (CNS)
- cephalgia (seff **AL** jee ah)
- cerebellar (ser eh **BELL** ar)
- cerebellitis (ser eh bell **EYE** tis)
- cerebellum (ser eh **BELL** um)
- cerebral (seh **REE** bral)
- cerebral angiography (seh **REE** bral an jee **OG** rah fee)
- cerebral cortex (seh **REE** bral **KOR** teks)
- cerebral palsy (CP) (seh **REE** bral **PAWL** zee)
- cerebrospinal (ser eh broh **SPY** nal)
- cerebrospinal fluid (CSF) (ser eh broh **SPY** nal **FLOO** id)

- cerebrospinal fluid analysis (ser eh broh **SPY** nal **FLOO** id an **NAL** ih sis)
- cerebrospinal fluid shunts (ser eh broh **SPY** nal **FLOO** id)
- cerebrovascular accident (CVA) (ser eh broh **VASS** kyoo lar **AK** sih dent)
- cerebrum (**SER** eh brum)
- chorea (koh **REE** ah)
- coma (**COH** mah)
- computerized axial tomography (CAT, CT) (**AK** see al toh **MOG** rah fee)
- concussion (kon **KUSH** un)
- conscious (**KON** shus)
- convulsion (kon **VULL** shun)
- cordectomy (kor **DEK** toh mee)
- cranial nerves (**KRAY** nee al)
- craniocele (**KRAY** nee oh seel)
- craniotomy (kray nee **OTT** oh mee)
- cryosurgery (cry oh **SER** jer ee)
- dementia (dee **MEN** she ah)
- dendrites (**DEN** drights)
- diencephalon (dye en **SEFF** ah lon)
- dura mater (**DOO** rah **MATE** er)
- dysphasia (dis **FAY** zee ah)
- echoencephalogram (ek oh en **SEFF** ah loh gram)
- efferent neurons (**EFF** er ent)
- electroencephalogram (EEG) (ee lek troh en **SEFF** ah loh gram)
- electroencephalograph (ee lek troh en **SEFF** ah loh graf)
- electroencephalography (EEG) (ee lek troh en seff ah **LOG** rah fee)
- electromyogram (EMG) (ee lek troh **MY** oh gram)
- embolism (**EM** boh lizm)
- encephalitis (en seff ah **LYE** tis)
- encephalocele (en **SEFF** ah loh seel)
- encephalomalacia (en seff ah loh mah **LAY** she ah)
- encephalosclerosis (en seff ah loh skleh **ROH** sis)
- epidural hematoma (ep ih **DOO** ral hee mah **TOH** mah)
- epilepsy (**EP** ih lep see)

- fissures (**FISH** ers)
- frontal lobe
- ganglion (**GANG** lee on)
- gastric glands (**GAS** trik)
- glioma (glee **OH** mah)
- grand mal (**GRAND MALL**)
- gray matter
- gyri (**JYE** rye)
- hematoma (hee mah **TOH** mah)
- hemiparesis (hem ee par **EE** sis)
- hemiplegia (hem ee **PLEE** jee ah)
- hemisphere (**HEM** is feer)
- herniated nucleus pulposus (HNP) (**HER** nee ay ted **NOO** klee us pul **POH** sus)
- Huntington's chorea (**HUNT** ing tonz koh **REE** ah)
- hydrocephalus (high droh **SEFF** ah lus)
- hyperesthesia (high per ess **THEE** zee ah)
- hypothalamus (high poh **THAL** ah mus)
- idiopathic (id ee oh **PATH** ik)
- impulse
- laminectomy (lam ih **NEK** toh mee)
- lethargy (**LETH** ar jee)
- lumbar puncture (LP) (**LUM** bar **PUNK** chur)
- magnetic resonance imaging (MRI) (mag **NEH** tik **REHZ** oh nance)
- medulla oblongata (meh **DULL** ah ob long **GAH** tah)
- meninges (men **IN** jeez)
- meningioma (meh nin jee **OH** mah)
- meningitis (men in **JYE** tis)
- meningocele (men **IN** goh seel)
- midbrain
- monoparesis (mon oh pah **REE** sis)
- monoplegia (mon oh **PLEE** jee ah)
- multiple sclerosis (MS) (**MULL** tih pl skleh **ROH** sis)
- myasthenia (my ass **THEE** nee ah)
- myasthenia gravis (my ass **THEE** nee ah **GRAV** iss)
- myelin (**MY** eh lin)
- myelinated (**MY** eh lih nayt ed)
- myelogram (**MY** eh loh gram)
- myelography (my eh **LOG** rah fee)
- myelomalacia (my eh loh mah **LAY** she ah)
- myelomeningocele (my eh loh meh **NIN** goh seel)
- narcolepsy (**NAR** koh lep see)
- nerve block
- nerves
- neuralgia (noo **RAL** jee ah)
- neurasthenia (noor ass **THEE** nee ah)
- neurectomy (noo **REK** toh mee)
- neuritis (noo **RYE** tis)
- neuroblastoma (noo roh blass **TOH** mah)
- neurologist (noo **RAL** oh jist)
- neurology (nu **RAL** oh jee)
- neurolysis (noo **ROL** ih sis)
- neuroma (noo **ROH** mah)
- neuron (**NOO** ron)
- neuroplasty (**NOOR** oh plas tee)
- neurorrhaphy (noo **ROR** ah fee)
- neurosurgeon (noo roh **SIR** jun)
- neurotomy (noo **ROT** oh mee)
- occipital lobe (ock **SIP** ih tal)
- palsy (**PAWL** zee)
- panplegia (pan **PLEE** jee ah)
- paralysis (pah **RAL** ih sis)
- paraplegia (pair ah **PLEE** jee ah)
- parasympathetic (pair ah sim pah **THET** ik)
- parietal lobe (pah **RYE** eh tal)
- Parkinson's disease (**PARK** in sons dih **ZEEZ**)
- peripheral nervous system (PNS) (per **IF** er al)
- petit mal (pet **EE MALL**)
- pia mater (**PEE** ah **MATE** er)
- pica (**PYE** kah)
- pneumoencephalography (noo moh en seff ah **LOG** rah fee)
- poliomyelitis (poh lee oh my ell **EYE** tis)
- polyneuritis (pol ee noo **RYE** tis)
- pons (**PONZ**)
- positron emission tomography (PET) (**PAHZ** ih tron ee **MISH** un toh **MOG** rah fee)
- quadriplegia (kwod rih **PLEE** jee ah)
- radiculitis (rah dick yoo **LYE** tis)
- Reye's syndrome (**RISE SIN** drohm)
- Romberg's test (**ROM** bergs)
- salivary glands (**SAL** ih vair ee)
- seizure (**SEE** zyoor)
- shingles (**SHING** lz)
- sleep disorder
- spina bifida (**SPY** nah **BIFF** ih dah)
- spinal canal
- spinal cord
- spinal nerves
- spinal puncture
- stimulus (**STIM** yoo lus)
- subarachnoid space (sub ah **RAK** noyd)
- subdural (sub **DOO** ral)
- subdural hematoma (sub **DOO** ral hee mah **TOH** mah)
- subdural space (sub **DOO** ral)
- sulci (**SULL** kye)
- sweat glands
- sympathectomy (sim pah **THEK** toh mee)
- sympathetic (sim pah **THET** ik)
- syncope (**SIN** koh pee)
- temporal lobe (**TEM** por al)
- tetraplegia (tet rah **PLEE** jee ah)
- thalamus (**THAL** ah mus)
- tic (**TIK**)
- tic douloureux (**TIK** doo loo **ROO**)
- tract
- transcutaneous electrical nerve stimulation (TENS) (tranz kyoo **TAY** nee us ee **LEK** trih kl nerve stim yoo **LAY** shun)
- transient ischemic attack (TIA) (**TRAN** shent iss **KEM** ik)
- tremor (**TREM** or)
- trephination (treff ih **NAY** shun)
- unconscious (un **KON** shus)
- vagotomy (vah **GOT** oh mee)
- ventricles (**VEN** trik lz)
- vertebra (**VER** teh brah)
- vertebral canal (**VER** teh bral)
- vertebral column (**VER** teh bral)
- white matter

Case Study

DISCHARGE SUMMARY

Admitting Diagnosis: Paraplegia following motorcycle accident.

Final Diagnosis: Comminuted L2 fracture with epidural hematoma and spinal cord damage resulting in complete paraplegia at the L2 level.

History of Present Illness: Patient is a 23-year-old male who was involved in a motorcycle accident. He was unconscious for 35 minutes but was fully aware of his surroundings upon regaining consciousness. He was immediately aware of total anesthesia and paralysis below the waist.

Summary of Hospital Course: CT scan revealed extensive bone destruction at the fracture site and that the spinal cord was severed. Lumbar puncture revealed sanguinous cerebrospinal fluid. Patient was unable to voluntarily contract any lower extremity muscles and was not able to feel touch or pinpricks. Lumbar laminectomy with spinal fusion was performed to stabilize the fracture and remove the epidural hematoma. The immediate post-operative recovery period proceeded normally with one incidence of pneumonia due to extended bed rest. It responded to antibiotics and respiratory therapy treatments. Patient began intensive rehabilitation with physical therapy and occupational therapy to strengthen upper extremities, and transfer and ADL training. After two months, X-rays indicated full healing of the spinal fusion and patient was transferred to a rehabilitation institute.

Discharge Plans: Patient was transferred to a rehabilitation institute to continue intensive PT and OT. He will require skilled nursing care to evaluate his skin for the development of decubitus ulcers and intermittent urinary catheterization for incontinence. Since spinal cord was severed, it is not expected that this patient will regain muscle function and sensation. However, long-term goals include independent transfers, independent mobility with a wheelchair, and independent ADLs.

CRITICAL THINKING QUESTIONS

1. The final diagnosis of "paraplegia at the L2 level" is not specifically defined by your text. Explain what you believe it to mean in the context of this discharge summary.

2. Is this patient expected to regain use of his muscles? Explain why or why not.

3. The following medical terms are not specifically referred to in this chapter. Using your text as a dictionary, define each term in your own words.

   a. comminuted

   b. sanguinous

   c. decubitus ulcer

   d. catheterization

4. Which of the following is NOT part of this patient's rehabilitation therapy?

   a. arm strengthening

   b. transfer training

   c. instruction in activities of daily living

   d. leg strengthening

5. Describe in your own words, the patient's long-term goals.

6. Name and describe the complete surgical procedure this patient underwent. Then describe the purpose for this surgery.

Chart Note Transcription

Chart Note

The chart note below contains eleven phrases that can be reworded with a medical term that you learned in this chapter. Each phrase is identified with an underline. Determine the medical term and write your answers in the space provided.

Current Complaint: Patient is a 38-year-old female referred to the specialist in the treatment of diseases of the nervous system[1] by her family physician with complaints of difficulty with speech,[2] loss of motion on one side of the body,[3] and severe involuntary muscle contractions.[4]

Past History: Patient is married and nulliparous. Has been well prior to current symptoms.

Signs and Symptoms: Her husband reports he first noted loss of motion on one side of the body when she began to drag her left foot. It has progressed to involve both left upper and lower extremities, with approximately a 50% loss in control of left lower extremity and a 25% loss of control in left upper extremity. Difficulty with speech is mild and mainly with recalling the names of common objects. Severe involuntary muscle contractions appear to be triggered by stress and last approximately 2 minutes. Results of a recording of the electrical activity of the brain[5] and a puncture with a needle into the low back to withdraw fluid for examination[6] were normal. However an image produced by the use of electromagnetic energy[7] revealed the presence of a mass in the right outer layer of the largest section of the brain.[8]

Diagnosis: Astrocyte tumor[9] in the right outer layer of the largest section of the brain.

Treatment: A right skull incision[10] was performed to permit the use of extreme cold to destroy[11] the tumor. Patient experienced moderate improvement in loss of motion on one side of the body and severe involuntary muscle contractions, but difficulty with speech was unchanged.

1 _____

2 _____

3 _____

4 _____

5 _____

6 _____

7 _____

8 _____

9 _____

10 _____

11 _____

Practice Exercises

A. COMPLETE THE FOLLOWING STATEMENTS.

1. The study of the nervous system is called _____ .
2. The organs of the nervous system are the _____ , _____ , and
   _____ .
3. The three divisions of the nervous system are the _____ , _____ , and
   _____ .
4. The neurons that carry impulses away from the brain and spinal cord are called _____ neurons.
5. The neurons that carry impulses to the brain and spinal cord are called _____ neurons.
6. The disease, caused by a virus, that attacks the gray matter of the spinal cord is _____ .
7. The largest portion of the brain is the _____ .
8. The second largest portion of the brain is the _____ .
9. The occipital lobe controls the _____ .
10. The temporal lobe controls the _____ and _____ .
11. A CVA on the left side of the brain will affect the _____ side of the patient.
12. The two divisions of the autonomic nervous system are the _____ and _____ .

B. STATE THE DESCRIBED TERMS USING THE COMBINING FORMS PROVIDED.

The combining form neur/o refers to the nerve. Use it to write a term that means

1. inflammation of the nerve _____
2. developing nerve cell _____
3. pain in the nerve _____
4. nerve weakness _____
5. excision of a nerve _____
6. surgical repair of a nerve _____
7. incision into a nerve or nerves _____
8. suture of a nerve _____

The combining form mening/o refers to the meninges or membranes. Use it to write a term that means

9. inflammation of the meninges _____
10. protrusion of the meninges through a defect _____
11. tumor of the meninges _____

The combining form encephal/o refers to the brain. Use it to write a term that means

12. X-ray examination of the brain _____
13. disease of the brain _____
14. inflammation of the brain _____
15. pertaining to the brain _____
16. acute inflammation of brain and spinal cord _____

The combining form cerebr/o refers to the brain. Use it to write a term that means

17. fluid in the brain and spinal cord _____
18. hardening of the brain _____
19. any disease of the brain _____
20. inflammation of the brain and its membranes _____
21. relating to the brain _____
22. relating to the brain and blood vessels _____

C. MATCH THE TERMS IN COLUMN A WITH THE DEFINITIONS IN COLUMN B.

A

1. _____ chorea
2. _____ meningitis
3. _____ palsy
4. _____ shingles
5. _____ syncope
6. _____ pica
7. _____ petit mal
8. _____ grand mal
9. _____ meningocele

B

a. eating disorder
b. bizarre movements
c. convulsion
d. congenital hernia of membranes
e. mild epilepsy
f. inflammation of meninges
g. shaking, tremors
h. painful virus on nerves
i. fainting

D. IDENTIFY THE FOLLOWING ABBREVIATIONS.

1. TIA _____
2. MS _____
3. CAT _____
4. CNS _____
5. PNS _____
6. MRI _____
7. CP _____
8. LP _____
9. ALS _____
10. ANS _____

E. MATCH THE CRANIAL NERVES IN COLUMN A WITH THE FUNCTIONS THEY CONTROL IN COLUMN B.

A

1. _____ olfactory
2. _____ optic
3. _____ oculomotor
4. _____ trochlear
5. _____ trigeminal
6. _____ abducens
7. _____ facial
8. _____ acoustic
9. _____ glossopharyngeal
10. _____ vagus
11. _____ spinal accessory
12. _____ hypoglossal

B

a. eyes, upper jaw, lower jaw
b. turn eye to side
c. taste and salivary glands
d. eye muscles control pupils
e. swallowing
f. muscles of tongue
g. eyeball muscle
h. smell
i. sensory nerve of head/neck
j. hearing and balance
k. vision
l. organs in lower cavities

F. DEFINE THE FOLLOWING PROCEDURES AND TESTS.

1. myelogram _____
2. cerebral angiography _____
3. Babinski's reflex _____
4. Romberg's test _____
5. cerebrospinal fluid analysis _____
6. PET scan _____
7. echoencephalography _____
8. spinal puncture _____

G. Define each suffix and provide an example of its use.

		Meaning	Example
1.	-lepsy		
2.	-plegia		
3.	-taxia		
4.	-algesia		
5.	-sthenia		
6.	-trophy		

H. Define the following combining forms.

1. mening/o
2. encephal/o
3. cerebell/o
4. myel/o
5. cephal/o
6. phas/o
7. gli/o
8. spondyl/o
9. cerebr/o

I. Define the following terms.

1. glioma
2. epilepsy
3. anesthesia
4. hemiparesis
5. neuralgia
6. analgesia
7. neurasthenia

J. Match the terms in column A with the definitions in column B.

A	B
1. _____ neurologist	a. seizures
2. _____ idiopathic	b. sleep disorder
3. _____ lethargy	c. Alzheimer's disease
4. _____ aphasia	d. physician who treats nervous problem
5. _____ narcolepsy	e. no known cause
6. _____ epilepsy	f. sluggishness
7. _____ dementia	g. loss of ability to speak

K. **BREAK THE FOLLOWING WORDS INTO THEIR COMPONENTS USING THE FOLLOWING SYMBOLS: WR = WORD ROOT, P = PREFIX, AND S = SUFFIX. DEFINE EACH COMPONENT AND THE TERM.**

For example: vagotomy
components: WR = vag/o, S = otomy
Definition of parts   *Vag/o means vagus nerve*
                                -otomy means to cut into

Definition of term: *cutting into the vagus nerve*

1. meningitis
   components: _____
   definition of parts: _____
   definition of term: _____

2. electroencephalography
   components: _____
   definition of parts: _____
   definition of term: _____

3. astrocytoma
   components: _____
   definition of parts: _____
   definition of term: _____

4. cerebrovascular
   components: _____
   definition of parts: _____
   definition of term: _____

5. hemiplegia
   components: _____
   definition of parts: _____
   definition of term: _____

6. hydrocephalus
   components: _____
   definition of parts: _____
   definition of term: _____

7. hematoma
   components: _____
   definition of parts: _____
   definition of term: _____

8. encephalitis
   components: _____
   definition of parts: _____
   definition of term: _____

9. craniocele
   components: _____
   definition of parts: _____
   definition of term: _____

10. meningocele
   components: _____
   definition of parts: _____
   definition of term: _____

11. cerebrospinal

    components: _____

    definition of parts: _____

    definition of term: _____

12. quadriplegia

    components: _____

    definition of parts: _____

    definition of term: _____

13. cryosurgery

    components: _____

    definition of parts: _____

    definition of term: _____

Getting Connected

Multimedia Extension Activities

CD-ROM

Use the CD-ROM enclosed with your textbook to gain additional reinforcement through interactive word building exercises, spelling games, labeling activities, and additional quizzes.

www.prenhall.com/fremgen

Use the above address to access the free, interactive Companion Website created for this textbook. Get hints, instant feedback, and textbook references to chapter-related multiple choice questions, and labeling and matching exercises. In addition, you will find an audio glossary, case studies, Internet exploration exercises, flashcards, and a comprehensive exam.

Answers

CASE STUDY (CRITICAL THINKING QUESTIONS)

1. the muscles that receive nerve supply from or below the 2nd lumbar vertebra are paralyzed   2. no, the spinal cord was completely severed   3. comminuted—shattered bone; sanguinous—bloody; decubitus ulcer—pressure sore; catheterization—thin, flexible tube inserted into the bladder   4. d—leg strengthening   5. independent transfers, independent wheelchair mobility, independent ADLs.   6. lumbar laminectomy with spinal fusion; stabilize the fracture and remove the epidural hematoma

CHART NOTE

1. neurologist—specialist in the treatment of diseases of the nervous system   2. dysphasia—difficulty with speech   3. hemiparesis—loss of motion on one side of the body   4. convulsions—severe involuntary muscle contractions   5. electroencephalography (EEG)—recording of the electrical activity of the brain   6. lumbar puncture (LP)—puncture with a needle into the low back to withdraw fluid for examination   7. magnetic resonance imaging (MRI)—an image produced by the use of electromagnetic energy   8. cerebral cortex—outer layer of the largest section of the brain   9. astrocytoma—astrocyte tumor   10. craniotomy—skull incision   11. cryosurgery—the use of extreme cold to destroy

PRACTICE EXERCISES

A. 1. neurology   2. brain, spinal cord, nerves   3. peripheral nervous system, central nervous system, autonomic nervous system   4. efferent   5. afferent   6. poliomyelitis   7. cerebrum   8. cerebellum   9. eyesight   10. hearing, smell   11. right   12. parasympathetic, sympathetic

B. 1. neuritis   2. neuroblast   3. neuralgia   4. neurasthenia   5. neurectomy   6. neuroplasty   7. neurotomy   8. neurorrhaphy   9. meningitis   10. meningocele   11. meningioma   12. encephalography   13. encephalopathy   14. encephalitis   15. encephalic   16. encephalomyelitis   17. cerebrospinal fluid   18. cerebrosclerosis   19. cerebropathy   20. cerebromeningitis   21. cerebral   22. cerebrovascular

C. 1. b   2. f   3. g   4. h   5. i   6. a   7. e   8. c   9. d

D. 1. transient ischemic attack   2. multiple sclerosis   3. computerized axial tomography   4. central nervous system   5. peripheral nervous system   6. magnetic resonance imaging   7. cerebral palsy   8. lumbar puncture   9. amyotropic lateral sclerosis   10. autonomic nervous system

E. 1. h   2. k   3. d   4. g   5. a   6. b   7. c   8. j   9. e   10. l   11. i   12. f

F. 1. Injecting radiopaque dye into spinal canal to examine under X-ray the outlines made by the dye.   2. X-ray of the blood vessels of the brain after the injection of radiopaque dye.   3. Reflex test on bottom of foot to detect lesion and abnormalities of nervous system.   4. Test of balance to determine neurological function.   5. Laboratory examination of fluid taken from the brain and spinal cord.   6. Positron emission tomography to measure cerebral blood flow, blood volume, oxygen, and glucose uptake.   7. Recording the ultrasonic echos of the brain.   8. Needle puncture into the spinal cavity to withdraw fluid.

G. 1. seizures   2. paralysis   3. muscular coordination   4. pain sensitivity   5. strength   6. development

H. 1. meninges   2. brain   3. cerebellum   4. spinal cord   5. head   6. speech   7. glue   8. vertebra   9. brain

I. 1. gluelike tumor of nervous cells   2. seizure   3. without sensation   4. paralysis of one-half of body   5. nerve pain   6. without pain sensitivity   7. lack of nervous strength

J. 1. d   2. e   3. f   4. g   5. b   6. a   7. c

K. 1. WR = mening/o s = -itis
        meninges, inflammation
        inflammation of meninges
   2. WR = electr/o WR = encephal/o
        s = -graphy
        electricity, brain, process of recording
        process of recording electrical activity of the
        brain
   3. WR = astr/o WR = cyt/o
        s = -oma
        star cell tumor
        tumor of star-shaped cells
   4. WR = cerebr/o WR = vascul/o
        s = -ar
        brain, blood vessels, pertaining to
        pertaining to brain blood vessels
   5. P = hemi- S = -plegia
        half, paralysis
        paralysis of half the body
   6. P = hydro- WR = cephal/o
        S = -us
        water, head
        converts word root into a noun
        water in the head

   7. WR = hemat/o s = -oma
        blood tumor, swelling
        swelling of blood
   8. WR = encephal/o s = -itis
        brain, inflammation
        inflammation of the brain
   9. WR = crani/o s = -cele
        skull, protrusion
        protrusion through the skull
  10. WR = mening/o s = -cele
        meninges, protrusion
        protrusion of the meninges
  11. WR = cerebr/o WR = spin/o s = -al
        brain, spine, pertaining to
        pertaining to the brain and spine
  12. P = quadri- s = plegia
        four, paralysis
        paralysis of four (limbs)
  13. P = cryo- s = surgery
        cold, surgery
        surgery using cold

Chapter 13

SPECIAL SENSES: THE EYE AND THE EAR

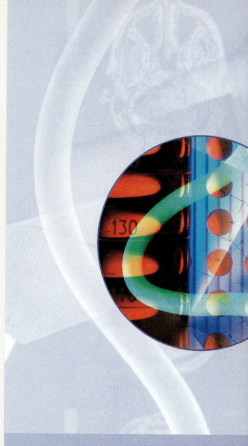

LEARNING OBJECTIVES

Upon completion of this chapter, you will be able to:

- Recognize the combining forms and suffixes introduced in this chapter.

- Gain the ability to pronounce medical terms and major anatomical structures.

- List the major organs of the eye and ear and their functions.

- Describe how we see.

- Describe the path of sound vibration.

- Build eye and ear medical terms from word parts.

- Define vocabulary, pathology, diagnostic, and therapeutic medical terms relating to the eye and ear.

- Interpret abbreviations associated with the eye and ear.

Overview

ORGANS OF THE SPECIAL SENSES

ear

eye

The organs of smell, taste, and touch are also considered special senses. However, these organs are discussed in other chapters.

PART I: *The Eye*

STRUCTURES RELATING TO THE EYE

choroid	lacrimal ducts
conjunctiva	lacrimal glands
cornea	lens
eye muscles	orbit
eye socket	pupil
eyeball	retina
eyelids	sclera
iris	

COMBINING FORMS RELATING TO THE EYE

ambly/o	dull or dim	ocul/o	eye
aque/o	water	ophthalm/o	eye
blephar/o	eyelid	opt/i	eye, vision
conjunctiv/o	conjunctiva	opt/o	eye, vision
cor/o	pupil	optic/o	eye
corne/o	cornea	palpebr/o	eyelid
cycl/o	ciliary/muscle	papill/o	optic disc
dacry/o	tear; tear duct	phac/o	lens
dipl/o	double	phot/o	light
glauc/o	gray	presby/o	old age
ir/o	iris	pupill/o	pupil
irid/o	iris	retin/o	retina
kerat/o	cornea	scler/o	sclera
lacrim/o	tears	uve/o	vascular
mi/o	smaller, less	vitre/o	glassy
mydr/o	larger, widen		

Suffix	Meaning	Example
-chalasis	relaxation	blepharochalasis
-opia	vision	hyperopia
-tropia	to turn	esotropia

ANATOMY AND PHYSIOLOGY OF THE EYE

conjunctiva	lacrimal glands	pupil
eye muscles	lens	retina
eyelids	ophthalmology (Ophth.)	
lacrimal ducts	orbit	

The study of the eye is known as **ophthalmology** (off thal **MALL** oh gee) **(Ophth.).** The eye is the incredible organ of sight that combines the functions of its many parts to transmit an external image by way of the nervous system (optic nerve) to the brain. The brain then translates these sensory impulses into what we understand as *sight* with a computerlike accuracy.

MED TERM TIP

Think of the eye as working much like a camera. The light rays pass through a very small opening (the **pupil**) in the eye and are focused by the **lens** on a surface that is receptive to these rays. This surface is called the **retina** (**RET** in ah). In your camera, the film would be similar to the retina. In both a camera and the eye, the lens inverts the image. The brain turns it right-side up again (see Figure 13.1).

The external structures of the eye consist of the **orbit, eye muscles, eyelids, conjunctiva** (kon **JUNK** tih vah), and **lacrimal** (**LAK** rim al) **glands** and **ducts** (see Figure 13.2 for anatomy of the eye).

THE ORBIT

eye socket	ophthalmic artery
eyeball	optic nerve

The orbit or **eye socket** is a cavity in the front of the skull containing the **eyeball.** It is formed from several bones and has a soft fatty tissue lining. The orbit of the eye has openings through which the **optic** (**OP** tik) **nerve** and **ophthalmic** (off **THAL** mik) **artery** enter the eyeball.

MUSCLES OF THE EYE

oblique muscles	strabismus
rectus muscles	

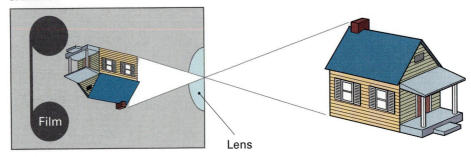

Film

Lens

EYE

Retina

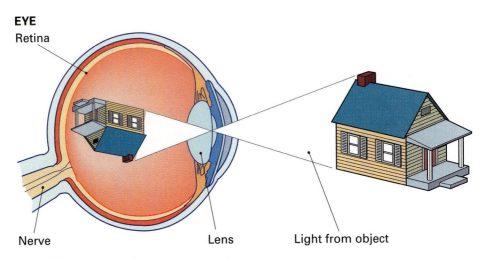

Nerve   Lens   Light from object

FIGURE 13.1 The eye mechanism is similar to a camera.

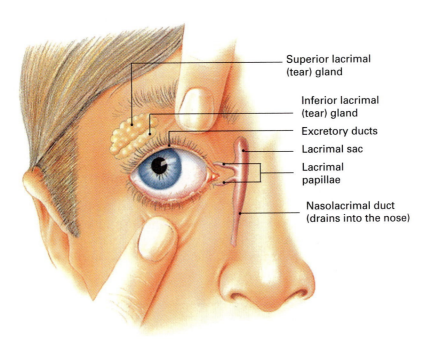

Superior lacrimal
(tear) gland

Inferior lacrimal
(tear) gland

Excretory ducts

Lacrimal sac

Lacrimal
papillae

Nasolacrimal duct
(drains into the nose)

FIGURE 13.2 Anatomy of the eye.

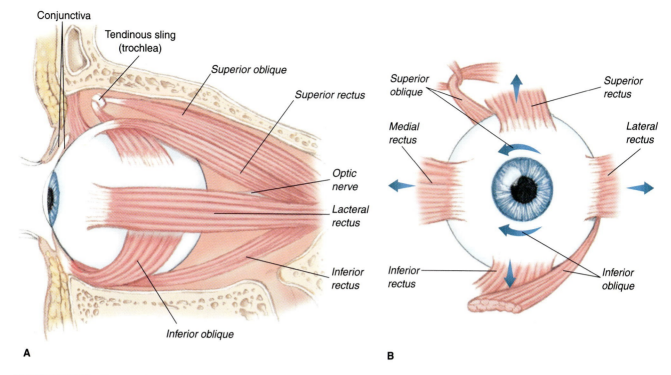

FIGURE 13.3 Eye muscles. (A) Lateral view, left eye. (B) Anterior view, left eye.

There are six muscles that connect the actual eyeball to the orbital cavity (see Figure 13.3). These muscles allow for rotation of the eyeball to assist with vision. In addition, they provide support for the eyeball in the eye socket or orbit. Children may be born with a weakness in some of these muscles and may require conservative treatment such as eye exercises or even surgery to correct this problem. This problem is commonly referred to as *crossed eyes* or **strabismus** (strah **BIZ** mus) (see Figure 13.4). The muscles involved are the four **rectus** (**REK** tus) or *straight* **muscles** and two **oblique** (oh **BLEEK**) or *slanted* **muscles.**

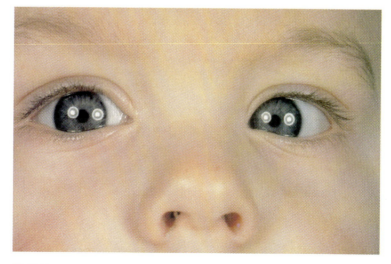

FIGURE 13.4 Strabismus in young child. (Barts Medical Library/Phototake NYC)

THE EYELIDS

chalazion   **sebaceous glands**

cilia

A pair of eyelids over each eye provides protection from foreign particles, injury from the sun and intense light, and trauma. Both the upper and lower edges of the eyelids have small hairs or **cilia** (**SIL** ee ah) called eyelashes that protect the eye from foreign particles. In addition, **sebaceous** (see **BAY** shus) or *oil* glands are located in the eyelids. These secrete a lubricating oil onto the eyeball. A small hard mass called a **chalazion** (kah **LAY** zee on), or stye, can develop on the eyelid when the sebaceous glands become clogged.

THE CONJUNCTIVA

conjunctivitis

The conjunctiva of the eye is the mucous membrane lining on the underside of each eyelid and across the anterior surface of each eyeball. This serves as a protection for the eye.

MED TERM *TIP*

Conjunctivitis (kon junk tih **VYE** tis) or *inflammation of the conjunctiva*, also called *pinkeye*, is a common problem caused by infection of the eyelid.

THE LACRIMAL GLAND AND DUCTS

lacrimal sac

The lacrimal gland is located in the outer corner of each eyelid. It serves the important function of washing the anterior surface of the eye with fluid or *tears*. Lacrimal ducts located in the inner corner of the eye socket then collect the fluid or tears and drain them into the **lacrimal** (**LAK** rim al) **sac.**

THE EYEBALL

aqueous humor	**iris**	**pupil**
choroid	**jaundice**	**retina**
ciliary body	**lens**	**retinal blood vessels**
cornea	**macula lutea**	**sclera**
fovea centralis	**optic disk**	**vitreous humor**

The actual eye is composed of three layers:

1. **Sclera** (**SKLAIR** ah)
2. **Choroid** (**KOR** oyd)
3. **Retina** (**RET** in ah)

The outer layer, the sclera, provides a tough protective layer for the inner structures of the eye. Another term for the sclera is the *white of the eye*.

The anterior portion of the sclera is called the **cornea** (**COR** nee ah). This is the clear, transparent part of the sclera and is responsible for allowing light to enter the interior of the eye. The cornea, often referred to as *the window of the eye,* actually bends the light rays (see Figure 13.5 for illustration of the eyeball).

Behind the cornea are the other structures of the anterior eye, the **iris, pupil, lens, and ciliary** (**SIL** ee ar ee) **body.** The iris is the colored portion of the eye and contains muscle. The pupil is the opening in the center of the iris that allows light rays to enter the eyeball. The iris muscle contracts or relaxes to change the size of the pupil, thereby controlling how much light enters the interior of the eyeball. Behind the iris is the lens. The edge of the lens is attached to the muscular ciliary body. By pulling on the edge of the lens, these muscles change the shape of the lens so it can focus incoming light onto the retina.

The second layer or middle layer of the eye is called the choroid. This layer provides the blood supply for the eye and is opaque.

The third, innermost layer, of the eyeball is the retina. It contains the sensory receptor cells that respond to light rays. When the lens projects an image onto the retina, it strikes an area called the **macula lutea** (yellow spot). In the center of the macula lutea

FIGURE 13.5 Eyeball.

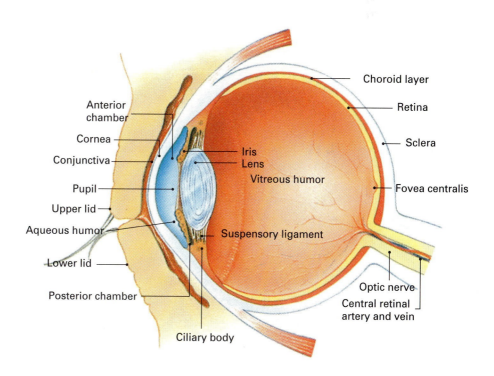

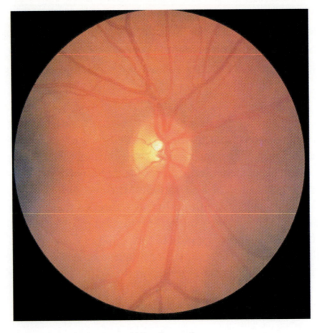

FIGURE 13.6 Retinal blood vessels.

is a depression called the **fovea centralis** (central pit). This pit contains a high concentration of sensory receptor cells and, therefore, is the point of clearest vision. Also visible on the retina is the **optic disk.** This is the point where the optic nerve leaves the eyeball. There are no sensory receptor cells in the optic disk and therefore it causes a blind spot in each eye's field of vision. The interior spaces of the eyeball are not empty. The spaces between the cornea and lens are filled with **aqueous** (**AY** kwee us) **humor,** a watery fluid, and the large open area between the lens and retina contains **vitreous** (**VIT** ree us) **humor,** a semi-solid gel. Figure 13.6 is a photo taken through the pupil of the eye. It shows the **retinal blood vessels.**

HOW WE SEE

cones   **rods**

Light passes through the cornea, pupil, lens, and vitreous humor. This light then stimulates the sensory receptors, called **rods** and **cones,** on the retina. The rods are active in dim light and do not perceive color. The cones are active in bright light and see in color. When the light rays hit the retina, an upside-down image is sent along nerve impulses in the rods and cones. The optic nerve transmits these impulses to the brain, where the upside-down image is translated into the right-side up image we are looking at (see Figures 13.7 and 13.8).

Vision requires four mechanisms to be working:

1. Coordination of the external eye muscles so that both eyes move together.
2. The correct amount of light admitted by the pupil.
3. The correct focus of light upon the retina by the lens.
4. The optic nerve transmitting sensory images to the brain.

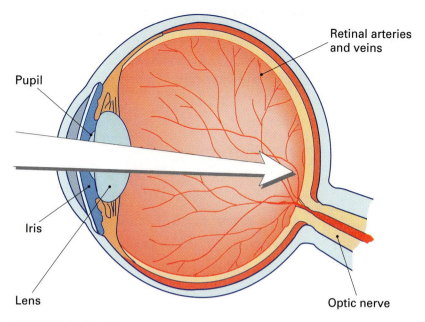

FIGURE 13.7 Light entering the eye.

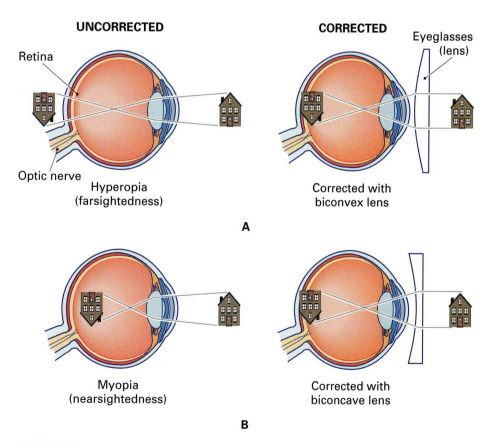

FIGURE 13.8 How lenses correct visual problems. (A) Hyperopia. (B) Myopia.

Word Building Relating to the Eye

The following list contains examples of medical terms built directly from word parts. The definitions of these terms can be determined by a straightforward translation of the word parts.

Combining Form	Combined With	Medical Term	Definition
blephar/o	-itis	blepharitis (blef ah **RYE** tis)	eyelid inflammation
	-plasty	blepharoplasty (**BLEF** ah roh plass tee)	surgical repair of eyelid
	-ptosis	blepharoptosis (blef ah rop **TOH** sis)	drooping eyelid
conjuctiv/o	-itis	conjunctivitis (kon junk tih **VYE** tis)	conjunctiva inflammation
dacry/o	cyst/o -itis	dacryocystitis (dak ree oh sis **TYE** tis)	tear bladder inflammation
dipl/o	-opia	diplopia (dip **LOH** pee ah)	double vision
iri/o	-itis	iritis (ih **RYE** tis)	iris inflammation
irid/o	-ectomy	iridectomy (ir id **EK** toh mee)	excision of iris
	-plegia	iridoplegia (ir id oh **PLEE** jee ah)	paralysis of iris
	scler/o-otomy	iridosclerotomy (ir ih doh skleh **ROT** oh mee)	incision into iris and sclera
kerat/o	-itis	keratitis (kair ah **TYE** tis)	cornea inflammation
	-plasty	keratoplasty (**KAIR** ah toh plass tee)	surgical repair of cornea
lacrim/o	-al	lacrimal (**LAK** rim al)	pertaining to tears
ocul/o	bi- -ar	binocular (bih **NOK** yoo lar)	pertaining to two eyes
	intra- -ar	intraocular (in trah **OCK** yoo lar)	pertaining to within the eye
	myc/o -osis	oculomycosis (ok yoo loh my **KOH** sis)	abnormal condition of eye fungus
ophthalm/o	-algia	ophthalmalgia (off thal **MAL** jee ah)	eye pain
	endo- -itis	endophthalmitis (en dof thal **MY** tis)	inflammation within the eye
	-ic	ophthalmic (off **THAL** mik)	pertaining to the eye
	-ologist	ophthalmologist (off thal **MALL** oh jist)	specialist in the eye
	-ology	ophthalmology (off thal **MALL** oh jee)	study of the eye
	-plegia	ophthalmoplegia (off thal moh **PLEE** jee ah)	eye paralysis
	-rrhagia	ophthalmorrhagia (off thal moh **RAH** jee ah)	rapid bleeding from the eye
	-scope	ophthalmoscope (off **THAL** moh scope)	instrument to view inside the eye
	-scopy	ophthalmoscopy (off thal **MOSS** koh pee)	process of viewing the eye
opt/o	-ic	optic (**OP** tik)	pertaining to the eye or vision
	-meter	optometer (op **TOM** eh ter)	instrument to measure vision
	-metry	optometry (op **TOM** eh tree)	process of measuring vision
phot/o	-phobia	photophobia (foh toh **FOH** bee ah)	fear of light
presby/o	-opia	presbyopia (prez bee **OH** pee ah)	old age vision

retin/o	-al	retinal (**RET** in al)	pertaining to the retina
	-pathy	retinopathy (ret in **OP** ah thee)	retina disease
scler/o	-malacia	scleromalacia (sklair oh mah **LAY** she ah)	softening of the sclera
	-otomy	sclerotomy (skleh **ROT** oh mee)	incision into the sclera
Prefix	**Suffix**	**Medical Term**	**Definition**
exo-	-tropia	exotropia (eks oh **TROH** pee ah)	turning outward
hemi- an-		hemianopia (hem ee ah **NOP** pee ah)	half no vision
hyper-	-opia	hyperopia (high per **OH** pee ah)	excessive (far) vision

Vocabulary Relating to the Eye

accommodation (Acc) (ah kom oh **DAY** shun)	Ability of the eye to adjust to variations in distance.
convergence (kon **VER** jens)	The moving inward of the eyes to see an object close to the face.
ectropion (ek **TROH** pee on)	Term referring to eversion (turning outward) of the eyelid.
emmetropia (EM) (em eh **TROH** pee ah)	State of normal vision.
entropion (en **TROH** pee on)	Term referring to inversion (turning inward) of the eyelid.
exophthalmos (eks off **THAL** mohs)	Abnormal protrusion of the eyeball. Can be due to hyperthyroidism.
laser	Device that emits intense, small beams of light capable of destroying or fixing tissue in place.
miotic (my **OT** ik)	Any substance that causes the pupil to constrict.
mydriatic (mid ree **AT** ik)	Any substance that causes the pupil to dilate.
ophthalmologist (off thal **MALL** oh jist)	A physician specialized in treating conditions and diseases of the eye.
ophthalmology (Ophth.) (off thal **MALL** oh jee)	The study of the eye.
optician (op **TISH** an)	Specialist in grinding corrective lenses.
optometrist (op **TOM** eh trist)	A doctor of optometry specializing in testing visual acuity and prescribing corrective lenses.
refraction (ree **FRAK** shun)	Eye examination performed by a physician to determine and correct refractive errors in the eye.
refractive (ree **FRAK** tiv) **error**	Defect in the ability of the eye to accurately focus the image that is hitting it. Occurs in farsightedness and nearsightedness (see Figure 13.9).

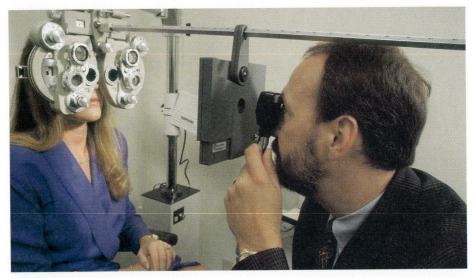

Pathology of the Eye

achromatopsia (ah kroh mah TOP see ah)	Condition of color blindness; more common in males.
astigmatism (Astigm) (ah STIG mah tizm)	A condition in which light rays are focused unevenly on the eye, which causes a distorted image, due to an abnormal curvature of the cornea.
blepharitis (blef ah RYE tis)	Inflammatory condition of the eyelash follicles and glands of the eyelids that results in swelling, redness, and crusts of dried mucus on the lids. Can be the result of allergy or infection.
blepharochalasis (blef ah roh KAL ah sis)	In this condition, the upper eyelid increases in size due to a loss of elasticity, which is followed by swelling and recurrent edema of the lids. The skin may droop over the edges of the eyes when the eyes are open.
cataract (KAT ah rakt)	Diminished vision resulting from the lens of the eye becoming opaque or cloudy. Treatment is usually surgical removal of the cataract.
chalazion (kah LAY zee on)	Small hard tumor or mass, similar to a sebaceous cyst, developing on the eyelids. May require incision and drainage (I & D).
conjunctivitis (kon junk tih VYE tis)	Also referred to as *pinkeye*, an inflammation of the conjunctiva.
diabetic retinopathy (dye ah BET ik re tin OP ah thee)	These small hemorrhages and edema in the eye develop in the retina as a result of diabetes mellitus. Laser surgery and vitrectomy may be necessary for treatment.
esotropia (ess oh TROH pee ah)	Inward turning of the eye. An example of a form of *strabismus* (muscle weakness of the eye).
exotropia (eks oh TROH pee ah)	Outward turning of the eye. Also an example of strabismus (muscle weakness of the eye).
glaucoma (glau KOH mah)	Increase in intraocular pressure, which, if untreated, may result in atrophy (wasting away) of the optic nerve and blindness. Glaucoma is treated with medication and surgery. There is an increased risk of developing glaucoma in persons over sixty years of age, in people of African ancestry, in persons who have sustained a serious eye injury, and in anyone with a family history of diabetes or glaucoma (see Figure 13.10).

hemianopia (hem ee ah **NOP** ee ah)	Loss of vision in half of the visual field. A stroke patient may suffer from this disorder.
hordeolum (hor **DEE** oh lum)	Refers to a *stye* (or *sty*), a small purulent inflammatory infection of a sebaceous gland of the eye; treated with hot compresses and surgical incision.
hyperopia (high per **OH** pee ah)	With this condition a person can see things in the distance but has trouble reading material at close range (see also Figure 13.8). Also known as *farsightedness*.
keratitis (kair ah **TYE** tis)	Inflammation of the cornea.
macular (**MAK** yoo lar) **degeneration**	Deterioration of the macular area of the retina of the eye. May be treated with laser surgery to destroy the blood vessels beneath the macula.
myopia (MY) (my **OH** pee ah)	With this condition a person can see things close up but distance vision is blurred (see also Figure 13.8). Also known as *near-sightedness*.
nystagmus (niss **TAG** mus)	Jerky-appearing involuntary eye movement.
presbyopia (prez bee **OH** pee ah)	Visual loss due to old age, resulting in difficulty in focusing for near vision (such as reading).
retinal (**RET** in al) **detachment**	Occurs when the retina becomes separated from the choroids layer. This separation seriously damages blood vessels and nerves resulting in blindness.
retinitis pigmentosa (ret in **EYE** tis pig men **TOH** sah)	Progressive disease of the eye that results in the retina becoming hard (sclerosed) and pigmented (colored), and atrophying (wasting away). There is no known cure for this condition.
strabismus (strah **BIZ** mus)	An eye muscle weakness resulting in the eyes looking in different directions at the same time. May be corrected with glasses, eye exercises, and/or surgery. Also called *lazy eye* or *crossed eyes*.
trachoma (tray **KOH** mah)	Chronic infectious disease of the conjunctiva and cornea caused by bacteria. Occurs more commonly in people living in hot, dry climates. Untreated, it may lead to blindness when the scarring invades the cornea. Trachoma can be treated with antibiotics.

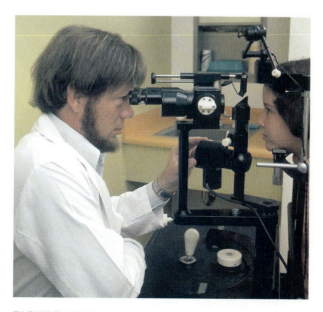

FIGURE 13.10 Examination for glaucoma.

Diagnostic Procedures Relating to the Eye

color vision tests	Use of polychromic (multi-colored) charts to determine the ability of the patient to recognize color (see Figure 13.11).
fluorescein angiography (floo oh RESS ee in an jee OG rah fee)	Process of injecting a dye (fluorescein) to observe the movement of blood and detect lesions in the macular area of the retina. Used to determine if there is a detachment of the retina.
gonioscopy (goh nee OSS koh pee)	Use of an instrument called a gonioscope to examine the anterior chamber of the eye and determine ocular mobility and rotation.
keratometry (kair ah TOM eh tree)	Measurement of the curvature of the cornea using an instrument called a keratometer.
ophthalmoscopy (off thal MOSS koh pee)	Examination of the interior of the eyes using an instrument called an ophthalmoscope. The physician dilates the pupil in order to see the cornea, lens, and retina. Used to identify abnormalities in the blood vessels of the eye and some systemic diseases.
slit lamp microscope	Instrument used in ophthalmology for examining the posterior surface of the cornea.
Snellen's (SNEL enz) chart	Chart used for testing distance vision named for Hermann Snellen, a Dutch ophthalmologist. It contains letters of varying size and it is administered from a distance of 20 feet. A person who can read at 20 feet what the average person can read at this distance is said to have 20/20 vision.
tonometry (tohn OM eh tree)	Measurement of the intraocular pressure of the eye using a tonometer to check for the condition of glaucoma. After a local anesthetic is applied, the physician places the tonometer lightly upon the eyeball and a pressure measurement is taken. Generally part of a normal eye exam for adults.
visual acuity (VA) (VIZH oo al ah KYOO ih tee)	Measurement of the sharpness of a patient's vision. Usually, a Snellen's chart is used for this test in which the patient identifies letters from a distance of 20 feet.

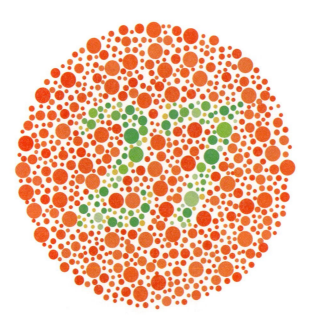

FIGURE 13.11 Color vision chart.

Treatment Procedures Relating to the Eye

cryoextraction (cry oh eks RAJ shun)	Procedure in which cataract is lifted from the lens with an extremely cold probe.
cryoretinopexy (cry oh RET ih noh pek see)	Surgical fixation of the retina by using extreme cold.
keratoplasty (KAIR ah toh plass tee)	Surgical repair of the cornea (corneal transplant).
laser-assisted in-situ keratomileusis (in SIH tyoo kair ah toh mih LOO sis) (LASIK)	Correction of myopia using laser surgery to remove corneal tissue.
phacoemulsification (fak oh ee mull sih fih KAY shun)	Use of high frequency sound waves to emulsify (liquefy) a lens with a cataract, which is then aspirated (removed by suction) with a needle.
photo refractive keratectomy (PRK) (foh toh ree FRAK tiv kair ah TEK toh mee)	Use of a laser to reshape the cornea and correct errors of refraction.
scleral (SKLAIR al) buckling	Placing a band of silicone around the outside of the sclera, which stabilizes a detaching retina.
strabotomy (strah BOT oh mee)	Incision into the eye muscles in order to correct strabismus.
vitrectomy (vih TREK toh mee)	Surgical procedure for replacing the contents of the vitreous chamber of the eye.

Professional Profile

Optometry

Optometry is the professional practice that provides care for the eyes. This includes diagnostic and visual acuity tests, prescriptive lenses, surgical procedures, and patient education. Optometry services are found in private offices, acute care facilities, and clinics.

Doctor of Optometry (OD)

- **Also referred to as an optometrist**
- **Assesses visual acuity and prescribes corrective lenses**

- **Graduates from an approved four-year college of optometry after attending at least two years of undergraduate college**
- **Licensed by the state of employment**

Optician

- **Grinds and fits prescription lenses and contacts as prescribed by a physician or optometrist**
- **Completes a four-to-five year apprenticeship**
- **Licensure required by some states**

Abbreviations Relating to the Eye

Acc	accommodation	**NVA**	near visual acuity
ARMD	age-related macular degeneration	**OD**	right eye (oculus dexter)
Astigm.	astigmatism	**Ophth.**	ophthalmology
c.gl.	correction with glasses	**OS**	left eye (oculus sinister)
cyl	cylindrical lens	**OU**	each eye
D	diopter (lens strength)	**PERRLA**	pupils equal, round, react to light and accommodation
DVA	distance visual acuity		
ECCE	extracapsular cataract extraction	**PRK**	photo refractive keratectomy
EM	emmetropia (normal vision)	**RE**	right eye
EOM	extraocular movement	**REM**	rapid eye movement
ICCE	intracapsular cataract cryoextraction	**s.gl.**	without correction or glasses
IOL	intraocular lens	**SMD**	senile macular degeneration
IOP	intraocular pressure	**VA**	visual acuity
L&A	light and accommodation	**VF**	visual field
LASIK	laser-assisted in-situ keratomileusis	**WNL**	within normal limits
LE	left eye	**+**	plus/convex
MY	myopia	**–**	minus/concave

MED TERM TIP

The terms for right (OD) and left eye (OS) are easy to remember when we know their origins. OD stands for *oculus* (eye) *dexter* (right). OS has its origin in oculus (eye) sinister (left). At one time in history it was considered to be sinister if a person looked at another from only the left side. Hence the term *oculus sinister* (OS) means left eye.

KEY TERMS

- accommodation (Acc) (ah kom oh **DAY** shun)
- achromatopsia (ah kroh mah **TOP** see ah)
- aqueous humor (**AY** kwee us)
- astigmatism (Astigm.) (ah **STIG** mah tizm)
- binocular (bih **NOK** yoo lar)
- blepharitis (blef ah **RYE** tis)
- blepharochalasis (blef ah roh **KAL** ah sis)
- blepharoplasty (**BLEF** ah roh plass tee)
- blepharoptosis (blef ah rop **TOH** sis)
- cataract (**KAT** ah rakt)

- chalazion (kah **LAY** zee on)
- choroid (**KOR** oyd)
- cilia (**SIL** ee ah)
- ciliary body (**SIL** ee ar ee)
- color vision tests
- cones
- conjunctiva (kon **JUNK** tih vah)
- conjunctivitis (kon junk tih **VYE** tis)
- convergence (kon **VER** jens)
- cornea (**COR** nee ah)

- cryoextraction (cry oh eks **TRAK** shun)
- cryoretinopexy (cry oh **RET** ih noh pek see)
- dacryocystitis (dak ree oh sis **TYE** tis)
- diabetic retinopathy
  (dye ah **BET** ik reh tin **OP** ah thee)
- diplopia (dip **LOH** pee ah)
- ectropion (ek **TROH** pee on)
- emmetropia (EM) (em eh **TROH** pee ah)
- endophthalmitis (en dof thal **MY** tis)
- entropion (en **TROH** pee on)
- esotropia (ess oh **TROH** pee ah)
- exophthalmos (eks off **THAL** mohs)
- exotropia (eks oh **TROH** pee ah)
- eye
- eye muscles
- eye socket
- eyeball
- eyelids
- fluorescein angiography
  (floo oh **RESS** ee in an jee **OG** rah fee)
- fovea centralis (**FOH** vee ah sen **TRAH** lis)
- glaucoma (glau **KOH** mah)
- gonioscopy (goh nee **OSS** koh pee)
- hemianopia (hem ee ah **NOP** ee ah)
- hordeolum (hor **DEE** oh lum)
- hyperopia (high per **OH** pee ah)
- intraocular (in trah **OCK** yoo lar)
- iridectomy (ir id **EK** toh mee)
- iridoplegia (ir id oh **PLEE** jee ah)
- iridosclerotomy (ir ih doh skleh **ROT** oh mee)
- iris (**EYE** ris)
- iritis (ih **RYE** tis)
- jaundice (**JAWN** diss)
- keratitis (kair ah **TYE** tis)
- keratometry (kair ah **TOM** eh tree)
- keratoplasty (**KAIR** ah toh plass tee)
- lacrimal (**LAK** rim al)
- lacrimal ducts (**LAK** rim al)
- lacrimal glands (**LAK** rim al)
- lacrimal sac (**LAK** rim al)
- laser
- laser-assisted in-situ keratomileusis (LASIK)
  (in **SIH** tyoo kair ah toh mih **LOO** sis)
- lens
- macula lutea (**MAK** yoo lah loo TEE ah)
- macular degeneration (**MAK** yoo lar)
- miotic (my **OT** ik)
- mydriatic (mid ree **AT** ik)
- myopia (MY) (my **OH** pee ah)
- nystagmus (niss **TAG** mus)
- oblique muscle (oh **BLEEK**)

- oculomycosis (ok yoo loh my **KOH** sis)
- ophthalmalgia (off thal **MAL** jee ah)
- ophthalmic (off **THAL** mik)
- ophthalmic artery (off **THAL** mik)
- ophthalmologist (off thal **MALL** oh jist)
- ophthalmology (Ophth.) (off thal **MALL** oh jee)
- ophthalmoplegia (off thal moh **PLEE** jee ah)
- ophthalmorrhagia (off thal moh **RAH** jee ah)
- ophthalmoscope (off **THAL** moh scope)
- ophthalmoscopy (off thal **MOSS** koh pee)
- optic (**OP** tik)
- optic disk (**OP** tik)
- optic nerve (**OP** tik)
- optician (op **TISH** an)
- optometer (op **TOM** eh ter)
- optometrist (op **TOM** eh trist)
- optometry (op **TOM** eh tree)
- orbit (**OR** bit)
- phacoemulsification
  (fak oh ee mull sih fih **KAY** shun)
- photo refractive keratectomy
  (foh toh ree **FRAK** tiv kair ah **TEK** toh mee)
- photophobia (foh toh **FOH** bee ah)
- presbyopia (prez bee **OH** pee ah)
- pupil
- rectus muscle (**REK** tus)
- refraction (ree **FRAK** shun)
- refractive error (ree **FRAK** tiv)
- retina (**RET** in ah)
- retinal (**RET** in al)
- retinal blood vessels (**RET** in al)
- retinal detachment (**RET** in al)
- retinitis pigmentosa
  (ret in **EYE** tis pig men **TOH** sah)
- retinopathy (ret in **OP** ah thee)
- rods
- sclera (**SKLAIR** ah)
- scleral buckling (**SKLAIR** al)
- scleromalacia (sklair oh mah **LAY** she ah)
- sclerotomy (skleh **ROT** oh mee)
- sebaceous glands (see **BAY** shus)
- slit lamp microscope
- Snellen's chart (**SNEL** enz)
- strabismus (strah **BIZ** mus)
- strabotomy (strah **BOT** oh mee)
- tonometry (tohn **OM** eh tree)
- trachoma (tray **KOH** mah)
- visual acuity (VA) (**VIZH** oo al ah **KYOO** ih tee)
- vitrectomy (vih **TREK** toh mee)
- vitreous humor (**VIT** ree us)

Case Study I

OPHTHALMOLOGY CONSULTATION REPORT

Reason for Consultation: Evaluation of progressive loss of vision in right eye.

History of Present Illness: Patient has noted gradual deterioration of vision and increasing photophobia over the past one year, particularly in the right eye. She states that it feels like there is a film over her right eye. Denies any change in vision in her left eye.

Past Medical History: Patient has used corrective lenses her entire adult life to correct hyperopia. She is not married and is nulligravida. Past medical history includes left breast cancer successfully treated with left breast mastectomy 10 years ago and cholelithiasis necessitating a cholecystectomy 2 years ago. She has no history of cardiac problems or hypertension.

Results of Physical Examination: Visual acuity test showed no change in this patient's long-standing hyperopia. The eye muscles function properly and there is no evidence of conjunctivitis or nystagmus. The pupils react properly to light. Intraocular pressure is WNL. Ophthalmoscopy after application of mydriatic drops revealed presence of large opaque cataract in lens of right eye. There is a very small cataract forming in the left eye. There is no evidence of retinopathy, macular degeneration, or keratitis.

Assessment: Diminished vision in OD secondary to cataract.

Recommendations: Phacoemulsification of cataract followed by aspiration of lens and prosthetic lens implant.

CRITICAL THINKING QUESTIONS FOR THE EYE

1. The results of the physical exam state that the patient's pupils react properly to light. What does this mean? How do pupils react in bright and dim light? Why is this important?

2. Carefully read the results of the physical examination and list the eye *structures* that do not have any problems.

3. Briefly describe the pathologies that form the patient's past medical history that required surgery, and the surgeries.

4. The ophthalmologist placed mydriatic drops in her eyes. For what purpose? What is the general name for drops with the opposite effect?

5. This patient wears corrective lenses for which condition?

   a. farsightedness

   b. nearsightedness

   c. abnormal curvature of the cornea

6. Her cataract was removed by phacoemulsification. Using your text as a reference, what other procedure could have been used to remove a cataract?

Chart Note Transcription I

Chart Note

The chart note below contains ten phrases that can be reworded with a medical term that you learned in this chapter. Each phrase is identified with an underline. Determine the medical term and write your answers in the space provided.

Current Complaint: A 56-year-old male made an appointment with the specialist in the treatment of eye diseases[1] because of increasing difficulty reading.

Past History: Patient wears corrective lenses for near-sightedness[2] and abnormal curvature of the cornea.[3]

Signs and Symptoms: The innermost layer of the eye[4] appears normal when inspected using an instrument to examine the interior of the eye.[5] No evidence of deterioration of the macular area[6] was observed with dye injected into blood vessels in order to study the retina.[7] However, a procedure to measure the pressure inside the eye[8] revealed increased intraocular pressure, especially on the right.

Diagnosis: Atrophy of the optic nerve due to increased intraocular pressure.[9]

Treatment: Patient was treated with surgery performed with an intense small beam of light.[10]

1 _____

2 _____

3 _____

4 _____

5 _____

6 _____

7 _____

8 _____

9 _____

10 _____

Practice Exercises I

A. COMPLETE THE FOLLOWING STATEMENTS.

1. The study of the eye is _____ .

2. The external structures of the eye consist of the _____ , _____ , _____ , _____ , _____ , and _____ .

3. The medical term for *crossed eyes* is _____ .

4. Another term for eyelashes is _____ .

5. Extremely pale conjunctiva could indicate _____ .

6. The glands responsible for tears are called _____ glands.

7. A yellowish cast to the sclera of the eye could indicate _____ .

8. The clear, transparent portion of the sclera is called the _____ .

9. The innermost layer of the eye, which is composed of nerve endings, is the _____ .

10. The pupil of the eye is actually a hole in the _____ .

11. The ability of the eye to adjust to variations in distance vision is called _____ .

12. A normal state of vision is referred to as _____ .

13. The condition whereby two layers of the retina become separated is _____ .

14. An abnormal curvature of the cornea causing light rays to be focused unevenly on the eyes is called _____ .

15. A stroke patient suffering from loss of vision in only half of the visual field is suffering from _____ .

B. STATE THE TERMS DESCRIBED USING THE COMBINING FORMS PROVIDED.

The combining form blephar/o refers to the eyelid. Use it to write a term that means

1. inflammation of the eyelid _____

2. surgical repair of the eyelid _____

3. relaxation of the upper eyelid _____

4. paralysis of the eyelid _____

The combining form retin/o refers to the retina. Use it to write a term that means

5. a disease of the retina _____

6. surgical fixation of the retina _____

The combining form ophthalm/o refers to the eye. Use it to write a term that means

7. the study of the eye _____

8. pertaining to the eye _____

9. an eye examination using a scope _____

The combining form optic/o refers to the eye. Use it to write a term that means

10. a person who grinds and fits eyeglasses _____

11. relating to the eye _____

C. Write the suffix for each expression and provide an example of its use.

Suffix   Example

1. to turn _____
2. vision _____
3. inflammation of _____
4. the study of _____
5. incision into _____
6. surgical repair _____
7. surgical fixation _____
8. abnormal narrowing _____

D. Define the following combining forms.

1. dacry/o _____
2. cor/o _____
3. aque/o _____
4. optic/o _____
5. blephar/o _____
6. vitre/o _____
7. kerat/o _____
8. scler/o _____
9. presby/o _____
10. ambyl/o _____
11. ocul/o _____
12. ophthalm/o _____

E. Define the following terms.

1. amblyopia _____
2. diplopia _____
3. mydriatic _____
4. miotic _____
5. presbyopia _____

F. Match the terms in column A with the definitions in column B.

A	B
1. _____ accommodation	a. opacity of the lens
2. _____ sclera	b. muscle regulating size of pupil
3. _____ cataract	c. nearsightedness
4. _____ conjunctiva	d. protective membrane of eye
5. _____ iris	e. blind spot
6. _____ refraction	f. involuntary movements of eye
7. _____ myopia	g. white of eye
8. _____ nystagmus	h. eye changes for near and far vision
9. _____ optic disk	i. bend light rays
10. _____ vitreous humor	j. material filling eyeball
11. _____ emmetropia	k. normal refraction of eye
12. _____ ptosis	l. prolapse of eyelid

G. IDENTIFY THE FOLLOWING ABBREVIATIONS.

1. OS _____
2. OU _____
3. REM _____
4. Acc _____
5. SMD _____
6. PERLA _____
7. IOP _____
8. RE _____
9. OD _____
10. VF _____

H. USE THE FOLLOWING TERMS IN THE SENTENCES THAT FOLLOW.

emmetropia	hyperopia	esotropia	myopia
exophthalmos	conjunctivitis	hordeolum	glaucoma
ectropion	chalazion	cataract	keratitis
entropion	keratometry	tonometry	strabismus

1. Cheri is having a regular eye checkup. The pressure reading test that the physician will do to detect glaucoma is _____ .

2. Gracibel has developed a painful, hard mass on her eyelid. This is called a(n) _____ .

3. Carlos's ophthalmologist tells him that he has normal vision. This is called _____ .

4. Ana has been given an antibiotic eye ointment for pinkeye. The medical term for this condition is _____ .

5. Adrian is nearsighted and cannot read signs in the distance. This is called _____ .

6. Ivan is scheduled to have surgery to have the opaque lens of his right eye removed. This condition is a(n) _____ .

7. Roberto has developed a sty on the corner of his left eye. He has been told to treat it with hot compresses. This condition is called a(n) _____ .

8. Lorenzo has an uncomfortable disorder in which his eyelashes are rubbing his cornea, due to inversion of his eyelid. This condition is called _____ .

9. Judith has twin boys with crossed eyes that will require surgical correction. The medical term for this condition is _____ .

10. Beth is farsighted and has difficulty reading textbooks. Her eyeglass correction will be for _____ .

11. Tina suffered from a lack of iodine in her diet and developed a thyroid problem. After her thyroid problem was corrected, she still had protruding eyeballs. This is called _____ .

Overview

PART II: *The Ear*

STRUCTURES OF THE EAR

auditory canal	mastoid bone
auricle	oval window
cochlea	semicircular canals
eustachian tube	stapes
incus	tympanic membrane (ear drum)
labyrinth	
malleus	

COMBINING FORMS RELATING TO THE EAR

acous/o	hearing	**labyrinth/o**	labyrinth
audi/o	hearing	**mastoid/o**	mastoid process
audit/o	hearing	**myring/o**	eardrum
aur/o	ear	**ot/o**	ear
auricul/o	ear	**staped/o**	stapes
cochle/o	cochlea	**tympan/o**	eardrum, middle ear

SUFFIXES RELATING TO THE EAR

Suffix	Meaning	Example
-cusis	hearing	anacusis
-mycosis	fungal infection	otomycosis
-otomy	incision into	myringotomy
-pyorrhea	discharge of pus	otopyorrhea
-rrhexis	rupture	tympanorrhexis

ANATOMY AND PHYSIOLOGY OF THE EAR

cochlear nerve	inner ear	vestibular nerve
equilibrium	middle ear	vestibulocochlear nerve
external ear	otology	

The study of the ear is referred to as **otology** (Oto) (oh **TOL** oh jee). The ear is responsible for both hearing and **equilibrium** (ee kwih **LIB** ree um) or our sense of balance. Hearing and equilibrium sensory information is carried to the brain by cranial nerve VIII, the **vestibulocochlear** (ves tib yoo loh **KOK** lee ar) **nerve.** This nerve is divided into two major branches. The **cochlear** (**KOK** lee ar) **nerve** carries hearing information and the **vestibular** (ves **TIB** yoo lar) **nerve** carries equilibrium information. Sound vibrations are

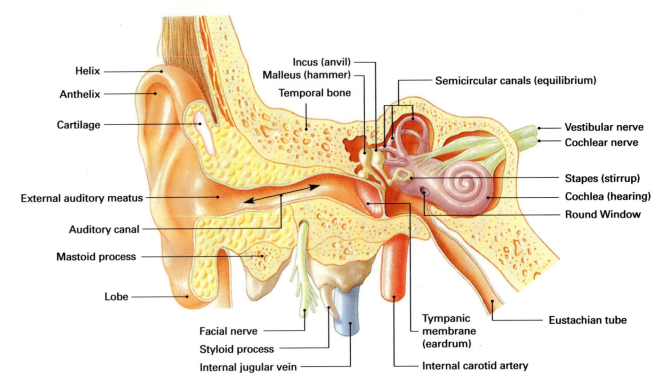

FIGURE 13.12 Anatomy of the ear.

picked up by the external apparatus of the ear, relayed by conduction through the middle ear, and converted to electrical stimuli by passing through the inner ear to the brain.

The ear can be described in terms of its three areas:

1. The **external** or outer **ear**
2. The **middle ear**
3. The **inner ear**

See Figure 13.12 for an illustration of the anatomy of the ear.

THE EXTERNAL EAR

auditory canal	**otoscope**	**tympanic membrane**
auricle	**otoscopy**	
cerumen	**pinna**	

The external ear consists of three parts: the **auricle** (AW rih k'l), the **auditory canal,** and the eardrum or **tympanic** (tim **PAN** ik) **membrane.** The auricle or **pinna** (**PIN** ah) is commonly referred to as the *ear* and contains the earlobe. The auricle has a unique shape in each person and functions like a funnel to capture sound waves as they go past the outer ear. The sound then moves along the auditory canal and causes the tympanic membrane to vibrate. The tympanic membrane or eardrum actually separates the external ear from the middle ear. Ear wax or **cerumen** (seh **ROO** men) is produced in oil glands in the auditory canal. This wax helps to protect and lubricate the ear. The ear canal is normally self-cleaning.

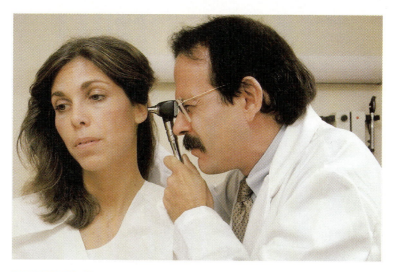

FIGURE 13.13   Examination of ear using otoscope.

THE MIDDLE EAR

eustachian tube	**mastoid process**	**otitis media**
incus	**mastoiditis**	**oval window**
malleus	**ossicles**	**stapes**

The middle ear is located in a small cavity in the temporal bone of the skull. It contains three tiny bones called **ossicles** (**OSS** ih kls). These three bones, the **malleus** (**MAL** ee us), **incus** (**ING** kus), and **stapes** (**STAY** peez), are vital to the hearing process. They amplify the vibrations in the middle ear and transmit them to the inner ear from the malleus to the incus and finally to the stapes. The stapes, the last of the three ossicles, is attached to a very thin membrane that covers the opening to the inner ear called the **oval window.** The middle ear transfers sound vibrations from the ossicles by transferring sound energy from the air to the fluids of the inner ear.

The **eustachian** (yoo **STAY** kee en) **tube** or auditory tube connects the nasopharynx with the middle ear. Pressure within the middle ear is equalized or balanced here.

The middle ear cavity has several openings that are lined with mucous membranes. These membranes can carry infections from the throat to the middle ear, resulting in **otitis** (oh **TYE** tis) **media** or middle ear infection. The ear structures are in close proximity to

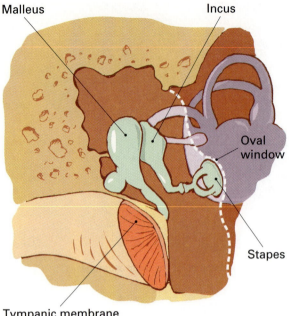

Malleus

Incus

Oval
window

Stapes

Tympanic membrane

FIGURE 13.14 Bones in the ear: malleus, stapes, and incus.

the **mastoid** (**MASS** toyd) **process,** the bony prominence felt behind the ear. An infection traveling into the mastoid cells results in **mastoiditis** (mass toyd **EYE** tis) or infection of the mastoid bone.

Thus the middle ear has a threefold job: carrying sound vibrations along to the inner ear, regulating air pressure on the tympanic membrane, and preventing some of the loud sounds from causing hearing damage.

THE INNER EAR

cochlea	**organ of Corti**	**utricle**
labyrinth	**saccule**	
Ménière's disease	**semicircular canals**	

The inner ear is also located in a cavity within the temporal bone (see also Figure 13.12). This cavity is referred to as the **labyrinth** (**LAB** ih rinth) because of its shape. The labyrinth contains the hearing and equilibrium sensory organs: the **cochlea** (**KOK** lee ah) for hearing and the **semicircular canals, utricle** (**YOO** trih k'l), and **saccule** (**SAK** yool) for equilibrium. Each of these organs contains hair cells, the actual sensory receptors cells. In the cochlea, the hair cells are collectively referred to as the **organ of Corti** (**KOR** tee).

Frequently, children will twirl in circles and fall or stumble from dizziness when they stop. This is caused from a temporary imbalance in the inner ear. However, more serious inner ear problems develop in adults, such as **Ménière's disease** (may nee **ARZ** dih **ZEEZ**), named for Prosper Ménière, a French physician. This disease, which can become completely disabling, makes air travel a problem for many people.

Path of sound vibrations

Outer ear | Middle ear | Inner ear

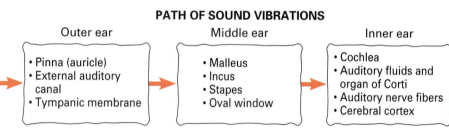

PATH OF SOUND VIBRATIONS

Outer ear | Middle ear | Inner ear

- Pinna (auricle)
- External auditory canal
- Tympanic membrane

- Malleus
- Incus
- Stapes
- Oval window

- Cochlea
- Auditory fluids and organ of Corti
- Auditory nerve fibers
- Cerebral cortex

FIGURE 13.15 Path of sound vibrations.

HOW WE HEAR

conductive hearing loss   **sensorineural hearing loss**

Figure 13.15 outlines the path of sound through the outer ear and middle ear and into the cochlea of the inner ear. Sound waves traveling down the external auditory canal strike the eardrum, causing it to vibrate. The ossicles conduct these vibrations across the middle ear from the eardrum to the oval window. Oval window movements initiate vibrations in the fluid that fills the cochlea. As the fluid vibrations strike a hair cell it bends the small hairs and stimulates the nerve ending. The nerve ending then sends an electrical impulse to the brain on the cochlear portion of the vestibulo-cochlear cranial nerve.

Hearing loss can be divided into two main categories: **conductive** (con **DUK** tiv) **hearing loss** and **sensorineural** (sen soh ree **NOO** ral) **hearing loss.** Conductive refers to disease or malformation of the outer or middle ear. All sound is weaker and muffled in conductive hearing loss since sound is not conducted efficiently. Sensorineural hearing loss is the result of damage or malformation of the inner ear (cochlea) or the auditory nerve. In this hearing loss, some sounds are distorted and heard incorrectly. There can also be a combination of both conductive and sensorineural hearing loss.

Word Building Relating to the Ear

The following list contains examples of medical terms built directly from word parts. The definitions of these terms can be determined by a straightforward translation of the word parts.

Combining Form	Combined With	Medical Term	Definition
acous/o	-tic	acoustic (ah **KOOS** tik)	pertaining to hearing
audi/o	-gram	audiogram (**AW** dee oh gram)	record of hearing
	-meter	audiometer (aw dee **OM** eh ter)	instrument to measure hearing
	-metry	audiometry (aw dee **OM** eh tree)	process of measuring hearing
	-ologist	audiologist (aw dee **OL** oh jist)	hearing specialist
	-ology	audiology (aw dee **OL** oh jee)	study of hearing
aur/o	-al	aural (**AW** ral)	pertaining to the ear
cochle/o	-ar	cochlear (**KOK** lee ar)	pertaining to the cochlea
labyrinth/o	-ectomy	labyrinthectomy (lab ih rin **THEK** toh mee)	excision of the labyrinth
	-itis	labyrinthitis (lab ih rin **THIGH** tis)	labyrinth inflammation
mastoid/o	-ectomy	mastoidectomy (mass toyd **ECK** toh mee)	excision of the mastoid bone
	-itis	mastoiditis (mass toyd **EYE** tis)	mastoid bone inflammation
	-otomy	mastoidotomy (mass toy **DOT** oh mee)	incision into mastoid bone
myring/o	-itis	myringitis (mir ing **JYE** tis)	eardrum inflammation
	-otomy	myringotomy (mir in **GOT** oh mee)	incision into eardrum
	-plasty	myringoplasty (mir **IN** goh plass tee)	surgical repair of eardrum
ot/o	-algia	otalgia (oh **TAL** jee ah)	ear pain
	-ic	otic (**OH** tik)	pertaining to the ear
	-itis	otitis (oh **TYE** tis)	ear inflammation
	myc/o -osis	otomycosis (oh toh my **KOH** sis)	abnormal condition of ear fungus
	-ologist	otologist (oh **TOL** oh jist)	ear specialist
	-ology	otology (oh **TOL** oh jee)	study of the ear
	py/o -rrhea	otopyorrhea (oh toh pye oh **REE** ah)	pus discharge from ear
	-sclerosis	otosclerosis (oh toh sklair **OH** sis)	ear hardening
	-scope	otoscope (**OH** toh scope)	instrument to view inside the ear
	-scopy	otoscopy (oh **TOSS** koh pee)	process of viewing the ear
presby/o	-cusis	presbycusis (pres bih **KYOO** sis)	old age hearing
staped/o	-ectomy	stapedectomy (stay pee **DEK** toh mee)	excision of stapes
tympan/o	-ic	tympanic (tim **PAN** ik)	pertaining to the eardrum
	-itis	tympanitis (tim pan **EYE** tis)	eardrum inflammation
	-meter	tympanometer (tim pah **NOM** eh ter)	instrument to measure eardrum
	-metry	tympanometry (tim pah **NOM** eh tree)	process of measuring eardrum
	-plasty	tympanoplasty (tim pan oh **PLASS** tee)	surgical repair of eardrum
	-rrhexis	tympanorrhexis (tim pan oh **REK** sis)	eardrum rupture

Vocabulary Relating to the Ear

American Sign Language (ASL)	Nonverbal method of communicating in which the hands and fingers are used to indicate words and concepts. Used by both deaf and speech-impaired persons (see Figure 13.16).
audiologist (aw dee OL oh jist)	Medical professional trained to perform hearing tests using such equipment as an audiometer, to fit and test hearing aids, and to provide auditory rehabilitation.
cerumen (seh ROO men) block	Ear wax causing a blockage in the external canal of the ear.
conductive hearing loss	Loss of hearing as a result of the blocking of sound transmission in the middle ear and outer ear.
decibel (dB) (DES ih bel)	Measures the intensity or loudness of a sound. Zero dB is the quietest sound measured and 120 dB is the loudest sound commonly measured.
eustachian (yoo STAY kee en) tube	Tube or canal that connects the middle ear with the nasopharynx and allows for a balance of pressure between the outer and middle ear. Infection can travel via the mucous membranes of the eustachian tube, resulting in middle ear infections.
fingerspelling	Use of various hand and finger shapes and positions that represent the written alphabet. These positions can be strung together to form words.
hertz (Hz)	Measurement of the frequency or pitch of sound. The lowest pitch on an audiogram is 250 Hz. The measurement can go as high as 8,000 Hz, which is the highest pitch measured.
interpreter	Person with training in areas such as sign language, fingerspelling, and speech, who can transmit verbal or written messages to the hearing-impaired person.
otorhinolaryngologist (oh toh rih noh lair in GOL oh jist)	A physician who specializes in the treatment of diseases of the ear, nose, and throat.
otorhinolaryngology (oh toh rih noh lair in GOL oh jee)	Branch of medicine that treats diseases of the ears, nose, and throat. Also referred to as *ENT*.
presbycusis (pres bih KYOO sis)	Loss of hearing that can accompany the aging process.
residual hearing	Amount of hearing that is still present after damage has occurred to the auditory mechanism.
sensorineural (sen soh ree NOO ral) hearing loss	Type of hearing loss in which the sound is conducted normally through the external and middle ear, but there is a defect in the inner ear or with the cochlear nerve, resulting in the inability to hear. A hearing aid may help (see Figure 13.17).
Signing Exact English (SEE-2)	Translation of English into signs. American Sign Language (ASL) is used in combination with other sign languages and fingerspelling to correspond exactly to the spoken English.
speech pathologist (pah THOL oh jist)	Medical professional trained to evaluate and train the person who is hearing impaired in using any one, or all, of the following: speech, sign language, fingerspelling, and residual hearing.
speechreading	Ability to watch a person's mouth and word formation during speaking to interpret what they are saying. Also referred to as *lipreading*.
tinnitus (tin EYE tus)	Ringing in the ears.
vertigo (VER tih goh)	Dizziness.
vestibular (ves TIB yoo lar) apparatus	Part of the inner ear responsible for equilibrium. Conditions resulting in loss of balance may arise from this area.

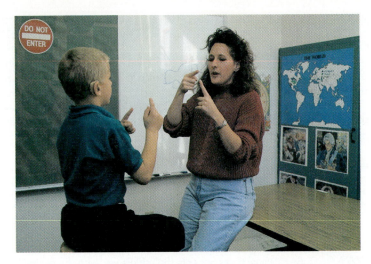

FIGURE 13.16 Sign-language teacher with child who is hearing impaired wearing behind-the-ear hearing aid. (Trevon Baker/About Faces)

FIGURE 13.17 (A) Small hearing aid in ear canal (Jane Schemilt/Science Photo Library/Photo Researchers, Inc.); (B) large hearing aid in ear canal (Jane Schemilt/Science Photo Library/Photo Researchers, Inc.); (C) hearing aid attached to glasses. (Jane Schemilt/Science Photo Library/Photo Researchers, Inc.)

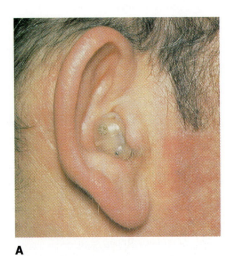

A

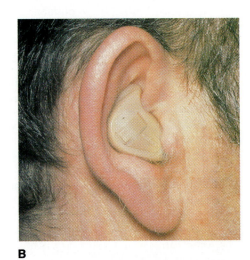

B

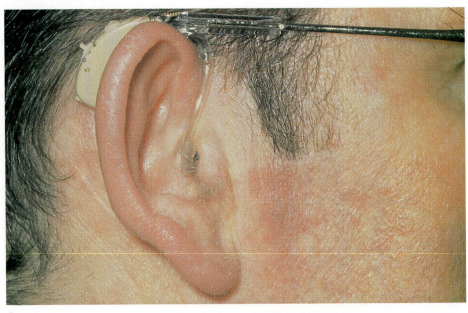

C

446

Pathology of the Ear

acoustic neuroma (ah KOOS tik noor OH mah)	Benign tumor of the eighth cranial nerve sheath. The pressure causes symptoms such as tinnitus, headache, dizziness, and progressive hearing loss.
anacusis (an ah KOO sis)	Total absence of hearing; inability to perceive sound. Also called *deafness*.
deafness	The inability to hear or having some degree of hearing impairment.
hearing impairment	Loss of hearing sufficient to interfere with a person's ability to communicate.
Ménière's disease (may nee ARZ dih ZEEZ)	Abnormal condition within the labyrinth of the inner ear that can lead to a progressive loss of hearing. The symptoms are dizziness or vertigo, hearing loss, and tinnitus (ringing in the ears). Named for Prosper Ménière, a French physician.
otitis media (OM) (oh TYE tis MEE dee ah)	Commonly referred to as *middle ear infection*; seen frequently in children. Often preceded by an upper respiratory infection.
otomycosis (oh toh my KOH sis)	Fungal infection of the ear, usually in the auditory canal.
otosclerosis (oh toh sklair OH sis)	Progressive hearing loss caused by immobility of the stapes bone.

MED TERM TIP Hearing impairment is becoming a greater problem for the general population for several reasons. First, people are living longer. Hearing loss can accompany old age, and there are a greater number of people over fifty years of age requiring hearing assistance. In addition, sound technology has been able to produce music quality that was never available before. However, listening to loud music either naturally or through earphones can cause gradual damage to the hearing mechanism.

Diagnostic Procedures Relating to the Ear

audiogram **(AW dee oh gram)**	Chart that shows the faintest sounds a patient can hear during audiometry testing (see Figure 13.18).
audiometric **(aw dee oh MET rik)** **test**	Test of hearing ability by determining the lowest and highest intensity (decibels) and frequencies (hertz) that a person can distinguish. The patient may sit in a soundproof booth and receive sounds through earphones as the technician decreases the sound or lowers the tones (see also Figure 13.18).
falling test	Test used to observe balance and equilibrium. The patient is observed balancing on one foot, then with one foot in front of the other, and then walking forward with eyes open. The same test is conducted with the patient's eyes closed. Swaying and falling with the eyes closed can indicate an ear and equilibrium malfunction.
hearing level	Audiometer reading in decibels (dB) corresponding to the listener's hearing threshold ratio that corresponds to the softest sound the listener can hear.
mastoid (MASS toyd) **X-ray**	X-ray taken of the mastoid bone to determine the presence of an infection, which can be an extension of a middle ear infection.
otoscopy **(oh TOSS koh pee)**	Use of a lighted otoscope to examine the auditory canal and middle ear (see Figure 13.19).
Rinne (RIN eh) and **Weber tuning-fork** **tests**	The physician holds a tuning fork, which is an instrument that produces a constant pitch when it is struck, against or near the bones on the side of the head. These tests assess both nerve and bone conduction of sound. Friedrich Rinne was a German otologist, and Ernst Weber was a German physiologist.
tympanometry **(tim pah NOM eh tree)**	Measurement of the movement of the tympanic membrane. Can indicate the presence of pressure in the middle ear.

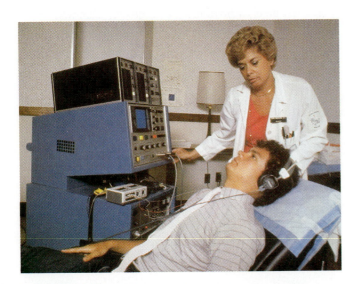

FIGURE 13.18 Technician performing a hearing test with audiometer. (Ann Chwatsky/Phototake NYC)

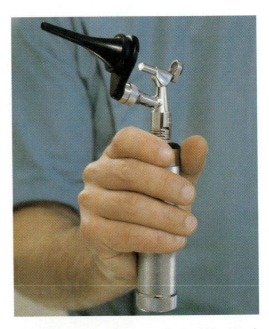

FIGURE 13.19 Otoscope. (Richard Hutchings/ Photo Researchers, Inc.)

Treatment Procedures Relating to the Ear

amplification (am plih fih KAY sun) device	Used to increase certain sounds for the hearing impaired person. Also known as *hearing aid*.
cochlear (KOK lee ar) implant	Mechanical device surgically placed under the skin behind the outer ear (pinna) that converts sound signals into magnetic impulses to stimulate the auditory nerve. Can be beneficial for those with profound sensorineural hearing loss.
hearing aid	Apparatus or mechanical device used by persons with impaired hearing to amplify sound. Same as *amplification device*.
mastoid antrotomy (MASS toyd an TROT oh mee)	Surgical opening made in the cavity within the mastoid process to alleviate pressure from infection and allow for drainage.
myringoplasty (mir IN goh plass tee)	Surgical reconstruction of the eardrum. Also called *tympanoplasty*.
myringotomy (mir in GOT oh mee)	Surgical puncture of the eardrum with removal of fluid and pus from the middle ear, to eliminate a persistent ear infection and excessive pressure on the tympanic membrane. A polyethylene tube is placed in the tympanic membrane to allow for drainage of the middle ear cavity.
otoplasty (OH toh plass tee)	Corrective surgery to change the size of the external ear or pinna. The surgery can either enlarge or decrease the size of the pinna.
otoscopy (oh TOSS koh pee)	Examination of the ear canal, eardrum, and outer ear using the otoscope. Foreign material can be removed from the ear canal with this procedure (see Figure 13.19).
polyethylene (pol ee ETH ih leen) tube (PE tube)	Small tube surgically placed in a child's ear to assist in drainage of infection.
stapedectomy (stay pee DEK toh mee)	Removal of the stapes bone to treat otosclerosis (hardening of the bone). A prosthesis or artificial stapes may be implanted.
tympanoplasty (tim pan oh PLASS tee)	Another term for the surgical reconstruction of the eardrum. Also called myringoplasty.

Professional Profile

Audiologists

Audiologists perform diagnostic hearing tests, fit patients/clients with hearing aids, and rehabilitate persons with hearing loss. They plan courses of treatment so individuals with hearing loss are able to regain their hearing ability, and conduct research to develop new and innovative hearing devices. Audiology services are found in hospitals, schools, and private offices. To become an audiologist, students must graduate from an accredited five-year master's degree program in audiology and pass a national certification exam. For more information regarding a career in audiology, visit the American Academy of Audiology's web site at www.audiology.org.

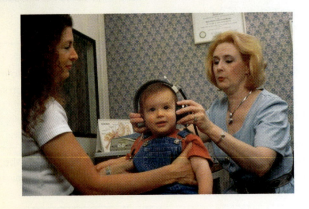

Certificate of Clinical Competence in Audiology (CCC-A)

- **Graduates from an accredited five-year master's degree audiology program**
- **Passes a certification examination**

Abbreviations Relating to the Ear

AC	air conduction		**HEENT**	head, ears, eyes, nose, throat
AD	right ear		**Hz**	Hertz
AS	left ear		**OM**	otitis media
ASL	American Sign Language		**Oto**	otology
AU	both ears		**PE tube**	polyethylene tube placed in the eardrum
BC	bone conduction		**SEE-2**	Signing Exact English
dB	decibel		**SOM**	serous otitis media
EENT	eyes, ears, nose, throat		**UCHD**	usual childhood diseases
ENT	ear, nose, and throat			

KEY TERMS

- acoustic (ah **KOOS** tik)
- acoustic neuroma (ah **KOOS** tik noor **OH** mah)
- American Sign Language
- amplification device (am plih fih **KAY** shun)
- anacusis (an ah **KOO** sis)
- audiogram (**AW** dee oh gram)
- audiologist (aw dee **OL** oh jist)
- audiology (aw dee **OL** oh jee)
- audiometer (aw dee **OM** eh ter)
- audiometric test (aw dee oh **MET** rik)
- audiometry (aw dee **OM** eh tree)
- auditory canal (**AW** dih tor ee)
- aural (**AW** ral)
- auricle (**AW** rih k'l)
- cerumen (seh **ROO** men)
- cochlea (**KOK** lee ah)
- cochlear (**KOK** lee ar)
- cochlear implant (**KOK** lee ar)
- cochlear nerve (**KOK** lee ar)
- conductive hearing loss (kon **DUK** tiv)
- deafness
- decibel (dB) (**DES** ih bel)
- ear
- equilibrium (ee kwih **LIB** ree um)
- eustachian tube (yoo **STAY** kee en)
- external ear
- falling test
- fingerspelling
- hearing aid
- hearing impairment
- hearing level
- hertz (Hz)
- incus (**ING** kus)
- inner ear
- interpreter
- labyrinth (**LAB** ih rinth)
- labyrinthectomy (lab ih rin **THEK** toh mee)
- labyrinthitis (lab ih rin **THIGH** tis)
- malleus (**MAL** ee us)
- mastoid antrotomy (**MASS** toyd an **TROT** oh mee)
- mastoid bone (**MASS** toyd)
- mastoid process (**MASS** toyd)
- mastoid X-ray (**MASS** toyd)
- mastoidectomy (mass toyd **ECK** toh mee)
- mastoiditis (mass toyd **EYE** tis)
- mastoidotomy (mass toy **DOT** oh mee)
- Ménière's disease (may nee **ARZ** dih **ZEEZ**)
- middle ear

- myringitis (mir ing **JYE** tis)
- myringoplasty (mir **IN** goh plass tee)
- myringotomy (mir in **GOT** oh mee)
- organ of Corti (**KOR** tee)
- ossicles (**OSS** ih kls)
- otalgia (oh **TAL** jee ah)
- otic (**OH** tik)
- otitis (oh **TYE** tis)
- otitis media (OM) (oh **TYE** tis **MEE** dee ah)
- otologist (oh **TOL** oh jist)
- otology (Oto) (oh **TOL** oh jee)
- otomycosis (oh toh my **KOH** sis)
- otoplasty (**OH** toh plass tee)
- otopyorrhea (oh toh pye oh **REE** ah)
- otorhinolaryngologist
  (oh toh rih noh lair in **GOL** oh jist)
- otorhinolaryngology
  (oh toh rih noh lair in **GOL** oh jee)
- otosclerosis (oh toh sklair **OH** sis)
- otoscope (**OH** toh scope)
- otoscopy (oh **TOSS** koh pee)
- oval window
- pinna (**PIN** ah)
- polyethylene tube (PE tube) (pol ee **ETH** ih leen)
- presbycusis (pres bih **KYOO** sis)
- residual hearing (rih **ZID** yoo al)
- Rinne and Weber tuning-fork test (**RIN** eh)
- saccule (**SAK** yool)
- semicircular canals
- sensorineural hearing loss (sen soh ree **NOO** ral)
- Signing Exact English (SEE-2)
- speech pathologist (pah **THOL** oh jist)
- speechreading
- stapedectomy (stay pee **DEK** toh mee)
- stapes (**STAY** peez)
- tinnitus (tin **EYE** tus)
- tympanic (tim **PAN** ik)
- tympanic membrane (tim **PAN** ik)
- tympanitis (tim pan **EYE** tis)
- tympanometer (tim pah **NOM** eh ter)
- tympanometry (tim pah **NOM** eh tree)
- tympanoplasty (tim pan oh **PLASS** tee)
- tympanorrhexis (tim pan oh **REK** sis)
- utricle (**YOO** trih k'l)
- vertigo (**VER** tih goh)
- vestibular apparatus (ves **TIB** yoo lar)
- vestibular nerve (ves **TIB** yoo lar)
- vestibulocochlear nerve (ves tib yoo loh **KOK** lee ar)

Case Study II

OTORHINOLARYNGOLOGY CONSULTATION REPORT

Reason for Consultation: Evaluation of progressive hearing loss.

History of Present Illness: Patient is a 35-year-old female who presents with tinnitus that began intermittently and very low. It has now progressed to the point she has difficulty hearing and is more severe on the left. She also has vertigo with almost constant nausea and occasional vomiting.

Past Medical History: Patient required bilateral myringotomy with tubes as an 8-year-old for chronic otitis media, but this resolved within 2 years and she has had no hearing problems since that time. Her only other surgery has been an appendectomy at 16. She has had no serious health problems up to this point. She is married, a school teacher and multipara with a 6-year-old daughter and a 2-year-old son. Her parents are alive and well.

Results of Physical Examination: Otoscopy of both ears showed normal ear canals and tympanic membranes. Audiometric tests indicate moderate hearing loss on the left and mild hearing loss on the right. Results of both the Rinne and Weber tuning-fork tests indicate patient has sensorineural hearing loss but not conductive hearing loss. This hearing loss is more pronounced on the left than the right. She was unable to complete a falling test due to excessive swaying with eyes closed. MRI was negative for an acoustic neuroma.

Assessment: Ménière's disease with edema of labyrinth causing sensorineural hearing loss, vertigo, and tinnitus.

Recommendations: Short course of steroids to reduce labyrinth inflammation, Antivert for dizziness, and Compazine to control vomiting. Patient is to restrict driving or other activities that require balance and avoid exposure to any loud noises. Make appointment for follow-up evaluation in one week.

CRITICAL THINKING QUESTIONS FOR THE EAR

1. The physician writing this consultation report is an otorhinolaryngologist. What is the literal translation for this term? What is the more common (although technically incorrect) name for this physician? What abbreviation is used for this medical specialty?

2. Explain the difference between sensorineural and conductive hearing loss.

3. The patient was placed on three medications. List them and explain what each is for.

4. Which of the following is NOT part of this patient's past medical history?

   a. has given birth to two children

   b. gallbladder surgery

   c. long-standing middle ear infections

   d. surgical removal of her appendix

5. What tests were used to distinguish between sensorineural hearing loss and conductive hearing loss? Which type does this patient have?

6. What diagnostic imaging procedure did this patient have? What pathology did this imaging procedure rule out?

Chart Note Transcription II

Chart Note

The chart note below contains ten phrases that can be reworded with a medical term that you learned in this chapter. Each phrase is identified with an underline. Determine the medical term and write your answers in the space provided.

Current Complaint: An 8-year-old female was referred to the specialist in the treatment of diseases of the ear, nose, and throat[1] by her pediatrician for evaluation of chronic left middle ear infection.[2]

Past History: Patient's mother reports that her daughter began to experience recurrent ear infections at approximately 6 months of age. Frequency of the infections has increased over the past two years and she is missing school. Mother also reports the child's teacher feels she is having difficulty hearing in the classroom.

Signs and Symptoms: Visual examination of the external ear canal and eardrum[3] of both ears[4] revealed that the membrane between the external ear canal and middle[5] ear is normal on the right and bulging on the left. An excessive amount of ear wax[6] was noted in both ears. Measurement of the movement of the eardrum[7] indicates that there is a build-up of fluid in the left middle ear. Tests of hearing ability[8] report normal hearing on the right and loss of hearing as a result of the blocking of sound transmission in the middle ear[9] on the left. Patient also noted to have acute pharyngitis with purulent drainage at time of evaluation.

Diagnosis: Hearing loss secondary to chronic left middle ear infection.

Treatment: Left eardrum incision[10] with placement of polyethylene tube for drainage.

1 _____

2 _____

3 _____

4 _____

5 _____

6 _____

7 _____

8 _____

9 _____

10 _____

Practice Exercises II

A. COMPLETE THE FOLLOWING STATEMENTS.

1. The three bones in the middle ear are the _____ , _____ , and _____ .

2. The study of the ear is called _____ .

3. Another term for the eardrum is _____ .

4. _____ is produced in the oil glands in the auditory canal.

5. The _____ tube connects the nasopharynx with the middle ear.

6. The inner ear is located in a cavity within the _____ bone.

7. The _____ is responsible for conducting impulses from the ear to the brain.

8. _____ hearing loss is the result of blocking sound transmission in the middle ear.

B. MATCH THE TERMS IN COLUMN A WITH THE PROCEDURES IN COLUMN B.

A	B
1. _____ myringoplasty	a. removal of stapes bone
2. _____ otoplasty	b. reconstruction of eardrum
3. _____ stapedectomy	c. surgical puncture of eardrum
4. _____ tympanoplasty	d. change size of pinna
5. _____ mastoid antrotomy	e. using a scope for viewing
6. _____ myringotomy	f. surgical opening in bone to relieve pressure

C. MATCH THE TERMS IN COLUMN A WITH THE DEFINITIONS IN COLUMN B.

A	B
1. _____ tinnitus	a. ossicle of ear
2. _____ stapes	b. inner ear
3. _____ tympanometry	c. middle ear infection
4. _____ eustachian tube	d. ringing in ears
5. _____ labyrinth	e. auditory tube
6. _____ audiogram	f. measure movement in eardrum
7. _____ otitis media	g. results of hearing test

D. WRITE THE ABBREVIATIONS FOR THE FOLLOWING TERMS.

1. otology _____
4. serous otitis media _____

2. left ear _____
5. usual childhood diseases _____

3. right ear _____
6. ear, nose, throat _____

E. IDENTIFY THE FOLLOWING ABBREVIATIONS.

1. PE tube _____

2. EENT _____

3. BC _____

4. AU _____

5. OM _____

F. USE THE FOLLOWING SUFFIXES TO FORM A TERM RELATING TO THE EAR.

-otomy   -itis   -pyorrhea   -cusis   -mycosis

1. fungal infection of the ear _____
2. incision into tympanic membrane to relieve pressure _____
3. inflammation of the middle ear _____
4. discharge of pus from the ear _____
5. deafness _____

G. USE THE FOLLOWING TERMS IN THE SENTENCES THAT FOLLOW.

otolaryngologist   falling test   presbycusis   Ménière's disease
oculist   vestibular   vertigo   acoustic neuroma

1. Grace was told by her physician that her hearing loss was a part of the aging process. The term for this is _____ .

2. Stacey is having frequent middle ear infections and wishes to be treated by a specialist. She would go to a(n) _____ .

3. Warren was told that his dizziness may be caused by a problem in the _____ area.

4. Shantel is suffering from an abnormal condition of the inner ear that results in tinnitus, dizziness, and hearing loss. Her diagnosis may be _____ .

5. Keisha was told that her tumor of the eighth cranial nerve was benign, but she still experienced a hearing loss as a result of the tumor. This tumor is called a(n) _____ .

H. THE COMBINING FORM OT/O REFERS TO EAR. WRITE A WORD THAT MEANS:

1. ear repair   _____
2. presence of pus in the ear   _____
3. pain in the ear   _____
4. discharge from the ear   _____
5. hardening in the bony labyrinth of the ear   _____
6. study of the ear   _____

Getting Connected

Multimedia Extension Activities

CD-ROM
Use the CD-ROM enclosed with your textbook to gain additional reinforcement through interactive word building exercises, spelling games, labeling activities, and additional quizzes.

www.prenhall.com/fremgen
Use the above address to access the free, interactive Companion Website created for this textbook. Get hints, instant feedback, and textbook references to chapter-related multiple choice questions, and labeling and matching exercises. In addition, you will find an audio glossary, case studies, Internet exploration exercises, flashcards, and a comprehensive exam.

Answers

CASE STUDY I (CRITICAL THINKING QUESTIONS)

1. Pupils open and close correctly when the physician shines a light into the eye; pupils become smaller in bright light and larger in dim light; it is important to prevent too much light from reaching the inside of the eyeball.   2. eye muscles, conjunctiva, iris/pupil, retina, macular area of the retina, cornea   3. breast cancer with a mastectomy, cholelithiasis with a cholecystectomy   4. dilate the pupil, miotic drops   5. a —farsightedness (hyperopia)
6. cryoextraction

CHART NOTE I

1. ophthalmologist—specialist in the treatment of eye diseases   2. myopia—nearsightedness   3. astigmatism—abnormal curvature of the cornea   4. retina—innermost layer of the eye   5. ophthalmoscope—instrument to examine the interior of the eye   6. macular degeneration—deterioration of the macular area   7. fluorescein angiography—dye injected into blood vessels in order to study the retina   8. tonometry—procedure to measure the pressure inside the eye   9. glaucoma—atrophy of optic nerve due to increased intraocular pressure   10. laser surgery—surgery performed with an intense small beam of light

PRACTICE EXERCISES I

A. 1. ophthalmology   2. orbit, muscles, eyelids, conjunctiva, lacrimal gland, and ducts   3. strabismus   4. cilia
5. bleeding problem/anemia   6. lacrimal   7. jaundice   8. cornea   9. retina   10. iris   11. accommodation
12. emmetropia   13. detached retina   14. astigmatism   15. hemianopia
B. 1. blepharitis   2. blepharoplasty   3. blepharochalasis   4. blepharoplegia   5. retinopathy   6. retinopexy
7. ophthalmology   8. ophthalmic   9. ophthalmoscopy   10. optician   11. optical
C. 1. -tropia,   2. -opia, -opsia;   3. -itis   4. -ology   5. -otomy   6. -plasty   7. -pexy   8. -stenosis
D. 1. tear   2. pupil   3. water   4. eye   5. eyelid   6. glassy   7. cornea   8. sclera   9. old age   10. dull or dim   11. eye
12. eye
E. 1. dull/dim vision   2. double vision   3. enlarge or widen pupil   4. constrict pupil   5. diminished vision of old age
F. 1. h   2. g   3. a   4. d   5. b   6. i   7. c   8. f   9. e   10. j   11. k   12. l
G. 1. left eye   2. each eye   3. rapid eye movement   4. accommodation   5. senile macular degeneration   6. pupils equal, react to light and accommodation   7. intraocular pressure   8. right eye   9. right eye   10. visual field
H. 1. tonometry   2. chalazion   3. emmetropia   4. conjunctivitis   5. myopia   6. cataract   7. hordeolum
8. entropion   9. strabismus   10. hyperopia   11. exopthalmos

CASE STUDY II (CRITICAL THINKING QUESTIONS)

1. ear, nose, voice box specialist; ear, nose, and throat doctor; ENT   2. sensorineural—sound is conducted normally through external and middle ear, but there is a defect with the inner ear or auditory nerve;   conductive—sound is blocked from passing (being conducted) through the outer or middle ear   3. steroids to reduce inflammation, Antivert to stop dizziness, Compazine to control vomiting   4. b—gallbladder surgery   5. Rinne and Weber tuning-fork tests; sensorineural hearing loss   6. magnetic resonance imaging (MRI); acoustic neuroma

CHART NOTE II

1. otorhinolaryngologist (ENT)—specialist in the treatment of diseases of the ear, nose, and throat   2. otitis media (OM)—middle ear infection   3. otoscopy—visual examination of the external ear canal and eardrum   4. AU—both ears   5. tympanic membrane—membrane between the outer and middle ear   6. cerumen—ear wax
7. tympanometry—measurement of the movement of the eardrum   8. audiometric test—test of hearing ability
9. conductive hearing loss—loss of hearing as the result of the blocking of sound transmission in the middle ear
10. myringotomy—eardrum incision

A. 1. malleus, incus, stapes   2. otology   3. tympanic membrane   4. cerumen   5. eustachian   6. temporal
7. eighth cranial nerve   8. conductive

B. 1. b   2. d   3. a   4. b   5. f   6. c

C. 1. d   2. a   3. f   4. e   5. b   6. g   7. c

D. 1. Oto   2. AS   3. AD   4. SOM   5. UCHD   6. ENT

E. 1. polyethylene tube placed in eardrum   2. eyes, ears, nose, throat   3. bone conduction   4. both ears   5. otitis media

F. 1. otomycosis   2. tympanotomy   3. otitis media   4. otopyorrhea   5. anacusis

G. 1. presbycusis   2. otolaryngologist   3. vestibular   4. Ménière's disease   5. acoustic neuroma

H. 1. otoplasty   2. otopyorrhea   3. otalgia   4. otorrhea   5. otosclerosis   6. otology

Chapter 14

PHARMACOLOGY

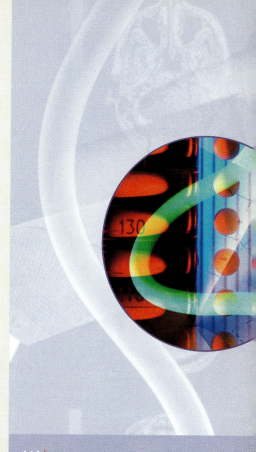

LEARNING OBJECTIVES

Upon completion of this chapter, you will be able to:

- Recognize the combining forms introduced in this chapter.

- Gain the ability to pronounce pharmacology terms.

- Describe the three names by which a drug can be known.

- Discuss the legal classifications of drugs.

- Recognize the different classes of drugs, their uses, and common examples.

- Identify the different routes of drug administration.

- Discuss the general rules for administering medications.

- Read a prescription.

- Define vocabulary medical terms relating to pharmacology.

- Interpret abbreviations associated with pharmacology.

Overview

COMBINING FORMS RELATING TO PHARMACOLOGY

aer/o	air	**lingu/o**	tongue
algesi/o	pain	**narc/o**	numb, stupor
bi/o	life	**pharmac/o**	drug
chem/o	drug	**pyret/o**	fever
cutane/o	skin	**tox/o**	poison
derm/o	skin	**toxic/o**	poison
esthesi/o	feeling	**ven/o**	vein
hypn/o	sleep		

Pharmacology (far ma **KALL** oh jee) is the study of the origin, characteristics, and effects of drugs. Drugs are obtained from many different sources.

Some drugs, such as vitamins, are found naturally in the foods we eat. Others, such as hormones, are obtained from animals. Penicillin and some of the other antibiotics are developed from mold, which is a fungus. Many drugs, such as those used in chemotherapy, are synthetic, which means they are developed by artificial means in the laboratory.

MED TERM TIP

The terms *drug* and *medication* have the same meaning. However, the general public often uses the term *drug* to refer to a narcotic type of medication. The term can also mean illegal chemical substances. For purposes of medical terminology, use of the word *drug* means medication.

DRUG NAMES

brand name	**nonproprietary name**	**proprietary name**
chemical name	**pharmaceutical**	**trade name**
generic name	**pharmacist**	

Every drug has three different names:

1. **Chemical** (**KEM** ih cal) **name**
2. **Generic,** or **nonproprietary name**
3. **Brand, trade,** or **proprietary** (proh **PRYE** ah tair ee) **name**

All drugs are chemicals. The chemical name describes the chemical formula or molecular structure of a particular drug. For example, the chemical name for ibuprofen, an over-the-counter pain medication, is 2-p-isobutylphenyl propionic acid. Just as in this case, chemical names are usually very long, so a shorter name is given to the drug. This name is the generic or nonproprietary name, and it is recognized and accepted as the official name for a drug.

Each drug has only one generic name, such as ibuprofen, and this name is not subject to trademark, so any pharmaceutical manufacturer may use it. However, the **pharmaceutical** company that originally developed the drug has exclusive rights to produce it for seventeen years. After that time, any manufacturer may produce and sell the drug. When a company manufactures a drug for sale, it must choose a brand, or proprietary, name for its product. This is the company's trademark for the drug. For

Table 14.1	Examples of Different Drug Names		
Chemical Name	**Generic Name**	**Brand Names**
2-p-isobutyl phenyl propionic acid	ibuprofen	Motrin Advil Nuprin
acetylsalicylic acid	aspirin	Anacin Bufferin Excedrin
S-2-[1-(methylamino) ethyl] benzenemethanol hydrochloride	pseudoephedrine hydrochloride	Sudafed Actifed Nucofed

example, ibuprofen is known by several brand names, including Motrin, Advil, and Nuprin. All three are the same ibuprofen; they are just marketed by different pharmaceutical companies. (See Table 14.1 for examples of different drug names.)

Generic drugs are usually priced lower than brand name drugs. A physician can indicate on the prescription if the **pharmacist** may substitute a generic drug for a brand name. The physician may prefer that a particular brand name drug be used if he or she believes it to be more effective than the generic drug.

REGULATIONS AND STANDARDS

Federal Food and Drug Administration

Federal Food, Drug, and Cosmetic Act of 1938

Controlled Substance Act of 1970

The **Federal Food and Drug Administration (FDA),** which is a branch of the Federal Department of Health and Human Services, ultimately enforces drug sales and distribution. The **Federal Food, Drug, and Cosmetic Act of 1938** stipulates the actual control of drugs. This act was initiated to ensure the safety of food, drugs, and cosmetics that are sold within U.S. borders. The **Controlled Substance Act of 1970** regulates the manufacture and distribution of drugs that are capable of causing dependence.

REFERENCES

Hospital Formulary

Physician's Desk Reference

United States Pharmacopeia-National Formulary

There are two major resources for drug information: the *Hospital Formulary* (**FORM** yoo lair ee) and the *Physician's Desk Reference (PDR).* The *Hospital Formulary* contains up-to-date information about drugs and their use. It is published by the American Hospital Formulary Service and used extensively by pharmacists. The *Physician's Desk Reference* or PDR is an easy-to-use resource and should be in every physician's office or medical facility. The PDR is published by a private company and is sent free of charge to medical offices and hospitals. It lists drug products with addresses of manufacturers, generic and chemical names, and other valuable information.

Another helpful reference is the *United States Pharmacopeia—National Formulary* (*USP—NF*). It lists all the official drugs authorized for use in the United States.

LEGAL CLASSIFICATION OF DRUGS

PRESCRIPTION DRUGS

prescription   **prescription drug**

A **prescription** (prih **SKRIP** shun) **drug** can only be ordered by a licensed physician, dentist, or veterinarian. These drugs must include the words *"Caution: Federal law prohibits dispensing without prescription"* on their labels. Antibiotics, such as penicillin, and heart medications, such as digoxin, are available only by prescription. A **prescription** (prih **SKRIP** shun) is the written explanation to the pharmacist regarding the name of the medication, the dosage, and the times of administration. A licensed physician can also give a prescription order orally to the pharmacist.

NONPRESCRIPTION DRUGS

antacids   **over-the-counter**

nonprescription drug

A **nonprescription** drug is also referred to as an **over-the-counter (OTC)** drug. They are accessible in drugstores without a prescription. Many medications or drugs can be purchased without a prescription; for example aspirin, **antacids** (ant **ASS** ids), and antidiarrheal medications.

However, taking aspirin along with an anticoagulant, such as coumadin, can cause internal bleeding in some people, and OTC antacids interfere with the absorption of the prescription drug tetracycline into the body. It is better for the physician or pharmacist to advise the patient on the proper OTC drugs to use with prescription drugs.

CONTROLLED SUBSTANCES

controlled substances   **Drug Enforcement Agency**

Certain drugs are **controlled substances** if they have a potential for being addictive (habit-forming) or can be abused. The **Drug Enforcement Agency (DEA)** enforces the control of these drugs. Some of the more commonly prescribed controlled substances are:

- anabolic steroids
- APC with codeine
- butabarbital
- chloral hydrate
- cocaine
- codeine
- diazepam

- heroin
- LSD
- marijuana
- morphine
- opium
- phenobarbital
- secobarbital

Table 14.2	*Schedule for Controlled Substances*
Classification	**Meaning**
Schedule I	Drugs with the highest potential for addiction and abuse. They are not accepted for medical use. Examples are heroin and LSD.
Schedule II	Drugs with a high potential for addiction and abuse accepted for medical use in the United States. Examples are codeine, cocaine, morphine, opium, and secobarbital.
Schedule III	Drugs with a moderate to low potential for addiction and abuse. Examples are butabarbital, anabolic steroids, and APC with codeine.
Schedule IV	Drugs with a lower potential for addiction and abuse than Schedule III drugs. Examples are chloral hydrate, phenobarbital, and diazepam.
Schedule V	Drugs with a low potential for addiction and abuse. An example is low-strength codeine combined with other drugs to suppress coughing.

The controlled drugs are classified in Schedule I through Schedule V, which indicates their potential for abuse. They are listed in Table 14.2.

Vocabulary Relating to Pharmacology

addiction (ah DICK shun)	Acquired dependence on a drug.
anaphylactic shock (an ah fih LAK tik)	Life-threatening reaction to certain foods and drugs in some people. This can cause respiratory distress, edema, rash, convulsions, and eventually unconsciousness and death if emergency treatment is not given.
antidote (AN tih doht)	Substance that will neutralize poisons or their side effects.
broad spectrum	Ability of a drug to be effective against a wide range of microorganisms.
chemotherapy (kee moh THAIR ah pee)	Use of chemicals (drugs) to treat cancer by killing the cells.
contraindication (kon trah in dih KAY shun)	Condition in which a particular drug should not be used.
cumulative action	Action that occurs in the body when a drug is allowed to accumulate or stay in the body.
dilute	To weaken the strength of a substance by adding something else.
drug tolerance (TAHL er ans)	Decrease in susceptibility to a drug after continued use of the drug.
habituation (hah bich yoo AY shun)	Development of an emotional dependence on a drug due to repeated use.
hemostatic (hee moh STAH tik)	Any drug, medicine, or clotting protein from blood that stops bleeding, such as vitamin K or factor VIII (the clotting factor missing in hemophiliacs).

(continued)

idiosyncrasy (id ee oh **SIN** krah see)	Unusual or abnormal response to a drug or food.
parenteral (par EN ter al)	A route for introducing medication other than through the gastrointestinal tract; most commonly involves injection into the body through a needle and syringe.
pharmacist (FAR mah sist)	One who is licensed to prepare and dispense drugs.
pharmacology (far mah **KALL** oh jee)	Study of the origins, nature, properties, and effects of drugs on the living organism.
placebo (plah SEE boh)	Inactive, harmless substance used to satisfy a patient's desire for medication. This is also used in research when given to a control group of patients in a study in which another group receives a drug. The effect of the placebo versus the drug is then observed.
prophylaxis (proh fih **LAK** sis)	Prevention of disease. For example, an antibiotic can be used to prevent the occurrence of a disease.
side effect	Response to a drug other than the effect desired.
tolerance (TAHL er ans)	Development of a capacity for withstanding a large amount of a substance, such as foods, drugs, or poison, without any adverse effect. A decreased sensitivity to further doses will develop.
toxicity (tok SISS ih tee)	Extent or degree to which a substance is poisonous.
unit dose	Drug dosage system that provides prepackaged, prelabeled, individual medications that are ready for immediate use by the patient.

GENERAL CLASSES OF DRUGS

The classification of drugs relates to their action on the body. Table 14.3 presents a comprehensive list of drug classifications. Table 14.4 contains examples of drugs classified by their use.

Table 14.3 Types of Drugs

Name	Use
analgesic (an al **JEE** zik)	Relieves pain without the loss of consciousness. May be either narcotic or nonnarcotic. Narcotic drugs are derived from the opium poppy and act on the brain to cause pain relief and drowsiness.
anesthetic (an ess **THET** ik)	Produces a lack of feeling that may be of local or general effect, depending on the type of administration.
antacid (ant **ASS** id)	Neutralizes acid in the stomach.
antianxiety (an tih ang **ZIGH** ah tee)	Relieves or reduces anxiety and muscle tension. Used to treat panic disorders, anxiety, and insomnia.
antiarrhythmic (an tih ah **RITH** mik)	Controls cardiac arrhythmias by altering nerve impulses within the heart.
antibiotic (an tih bye **OT** ik)	Destroys or prohibits the growth of microorganisms. Used to treat bacterial infections. Has not been found to be effective in treating viral infections. To be effective must be taken regularly for a specified period.
anticholinergic (an tih koh lin **ER** jik)	Blocks the function of the parasympathetic nervous system. Used to treat intestinal, bladder, and bronchial spasms.
anticoagulant (an tih koh **AG** yoo lant)	Prevents or delays blood clotting; also called a blood thinner. Some drugs such as warfarin, are administered orally; others, such as heparin, are administered parenterally.
anticonvulsant (an tih con **VULL** sant)	Prevents or relieves convulsions. Drugs such as phenobarbital reduce excessive stimulation in the brain to control seizures and other symptoms of epilepsy.
antidepressant (an tih dee **PRESS** ant)	Prevents or relieves the symptoms of depression. Also used in the prevention of migraine headaches.
antidiabetic (an tih dye ah **BET** ik)	Insulin drug that controls diabetes by regulating the level of glucose in the blood and the metabolism of carbohydrates and fat.
antidiarrheal (an tih dye ah **REE** al)	Prevents or relieves diarrhea.
antidote (**AN** tih doht)	Counteracts the effects of poisons.
antiemetic (an tih ee **MET** ik)	Controls nausea and vomiting.
antihistamine (an tih **HISS** tah meen)	Acts to control allergic symptoms by counteracting histamine, which exists naturally in the body and is released in allergic reactions.
antihypertensive (an tih high per **TEN** siv)	Prevents or controls high blood pressure. Some of these drugs act to block nerve impulses that increase the blood pressure by causing arteries to constrict. Other drugs slow the heart rate and decrease its force of contraction. Still others may reduce the amount of the hormone aldosterone in the blood that is causing the blood pressure to rise.
anti-inflammatory (an tih in **FLAM** ah tor ee)	Acts to counteract inflammation.
antipyretic (an tih pye **RET** ik)	Used to reduce fever.
antitussive (an tih **TUSS** iv)	Controls or relieves coughing. Codeine is an ingredient in many prescription cough medicines that acts upon the brain to control coughing.
astringent (ah **STRIN** jent)	Substance that causes tissues to dry up and contract; also may be used to stop bleeding.
bronchodilator (brong koh **DYE** lay tor)	Dilates or opens the bronchi (airways in the lungs) to improve breathing.
cardiotonic (kar dee **TON** ik)	Strengthens the heart muscle.

(continued)

Name	Use
cathartic (kah **THAR** tik)	Causes bowel movements to occur.
contraceptive (con trah **SEP** tiv)	Used to prevent conception.
decongestant (dee kon **JESS** tant)	Reduces nasal congestion and swelling.
diuretic (dye yoor **RET** ik)	Increases the excretion of urine, which promotes the loss of water and salt from the body. Can assist in lowering blood pressure; therefore, these drugs are used to treat hypertension. Potassium in the body may be depleted with continued use of diuretics. Potassium-rich foods such as bananas, kiwi, and orange juice can help correct this deficiency.
emetic (ee **MET** ik)	Induces vomiting.
estrogen (**ESS** troh jen)	Hormone used to replace natural estrogen lost during menopause. Estrogen is responsible for the development of secondary sexual characteristics and is produced by the ovaries.
expectorant (ek **SPEK** toh rant)	Assists in the removal of secretions from the bronchopulmonary membranes.
hemostatic (hee moh **STAH** tik)	Used to control bleeding.
Hormone (**HOR** mohn)	Given to replace the loss of natural hormones or to treat disease by simulating hormonal effects.
hypnotic (hip **NOT** ik)	Used to produce sleep or hypnosis.
hypoglycemic (high poh glye **SEE** mik)	Lowers blood glucose level.
immunosuppressive (im yoo noh suh **PRESS** iv)	Suppresses the body's natural immune response to an antigen. This is used to control autoimmune diseases such as multiple sclerosis and rheumatoid arthritis.
laxative (**LACK** sah tiv)	A mild cathartic.
miotic (my **OT** ik)	Constricts the pupils of the eye.
muscle relaxant	Produces the relaxation of skeletal muscle.
mydriatic (mid ree **AT** ik)	Dilates the pupils of the eye.
narcotic (nar **KOT** ik)	Produces sleep or stupor. In moderate doses this drug will depress the central nervous system and relieve pain. In excessive doses it will cause stupor, coma, and even death. Can become habit forming (addictive).
psychedelic (sigh kah **DELL** ik)	Drug such as lysergic acid diethylamide (LSD) that can produce visual hallucinations.
purgative (**PUR** gah tiv)	A strong cathartic.
sedative (**SED** ah tiv)	Produces relaxation without causing sleep.
stimulant (**STIM** yoo lant)	Speeds up the heart and respiratory system. Used to increase alertness.
tranquilizer (trang kwih **LIGH** zer)	Used to reduce mental anxiety and tensions.
vaccine (**VAK** seen)	Given to promote resistance to infectious diseases.
vasodilator (vas oh **DYE** lay tor)	Produces a relaxation of blood vessels to lower blood pressure.
vasopressor (vas oh **PRESS** or)	Produces the contraction of muscles in the capillaries and arteries that elevates the blood pressure.
vitamin (**VIGH** tah min)	Organic substance found naturally in foods that is essential for normal metabolism. Most have been produced synthetically to be taken in pill form.

Table 14.4	Examples of Drugs Classified by Usage	
Type/Usage	**Example**	
analgesic	Advil (ibuprofen)	
	Darvon [propoxyphene hydrochloride (HCl)]	
	Dilaudid (hydromorphine HCl)	
	Demerol (meperidine HCl)	
	Talwin (pentazocine HCl)	
	Tylenol (acetaminophen)	
anesthetic	Carbocaine (mepivacaine HCl)	
	Novocaine (procaine HCl)	
	Nupercaine (dibucaine HCl)	
	Xylocaine (lidocaine HCl)	
antacid	milk of magnesia (magnesia magma)	
	Mylanta (aluminum hydroxide)	
antianxiety	Valium (diazepam)	
antiarrhythmic	Norpace (disopyramide)	
	Pronestyl (procainamide HCl)	
antibiotic		
Aminogylcosides	Garamycin (gentamicin sulfate)	
	Kantrex (kanamycin)	
	Mycifradin Sulfate (neomycin sulfate)	
	Nebcin (tobramycin sulfate)	
	Neobiotic (neomycin sulfate)	
	Nystatin (mycostatin)	
Cephalosporins	Ancef (cefazolin sodium)	
	Anspor (cephradine)	
	Ceclor (cefaclor)	
	Duricef (cefadroxil)	
	Keflex (cephalexin)	
	Keflin (cephalothin sodium)	
Penicillins	Amoxil (amoxicillin)	
	Bicillin (penicillin G potassium)	
	Duracillin (penicillin G procaine)	
	Polycillin (ampicillin)	
Tetracyclines	Acromycin (tetracycline HCl)	
	Declomycin (democlocycline)	
	Terramycin (oxytetracycline)	
	Vibramycin (doxycycline hyclate)	

(continued)

Type/Usage	Example
anticholinergic	Atropine (atropine sulfate)
	Banthine (methantheline bromide)
	Donnatol (belladonna)
anticoagulant	Coumadin (warfarin sodium)
anticonvulsant	Dilantin (phenytoin sodium)
antidepressant	Elavil (amitriptyline HCl)
antidiabetic	insulin
antidiarrheal	Kaopectate (kaolin and pectin mixture)
	Lomotil (diphenoxylate)
antiemetic	Atarax (hydroxyzine HCl)
	Compazine (prochlorperazine)
	Dramamine (dimenhydrinate)
	Phenergan (promethazine HCl)
antihistamine	adrenalin (epinephrine)
	Benadryl (diphenhydramine)
	Chlor-Trimeton (chlorapheneramine maleate)
	Dimetane (brompheniramine maleate)
antihypertensive	Aldomet (methyldopa)
	Catapres (clonidine HCl)
	Lopressor (metoprolol tartrate)
	Minipress (prazosin HCl)
anti-inflammatory	aspirin (acetylsalicylic acid)
	Indocin (indomethacin)
	Motrin (naprosyn)
	Nalfon (fenoprofen calcium)
	Naproxen (naprosyn)
antipyretic	Advil (ibupropin)
	aspirin
	Tylenol (acetaminophen)
antitussive	codeine (codeine phosphate)
bronchodilator	Alupent (metaproterenol sulfate)
	Brethine (terbutaline sulfate)
	Isuprel (isoproterenol HCl)
	Theolair (theophylline)
cardiotonic	Lanoxin

Type/Usage	Example
contraceptive	Enovid-E 21 (estrogen with progestogen)
	Ortho-Novum 10/11-21 (estrogen with progestogen)
decongestant	Neosynephrine (phenylephrine HCl)
	Sudafed (pseudoephedrine HCl)
diuretic	Diuril (chlorothiazide)
	Hygroton (chlorthalidone)
	Lasix (furosemide)
emetic	Ipecac
estrogen (**ESS** troh jen)	Estrace (estrogen)
	Premarin
expectorant	Robitussin (guaifenesin)
hormone (**HOR** mohn)	testosterone
hypnotic	Seconal (secobarbital)
hypoglycemic	insulin
laxative	Dulcolax (bisacodyl)
muscle relaxant	Robaxin (methocarbamol)
	Valium (diazepam)
narcotic	Demerol (meperidine HCl)
psychedelic	LSD (lysergic acid diethylamide)
purgative	Ex-Lax (phenolphthalein)
sedative	Amytal (amobarbital)
	Butisol (butabarbital sodium)
	Nembutal Sodium (phenobarbital)
	Seconal Sodium (secobarbital sodium)
	Valium (diazepam)
stimulant	Dexedrine (dextroamphetamine sulfate)
tranquilizer	Haldol (haloperidol)
vasodilator	Isordil (isorbide dinitrate)
	Nitrobid (nitroglycerine)
	Nitrostat (nitroglycerine)
vasopressor	Levophed (norepinephrine)
vitamin	Vitamin A
	Vitamin C
	Vitamin D
	Vitamin K

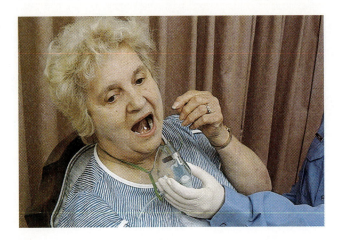

FIGURE 14.1 Place the nitroglycerin tablet under the tongue.

ROUTES AND METHODS OF DRUG ADMINISTRATION

The method by which a drug is introduced into the body is referred to as the route of administration. In general, the routes of administration are as follows:

1. **Oral** (**OR** al): This method includes all drugs that are given by mouth. The advantages are ease of administration and a slow rate of absorption via stomach and intestinal wall. The disadvantages include slowness of absorption and destruction of some chemical compounds by gastric juices. In addition, some medications, such as aspirin, can have a corrosive action on the stomach lining.

2. **Sublingual** (sub **LING** gwal): These are drugs that are held under the tongue and not swallowed. The medication is absorbed by the blood vessels on the underside of the tongue as the saliva dissolves it. The rate of absorption is quicker than the oral route. Nitroglycerin to treat angina or chest pain is administered by this route (see Figure 14.1).

3. **Parenteral** (par **EN** ter al): This is an invasive method of administering drugs since it requires the skin to be punctured by a needle. The needle with syringe attached is introduced either under the skin or into a muscle, vein, or body cavity. See Table 14.5

Table 14.5	*Methods for Parenteral Administration of Drugs*
Method	**Description**
intracavitary (in trah **KAV** ih tair ee)	Injection into a body cavity such as the peritoneal and chest cavity.
intradermal (ID) (in trah **DER** mal)	Very shallow injection just under the top layer of skin. Commonly used in skin testing for allergies.
intramuscular (IM) (in trah **MUSS** kyoo lar)	Injection directly into the muscle of the buttocks or upper arm. Used when there is a large amount of medication or it is irritating (see Figure 14.2).
intrathecal (in trah **THEE** kal)	Injection into the meninges space surrounding the brain and spinal cord.
intravenous (IV) (in trah **VEE** nus)	Injection into the veins. This route can be set up so that there is a continuous administration of medication.
subcutaneous (SC) (sub kyoo **TAY** nee us)	Injection into the skin, usually the upper, outer arm.

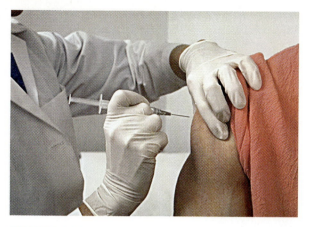
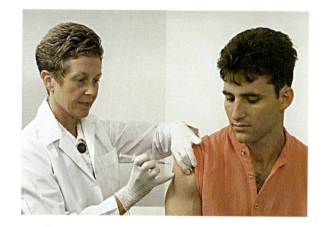

FIGURE 14.2 Intramuscular injections.

for a description of the methods for parenteral administration. See Figure 14.2 for illustrations of an injection into the muscle (intra muscular).

4. **Rectal** (**REK** tal): Introduced directly into the rectal cavity in the form of **suppositories** (suh **POZ** ih tor ees) or solution. Drugs may have to be administered by this route if the patient is unable to take them by mouth due to nausea, vomiting, and surgery.

5. **Inhalation** (in hah **LAY** shun): Includes drugs that are inhaled directly into the nose and mouth. **Aerosol** (**AIR** oh sol) sprays are administered by this route.

6. **Topical** (**TOP** ih kal): Applied directly to the skin or mucous membranes. They are distributed in ointment, cream, or lotion form. Used to treat skin infections and eruptions.

7. **Vaginal** (**VAJ** in al): Tablets and suppositories inserted vaginally used to treat vaginal yeast infections and other irritations.

8. **Eye drops:** Used during eye examinations to dilate the pupil of the eye for better examination of the interior of the eye. Also placed into the eye to control eye pressure in glaucoma.

9. **Ear drops:** Placed directly into the ear canal for the purpose of relieving pain or treating infection.

10. **Buccal** (**BUCK** al): Drugs that are placed under the lip or between the cheek and gum.

In order to be effective, drugs must be administered by a particular route. In some cases, there may be a variety of routes by which a drug can be administered. For instance, the female hormone estrogen can be administered orally in pill form or on a patch applied to the skin.

SIDE EFFECTS OF MEDICATIONS

In addition to the desirable effects for which drugs are prescribed, there are undesirable side effects for almost all medications. In some cases these side effects can be lethal for the patient, so it is important to take them seriously.

Some side effects are simply an individual patient's reaction to medication. In some cases the effects are quite obvious, such as a rash indicating an allergy to a medication. In other cases the side effects are hidden and may require laboratory testing to detect. In general, side effects range from a rash and/or itching, to drowsiness, runny nose, constipation, dizziness, headache, temporary ringing in the ears (tinnitus), blurred vision, loss of appetite, and nausea.

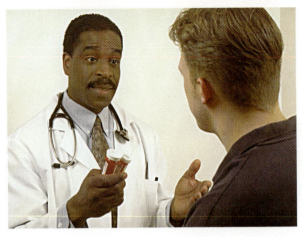

FIGURE 14-3 Provide patient instruction as needed.

Patients should be instructed to call their physician if side effects are persistent or troublesome. The physician may adjust the medication dosage or change to a similar medication with fewer side effects. In all cases, the patients should be instructed not to adjust the dosage themselves or stop taking the medication without consulting the physician (see Figure 14.3).

GENERAL RULES FOR THE ADMINISTRATION OF MEDICATIONS

1. Medications/drugs can be administered to a patient only under the supervision of a licensed physician. To do otherwise is considered *practicing medicine without a license*. The medication order *must be* written on the patient's chart by the physician.

2. The medical assistant acts as the liaison or intermediary between the physician and the patient. Some of the duties include ordering, storing, rotating medications, and checking expiration dates.

3. Remember the *six rights* in administering medications:
   a. Right patient
   b. Right medication
   c. Right dosage
   d. Right route
   e. Right time
   f. Right documentation

4. Keep a record on the patient's chart of all allergies. In many offices these allergies are noted on the front of the chart as well as within the chart.

5. The documentation on the patient's chart must include the following:
   a. Name of the medication
   b. Dosage
   c. Route of administration
   d. Date of administration
   e. Site of administration
   f. Signature of the person administering the medication together with initials designating the status (i.e., CMA, RN)

6. Medications must be checked three times before administration.
   a. When they are removed from the medication cabinet
   b. Before they are poured or drawn up into a syringe
   c. Before the medication is returned to the cabinet

7. Medications cannot be returned to the container once they have been removed. If they are not administered, they must be discarded.

8. All narcotics must be recorded into a record maintained for that purpose. This is referred to as *logging a narcotic*. Every narcotic must be accounted for.

9. Be careful that you administer the medication by the correct route. Methods of administration include the following:
   a. Oral (by mouth)
   b. Sublingual (under the tongue)
   c. Parenteral (by injection)
   d. Rectal (inserted into the anal cavity)
   e. Inhalation (by breathing the medication)
   f. Topical (applied to the skin)
   g. Vaginal (inserted into the vagina)
   h. Eye drops (placed in the eye)
   i. Ear drops (placed in the ear)
   j. Buccal (in the cheek)

10. Medication labels should be clean and readable. If they become soiled, unreadable, or fall off the container, they must be discarded.

11. If you are not familiar with a particular medication, you must look it up in PDR. *Never* violate this rule.

12. Know the side effects for the medication you are administering.

13. Always advise the patient to take the complete number of dosages ordered in the prescription. This is especially important when using antibiotics.

14. Advise the patient to use medication only for the member of the family or person for whom it was prescribed.

How to Read a Prescription

A prescription is not difficult to read once you understand the symbols that are used. Symbols and abbreviations based on Latin and Greek words are used to save time for the physician. For example, the abbreviation *po*, meaning *to be taken by mouth*, comes from the Latin term *per os*, which means *by mouth*.

MED TERM TIP Many abbreviations have multiple meanings, such as *od*, which can mean once a day (od), overdose (OD), or right eye (OD), depending on whether the letters are lowercase or capitalized. Care must be taken when reading abbreviations since some may be written too quickly, making them difficult to decipher. Never create your own abbreviations. Some of the most common abbreviations are listed on pages 476 and 477.

See Figure 14.4 for an example of a prescription. In this example the physician has ordered the medication Estrace, which is a form of the hormone estrogen. The prescription is telling the pharmacist to give 100 (dtd C) tablets, and orders a 1-mg dosage, which is to be taken once a day (1 q am). The instruction to the pharmacist is to refill the prescription three times and not to substitute with another (generic) medication.

```
Melvin A. Brown, M.D.
Chicago, IL 60000


DEA# 123456789      Phone# 123-0000
NAME  (patient name here)   AGE _____
ADDRESS _____        DATE _____
Rx        Estrace 1 mg.
          dtd C
          Sig: 1 q am
[x]  LABEL
REFILL   3   TIMES
[ ] MAY SUBSTITUTE
[x] MAY NOT SUBSTITUTE        (physician signature here) M.D.

_____
```

FIGURE 14.4 Sample prescription.

On some prescriptions the physician will give a *prn* refill order, meaning that the prescription can be refilled as needed. The physician will fill in the name, address, age of the patient, and date. He or she must also sign his or her name at the bottom of the prescription. A blank prescription cannot be handed to a patient.

The physician's instruction to the patient will be placed on the label. The pharmacist will also include instructions about the medication and alert the patient to side effects that may need to be reported to the physician. In addition, any special instructions regarding the medication (i.e., take with meals, do not take along with dairy products) will also be supplied by the pharmacist.

The label on the medication container must always be checked to match the prescription. If in doubt, always question the pharmacist (see Figure 14.5).

FIGURE 14.5 Speak with the pharmacist about any questions you have concerning prescription medications.

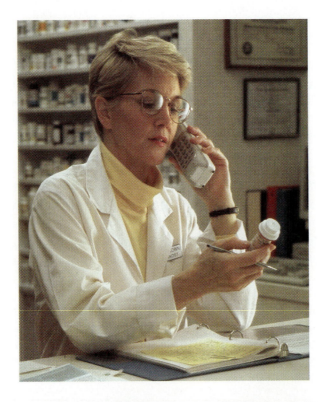

Pharmacy workers prepare and dispense drugs. They also review patients' medications for drug interactions, provide health care workers with information regarding drugs, and educate the public concerning their drugs. Pharmacy workers are found in acute and long-term care facilities, clinics, community-based pharmacies, health departments, and pharmaceutical companies.

Pharmacy Technician

Pharmacy technicians support the pharmacist in dispensing medications under physician's orders. The pharmacy technician's job duties include receiving the drug request made by the physician as well as gathering pertinent information that would affect the dispensing of certain drugs, such as allergies, previous drug interactions, and patient history. Other job responsibilities include typing the labels for the medications and keeping orderly and accurate records in the pharmacy log. Pharmacy technicians are able to work in a wide variety of settings including acute and long-term care facilities, clinics, pharmacies, and pharmaceutical companies. To become a pharmacy technician, a one-to-two year junior college program is required along with two-to-twelve months of on-the-job training. Some states award a pharmacy technician certification upon the passage of a certification examination. For more information regarding a career as a pharmacy technician, visit the American Association of Colleges of Pharmacy's web site at www.aacp.org.

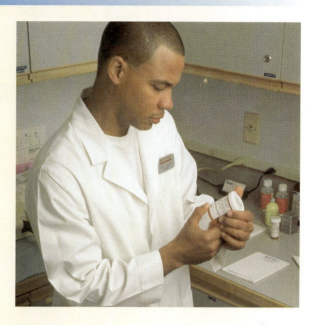

Pharmacist (RPh)

- **Fills prescriptions as written by physicians, dentists, and other doctors**
- **Graduates from an accredited five-year pharmacy program**
- **Licensed by the state of employment**

Pharmacy Technician

- **Works under the supervision of a pharmacist**
- **Completes a one-to-two year junior college program and receives two-to-twelve months on-the-job training**
- **Some states offer certification**

Abbreviations Relating to Pharmacology

@	at		gtt	drop
3x	three times		H	hour/hypodermic
ā	before		HRT	hormone replacement therapy
aa	of each		hs	hour of sleep
ac	before meals		i	one
AD	right ear		ID	intradermal
ad lib	as desired		ii	two
alt dieb	alternate days		iii	three
alt hor	alternate hours		IM	intramuscular
alt noc	alternate nights		inj	injection
am, AM	morning		IU	international unit
amt	amount		IV	intravenous
ante	before		K	potassium
aq	aqueous (water)		kg	kilogram
AS	left ear		L	liter
AU	both ears		liq	liquid
bid	twice a day		mcg	microgram
C	100		mEq	milliequivalent
c	with		mg	milligram
cap(s)	capsule(s)		mL	milliliter
cc	cubic centimeter		mm	millimeter
d	day		noc	night
DC, disc	discontinue		noct	night
d/c, DISC	discontinue		non rep	do not repeat
DEA	Drug Enforcement Agency		no sub	no substitute
dil	dilute		NPO	nothing by mouth
disp	dispense		NS	normal saline
dr	dram		NSAID	non-steroidal anti-inflammatory drug
Dx	diagnosis		O	pint
elix	elixir		od	once a day/daily
emul	emulsion		OD	overdose
et	and		OD	right eye
ext	extract/external		oint., ung	ointment
FDA	Federal Drug Administration		om	every morning
Fe	iron		OS	left eye
fl	fluid		OTC	over the counter
gal	gallon		OU	each eye
GM, gm	gram		oz	ounce
gr	grain		p	after
gt	drop		pc	after meals

PDR	*Physicians Desk Reference*		**sol**	solution
per	with		**ss**	one-half
PM	evening		**stat**	at once/immediately
PO	phone order		**Subc, SubQ**	subcutaneous
po	by mouth		**subling**	sublingual
prn	as needed		**suppos, supp.**	suppository
pt	pint		**susp**	suspension
pulv	powder		**syr**	syrup
q	every		**T, tbsp**	tablespoon
qam	every morning		**tab**	tablet
qd	once a day/every day		**tid**	three times a day
qh	every hour		**tinc/tr**	tincture
qhs	every night		**TO**	telephone order
qid	four times a day		**top**	apply topically
qod	every other day		**t, tsp**	teaspoon
qs	quantity sufficient		**u**	unit
Rx	take		**ung**	ointment
s	without		**UT**	under the tongue
SC	subcutaneous		**ut dict, UD**	as directed
Sig	label as follows/directions		**VO**	verbal order
sl	under the tongue		**wt**	weight
SOB	shortness of breath		**x4**	four times

KEY TERMS

- addiction (ah **DICK** shun)
- aerosol (**AIR** oh sol)
- analgesic (an al **JEE** zik)
- anaphylactic shock (an ah fih **LAK** tik)
- anesthetic (an ess **THET** ik)
- antacid (ant **ASS** id)
- antianxiety (an tih ang **ZIGH** ah tee)
- antiarrhythmic (an tih ah **RITH** mik)
- antibiotic (an tih bye **OT** ik)
- anticholinergic (an tih koh lin **ER** jik)
- anticoagulant (an tih koh **AG** yoo lant)
- anticonvulsant (an tih kon **VULL** sant)
- antidepressant (an tih dee **PRESS** ant)

- antidiabetic (an tih dye ah **BET** ik)
- antidiarrheal (an tih dye ah **REE** al)
- antidote (**AN** tih doht)
- antiemetic (an tih ee **MET** ik)
- antihistamine (an tih **HISS** tah meen)
- antihypertensive (an tih high per **TEN** siv)
- anti-inflammatory (an tih in **FLAM** ah tor ee)
- antipyretic (an tih pye **RET** ik)
- antitussive (an tih **TUSS** iv)
- astringent (ah **STRIN** jent)
- brand name
- broad spectrum
- bronchodilator (brong koh **DYE** lay tor)

- buccal (**BUCK** al)
- cardiotonic (kar dee oh **TON** ik)
- cathartic (kah **THAR** tik)
- chemical name (**KEM** ih cal)
- chemotherapy (kee moh **THAIR** ah pee)
- contraceptive (con trah **SEP** tiv)
- contraindication (kon trah in dih **KAY** shun)
- Controlled Substance Act of 1970
- controlled substances
- cumulative action
- decongestant (dee kon **JESS** tant)
- dilute
- diuretic (dye yoor **RET** ik)
- Drug Enforcement Agency (DEA)
- drug tolerance (**TAHL** er ans)
- ear drops
- emetic (ee **MET** ik)
- estrogen (**ESS** troh jen)
- expectorant (ek **SPEK** toh rant)
- eye drops
- Federal Food and Drug Administration (FDA)
- Federal Food, Drug, and Cosmetic Act of 1938
- generic name
- habituation (hah bich yoo **AY** shun)
- hemostatic (hee moh **STAH** tik)
- hormone (**HOR** mohn)
- *Hospital Formulary* (**FORM** yoo lair ee)
- hypnotic (hip **NOT** ik)
- hypoglycemic (high poh glye **SEE** mik)
- idiosyncrasy (id ee oh **SIN** krah see)
- immunosuppressive (im yoo noh suh **PRESS** iv)
- inhalation (in hah **LAY** shun)
- intracavitary (in trah **KAV** ih tair ee)
- intradermal (ID) (in trah **DER** mal)
- intramuscular (IM) (in trah **MUSS** kyoo lar)
- intrathecal (in trah **THEE** kal)
- intravenous (IV) (in trah **VEE** nus)
- laxative (**LACK** sah tiv)
- miotic (my **OT** ik)

- muscle relaxant
- mydriatic (mid ree **AT** ik)
- narcotic (nar **KOT** ik)
- nonprescription drug
- nonproprietary name
- oral (**OR** al)
- over-the-counter (OTC)
- parenteral (par **EN** ter al)
- pharmaceutical (far mih **SOO** tih kal)
- pharmacist (**FAR** mah sist)
- pharmacology (far mah **KALL** oh jee)
- *Physician's Desk Reference* (PDR)
- placebo (plah **SEE** boh)
- prescription (prih **SKRIP** shun)
- prescription drug (prih **SKRIP** shun)
- prophylaxis (proh fih **LAK** sis)
- proprietary name (proh **PRYE** ah tair ee)
- psychedelic (sigh kah **DELL** ik)
- purgative (**PUR** gah tiv)
- rectal (**REK** tal)
- sedative (**SED** ah tiv)
- side effect
- stimulant (**STIM** yoo lant)
- subcutaneous (SC) (sub kyoo **TAY** nee us)
- sublingual (sub **LING** gwal)
- suppositories (suh **POZ** ih tor ees)
- tolerance (**TAHL** er ans)
- topical (**TOP** ih kal)
- toxicity (tok **SISS** ih tee)
- trade name
- tranquilizer (**TRANG** kwih ligh zer)
- unit dose
- *United States Pharmacopeia-National Formulary (USP-NF)*
- vaccine (**VAK** seen)
- vaginal (**VAJ** in al)
- vasodilator (vas oh **DYE** lay tor)
- vasopressor (vas oh **PRESS** or)
- vitamin (**VIGH** tah min)

Practice Exercises

A. COMPLETE THE FOLLOWING STATEMENTS:

1. The governmental agency that enforces drug sales and distribution is the _____ .

2. A person specializing in the dispensing of medications is a _____ .

3. The legal name for a drug is the _____ name.

4. The commercial name for a drug is the _____ name.

5. What does the chemical name represent? _____

6. List precautions to observe when administering medications.

   a. _____

   b. _____

   c. _____

   d. _____

   e. _____

   f. _____

   g. _____

   h. _____

   i. _____

7. A reference book that is one of the most frequently used sources of information when administering medications in the physician's office is the _____ .

8. What federal law controls the use of drugs causing dependency?

   _____

9. What are the *six rights* in medication administration?

   a. _____

   b. _____

   c. _____

   d. _____

   e. _____

   f. _____

10. How many times must a drug be checked before it is administered? _____ State when these checks take place.

    a. _____

    b. _____

    c. _____

11. What procedure do you follow if a patient has a drug allergy?

    _____

    _____

12. State when a medical assistant may administer a medication.

    _____

13. Define "logging a narcotic."

    _____

14. List the information that must be charted when administering a medication.

    a. _____

    b. _____

    c. _____

    d. _____

    e. _____

    f. _____

B. USE THE FOLLOWING COMBINING FORMS TO CREATE A MEDICAL TERM RELATING TO PHARMACOLOGY.

Combining Form	Meaning	Term
1. cutane/o	under the skin	_____
2. alges/o	sensitive to pain	_____
3. ven/o	into the vein	_____
4. pharmac/o	study of drugs	_____
5. narc/o	producing a stupor	_____
6. hypn/o	producing sleep	_____
7. aer/o	combine air in solution	_____
8. chem/o	drug therapy	_____
9. vas/o	dilates vessels	_____
10. toxic/o	study of poisons	_____

C. EXPLAIN THE FUNCTIONS OF THE FOLLOWING TYPES OF MEDICATION.

1. diuretic _____
2. bronchodilator _____
3. antiemetic _____
4. hypnotic _____
5. sedative _____
6. anti-inflammatory agent _____
7. vasodilator _____
8. anticonvulsive _____
9. anesthetic _____
10. analgesic _____
11. antacid _____
12. antibiotic _____
13. anticoagulant _____
14. antihistamine _____

D. NAME THE ROUTE OF DRUG ADMINISTRATION FOR THE FOLLOWING DESCRIPTIONS.

1. under the tongue _____
2. into the anus or rectum _____
3. applied to the skin _____
4. injected under the first layer of skin _____
5. injected into a muscle _____
6. injected into the skin _____
7. by mouth _____

E. DEFINE THE FOLLOWING TERMS IN THE SPACE PROVIDED.

1. idiosyncrasy _____
2. parenteral _____
3. placebo _____
4. toxicity _____
5. side effect _____
6. unit dose _____
7. habituation _____
8. antidote _____
9. contraindication _____
10. prophylaxis _____

F. MATCH THE TERMS IN COLUMN A WITH THE DEFINITIONS IN COLUMN B.

A	B
1. _____ antacid	a. lowers blood glucose level
2. _____ diuretic	b. produces sleep or hypnosis
3. _____ hypoglycemic	c. dilates pupils of eye
4. _____ anesthetic	d. destroys microorganisms
5. _____ hypnotic	e. strengthens heart muscle
6. _____ antianxiety	f. neutralizes acid
7. _____ mydriatic	g. produces vomiting
8. _____ emetic	h. increases urine excretion
9. _____ cardiogenic	i. produces lack of feeling
10. _____ antibiotic	j. relieves tension

G. WHAT ARE THE FOLLOWING DRUGS/MEDICATIONS USED FOR?

1. Milk of Magnesia _____
2. Insulin _____
3. Amoxil _____
4. Coumadin _____
5. Novocaine _____
6. Lopressor _____
7. Codeine _____
8. Demerol _____
9. Valium _____
10. Levophed _____
11. Lanoxin _____
12. Premarin _____
13. Lasix _____
14. Ortho-Novum _____
15. Nitrostat _____

H. GIVE THE MEANING OF THE FOLLOWING ABBREVIATIONS IN THE SPACE PROVIDED.

1. gr _____
2. bid _____
3. tid _____
4. ad lib _____
5. prn _____
6. ante _____
7. ext _____
8. gt _____
9. Sig _____
10. stat _____
11. tinc _____
12. qd _____
13. noc _____
14. NPO _____
15. hs _____
16. ung _____
17. mm _____
18. gtt _____
19. C _____
20. d/c _____

I. MATCH THE ABBREVIATIONS IN COLUMN A WITH THE DEFINITIONS IN COLUMN B.

	A		B
1. _____	SOB	a.	dispense
2. _____	OTC	b.	before meals
3. _____	emul	c.	right eye
4. _____	disp	d.	apply topically
5. _____	ac	e.	shortness of breath
6. _____	Fe	f.	under the tongue
7. _____	OU	g.	over the counter
8. _____	OD	h.	iron
9. _____	top	i.	each eye
10. _____	UT	j.	emulsion

J. WRITE OUT THE FOLLOWING PRESCRIPTION INSTRUCTIONS IN THE SPACE PROVIDED.

1. Pravachol, 20 mg., Sig. i qd @ noc, 30, refill 3x, no sub.

   _____
   _____

2. Lanoxin 0.125 mg., Sig. iii stat, then ii q AM, C, refills prn.

   _____
   _____

3. Synthroid 0.075 mg., Sig. i qd, C, refill x4.

   _____
   _____

4. Norvasc 5 mg., i q am, 60, refillable.

   _____
   _____

Getting Connected

Multimedia Extension Activities

CD-ROM

Use the CD-ROM enclosed with your textbook to gain additional reinforcement through interactive word building exercises, spelling games, labeling activities, and additional quizzes.

www.prenhall.com/fremgen

Use the above address to access the free, interactive Companion Website created for this textbook. Get hints, instant feedback, and textbook references to chapter-related multiple choice questions, and labeling and matching exercises. In addition, you will find an audio glossary, case studies, Internet exploration exercises, flashcards, and a comprehensive exam.

Answers

PRACTICE EXERCISES

A. 1. Federal Food and Drug Administration (FDA)   2. pharmacist   3. generic   4. brand   5. the chemical formula
6. a. must be administered under supervision of licensed physician   b. *six rights*   c. note all allergies on the chart
d. check medication three times before administration   e. do not return medication to container once it has been
removed   f. record all narcotics in a log   g. keep labels clear and clean   h. look up all unfamiliar medications   i. know
the side effects for all medications   7. *Physician's Desk Reference* (PDR)   8. Controlled Substance Act of 1970   9. a. right
patient   b. right medication   c. right dosage   d. right route   e. right time   f. right documentation   10. three times
a. when medication is removed from cabinet   b. before being poured or drawn into syringe   c. before medication is
returned to cabinet   11. note it on the front of the chart and inside the chart   12. only under the direct supervision of a
physician   13. recording all narcotics on the narcotic record (log)   14. a. name of medication   b. dosage   c. route of
administration   d. date of administration   e. site of administration   f. signature of person administering the medication
and initials designating status

B. 1. subcutaneous   2. analgesic   3. intravenous   4. pharmacology   5. narcotic   6. hypnotic   7. aerosol
8. chemotherapy   9. vasodilator   10. toxicology

C. 1. increases the excretion of urine   2. dilates (opens) the bronchi   3. controls nausea and vomiting
4. produces sleep or hypnosis   5. produces relaxation   6. reduces or counteracts inflammation   7. relaxes blood
vessels to lower blood pressure   8. prevents or relieves convulsions   9. produces a lack of feeling   10. relieves
pain   11. neutralizes acid   12. destroys or prohibits the growth of microorganisms   13. prevents or delays blood
clotting   14. acts to control allergic reactions

D. 1. sublingual   2. rectal   3. topical   4. intradermal   5. intramuscular   6. subcutaneous   7. oral

E. 1. unusual or abnormal response to a drug   2. administration of a drug through a needle and syringe under the
skin, or into a muscle, vein, or body cavity.   3. harmless substance to satisfy patient's desire for medication
4. extent to which a substance is poisonous.   5. response to drug other than the expected response   6. prepackaged
and prelabeled method of medication distribution   7. emotional dependence on a drug   8. substance that neutralizes
poisons   9. condition under which a particular drug should not be used   10. prevention of disease

F. 1. f   2. h   3. a   4. i   5. b   6. j   7. c   8. g   9. e   10. d

G. 1. antacid   2. diabetes   3. infection   4. anticoagulant (prevent clotting)   5. anesthetic   6. antihypertensive
7. antitussive (prevent cough)   8. pain relief; analgesic   9. relaxant   10. vasopressor   11. cardiotonic
12. estrogen (hormone)   13. diuretic   14. hormone/contraception   15. vasodilator

H. 1. grain   2. two times a day   3. three times a day   4. as desired   5. as needed   6. before   7. extract
8. drop   9. label as follows/directions   10. immediately   11. tincture   12. every day   13. night   14. nothing by
mouth   15. hour of sleep   16. ointment   17. millimeter   18. drop   19. 100   20. discontinue

I. 1. e   2. g   3. j   4. a   5. b   6. h   7. i   8. c   9. d   10. f

J. 1. Pravachol, 20 milligrams each, take one every day at nighttime, supply with 30 tablets, refill three times with no
substitutions.   2. Lanoxin, 0.125 milligram each, take three pills now and then 2 pills every morning, supply with 100 pills
and may refill as needed.   3. Synthroid, 0.075 milligram each, take one every day, supply with 100 pills and may refill
four times.   4. Norvasc, 5—100 milligram dose each, take 1 every morning, supply with 60 pills and may refill.

Chapter 15

SPECIAL TOPICS

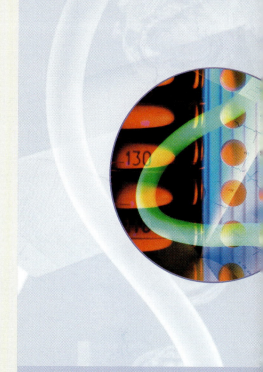

Overview

There are many specialized areas within medicine and each has specialized vocabularies relating to that field. This chapter presents medical terminology from eight of these fields:

1. Emergency medicine
2. Gerontology
3. Radiology
4. Oncology
5. Rehabilitation services
6. Surgery
7. Mental health
8. Pediatrics

EMERGENCY MEDICINE

Emergency medicine is the branch of medicine that specializes in emergency care of the acutely ill and injured. It has been determined that if injured patients are treated immediately, even before transport to a hospital, they have a much better chance of surviving their injuries. To be certified in emergency medicine, a physician has to complete a residency and an examination.

Emergency medical technicians (**EMTs**) are trained professionals who can handle a variety of emergencies, including cardiac arrest, heart attack, and trauma. In many cities EMTs communicate directly with the hospital from the accident site and are able to transmit electrocardiograms (ECGs) to the hospital for interpretation by a physician (see Figure 15.1).

The emergency medical services (EMS) system was established in the 1960s to provide rescue operations, ambulance transportation, emergency department services, and public education for the acutely ill or injured. In addition, a centralized emergency telephone number (911) was established for public access.

Emergency situations can develop relating to every system of the body. Some of the most frequent are those that involve accidents and childbirth.

FIGURE 15.1 EMS personnel with patient at hospital emergency center.

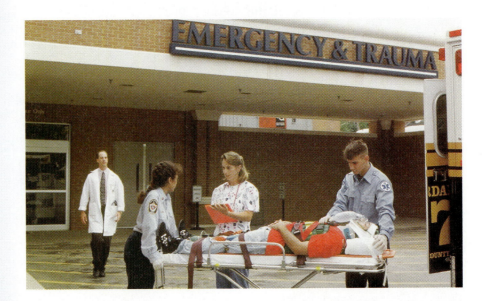

Vocabulary Relating to Emergency Medicine

airway	Includes the mouth, pharynx, larynx, trachea, bronchi, and lungs. These must remain patent (open) for respiration to take place.
artificial ventilation	Forcing air or oxygen into the lungs when breathing has stopped or is inadequate.
basic life support	Combination of cardiopulmonary resuscitation (CPR) and emergency cardiac care to maintain respiration and circulation of a victim until transported to a medical facility.
blood pressure	Measurement of the pressure exerted by the blood on the wall of large blood vessels.
cardiopulmonary resuscitation (CPR) (car dee oh PULL mon air ee ree suss ih TAY shun)	Method for artificially supplying blood to the brain and maintaining oxygen flow to the lungs by administering compressions over the heart and forcing air into the mouth at set intervals.
coronary care unit (CCU)	Specialized hospital unit equipped to care for and monitor patients who have suffered a heart attack.
crash cart	Emergency cart on wheels that contains medications and equipment needed in emergency situations. The cart can be moved to the patient's bedside or from one office to another.
crepitation (crep ih TAY shun)	Sound of broken bones rubbing together.
defibrillator (dee FIB rih lay tor)	Equipment that sends an electrical charge through a person's body in an attempt to enable the heart to start beating in a normal manner.
emergency medical technician (EMT)	Person trained in techniques of administering emergency care.
emergency room	Area of a hospital or a free-standing unit that is prepared to care for the severely ill and injured.
first aid	Providing emergency care to the injured or disabled before the physician arrives or the patient can be transported to a hospital.
Heimlich maneuver (HYME lik)	Technique for removing a foreign body or food from the trachea or pharynx when it is choking a person. The maneuver, named after Harry Heimlich, an American thoracic surgeon, consists of applying pressure just under the diaphragm to pop the obstruction out.
intensive care unit (ICU)	Specialized hospital unit equipped to care for and monitor patients who have suffered severe injuries and illnesses and require constant supervision and lifesaving measures (see Figure 15.2).
intubation (in too BAY shun)	Insertion of a thin, flexible tube into a hollow organ such as the trachea.
residency	Time spent by a physician in training after the internship.
stabilize	Maintaining a victim's condition without allowing it to worsen. In most cases the vital signs remain unchanged when a patient is stabilized.
tourniquet (TOOR nih ket)	Device to restrict blood flow to and from an extremity. Used carefully when hemorrhage is present to prevent further bleeding.
trauma (TRAW mah)	Physical wound or injury caused by an external force or violence.
triage (tree AHZH)	Quick screening and classification of sick, wounded, or injured persons during a disaster or war. Priorities are determined for the efficient use of medical personnel, equipment, and facilities.
vital signs (VS)	Respiration, pulse, temperature, skin color, blood pressure, and reaction of pupils. These are signs of the condition of body functions.

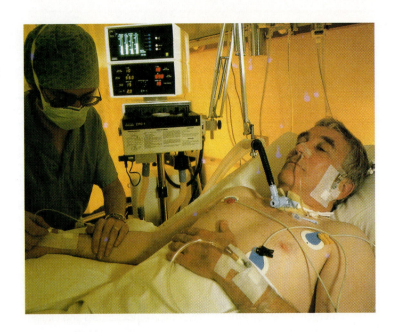

FIGURE 15.2 Nurse starting an IV on patient in intensive care unit (ICU). (Malcolm Fielding, The BOC Group PLC/Science Photo Library/Photo Researchers, Inc.)

Pathology Relating to Emergency Medicine

abdominal pain (ab DOM ih nal)	In an emergency situation this pain is usually acute. Requires immediate evaluation since there may be a need for surgery.
acute myocardial infarction (my oh CAR dee al in FARC shun) (AMI)	Occurs when a portion of the heart muscle dies due to the partial or complete closure of the coronary arteries. Also called a *heart attack*.
allergic reaction	Can be life threatening if there is a severe drop in blood pressure and swelling of the airway as a result of an allergy.
amputation (am pew TAY shun)	Surgical or traumatic removal of a limb or body part.
anaphylactic (an ah fih LAK tik) **shock**	Allergic reaction that can become life-threatening when the airway swells due to tissue inflammation and a drop in blood pressure.
apnea (AP nee ah)	Temporary stoppage of breathing.
asphyxia (as FIK see ah)	Condition caused by the insufficient intake of oxygen (see Figure 15.3).
asthmatic (az MAT ik) **attack**	Attack of difficulty in breathing (dyspnea) and wheezing due to bronchial constriction.
bite or sting	Puncture wound of the skin made by humans, animals, insects, ticks, bees, hornets, or wasps. There is a danger of infection. An emergency situation arises if the person is allergic to venom in stings.
burn	A full-thickness burn exists when all the layers are burned; also called a *third-degree burn*. A partial thickness burn exists when the first layer of skin, the epidermis, is burned, and the second layer of skin, dermis, is damaged; also called a *second-degree burn*.

cardiac (CAR dee ak) arrest	When the heart stops beating and circulation ceases.
cerebrovascular accident (ser eh broh VASS kyoo lar AK sih dent) (CVA)	Caused by a blockage or rupture of a blood vessel in the brain. Also referred to as a *stroke*.
choking	Obstruction within the respiratory passage that interferes with breathing and circulation. (See Figure 15.4 for the universal sign for choking.)
convulsion (kon VULL shun)	Sudden, violent, uncontrolled twitching and contraction of muscles. There are many causes of convulsions, ranging from high fevers to epilepsy.
diabetic (dye ah BET ik) coma	Abnormal deep stupor occurring as a result of lack of insulin. The person will have a sweet breath, from acidosis.
drowning	Asphyxiation due to immersion in water or a liquid.
epiglottitis (ep ih glot TYE tis)	Swelling of the epiglottis, causing an airway obstruction. A potentially life-threatening condition that can be caused by bacterial infection.
epilepsy (EP ih lep see)	Medical condition that can cause convulsions (seizures).
epistaxis (ep ih STAKS sis)	Also called *nosebleed*.
foreign bodies	Slivers, cinders, dirt, or small objects that lodge in the eyes, ears, nose, skin, or internally.
fracture	Break in a bone.
hemorrhage (HEM eh rij)	Abnormal, severe discharge of blood.
insulin (IN soo lin) reaction	Reaction that occurs when a diabetic patient receives too much insulin. Glucose in the form of juice or candy is administered if the patient is conscious.
near-drowning	When a person survives being underwater for a period of time that could have resulted in drowning. The person may require resuscitation to bring back a heartbeat or pulse.
open wounds	A wound that has penetrated the skin. Deep wounds due to abrasion, incision, laceration, and puncture may require emergency care and suturing.
pneumothorax (new moh THOH raks)	Collection of air or gas in the pleural cavity that can result in the collapse of a lung.
poisoning	Ingestion of harmful or toxic material into the body.
respiratory (RES pih rah tor ee) failure	Failure of the respiratory system to maintain adequate gas exchange in the lungs to sustain life.
shock	Situation in which not enough blood is flowing to the heart for normal function. The symptoms of shock are paleness, staring eyes, dilated pupils, weak and rapid pulse, increased shallow respirations, and decreased blood pressure.
sucking chest wound	Open wound in the chest that draws outside air into the chest cavity.
syncope (SIN koh pee)	Temporary loss of consciousness due to a lack of blood flow to the brain. Also called *fainting*.

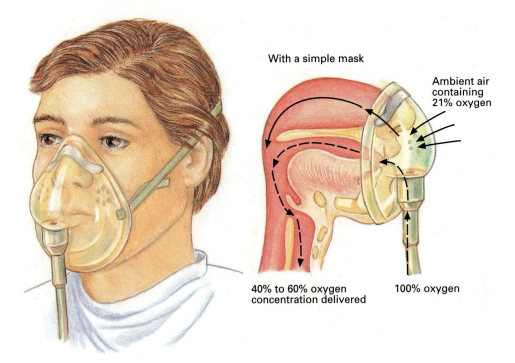

With a simple mask

Ambient air containing 21% oxygen

40% to 60% oxygen concentration delivered

100% oxygen

FIGURE 15.3   Emergency personnel administering oxygen to patient.

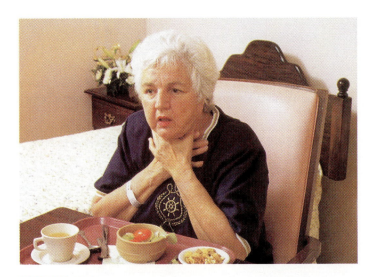

FIGURE 15.4   Woman demonstrating universal sign for choking.

Emergency Medical Service

Emergency medical services provide basic and advanced pre-hospital emergency care for traumatic or medical emergencies. They evaluate the patient's condition, relay the information to an emergency physician, initiate the medical care ordered by the physician, and stabilize and transport the patient to a hospital. Emergency medical services work out of rescue, police, and fire departments; hospital emergency rooms; and private ambulance services.

Emergency Medical Technician—Paramedic (EMT-P)

- Trained in advanced emergency medical techniques
- Completes an approved paramedic program
- Completes six months of field experience
- Passes a national certification examination

Emergency Medical Technician (EMT)

- Trained in basic life support and patient transportation
- Completes an approved emergency medical technician basic program
- Passes a national certification examination

Abbreviations Relating to Emergency Medicine

Ab	abortion		ER	emergency room
ACLS	advanced cardiac life support		fx	fracture
AMI	acute myocardial infarction		GSW	gunshot wound
ARDS	adult respiratory distress syndrome		IC	intracardiac
CCU	cardiac care unit		ICU	intensive care unit
c/o	complains of		LAC	laceration
COPD	chronic obstructive pulmonary disease		MI	myocardial infarction
CP	chest pain		MICU	mobile intensive care unit
CPR	cardiopulmonary resuscitation		MVA	motor vehicle accident
CVA	cerebrovascular accident		NAD	no apparent distress
CVP	central venous pressure		NICU	neonatal intensive care
D/C	discontinue		OD	overdose (also means right eye)
DOA	dead on arrival		OR	operating room
DOE	dyspnea on exertion		SICU	surgical intensive care unit
DT'S	delerium tremens		SIDS	sudden infant death syndrome
ECG, EKG	electrocardiogram		SOB	shortness of breath
EMS	emergency medical services system		STAT	immediately
EMT	emergency medical technician		VS	vital signs
EMT-P	paramedic			

Practice Exercises

A. COMPLETE THE FOLLOWING STATEMENTS.

1. The system established to provide rescue operations for people who are acutely ill or injured is called the _____ .

2. The medical professional who is trained to handle emergencies in the field under the supervision of a physician is a(n) _____ .

3. Another term for stroke is _____ .

4. Another term for heart attack is _____ .

5. Included under the term vital signs are _____ , _____ , _____ , _____ , and _____ .

6. A medical condition that causes convulsions or seizures is _____ .

7. The term for nosebleed is _____ .

8. A severe allergic reaction to food or drugs that results in a medical emergency is called _____ .

B. IDENTIFY THE FOLLOWING ABBREVIATIONS.

1. MI _____
2. NICU _____
3. CP _____
4. STAT _____
5. SOB _____
6. c/o _____
7. CVA _____
8. GSW _____
9. fx _____
10. SICU _____
11. CCU _____
12. DT's _____
13. SIDS _____

GERONTOLOGY

Gerontology (jer on **TALL** oh jee) is the scientific study of the effects of aging and age-related diseases. A gerontologist is a physician who has received special training in the care of the elderly.

In general, the same conditions that affect a younger population also affect the elderly. With some medical problems, such as fractures, the elderly require a longer healing time since some of the elasticity of the joints and muscles has diminished. However, there are a few disorders, such as Alzheimer's disease, that strike people over 50.

One means of assessing a person's ability to continue to care for himself or herself is to assess the **activities of daily living (ADL).** These are the normal functions that everyone performs during a normal day in order to live. Six items are assessed, based on a person's ability to do the tasks unaided. These are eating, toileting, dressing, bathing, mobility, and continence of bowels and urine (see Figure 15.5).

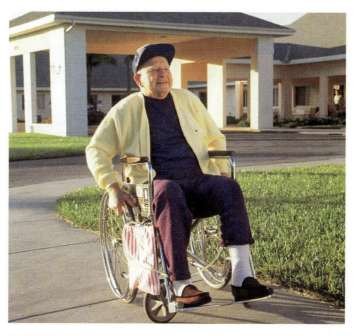

FIGURE 15.5 Maintaining mobility.

Vocabulary Relating to Gerontology

adaptive equipment	Equipment used by the elderly that has been structured to aid them in mobility, eating, and managing the other activities of daily living. This equipment includes special walkers and spoons for the stroke patient (see Figures 15.6 and 15.7).
aging	Gradual progressive changes that relate to the passage of time. There is no standard by which everyone ages.
ambulatory (AM byoo lah toh ree)	Able to walk.
anxiety (ang ZY eh tee)	A feeling of apprehension or worry.
aphasia (ah FAY zee ah)	Inability to communicate through speech. Often an aftereffect of a stroke (CVA).
assisted living	Living arrangement in which the person may have his or her own apartment space but will join other residents for meals and other activities.
discharge planning	Preparation made by the caregivers and family of a patient upon discharge from a hospital or nursing home.
elder abuse	Mistreatment of the elderly.
long-term care facility	Living environment for people who cannot take care of all their activities of daily living and need supervision and meals but who do not require hospitalization (see Figure 15.8).
nursing home	Type of long-term care facility.
restorative care	Care focused on assisting the individual to attain the highest level of physical and mental ability possible.
senile (SEE nyl)	Mental weakness associated with old age in some people.

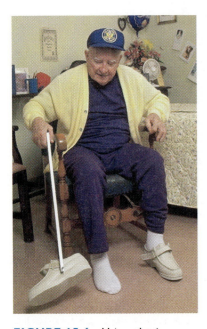

FIGURE 15.6 Using adaptive equipment to assist in putting on shoes.

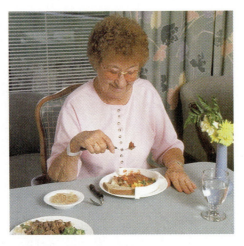

FIGURE 15.7 Nursing home resident dining with adaptive edge on plate.

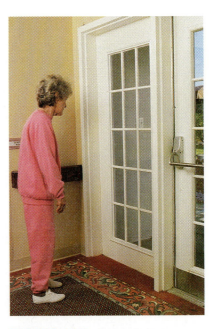

FIGURE 15.8 Patient in long-term facility.

Pathology Relating to Gerontology

acute illness	Illness that begins suddenly and does not last long.
Alzheimer's disease (ALTS high merz dih ZEEZ)	Chronic, organic, mental disorder named after Alois Alzheimer, a German neurologist. A progressive disease that can eventually result in irreversible memory loss, speech and walking disturbances, and disorientation.
arteriosclerosis (ar tee ree oh skleh ROH sis)	Thickening, hardening, and narrowing of the arterial walls. Can lead to heart conditions, elevated blood pressure, and senility.
arthritis (ar THRY tis)	Inflammation of a joint that is usually accompanied by pain and swelling. A chronic disease.
chronic disease (KRON ik dih ZEEZ)	Illness that comes on slowly and can be long-lasting.
osteoarthritis (oss tee oh ar THRY tis)	Inflammation of the bones and joints.
terminal illness	Illness from which one will not recover.

Special Equipment for the Infirm Elderly

bedside commode	Chairlike portable toilet that can be placed at the side of the bed for people who have difficulty walking.
Foley catheter (FOH lee CATH eh ter)	Indwelling, thin, sterile tubing placed into the urinary bladder to withdraw urine continuously. Developed by Frederic Foley, an American urologist.
fracture pan	Small bedpan with a flat edge that will go under the person who is bedridden.
gastrostomy (gas TROSS toh mee) tube	Thin tubing placed into the stomach for liquid feedings.
geriatric (jer ee AT rik) chair (geri-chair)	Wheeled chair that reclines and has a tray for meals. Provides security for a confused person since he or she is unable to get up from the chair without assistance.
quad cane	Walking cane with four prongs at the base to provide steady support.
shower chair	Waterproof chair that is placed inside the shower stall so that a weak person may sit during showering.
urinal (YOO rih nal)	Urine container for males.
walker	Aluminum device with or without wheels to provide support for someone who is having difficulty walking.

Practice Exercises

C. COMPLETE THE FOLLOWING STATEMENTS:

1. A _____ is an illness that comes on slowly and can be long-lasting.

2. _____ focuses on assisting the individual to attain the highest level of physical and mental ability possible.

3. Another term for a long-term care facility is _____ .

4. Another term for being able to walk is to _____ .

5. The term for an illness from which one will not recover is _____ .

D. ANSWER THE FOLLOWING QUESTIONS:

1. What does the abbreviation ADL stand for? _____

   _____

2. List the six items that are evaluated during an ADL assessment. _____

   _____

3. List and briefly describe at least five pathological conditions of particular importance in the older population.

   _____

E. MATCH THE FOLLOWING TYPES OF EQUIPMENT TO THEIR DEFINITION:

A	B
1. _____ fracture pan	a. urine container for males
2. _____ walker	b. wheeled chair that reclines and has a tray for meals
3. _____ urinal	c. small bedpan with a flat edge
4. _____ shower chair	d. aluminum device to provide support for walking
5. _____ geriatric chair	e. waterproof chair

RADIOLOGY

COMBINING FORMS RELATING TO RADIOLOGY

fluor/o	fluorescence, luminous	**radi/o**	X-ray
is/o	same	**roentgen/o**	X-ray
leth/o	death		

SUFFIXES RELATING TO RADIOLOGY

Suffix	Meaning	Example
-gram	record	myelogram
-graphy	recording	mammography
-opaque	nontransparent	radiopaque

Radiology (ray dee **ALL** oh jee) is the branch of medicine that uses radioactive substances such as X-rays, isotopes, and radiation to prevent, diagnose, and treat diseases. An older term for radiology is *roentgenology,* named after Wilhelm Roentgen, a German physicist, who discovered roentgen rays in 1895. This discovery revolutionized the diagnosis of disease. Specially trained technologists assist the physician with positioning the patients and taking the X-ray films. Common X-ray positions are as follows:

1. **AP view:** Stands for anteroposterior; positioning the patient so that the X-rays pass through the body from the anterior side to the posterior side.
2. **PA view:** Stands for posteroanterior; positioning the patient so that the X-rays pass through the body from the posterior side to the anterior side.
3. **Lateral view:** Positioning the patient so that the side of the body faces the X-ray machine.
4. **Oblique** (oh **BLEEK**) **view:** Positioning the patient so that the X-rays pass through the body on an angle.

Vocabulary Relating to Radiology

barium (Ba) (BAH ree um)	Soft metallic element from the earth used as a radiopaque X-ray dye.
cyclotron (SIGH kloh tron)	Equipment consisting of a particle accelerator in which the particles are rotated between magnets.
diagnostic (dye ag NOS tik)	Procedure to determine the cause and nature of a person's illness.
electron (ee LEK tron)	Minute particle with a negative electrical charge that is emitted from radioactive substances. These are called *rays.*
film	Thin sheet of cellulose material coated with a light-sensitive substance that is used in taking photographs. There is a special photographic film that is sensitive to X-rays.
film badge	Badge containing film that is sensitive to X-rays. This is worn by all personnel in radiology to measure the amount of X-rays to which they are exposed.
Geiger (GYE ger) counter	Instrument used for detecting radiation.

(continued)

radiation therapy (ray dee AY shun THAIR ah pee)	Use of X-rays to treat disease, especially cancer.
radioactive (ray dee oh AK tiv)	Substance capable of emitting or sending out radiant energy.
radiography (ray dee OG rah fee)	Making of X-ray pictures.
radioisotope (ray dee oh EYE soh tohp)	Radioactive form of an element.
radiologist (ray dee ALL oh jist)	Physician who practices diagnosis and treatment by using radiant energy. He or she is responsible for interpreting X-ray films.
radiopaque (ray dee oh PAYK)	Structures that are impenetrable to X-rays, appearing as a light area on the radiograph (X-ray).
roentgen (RENT gen)	Unit for describing an exposure dose of radiation.
roentgen (RENT gen) **ray**	The preferred term is *X-ray*.
roentgenologist (rent gen ALL oh jist)	Physician who is skilled in X-ray diagnosis and treatment. The preferred term is *radiologist*.
scan	Recording on a photographic plate the emission of radioactive waves after a substance has been injected into the body.
shield	Protective device used to protect against radiation.
tagging	Attaching a radioactive material to a chemical, and tracing it as it moves through the body.
therapeutic (thair ah PEW tik)	Treating disease by applying specified remedies.
uptake	Absorption of radioactive material and medicines into an organ or tissue.
X-ray	High-energy wave that can penetrate most solid matter and present the image on photographic film (see Figure 15.9).

FIGURE 15.9 Enhanced color X-ray of normal chest in an eleven-year-old boy. (Science Photo Library/Photo Researchers, Inc.)

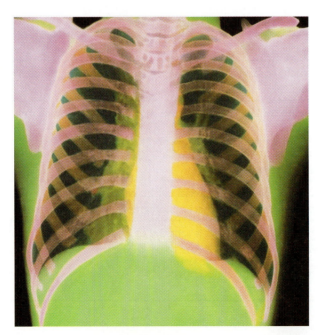

Diagnostic Procedures Relating to Radiology

angiocardiography (an jee oh kar dee OG rah fee)	X-ray of the heart and blood vessels after injecting a radiopaque dye.
angiogram (AN jee oh gram)	X-ray of a blood vessel that is taken in rapid sequence after injection of a radiopaque substance into the blood vessel.
angiography (an jee OG rah fee)	X-ray of blood or lymphatic vessels after injection of a radiopaque substance.
aortography (ay or TOG rah fee)	X-ray of the aorta after injection of a radiopaque material.
arteriography (ar tee ree OG rah fee)	X-ray of arteries after injection of a radiopaque dye.
barium enema (BaE) (BAH ree um EN eh mah)	Introduction of a barium solution into the rectum and colon to provide a visual picture of the lower bowel.
bronchography (brong KOG rah fee)	X-ray of the lung after a radiopaque substance has been placed into the trachea or bronchial tree.
cholangiogram (koh LAN jee oh gram)	X-ray picture of the bile ducts.
cholecystogram (koh lee SIS toh gram)	X-ray picture of the gallbladder.
echoencephalogram (ek oh en SEFF ah loh gram)	Recording of the ultrasound echoes of the brain.
fluoroscopy (floo ROS koh pee)	Use of a fluoroscope to picture the shadows of objects. Also referred to as *X-rays*.
hysterosalpingography (hiss ter oh sal ping OG rah fee)	X-ray of the uterus and oviducts after a radiopaque material is injected into the organs.
lymphangiography (lim fan jee OG rah fee)	X-ray of the lymph vessels after the injection of a radiopaque material.
magnetic resonance imaging (MRI) (mag NEH tik REHZ oh nance)	Use of electromagnetic energy to produce an image of the heart, blood vessels, brain, and soft tissues. Does not involve the use of radiation or an invasive procedure (see Figures 15.10 to 15.12).
mammography (mam OG rah fee)	Use of radiography of the breast to diagnose breast cancer.
myelogram (MY eh loh gram)	X-ray of the spinal canal after injecting a radiopaque dye.
positron emission tomography (PET) (PAHZ ih tron ee MISH un toh MOG rah fee)	Reconstruction of brain sections by using particles of radionuclides. Measurements can be taken of cerebral blood flow and volume, oxygen, and glucose uptake.
sonogram (SON oh gram)	The image produced by ultrasound waves bouncing off internal body structures.
thermograph (THER moh graf)	Technique that detects and records surface temperatures of the body. The hot and cold spots on the body are revealed, which assists in disease detection. Used to detect cancer of the breast and blood flow in the limbs.
ultrasound (US) (ULL trah sound)	Use of inaudible sound waves to outline shapes of tissues, organs, and the fetus. Also called *echography*.
venography (vee NOG rah fee)	X-ray tracing of a vein.

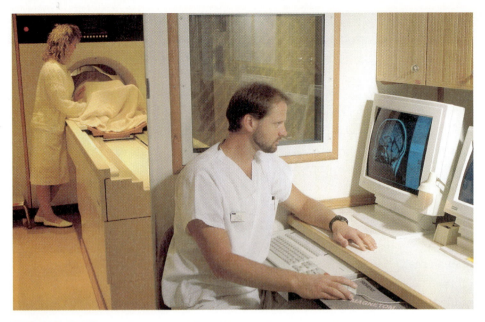

FIGURE 15.10   MRI lab. (Will and Demi McIntyre/Photo Researchers, Inc.)

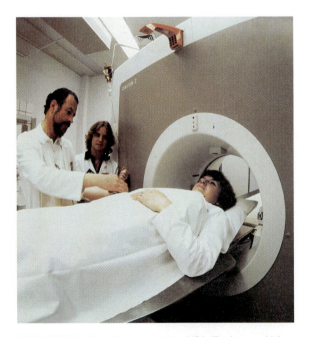

FIGURE 15.11   Open chamber MRI. (Dr. Lorenz H./
Mauritius GMBH/Phototake NYC)

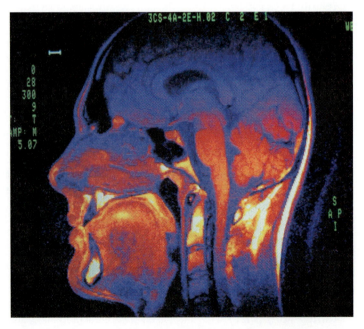

FIGURE 15.12   Enhanced color MRI of mid-sagittal of head and brain.
(Philippe Plailly/Science Photo Library/Photo Researchers, Inc.)

Radiologic Technologist

Radiologic technologists produce images of internal body parts through the use of X-ray, ultrasound, magnetic resonance imaging (MRI), or radionuclide slides. These images are then used by physicians and other health care personnel in diagnosing and planning patient treatment. For example, X-rays are important in diagnosing and treating fractures and blood clots. Radiologic technologists have career opportunities in acute care facilities, clinics, physician's offices, and private imaging services. To be a radiologic technologist, students must graduate from a four-year bachelor's degree program in radiology and pass a registration exam administered by the American Registry of Radiologic Technologies. For more information regarding a career in radiology, visit the American Registry of Radiologic Technologies' web site at www.arrt.org/index.asp.

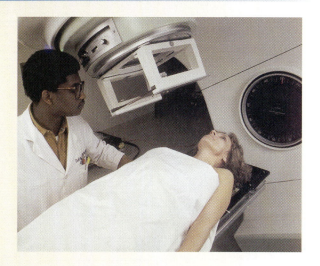

Registered Radiologic Technologist (RRT)

- Performs imaging procedures as ordered by a physician

- Operates at least two different types of imaging equipment

- Graduates from an approved radiologic program or a four-year bachelor's degree radiologic program

- Passes registration examination

Abbreviations Relating to Radiology

ACAT	automated computerized axial tomography		**kW**	kilowatt
Angio	angiography		**LAT**	lateral
AP	anteroposterior		**LGI**	lower gastrointestinal series
Ba	barium		**LL**	left lateral
BaE	barium enema		**mA**	milliampere
CAT	computerized axial tomography		**mCi**	millicurie
Ci	curie		**MRI**	magnetic resonance imaging
C-spine	cervical spine film		**NMR**	nuclear magnetic resonance
CT	computerized tomography		**PA**	posteroanterior
DSA	digital subtraction angiography		**PET**	positive emission tomography
ERCP	endoscopic retrograde cholangiopancreatography		**PTC**	percutaneous transhepatic cholangiography
ERT	external radiation therapy		**R**	roentgen
Fx	fracture		**Ra**	radium
GB	gallbladder X-ray		**rad**	radiation absorbed dose
IRT	internal radiation therapy		**RL**	right lateral
IVC	intravenous cholangiogram		**RRT**	registered radiologic technologist
IVP	intravenous pyelogram		**UGI**	upper gastrointestinal series
KUB	kidneys, ureters, bladder		**US**	ultrasound
kV	kilovolt			

Practice Exercises

F.   IDENTIFY THE FOLLOWING ABBREVIATIONS.

1. MRI   _____

2. Ba   _____

3. AP   _____

4. CT   _____

5. RL   _____

6. PA   _____

7. LL   _____

8. PET   _____

9. UGI   _____

10. LGI   _____

G.   IDENTIFY THE ORGAN OR STRUCTURE BEING STUDIED IN EACH OF THE FOLLOWING PROCEDURES:

1. hysterosalpingography   _____

2. aortography   _____

3. cholecystography   _____

4. lymphangiography   _____

5. mammography   _____

6. angiocardiography   _____

7. bronchography   _____

8. myelography   _____

H.   COMPLETE THE FOLLOWING STATEMENTS:

1. The radioactive form of an element is a _____ .

2. Another term for roentgen ray is _____ .

3. A _____ is an image produced after a radioactive substance has been injected into the body.

4. A _____ procedure is used to determine the cause of an illness, while a _____ procedure is used to treat a disease.

5. A piece of equipment that contains a particle accelerator is called a _____ .

6. An _____ produces an image using the echoes from high frequency sound waves.

7. A device that detects and records the amount of heat present is called a _____ .

ONCOLOGY

COMBINING FORMS RELATING TO ONCOLOGY

blast/o	primitive cell	**onc/o**	tumor
carcin/o	cancerous	**plas/o**	formation of cells
chem/o	chemical	**radi/o**	radiation, X-rays
mut/a	genetic change, mutation	**tox/o**	toxic

SUFFIXES RELATING TO ONCOLOGY

Suffix	Meaning	Example
-oma	tumor, mass	adenoma
-plakia	plate, patch	leukoplakia
-plasia	growth, formation	hyperplasia
-plasm	growth, formation	neoplasm
-therapy	treatment	chemotherapy

Oncology (ong **KALL** oh jee) is the branch of medicine dealing with **tumors** (**TOO** mors). A tumor can be classified as **benign** (bee **NINE**) or **malignant** (mah **LIG** nant). A benign tumor is one that is generally not progressive or recurring. Generally, a benign tumor will have the suffix *-oma* at the end of the term. On the other hand, a malignant tumor indicates that there is a cancerous growth present. These terms will usually have the word **carcinoma** (kar sin **NOH** mah) added. The medical specialty of oncology primarily treats patients who have cancer.

MED TERM TIP

Carcinoma or cancer (Ca) can affect almost every organ in the body. The medical term reflects the area of the body affected as well as the type of tumor cell. For example, there can be an esophageal carcinoma, gastric adenocarcinoma, or adenocarcinoma of the uterus.

The treatment for cancer can consist of a variety or a combination of treatments. The **protocol** (**PROH** toh kall) (prot) for a particular patient will consist of the actual plan of care, including the medications, surgeries, and treatments. Often, the entire health care team, including the physician, oncologist, radiologist, nurse, and patient, will assist in designing the treatment plan (see Figure 15.13).

Staging Tumors

The process of classifying tumors based on their degree of tissue invasion and the potential response to therapy is referred to as **staging.** The TNM staging system is frequently used. The T refers to the tumor's size and invasion, the N refers to lymph node involvement, and the M refers to the presence of **metastases (mets)** (meh **TASS** tah seez) of the tumor cells.

FIGURE 15.13 Elderly patient in a hospice setting. Hospice is an interdisciplinary program of care and supportive services. (John Moss/Science Source/Photo Researchers, Inc.)

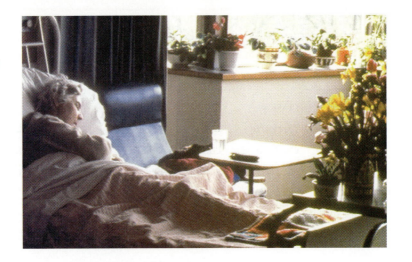

In addition, a tumor can be graded from grade I through grade IV. The **grade** is based on the microscopic appearance of the tumor cells. The **pathologist** (path **ALL** oh jist) rates or grades the cells based on whether the tumor resembles the normal tissue. The classification system is illustrated in Table 15.1. A grade I tumor is well differentiated and is easier to treat than the more advanced grades.

Table 15.1	Tumor Grade Classification
Grade	**Meaning**
GX	The grade cannot be determined
GI	The cells are well differentiated
GII	The cells are moderately differentiated
GIII	The cells are poorly differentiated
GIV	The cells are undifferentiated

Vocabulary Relating to Oncology

carcinogen (kar **SIN** oh jen)	Substance or chemical agent that produces or increases the risk of developing cancer. For example, cigarette smoke and insecticides are considered to be carcinogens.
encapsulated (en **CAP** soo lay ted)	Growth enclosed in a sheath of tissue that prevents tumor cells from invading surrounding tissue.
hyperplasia (high per **PLAY** zee ah)	Excessive development of normal cells within an organ.
invasive (in **VAY** siv) **disease**	Tendency of a malignant tumor to spread to immediately surrounding tissue and organs.
metastasis (mets) (meh **TASS** tah sis)	Movement and spread of cancer cells from one part of the body to another. *Metastases* is plural.
morbidity (mor **BID** ih tee)	Number that represents the number of sick persons in a particular population.
mortality (mor **TAL** ih tee)	Number that represents the number of deaths in a particular population.

mutation (mew TAY shun)	Change or transformation from the original.
neoplasm (NEE oh plazm)	New and abnormal growth or tumor. These can be benign or malignant.
oncogenic (ong koh JEN ik)	Cancer-causing.
primary site	Term that is used to designate where a malignant tumor first appeared.
protocol (prot) (PROH toh kall)	Plan of treatment for cancer patients developed by examining all the options available, including radiation therapy, chemotherapy, removal of entire organ with the tumor, removal of only the tumor, removal of surrounding lymph nodes, and others.
remission (rih MISH un)	Period during which the symptoms of a disease or disorder leave. Can be temporary.

Pathology Relating to Oncology

adenocarcinoma (ad eh noh kar sin NOH mah)	Malignant adenoma in a glandular organ.
adenoma (ad eh NOH mah)	Neoplasm of the glandular epithelium.
astrocytoma (ass troh sigh TOH mah)	Tumor of the brain or spinal cord composed of astrocytes.
basal cell carcinoma (BAY sal SELL kar sin NOH mah)	Malignancy of the skin that usually does not metastasize.
Burkitt's lymphoma (lim FOH mah)	Tumor of the lymph tissue that involves sites other than lymph nodes. Commonly found in the jaw and more common in Central Africa. Named after Denis Burkitt, a Ugandan physician.
carcinoma (kar sin NOH mah)	New growth or malignant tumor that occurs in epithelial tissue. It can spread to other organs through the blood or by direct extension from the organ.
carcinoma in situ (CIS) (kar sin NOH mah)	Malignant tumor that has not extended beyond the original site.
chondrosarcoma (kon droh sar KOH mah)	Sarcoma of cartilage tissue.
Ewing's sarcoma (YOO ingz sar KOH mah)	Myeloma forming on long bones, named after James Ewing, an American pathologist.
fibrosarcoma (figh broh sar KOH mah)	Sarcoma containing connective tissue.
glioblastoma (glee oh blas TOH mah)	Neurological tumor.
glioma (glee OH mah)	Sarcoma of neurological origin.
Hodgkin's disease (HD) (HOJ kins dih ZEEZ)	Solid tumor of the lymphatic system that usually begins in the supraclavicular lymph nodes. If untreated, it will invade other areas and organs. This disease is now curable in 70 percent of cases.
hypernephroma (high per neh FROH mah)	Renal or kidney cell carcinoma.

(continued)

Kaposi's sarcoma (KAP oh seez sar KOH mah)	Sarcoma seen in a number of areas, initially in the skin. It is common in AIDS patients. Named after Moritz Kaposi, an Austrian dermatologist.
leukemia (loo KEE mee ah)	Chronic or acute disease with a growth of the stem cells of the blood-forming tissues. This slow-growing disease does not allow blood cells to mature properly.
leukoplakia (loo koh PLAY kee ah)	Formation of white patches or spots on the mucous membranes of the cheek or tongue. These lesions may become malignant.
lymphoma (lim FOH mah)	Tumor arising out of the lymph system.
malignant melanoma (mah LIG nant mel ah NOH mah)	Malignant, darkly pigmented tumor or mole of the skin.
medulloblastoma (meh dull oh blas TOH mah)	Soft malignant tumor of the brain.
multiple myeloma (MULL tih pl my eh LOH mah)	Neoplasm that infiltrates the bone and bone marrow, and eventually forms multiple tumor masses. A progressive and highly lethal disease.
nephrosarcoma (nef roh sar KOH mah)	Cancer of the kidney. Also called *Wilm's tumor*, it occurs mainly in children.
neuroblastoma (noo roh blass TOH mah)	Malignant hemorrhagic tumor arising out of the sympathetic system, especially the adrenal medulla. This is found primarily in infants and children.
non-Hodgkin's lymphoma (NHL)	Malignant, solid tumors of lymphoid tissue.
retinoblastoma (ret ih noh blas TOH mah)	Malignant glioma of the retina.
sarcoma (sar KOH mah)	Cancer arising from the connective tissue, such as muscle or bone. May affect the kidneys, bladder, bones, liver, lungs, and spleen.

Diagnostic Procedures Relating to Oncology

biopsy (bx) (BYE op see)	Excision of a small piece of tissue for microscopic examination to assist in determining a diagnosis.
bone marrow biopsy (BYE op see)	Removal of a small amount of bone marrow for microscopic examination to determine the presence of malignant tumor cells.
cytologic (sigh toh LOG ik) testing	Examination of cells to determine their structure and origin. PAP smears are considered a form of cytologic testing.
exploratory surgery (ek SPLOR ah tor ee SER jer ee)	Surgery performed for the purpose of determining if there is cancer present or if a known cancer has spread. Biopsies are generally performed.
lumbar puncture (LUM bar PUNK chur)	Puncture made by placing a needle into the fourth intervertebral space of the lumbar area to remove spinal fluid for analysis.
needle biopsy (BYE op see)	Core of tissue is removed using a needle. The tissue cells are then tested for the abnormal cellular growth of cancer.
staging laparotomy (lap ah ROT oh mee)	Surgical procedure in which the abdomen is entered to determine the extent and staging of a tumor.

Treatment Procedures Relating to Oncology

chemotherapy (chemo) (kee moh THAIR ah pee)	Treating disease by using chemicals that have a toxic effect upon the body, especially cancerous tissue.
cryosurgery (cry oh SER jer ee)	Technique of exposing tissues to extreme cold to produce cell injury and destruction. Used in the treatment of malignant tumors to control pain and bleeding.
hormone therapy (HOR mohn THAIR ah pee)	Treatment of cancer with natural hormones or with chemicals that produce hormone-like effects.
immunotherapy (im yoo noh THAIR ah pee)	The production or strengthening of immunity.
palliative therapy (PAL ee ah tiv THAIR ah pee)	Treatment designed to reduce the intensity of painful symptoms, but does not produce a cure.
radical surgery	Extensive surgery to remove as much tissue associated with a tumor as possible.
radioactive (ray dee oh AK tiv) implant	Embedding a radioactive source directly into tissue to provide a highly localized radiation dosage to damage nearby cancerous cells. Also called *brachytherapy*.
radiation therapy (ray dee AY shun THAIR ah pee)	Exposing tumors and surrounding tissues to X-rays or gamma rays to interfere with their ability to multiply.

Abbreviations Relating to Oncology

Ba	barium	**mets**	metastases
bx	biopsy	**MTX**	methotrexate
Ca	cancer	**NED**	no evidence of disease
CCU	coronary care unit	**NHL**	non-Hodgkin's lymphoma
chemo	chemotherapy	**NPDL**	nodular, poorly differentiated lymphocytes
CIS	carcinoma in situ	**PAP**	Papanicolaou test
5-FU	5-fluorouracil	**prot**	protocol
GA	gallium	**PSA**	prostate specific antigen
geri-chair	geriatric chair	**st**	stage
HD	Hodgkin's disease	**TNM**	tumor, nodes, metastases

Chart Note Transcription

Chart Note

The chart note below contains eleven phrases that can be reworded with a medical term that you learned in this chapter. Each phrase is identified with an underline. Determine the medical term and write your answers in the space provided.

Current Complaint: A 56-year-old male was referred to a specialist in the treatment of cancer[1] for treatment of a suspicious right kidney mass discovered by his internist on a CT scan.

Past History: Patient had been aware of right side pain, difficulty urinating, and weight loss over the past 6 months.

Signs and Symptoms: A surgery performed to determine if cancer is present[2] was performed and small samples of tissue removed for examination under a microscope[3] were taken from the suspicious right kidney mass. After it was determined to be cancerous with a tendency to grow worse,[4] a right nephrectomy was performed. Reports indicate that the new and abnormal growth[5] was graded to be moderately differentiated[6] and well enclosed in a sheath of tissue[7] with no signs of spreading to another part of the body.[8]

Diagnosis: Cancer of the right kidney.[9]

Treatment: Post-surgery the patient began a plan of treatment[10] of the use of chemical agents with a specific toxic effect.[11]

1 _____

2 _____

3 _____

4 _____

5 _____

6 _____

7 _____

8 _____

9 _____

10 _____

11 _____

Practice Exercises

I. IDENTIFY THE LOCATION OF THE FOLLOWING CANCEROUS TUMORS:

1. Hodgkin's disease _____

2. leukemia _____

3. malignant melanoma _____

4. astrocytoma _____

5. chondrosarcoma _____

6. nephrosarcoma _____

7. basal cell carcinoma _____

8. fibrosarcoma _____

9. adenocarcinoma _____

10. Kaposi's sarcoma _____

J. MATCH THE FOLLOWING TERMS TO THEIR DEFINITIONS:

A	B
1. _____ oncogenic	a. examine cells to determine their structure and origin
2. _____ benign	b. the plan for care for any individual patient
3. _____ encapsulated	c. biopsy
4. _____ PAP	d. growth that is not recurrent or progressive
5. _____ primary site	e. placing a radioactive substance directly into the tissue
6. _____ protocol	f. where the malignant tumor first appeared
7. _____ staging laparotomy	g. growth is enclosed in a tissue sheath
8. _____ crytologic testing	h. cancer causing
9. _____ radioactive implant	i. abdominal surgery to determine extent of tumor
10. _____ bx	j. Papanicolaou test

COMBINING FORMS RELATING TO REHABILITATION SERVICES

cry/o	cold	**orth/o**	straight, correct
electr/o	electric current	**prosth/o**	addition
erg/o	work	**therm/o**	heat
hydr/o	water		

The goal of rehabilitation is to prevent disability and restore as much function as possible following disease, illness, or injury. Rehabilitation services include the medical specialties of **physical therapy** (PT) and **occupational therapy** (OT).

Physical Therapy

The medical specialty of physical therapy (PT) involves treating disorders using physical means and methods (see Figure 15.14). Physical therapy personnel assess joint motion, muscle strength and endurance, function of heart and lungs, and performance of activities required in daily living, and carry out other responsibilities (see Figure 15.15).

Physical therapy treatment includes gait training, therapeutic exercise, massage, joint and soft tissue mobilization, thermal and cryotherapy, electrical stimulation, ultrasound, and hydrotherapy. These methods strengthen muscles, improve motion and circulation, reduce pain, and increase function.

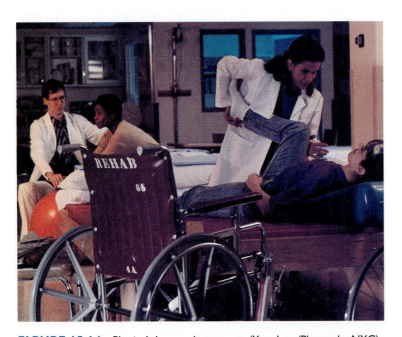

FIGURE 15.14 Physical therapy department. (Yoav Levy/Phototake NYC)

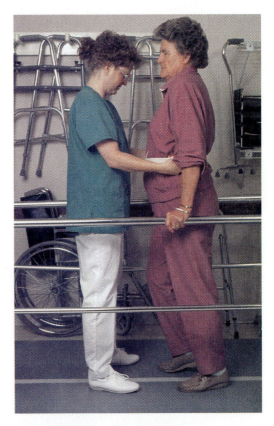

FIGURE 15.15 Physical therapist working with patient's ambulation on parallel bars.

Occupational Therapy

The medical specialty of occupational therapy (OT) assists patients to regain, develop, and improve skills that are important for independent functioning. Occupational therapy personnel work with people who, because of illness, injury, or developmental or psychological impairments, require specialized training in skills that will enable them to lead independent, productive, and satisfying lives. Occupational therapists instruct patients in the use of adaptive equipment and techniques, body mechanics, and energy conservation. They also employ modalities such as heat, cold, and therapeutic exercise.

Vocabulary Relating to Rehabilitation Services

activities of daily living (ADL)	The activities usually performed in the course of a normal day, such as eating, dressing, and washing (see Figure 15.16).
adaptive equipment	Modification of equipment or devices to improve the function and independence of a person with a disability.
body mechanics	Use of good posture and position while performing activities of daily living to prevent injury and stress on body parts.
ergonomics (er goh NOM iks)	The study of human work including how the requirements for performing work and the work environment affect the musculoskeletal and nervous system.
fine motor skills	The use of precise and coordinated movements in such activities such as writing, buttoning, and cutting.
gait (GAYT)	Manner of walking.
gross motor skills	The use of large muscle groups that coordinate body movements such as walking, running, jumping, and balance.
lower extremity (LE)	The leg.
mobility	State of having normal movement of all body parts.
orthotics (or THOT iks)	The use of equipment, such as splints and braces, to support a paralyzed muscle, promote a specific motion, or correct musculoskeletal deformities.
physiatrist (fiz ee AT rist)	Physician who specializes in physical medicine.
physical medicine	Use of natural methods, including physical therapy, to cure diseases and disorders.
prosthetics (pros THET iks)	Artificial devices, such as limbs and joints, that replace a missing body part (see Figure 15.17).
range of motion (ROM)	The range of movement of a joint, from maximum flexion through maximum extension. It is measured as degrees of a circle.
rehabilitation (ree hah bill ih TAY shun)	Process of treatment and exercise that can help a disabled person attain maximum function and well-being.
upper extremity (UE)	The arm.

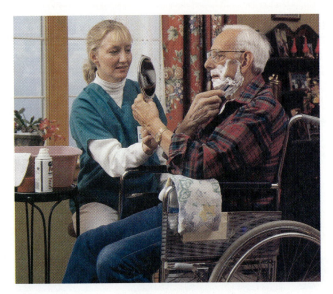

FIGURE 15.16 Occupational therapist assisting with activities of daily living (ADL).

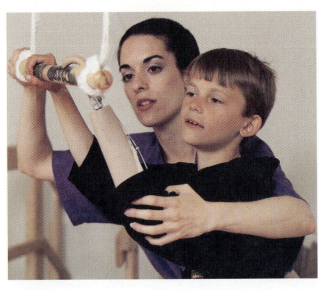

FIGURE 15.17 Physical therapist assisting child in use of prosthetic arm. (Yoav Levy/Phototake NYC)

Pathology Relating to Rehabilitation Services

amputation (am pew TAY shun)	Removal of an extremity due to injury or disease.
arthritis (ar THRY tis)	Inflammation of a joint, which usually occurs with pain and swelling.
burns	Damage to the skin as a result of first-, second-, and third-degree burns. Physical therapy is necessary to maintain mobility and avoid stiffness.
bursitis (bur SIGH tis)	Inflammation of a bursa between bony prominences and muscles or tendons. Common in the shoulder and knee.
carpal tunnel syndrome (CAR pul TUN el SIN drohm)	A painful disorder of the wrist and hand, induced by compression of the median nerve as it passes under ligaments on the palm side of the wrist. Symptoms include weakness, pain, burning, tingling, and aching in the forearm, wrist, and hand.
cerebral palsy (CP) (seh REE bral PAWL zee)	Nonprogressive paralysis that results from defects in the brain or birth trauma.
cerebrovascular accident (CVA) (ser eh broh VASS kyoo lar AK sih dent)	Brain damage as a result of blockage or rupture of a cerebral artery. It may result in unconsciousness and paralysis. This is also called a *stroke*.

developmental disabilities	A disorder that interferes with the normal growth and development of a child. This condition may affect muscles or mental abilities.
head injury	Blunt trauma to the skull causing bleeding and edema resulting in damage to the brain. Symptoms may include muscle paralysis and mental difficulties. Symptoms may be permanent or temporary depending on the severity of the injury.
herniated nucleus pulposus (HNP) (HER nee ay ted NOO klee us pul POH sus)	A rupture of the fibrocartilage disk between two vertebrae. This results in pressure on a spinal nerve and causes pain, weakness, and nerve damage. Also called a *slipped disk*.
multiple sclerosis (MS) (MULL tih pl skleh ROH sis)	Inflammatory disease of the central nervous system. Rare in children. Generally strikes adults between the ages of 20 and 40. There is progressive weakness and numbness.
muscular dystrophy (MUSS kew lar DIS troh fee)	Wasting disease of the muscles.
osteoporosis (oss tee oh por ROH sis)	Disease that results in a reduction of the bone mass. Occurs most frequently in postmenopausal women and can result in back pain and fractures.
paraplegia (pair ah PLEE jee ah)	Paralysis of the lower portion of the body, including the legs.
Parkinson's disease (PARK in sons dih ZEEZ)	Chronic nervous disease with fine tremors, slow gait, muscular weakness, and rigidity. Named after Sir John Parkinson, a British physician.
poliomyelitis (poh lee oh my ell EYE tis)	Acute viral disease that causes an inflammation of the gray matter of the spinal cord, resulting in paralysis in some cases. It has been brought under almost total control through vaccinations.
pressure sore	Open sore that is caused from excessive rubbing on the skin or lying too long in the same position. Also called a *decubitus ulcer*.
quadriplegia (kwod rih PLEE jee ah)	Paralysis of all four extremities.
repetitive motion injury	Musculoskeletal system damage that results from simple motions repeated many times within a given period of time. Often associated with assembly line work in which the worker performs one specialized task over and over.
rheumatoid arthritis (RA) (ROO mah toyd ar THRY tis)	Form of arthritis with inflammation of the joints, swelling, stiffness, and pain.
spinal cord injury (SCI)	Bruising or severing of the spinal cord from a blow to the vertebral column resulting in muscle paralysis and sensory impairment below the injury level.
sprain	Pain and disability caused by trauma to a joint. A ligament may be torn in severe sprains.
strain	Trauma to muscle from excessive stretching or pulling.
tendonitis (ten dun EYE tis)	Inflammation of a tendon.

Treatment Procedures Relating to Rehabilitation Services

active exercises	Exercises that a patient performs without assistance.
active range of motion (AROM)	Range of motion for joints that a patient is able to perform without the assistance of someone else.
active-resistive exercises	Exercises in which the patient works against an artificial resistance applied to a muscle, such as a weight. Used to increase strength (see Figure 15.18).
aided exercises	Exercises in which the patient has assistance in performing the exercise from someone or something else.
cryotherapy (cry oh THAIR ah pee)	Using cold for therapeutic purposes.
debridement (day breed MON)	Removal of dead or damaged tissue from a wound. Commonly performed for burn therapy.
electromyogram (EMG) (ee lek troh MY oh gram)	Graphic recording of the contraction of a muscle. The result of applying an electrical stimulation to the muscle.
heat application	Applying either dry or moist warmth to a body part to produce the slight dilation of blood vessels in the skin. Causes muscle relaxation in the deeper regions of the body and increases circulation, which aids healing.
heat hydrotherapy (high droh THAIR ah pee)	Application of warm water as a therapeutic treatment. Can be done in baths, swimming pools, and whirlpools.
hot moist compresses	Applying moist heat with wet pads.
hydrotherapy (high droh THAIR ah pee)	Using water for treatment purposes.
ice packs	Using ice in a bag or container to treat localized conditions.
massage (mah SAHZH)	Kneading or applying pressure by hands to a part of the patient's body to promote muscle relaxation and reduce tension.
nerve conduction velocity	A test to determine if nerves have been damaged by recording the rate at which an electrical impulse travels along a nerve. If the nerve is damaged, the velocity will be decreased.
pain control	Managing pain through a variety of means, including medications, biofeedback, and mechanical devices.
passive range of motion (PROM)	Therapist putting a patient's joints through a full range of motion without assistance from the patient.
percussion (per KUH shun)	Use of the fingertips to tap the body lightly and sharply. Aids in determining the size, position, and consistency of the underlying body part.
phonophoresis (foh noh foh REE sis)	The use of ultrasound waves to introduce medication across the skin and into the subcutaneous tissues.
postural drainage with clapping	Draining secretions from the bronchi or a lung cavity by having the patient lie so that gravity allows drainage to occur. Clapping is using the hand in a cupped position to perform percussion on the chest. Assists in loosening secretions and mucus.
therapeutic (thair ah PEW tik) exercise	Exercise planned and carried out to achieve a specific physical benefit, such as improved range of motion, muscle strength, or cardiovascular function.

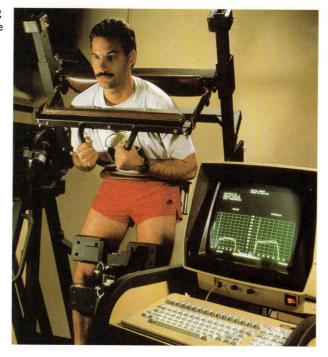

thermotherapy (ther moh THAIR ah pee)	Applying heat to the body for therapeutic purposes.
traction (TRAK shun)	Process of pulling or drawing, usually with a mechanical device. Used in treating orthopedic (bone and joint) problems and injuries.
transcutaneous electrical nerve stimulation (TENS) (tranz kyoo TAY nee us ee LEK trih kl nerve stim yoo LAY shun)	The application of an electric current to a peripheral nerve to relieve pain.
ultrasound (US) (ULL trah sound)	The use of high frequency sound waves to create heat in soft tissues under the skin. It is particularly useful for treating injuries to muscles, tendons, and ligaments, as well as muscle spasms.
whirlpool	Bath in which there are continuous jets of hot water reaching the body surfaces.

Abbreviations Relating to Rehabilitation Services

ADL	activities of daily living	OT	occupational therapy
AROM	active range of motion	PROM	passive range of motion
CP	cerebral palsy	PT	physical therapy
CVA	cerebrovascular accident	RA	rheumatoid arthritis
EMG	electromyogram	ROM	range of motion
e-stim	electrical stimulation	SCI	spinal cord injury
HNP	herniated nucleus pulposus	TENS	transcutaneous electrical stimulation
LE	lower extremity	UE	upper extremity
MS	multiple sclerosis	US	ultrasound

Practice Exercises

K. MATCH THE TERMS IN COLUMN A WITH THE DEFINITIONS IN COLUMN B.

A	B
1. _____ cerebral palsy	a. affects gray matter
2. _____ muscular dystrophy	b. paralysis of four extremities
3. _____ Parkinson's disease	c. paralysis from birth defect
4. _____ poliomyelitis	d. cerebrovascular accident
5. _____ quadriplegia	e. trauma to a joint
6. _____ paraplegia	f. wasting muscle disease
7. _____ osteoporosis	g. inflammation of joint
8. _____ CVA	h. paralysis of lower extremities
9. _____ arthritis	i. tremors, slow gait, rigidity
10. _____ sprain	j. reduction of bone mass

L. IDENTIFY THE FOLLOWING ABBREVIATIONS.

1. ROM   _____
2. CVA   _____
3. HNP   _____
4. LE   _____
5. EMG   _____
6. TENS   _____
7. MS   _____
8. SCI   _____
9. e-stim   _____
10. US   _____

M. IDENTIFY THE REHABILITATION PROCEDURE DESCRIBED BY EACH PHRASE.

1. kneading or applying pressure by hands _____
2. removal of dead and damaged tissue from a wound _____
3. using water for treatment purposes _____
4. drainage of secretions from the bronchi _____
5. exercises performed by a patient without resistance _____
6. medication introduced by ultrasound waves _____
7. use of cold for therapeutic purposes _____
8. pulling with a mechanical device _____

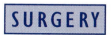

COMBINING FORMS RELATING TO SURGERY

asthesi/o	sensation, feeling	electr/o	electricity
cis/o	to cut	sect/o	cut
cry/o	cold		

Surgery is the branch of medicine dealing with operative procedures to correct deformities and defects, repair injuries, and diagnose and cure diseases. A **surgeon** is a physician who has completed additional training of five years or more in a surgical specialty area. These specialty areas include orthopedics; neurosurgery; gynecology; ophthalmology; urology; and thoracic, vascular, cardiac, plastic, and general surgery. The surgeon must complete an **operative report** for every procedure that he or she performs. This is a detailed description that includes the following:

- preoperative diagnosis
- indication for the procedure
- name of the procedure
- surgical techniques employed
- findings during surgery
- postoperative diagnosis
- name of the surgeon

This report also includes information pertaining to the patient such as name, address, age, patient number, and date of the procedure.

Surgical terminology includes terms related to anesthesiology, surgical instruments, surgical procedures, incisions, and suture materials. Specific surgical procedures are frequently named by using the combining form for the body part being operated on and adding a suffix that describes the procedure. For example, an incision into the chest is a **thoracotomy** (thor ah **KOT** oh mee), removal of the stomach is **gastrectomy** (gas **TREK** toh mee), and surgical repair of the skin is **dermatoplasty** (**DER** mah toh plas tee). A list of the most frequently used surgical suffixes is found in Chapter 1 and common surgical procedures are defined in each system chapter.

Anesthesia

An **anesthesiologist** (an es thee zee **OL** oh jist) is a physician who specializes in the practice of administering anesthetics (see Figure 15.19). A **nurse anesthetist** (ah **NES** the tist) is a registered nurse who has received additional training and education in the administration of anesthetic medications.

Anesthesia (an ess **THEE** zee ah) results in the loss of feeling or sensation. The most common types of anesthesia are general, regional, local, and topical anesthesia.

- **General anesthesia (GA)** produces a loss of consciousness including an absence of pain sensation. It is administered to a patient by either an **intravenous** (in trah **VEE** nus) **(IV)** (into the vein) or **inhalation** (in hah **LAY** shun) (breathing) **method.** The patient's **vital signs (VS)** (heart rate, breathing rate, pulse, and blood pressure) are carefully monitored when using a general anesthetic.
- **Regional anesthesia** is also referred to as a **nerve block.** This anesthetic interrupts a patient's pain sensation in a particular region of the body. The anesthetic is injected near the nerve that will be blocked from sensation. The patient usually remains conscious.
- **Local anesthesia** produces a loss of sensation in one localized part of the body. The patient remains conscious. The anesthetic is administered either **topically** (on the skin) or via a **subcutaneous** (sub kyoo **TAY** nee us) (into the skin) route.
- **Topical anesthesia** uses an anesthetic liquid or gel placed directly into a specific area. The patient remains conscious. This type of anesthetic is used on the skin, the cornea, and the mucous membranes in dental work.

FIGURE 15.19

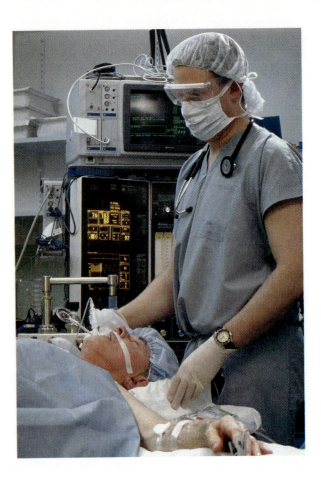

Instruments

Physicians have developed surgical instruments since the time of the early Egyptians. Instruments include surgical knives, saws, clamps, drills, and needles. Some of the more commonly used surgical instruments are listed in Table 15.2

Table 15.2	Common Surgical Instruments
Instrument	**Use**
aspirator (**AS** pih ray tor)	suctions fluid
clamp	grasps tissue; controls bleeding
curette (kyoo **RET**)	scrapes and removes tissue
dilator (dye **LAY** tor)	enlarges an opening by stretching
forceps (**FOR** seps)	grasps tissue
hemostat (**HEE** moh stat)	forceps to grasp blood vessel to control bleeding
probe	explores tissue
scalpel	cuts and separates tissue
speculum (**SPEK** yoo lum)	spreads apart walls of a cavity
tenaculum (teh **NAK** yoo lum)	long handled clamp
trephine (treh **FINE**)	saw that removes disc-shaped piece of tissue or bone

Vocabulary Relating to Surgery

analgesic (an al JEE zik)	Medication to relieve pain.
anesthetic (an ess THET ik)	Medication to produce partial to complete loss of sensation.
cauterization (kaw ter ih ZAY shun)	Using heat, cold, electricity, or chemicals to scar, burn, or cut tissues.
circulating nurse	Nurse who assists the surgeon and scrub nurse by providing needed materials during the procedure and by handling the surgical specimen. This person does not wear sterile clothing and may enter and leave the operating room during the procedure.
cryosurgery (cry oh SER jer ee)	Using extreme cold to destroy tissue.
day surgery	A type of outpatient surgery in which the patient is discharged on the same day he or she is admitted; also called *ambulatory surgery*.
dissection (dih SEK shun)	The surgical cutting of parts for separation and study.
draping	Process of covering the patient with sterile cloths that allow only the operative site to be exposed to the surgeon.
electrocautery (ee lek troh KAW ter ee)	Use of an electric current to stop bleeding by coagulating blood vessels.
endoscopic (en doh SKOP ik) surgery	Use of a lighted instrument to examine the interior of a cavity.
hemostasis (hee moh STAY sis)	Stopping the flow of blood using instruments, pressure, and/or medication.
laser surgery	Use of a controlled beam of light for cutting, hemostasis, or tissue destruction.
perioperative (per ee OP er ah tiv)	The period of time that includes before, during, and after a surgical procedure.
postoperative (post OP er ah tiv)	The period of time immediately following the surgery.
preoperative (preop, pre-op) (pree OP er ah tiv)	The period of time preceding surgery.
resection (ree SEK shun)	To surgically cut out; excision.
scrub nurse	Surgical assistant who hands instruments to the surgeon. This person wears sterile clothing and maintains the sterile operative field.
suture (SOO cher) material	Used to close a wound or incision. Examples are catgut, silk thread, or staples. They may or may not be removed when the wound heals, depending on the type of material that is used.

Surgical Positions

Patients are placed in specific positions so the surgeon is able to reach the area that is to be operated on. Table 15.3 describes some common surgical positions.

Table 15.3	*Common Surgical Positions*
Surgical Position	**Description**
Fowler	sitting with back positioned at a 45° angle
lateral recumbent (**LAT** er al ree **KUM** bent)	lying on either the left or right side
lithotomy (lith **OT** oh mee)	lying face up with hips and knees bent at 90° angles
prone (**PROHN**)	lying horizontal with face down
supine (soo **PINE**)	lying horizontal and face up; also called *dorsal recumbent*
Trendelenburg (**TREN** dee len berg)	lying face up and on an incline with head lower than legs

Abbreviations Relating to Surgery

D & C	dilation and curettage	**PARR**	postanesthetic recovery room
EAU	exam under anesthesia	**preop, pre-op**	preoperative
Endo	endoscopy	**prep**	preparation, prepared
GA	general anesthesia	**S/R**	suture removal
I & D	incision and drainage	**T & A**	tonsillectomy and adenoidectomy
MUA	manipulation under anesthesia	**TAH**	total abdominal hysterectomy
OR	operating room	**TURP**	transurethral resection of prostate

Practice Exercises

N. MATCH EACH TERM WITH ITS DEFINITION.

A		B	
1. _____ forceps		a.	scrapes and removes tissue
2. _____ tenaculum		b.	cuts and separates tissue
3. _____ Trendelenburg		c.	lying horizontal and face up
4. _____ lithotomy		d.	lying on either the left or right side
5. _____ curette		e.	long handled clamp
6. _____ aspirator		f.	explores tissue
7. _____ supine		g.	lying face up with hips and knees bent at 90° angle
8. _____ probe		h.	grasps tissue
9. _____ scalpel		i.	suctions fluid
10. _____ lateral recumbent		j.	lying face up and on an incline, head lower than legs

O. IDENTIFY THE TYPE OF ANESTHESIA FOR EACH DESCRIPTION.

1. produces loss of consciousness and absence of pain   _____

2. produces loss of sensation in one localized part of the body   _____

3. anesthetic applied directly onto a specific skin area   _____

4. also referred to as a nerve block   _____

COMBINING FORMS RELATING TO MENTAL HEALTH

ment/o	mind	**psych/o**	mind
neur/o	nerve	**schiz/o**	divided
pharmac/o	drugs	**somat/o**	body
phren/o	mind	**somn/o**	sleep

SUFFIXES RELATING TO MENTAL HEALTH

Suffix	Meaning	Example
-iatrist	physician	psychiatrist
-mania	excessive excitement	pyromania
-ology	study of	psychology
-philia	affinity for, craving for	pedophilia
-phobia	irrational fear	photophobia

Psychology

Psychology (sigh **KALL** oh jee) is the study of human behavior and thought process. This behavioral science is primarily concerned with understanding how human beings interact with their physical environment and with each other. Behavior can be divided into two categories, normal and abnormal. The study of normal psychology includes how the personality develops, how people handle stress, and the stages of mental development. On the other hand, **abnormal psychology** studies and treats behaviors that are outside of normal and that are detrimental to the person or society. These maladaptive behaviors range from occasional difficulty coping with stress, to bizarre actions and beliefs, to total withdrawal. A **clinical psychologist** (sigh **KALL** oh jist) is a specialist in evaluating and treating persons with mental and emotional disorders.

MED TERM TIP

All social interactions pose some problems for some people. These problems are not necessarily abnormal. One means of judging if behavior is abnormal is to compare one person's behavior with others in the community. Also, if a person's behavior interferes with the activities of daily living it is often considered abnormal.

Psychiatry

Psychiatry (sigh **KIGH** ah tree) is the branch of medicine that deals with the diagnosis, treatment, and prevention of mental disorders. A **psychiatrist** (sigh **KIGH** ah trist) is a medical physician specializing in the care of patients with mental, emotional, and behavioral disorders. Other health professions also have specialty areas in caring for clients with mental illness. Good examples are **psychiatric** (sigh kee **AT** rik) **nurses** and **psychiatric social workers.**

Mental Disorders

The legal definition of mental disorder is "impaired judgment and lack of self-control." The guide for terminology and classifications relating to psychiatric disorders is the *Diagnostic and Statistical Manual of Mental Disorders (DSM-IV, 1994)*, which is published by the American

Psychiatric Association. The DSM organizes mental disorders into sixteen major diagnostic categories of mental disorders. Some of these categories are described below.

Mental Disorders

Anxiety Disorders	characterized by persistent worry; includes **panic attacks, anxiety** (ang **ZY** eh tee), **phobias** (**FOH** bee ahs) (irrational fear, such as **photophobia** (foh toh **FOH** bee ah) (or fear of light), **obsessive-compulsive disorder** (ob **SESS** iv kom **PUHL** siv) (OCD) (performing repetitive rituals to reduce anxiety)
Cognitive Disorders	deterioration of mental functions due to temporary brain or permanent brain dysfunction; also called organic mental disease; includes **dementia** (dee **MEN** she ah) (progressive confusion and disorientation), and degenerative disorders such as **Alzheimer's disease** (**ALTS** high merz dih **ZEEZ**)
Disorders Diagnosed in Infancy and Childhood	mental disorders associated with childhood; includes **mental retardation, attention deficit disorder (ADD)** (attention **DEFF** ih sit dis **OR** der), **autism** (**AW** tizm) (extreme withdrawal)
Dissociative Disorders	disorders in which severe emotional conflict is so repressed that a split in the personality occurs; includes **amnesia** (am **NEE** zee ah) (loss of memory), and **multiple personality disorder** (**MULL** tih pl per son **AL** ih tee dis **OR** der)
Eating Disorders	abnormal behaviors related to eating; includes **anorexia nervosa** (an oh **REK** see ah ner **VOH** sah) (refusal to eat), **bulimia** (boo **LIM** ee ah) (binge eating and intentional vomiting)
Factitious Disorders	intentionally feigning illness symptoms in order to gain attention; includes **malingering,** which means to pretend illness or injury without apparent motive
Impulse Control Disorders	inability to resist an impulse to perform some act that is harmful to the individual or others; includes **kleptomania** (klep toh **MAY** nee ah) (stealing), **pyromania** (pie roh **MAY** nee ah) (setting fires), **explosive disorder** (ek **SPLOH** siv dis **OR** der) (violent rages), **pathological** (path ah **LOJ** ih kal) **gambling**
Mood Disorders	periods of deep depression with suicide potential, may alternate with **mania** (**MAY** nee ah) (extreme elation); includes **major depression** (**MAY** jer dee **PRES** shun), **bipolar disorder** (by**POHL** ar dis **OR** der) (**BPD**)(alternation between periods of deep depression and mania)
Personality Disorders	inflexible or maladaptive behavior patterns that affect person's ability to function in society; includes **paranoid personality disorder** (**PAIR** ah noyd per son **AL** ih tee dis **OR** der) (exaggerated feelings of persecution), **narcissistic personality disorder** (nar sis **SIST** ik per son **AL** ih tee dis **OR** der) (abnormal sense of self importance), **antisocial personality disorder** (an tih **SOH** shal per son **AL** ih tee dis **OR** der) (behaviors that are against legal or social norms), and **passive aggressive personality** (**PASS** iv ah **GRESS** iv per son **AL** ih tee) (indirect expression of hostility or anger)
Schizophrenia	mental disorders characterized by distortions of reality such as **delusions** (dee **LOO** zhuns) (a false belief held even in the face of contrary evidence) and **hallucinations** (hah loo sih **NAY** shuns) (perceiving something that is not there)
Sexual Disorders	disorders include aberrant sexual activity and sexual dysfunction; includes **pedophilia** (pee doh **FILL** ee ah) (sexual interest in children), **masochism** (**MAS** oh kizm) (gratification derived from being hurt or abused), **voyeurism** (**VOY** er izm) (gratification derived from observing others engaged in sexual acts), **low sex drive, premature ejaculation** (ee jak yoo **LAY** shun)
Sleeping Disorders	disorders relating to sleeping; includes **insomnia** (in **SOM** nee ah) (inability to sleep) and **sleepwalking**
Somatoform Disorders	patient has physical symptoms for which no physical disease can be determined; includes **hypochondria** (high poh **KON** dree ah) (a preoccupation with health concerns), and **conversion** (kon **VER** zhun) **reaction** (anxiety is transformed into physical symptoms such as heart palpitations, paralysis, or blindness)
Substance-Related Disorders	overindulgence or dependence on chemical substances including alcohol, illegal drugs, and prescription drugs

Treatments

Treatments for mental disorders include a variety of methods such as **psychotherapy** (sigh koh **THAIR** ah pee), **psychopharmacology** (sigh koh far mah **KALL** oh jee), and **electroconvulsive therapy (ECT)** (ee lek troh kon **VULL** siv **THAIR** ah pee).

Psychotherapy is a method of treating mental disorders by mental rather than chemical or physical means. It includes psychoanalysis, humanistic therapies, and family and group therapy.

- Psychoanalysis is a method of obtaining a detailed account of the past and present emotional and mental experiences from the patient to determine the source of the problem and eliminate the effects. It is a system developed by Sigmund Freud that encourages the patient to discuss repressed, painful, or hidden experiences with the hope of eliminating or minimizing the problem.

- Humanistic psychotherapy is also called *client-centered* or *nondirective psychotherapy.* The therapist does not delve into the patients' past when using these methods. Instead, it is believed that patients can learn how to use their own internal resources to deal with their problems. The therapist creates a therapeutic atmosphere, which builds patients' self-esteem and encourages them to discuss their problems, thereby gaining insight in how to handle them.

- Family and group psychotherapy is described as solution focused. The therapist places minimal emphasis on the patient's past history and strong emphasis on having the patient state and discuss their goals and then find a way to achieve them.

Psychopharmacology relates to the study of the effects of drugs on the mind and particularly the use of drugs in treating mental disorders. The main classes of drugs for the treatment of mental disorders are antipsychotic drugs, antidepressant drugs, *minor* tranquilizers, and lithium.

- Antipsychotic drugs are the major tranquilizers including chlorpromazine (Thorazine), haloperidol (Haldol), clozapine (Clozaril), and risperidone. These drugs have transformed the treatment of patients with psychoses and schizophrenia by reducing patient agitation and panic and shortening schizophrenic episodes. One of the side effects of these drugs is involuntary muscle movements, which approximately one-fourth of all adults who take the drugs develop.

- Antidepressant drugs are classified as stimulants and alter the patient's mood by affecting levels of neurotransmitters in the brain. Antidepressants, such as monoamine oxidase (MAO) inhibitors, are nonaddictive but they can produce unpleasant side effects such as dry mouth, weight gain, blurred vision, and nausea.

- *Minor* tranquilizers include Valium and Xanax. These are also classified as depressants and are prescribed for anxiety.

- Lithium is a special category of drug. It is used successfully to calm patients who suffer from bipolar disorder (depression alternating with manic excitement).

Electroconvulsive therapy (ECT) is a procedure occasionally used for cases of prolonged major depression. This is a controversial treatment in which an electrode is placed on one or both sides of the patient's head and a current is turned on briefly causing a convulsive seizure. A low level of voltage is used in modern ECT, and the patient is administered a muscle relaxant and anesthesia. Advocates of this treatment state that it is a more effective way to treat severe depression than using drugs. It is not effective with disorders other than depression, such as schizophrenia and alcoholism.

Word Building Relating to Mental Health

The following list contains examples of medical terms built directly from word parts. The definition for these terms can be determined by a straightforward translation of the word parts.

Combining Form	Combined With	Medical Term	Definition
psych/o	-genic	psychogenic (sigh koh **JEN** ik)	formed by the mind
	-ologist	psychologist (sigh **KALL** oh jist)	specialist in the mind
	-ology	psychology (sigh **KALL** oh jee)	study of the mind
	-pathy	psychopathy (sigh **KOP** ah thee)	mind disease

Vocabulary Relating to Mental Health

amnesia (am NEE zee ah)	Loss of memory in which people forget their identity as a result of a head injury or a disorder such as epilepsy, senility, or alcoholism. Can be either temporary or permanent.
delirium (dee LEER ee um)	State of mental confusion with a lack of orientation to time and place.
neurosis (noo ROH sis)	Mental disorder in which there are symptoms such as depression and anxiety.
psychiatrist (sigh KIGH ah trist)	Physician who specializes in the treatment and prevention of mental disorders.
psychiatry (sigh KIGH ah tree)	Branch of medicine that deals with the treatment of mental disorders.
psychologist (sigh KALL oh jist)	Specialist trained in the study of psychological analysis, therapy, and research.
psychology (sigh KALL oh jee)	Study of the mind and behavior.
psychosis (sigh KOH sis)	Severe mental disorder in which there are symptoms such as depression and anxiety, or the patient is not in touch with reality. He or she may withdraw into an inner world, as in schizophrenia, or become severely emotionally impaired, as in mania.
psychosomatic (sigh koh soh MAT ik)	Pertaining to the relationship between the mind and the body. Relates to physical disorders that are thought to originate in the emotional state of the patient.

Abbreviations Relating to Mental Health

ADD	attention deficit disorder		ECT	electroconvulsive therapy
ADHD	attention deficit hyperactivity disorder		MA	mental age
BPD	bipolar disorder		MAO	monoamine oxidase
CA	chronological age		OCD	obsessive-compulsive disorder
DSM	Diagnostic and Statistical Manual for Mental Disorders			

Practice Exercises

P. **MATCH THE MENTAL DISORDER CATEGORY WITH THE CORRECT EXAMPLE.**

A

1. _____ cognitive disorders
2. _____ factitious disorders
3. _____ dissociative disorders
4. _____ eating disorders
5. _____ sleeping disorders
6. _____ mood disorders
7. _____ impulse control disorders
8. _____ somatoform disorders
9. _____ personality disorders
10. _____ sexual disorders
11. _____ anxiety disorders

B

a. hypochondria
b. kleptomania
c. masochism
d. narcissistic personality
e. insomnia
f. bipolar disease
g. panic attacks
h. amnesia
i. dementia
j. anorexia nervosa
k. malingering

Q. **IDENTIFY EACH MENTAL HEALTH TREATMENT FROM ITS DESCRIPTION.**

1. depressant drugs prescribed for anxiety _____

2. client-centered psychotherapy _____

3. drug used to calm patients with bipolar disorder _____

4. reduces patient agitation and panic and shortens schizophrenic episodes _____

   _____

5. obtains a detailed account of the past and present emotional and mental experiences _____

   _____

6. stimulants that alter the patient's mood by affecting neurotransmitter levels _____

   _____

COMBINING FORMS RELATING TO PEDIATRICS

nat/o	birth
ped/o	child

Pediatrics (pee dee **AT** riks) is the branch of medicine specialized in caring for children. **Pediatricians** (pee dee ah **TRISH** ans) are physicians who are involved in the prevention and treatment of childhood diseases. **Neonatologists** (nee oh nay **TALL** oh jists) are even more specialized in the care of newborn infants. Because the needs of children differ in important ways from adults, there are many other pediatric health care professionals. These include pediatric anesthesiology, pediatric dentistry, pediatric neurology, pediatric nursing, and pediatric surgery.

Preventative Care

Pediatricians do not just see children in their offices when they are ill. Parents are encouraged to bring their children for **well-baby** or **well-child check-ups.** During these visits, the physician assesses the child's growth and development and looks for early signs of disease or abnormalities. Parents also receive education in topics such as nutrition and child development. Children also need to receive routine **immunization** (im yoo nih **ZAY** shun) or **vaccination** (vak sih **NAY** shun). Many childhood diseases that were once common are no longer a threat thanks to widespread immunization. Children can now be immunized for the following diseases:

- hepatitis B
- diphtheria, pertussis, tetanus (DPT)
- tetanus
- pertussis
- *Haemophilus influenza* type b (HiB)
- polio
- measles, mumps, rubella (MMR)
- chickenpox

Common Childhood Pathologies

Childhood diseases generally fall into four categories: pathological conditions, communicable diseases, congenital anomalies, and inherited conditions. Many of the common congenital anomalies and inherited conditions have been covered in the system chapters. The following list contains pathological conditions and communicable diseases that are closely associated with childhood.

acute glomerulonephritis (gloh mair yoo loh neh FRYE tis) (AGN)	A form of nephritis that usually follows a streptococcal infection of the upper respiratory tract.
asthma (AZ mah)	Sudden attacks of bronchospasms and swelling of the mucous membranes that narrow the airways. Asthma is found in all age groups, but most often appears during childhood or young adulthood (see Figure 15.20).

(continued)

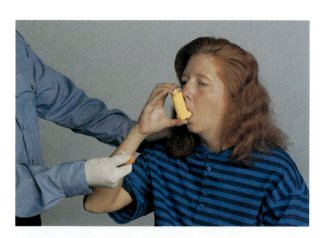

FIGURE 15.20 A prescribed inhaler may help a patient who has respiratory problems.

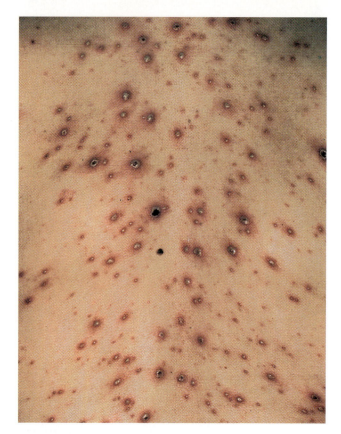

FIGURE 15.21 Chickenpox (varicella).

attention deficit disorder (attention DEFF ih sit dis OR der)	A syndrome affecting children that is characterized by learning and behavioral disabilities.
bronchitis (brong KIGH tis)	An acute or chronic inflammation of the lower respiratory tract that often occurs after other childhood infections such as measles.
cancer (Ca)	Malignant tumors are the leading cause of death in children between the ages of 3 and 15 years of age.
celiac disease (SEE lee ak dih ZEEZ)	The chronic inability to tolerate foods containing gluten (wheat). Symptoms include distended abdomen, diarrhea, vomiting, muscle wasting, and lethargy.
cerebral palsy (CP) (seh REE bral PAWL zee)	A group of disabilities caused by injury to the brain before or during birth or very early in infancy. This is the most common permanent disability in childhood.
chickenpox (varicella)	A contagious infection caused by a *Herpes* virus. It is characterized by a raised rash that turns into blisters and finally scabs over (see Figure 15.21).
congenital hip dysplasia (con JEN ih tal hip dis PLAY zee ah)	An orthopedic condition in which the head of the femur does not articulate with the acetabulum. The hip dislocation can be partial or complete.
croup (KROOP)	Acute viral respiratory infection common in infants and young children and characterized by a hoarse cough.

cryptorchidism (kript OR kid izm)	The failure of one or both of the testicles to descend into the scrotum.
cystic fibrosis (SIS tik fye BROH sis)	A chronic inherited disorder of the exocrine glands characterized by thick pulmonary and intestinal mucus secretions.
diphtheria (diff THEE ree ah)	A bacterial infection of the respiratory system characterized by severe inflammation that can form a membrane coating in the upper respiratory tract. This can cause marked difficulty breathing.
Duchenne muscular dystrophy (MD) (doo SHEN MUSS kew lar DIS troh fee)	An inherited disorder with progressive degeneration and weakness of skeletal muscles.
febrile convulsions (FEB rill kon VULL shuns)	Convulsions brought on by an elevated temperature.
fluid and electrolyte imbalance	Serious secondary development in young children with another illness or infection, particularly those with high fever, vomiting, and diarrhea.
German measles (rubella) (roo BELL lah)	A contagious viral disease that resembles measles (rubeola) but has a shorter course of infection and little fever.
hemophilia (hee moh FILL ee ah)	A hereditary bleeding disorder characterized by a deficiency in a blood clotting factor.
hypothyroidism (high poh THIGH roy dism)	A condition caused by a diminished production of thyroid hormone. In a child, hypothyroidism may result in dwarfism, mental retardation, dry skin, and muscular incoordination.
impetigo (im peh TYE goh)	A highly contagious staphylococcal skin infection, most commonly occurring on the faces of children. It begins as blisters that then rupture and dry into a thick, yellow crust.
intussusception (in tus suh SEP shun)	An intestinal condition in which one portion of the intestine telescopes into an adjacent portion causing an obstruction and gangrene if untreated.
juvenile rheumatoid arthritis (juvenile ROO mah toyd ar THRY tis)	A form of rheumatoid arthritis that usually affects the larger joints of children under the age of 16 years.
lead poisoning	Poisoning that occurs in children who ingest lead, often from paint chips.
leukemia (loo KEE mee ah)	A malignant neoplasm of the blood-forming tissues characterized by the replacement of bone marrow with immature white cells.
measles (rubeola) (roo bee OH lah)	A highly contagious viral disease characterized by fever, malaise, lung congestion, and rash. Also called seven-day measles or red measles.
meconium ileus (meh KOH nee um ILL ee us)	An obstruction of the small intestine in newborn infants that is caused by an impaction of thick meconium, a substance that collects in the intestines of a fetus and becomes the first stool of a newborn.
mental retardation	A disorder characterized by a diminished ability to process intellectual functions.
mumps	A contagious viral disease characterized by high fever and the inflammation and swelling of the parotid salivary glands.
nonorganic failure to thrive (NFTT)	A condition in infants in which the weight remains below the fifth percentile of weight for children of the same age. It is not associated with a particular disease.
otitis media	An inflammation or infection of the middle ear.

(continued)

pertussis (whooping cough) **(per TUH sis)**	A contagious bacterial infection of the larynx, trachea, and bronchi characterized by coughing attacks that end with a whooping sound.
Reye's syndrome **(RISE SIN drohm)**	A brain inflammation that occurs in children following a viral infection, usually the flu or chickenpox. It is characterized by vomiting and lethargy and may lead to coma and death.
roseola (roh zee OH lah)	A viral infection with a rosy red rash.
scarlet fever (scarlatina) **(SCAR let FEE ver)** **(scar lah TEE nah)**	A streptococcal infection characterized by fever and a dense bright red rash that is followed by peeling.
sudden infant death **syndrome (SIDS)**	The sudden, unexplained death of an infant in which a postmortem examination fails to determine the cause of death.
Type 2 diabetes mellitus **(dye ah BEE teez** **MELL ih tus)**	Severe form of diabetes mellitus that often appears before the age of twenty-one. It results from the destruction of the insulin producing tissue in the pancreas, and the patient is dependent on insulin injections.
Wilm's tumor **(VILMZ TOO mor)**	A malignant tumor of the kidney that occurs in young children, usually before the age of five.

Abbreviations Relating to Pediatrics

AGN	acute glomerulonephritis		**MMR**	measles, mumps, rubella
CP	cerebral palsy		**NFTT**	nonorganic failure to thrive
DPT	diphtheria, pertussis, tetanus		**OM**	otitis media
DS	Down syndrome		**SIDS**	sudden infant death syndrome
FTT	failure to thrive		**T & A**	tonsillectomy and adenoidectomy
HiB	*Haemophilus influenzae* type b		**URI**	upper respiratory infection
HMD	hyaline membrane disease		**VSD**	ventricular septal defect

Practice Exercises

R. **LIST THE DISEASES FOR WHICH CHILDREN CAN RECEIVE IMMUNIZATION.**

_____

_____

_____

_____

_____

_____

_____

S. **MATCH EACH DISEASE WITH ITS DESCRIPTION.**

A		B	
1. _____	cystic fibrosis	a.	inability to tolerate foods containing gluten
2. _____	celiac disease	b.	viral disease with fever, malaise, lung congestion, rash
3. _____	asthma	c.	weight remains below the fifth percentile
4. _____	attention deficit disorder	d.	sudden attacks of bronchospasms
5. _____	croup	e.	inflamed and swollen parotid salivary glands
6. _____	red measles	f.	hereditary bleeding disorder
7. _____	mumps	g.	malignant tumor of the kidney
8. _____	hemophilia	h.	inherited disorder with thick mucus secretions
9. _____	otitis media	i.	learning and behavior disabilities
10. _____	Reye's syndrome	j.	brain inflammation following viral infection
11. _____	Wilm's tumor	k.	middle ear infection
12. _____	failure to thrive	l.	viral infection with hoarse cough

- abdominal pain (ab **DOM** ih nal)
- abnormal psychology (sigh **KALL** oh jee)
- active exercises
- active range of motion (AROM)
- active-resistive exercises
- activities of daily living (ADL)
- acute glomerulonephritis (AGN)
  (gloh mair yoo loh neh **FRYE** tis)
- acute illness
- acute myocardial infarction (AMI)
  (my oh **CAR** dee al in **FARC** shun)
- adaptive equipment
- adenocarcinoma (ad eh noh kar sin **NOH** mah)
- adenoma (ad eh **NOH** mah)
- aging
- aided exercises
- airway
- allergic reaction
- Alzheimer's disease (**ALTS** high merz dih **ZEEZ**)
- ambulatory (**AM** byoo lah toh ree)
- amnesia (am **NEE** zee ah)
- amputation (am pew **TAY** shun)
- analgesic (an al **JEE** zik)
- anaphylactic shock (an ah fih **LAK** tik)
- anesthesia (an es **THEE** zee ah)
- anesthesiologist (an es thee zee **OL** oh jist)
- anesthetic (an ess **THET** ik)
- angiocardiography (an jee oh kar dee **OG** rah fee)
- angiogram (**AN** jee oh gram)
- angiography (an jee **OG** rah fee)
- anorexia nervosa (an oh **REK** see ah ner **VOH** sah)
- antisocial personality disorder (an tih **SOH** shal
  per son **AL** ih tee dis **OR** der)
- anxiety (ang **ZY** eh tee)
- aortography (ay or **TOG** rah fee)
- AP view
- aphasia (ah **FAY** zee ah)
- apnea (ap **NEE** ah)
- arteriography (ar tee ree **OG** rah fee)
- arteriosclerosis (ar tee ree oh skleh **ROH** sis)
- arthritis (ar **THRY** tis)
- artificial ventilation
- asphyxia (as **FIK** see ah)
- aspirator (**AS** pih ray tor)
- assisted living
- asthma (**AZ** mah)
- asthmatic attack (az **MAT** ik)
- astrocytoma (ass troh sigh **TOH** mah)
- attention deficit disorder (ADD)
  (attention **DEFF** ih sit dis **OR** der)
- autism (**AW** tizm)
- barium (Ba) (**BAH** ree um)
- barium enema (BaE) (**BAH** ree um **EN** eh mah)
- basal cell carcinoma
  (**BAY** sal **SELL** kar sin **NOH** mah)
- basic life support
- bedside commode

- benign (bee **NINE**)
- biopsy (**BYE** op see)
- bipolar disorder (by **POHL** ar dis **OR** der)
- bite or sting
- blood pressure
- body mechanics
- bone marrow biopsy (**BYE** op see)
- bronchitis (brong **KIGH** tis)
- bronchography (brong **KOG** rah fee)
- bulimia (boo **LIM** ee ah)
- Burkitt's lymphoma (lim **FOH** mah)
- burn
- bursitis (bur **SIGH** tis)
- cancer (Ca)
- carcinogen (kar **SIN** oh jen)
- carcinoma (kar sin **NOH** mah)
- carcinoma in situ (CIS) (kar sin **NOH** mah)
- cardiac arrest (**CAR** dee ak)
- cardiopulmonary resuscitation (CPR)
  (car dee oh **PULL** mon air ee ree suss ih **TAY** shun)
- carpal tunnel syndrome
  (**CAR** pul **TUN** el **SIN** drohm)
- cauterization (kaw ter ih **ZAY** shun)
- celiac disease (**SEE** lee ak dih **ZEEZ**)
- cerebral palsy (CP) (seh **REE** bral **PAWL** zee)
- cerebrovascular accident (CVA)
  (ser eh broh **VASS** kyoo lar **AK** sih dent)
- chemotherapy (chemo) (kee moh **THAIR** ah pee)
- chickenpox (varicella)
- choking
- cholangiogram (koh **LAN** jee oh gram)
- cholecystogram (koh lee **SIS** toh gram)
- chondrosarcoma (kon droh sar **KOH** mah)
- chronic disease (**KRON** ik dih **ZEEZ**)
- circulating nurse
- clamp
- clinical psychologist (sigh **KALL** oh jist)
- congenital hip dysplasia
  (con **JEN** ih tal hip dis **PLAY** zee ah)
- conversion reaction (kon **VER** zhun)
- convulsion (kon **VULL** shun)
- coronary care unit (CCU) (**KOR** ah nair ee)
- crash cart
- crepitation (crep ih **TAY** shun)
- croup (**KROOP**)
- cryosurgery (cry oh **SER** jer ee)
- cryotherapy (cry oh **THAIR** ah pee)
- cryptorchidism (kript **OR** kid izm)
- curette (kyoo **RET**)
- cyclotron (**SIGH** kloh tron)
- cystic fibrosis (**SIS** tik fye **BROH** sis)
- cytologic testing (sigh toh **LOG** ik)
- day surgery
- debridement (day breed **MON**)
- defibrillator (dee **FIB** rih lay tor)
- delirium (dee **LEER** ee um)
- delusions (dee **LOO** zhuns)

- dementia (dee **MEN** she ah)
- dermatoplasty (**DER** mah toh plas tee)
- developmental disabilities
- diabetic coma (dye ah **BET** ik)
- diagnostic (dye ag **NOS** tik)
- dilator (dye **LAY** tor)
- diphtheria (diff **THEE** ree ah)
- discharge planning
- dissection (dih **SEK** shun)
- draping
- drowning
- Duchenne muscular dystrophy
  (doo **SHEN MUSS** kew lar **DIS** troh fee)
- echoencephalogram (ek oh en **SEFF** ah loh gram)
- elder abuse
- electrocautery (ee lek troh **KAW** ter ee)
- electroconvulsive therapy (ECT)
  (ee lek troh kon **VULL** siv **THAIR** ah pee)
- electromyogram (ee lek troh **MY** oh gram)
- electron (ee **LEK** tron)
- emergency medical technician (EMT)
- emergency medicine (EM)
- emergency room
- encapsulated (en **CAP** soo lay ted)
- endoscopic surgery (en doh **SKOP** ik)
- epiglottitis (ep ih glot **TYE** tis)
- epilepsy (**EP** ih lep see)
- epistaxis (ep ih **STAKS** is)
- ergonomics (er goh **NOM** iks)
- Ewing's sarcoma (**YOO** ingz sar **KOH** mah)
- exploratory surgery (ek **SPLOR** ah tor ee **SER** jer ee)
- explosive disorder (ek **SPLOH** siv dis **OR** der)
- febrile convulsions (**FEB** rill kon **VULL** shuns)
- fibrosarcoma (figh broh sar **KOH** mah)
- film
- film badge
- fine motor skills
- first aid
- fluid and electrolyte imbalance
- fluoroscopy (floo **ROS** koh pee)
- Foley catheter (**FOH** lee **CATH** eh ter)
- forceps (**FOR** seps)
- foreign bodies
- Fowler
- fracture
- fracture pan
- gait (**GAYT**)
- gastrectomy (gas **TREK** toh mee)
- gastrostomy tube (gas **TROSS** toh mee)
- Geiger counter (**GYE** ger)
- general anesthesia (an ess **THEE** zee ah)
- geriatric chair (jer ee **AT** rik) (geri-chair)
- German measles (rubella) (roo **BELL** lah)
- gerontology (jer on **TALL** oh jee)
- glioblastoma (glee oh blas **TOH** mah)
- glioma (glee **OH** mah)
- grade
- gross motor skills
- hallucinations (hah loo sih **NAY** shuns)
- head injury

- heat application
- heat hydrotherapy (high droh **THAIR** ah pee)
- Heimlich maneuver (**HYME** lik)
- hemophilia (hee moh **FILL** ee ah)
- hemorrhage (**HEM** eh rij)
- hemostasis (hee moh **STAY** sis)
- hemostat (**HEE** moh stat)
- herniated nucleus pulposus
  (**HER** nee ay ted **NOO** klee us pul **POH** sus)
- Hodgkin's disease (HD) (**HOJ** kins dih **ZEEZ**)
- hormone therapy (**HOR** mohn **THAIR** ah pee)
- hot moist compresses
- hydrotherapy (high droh **THAIR** ah pee)
- hypernephroma (high per neh **FROH** mah)
- hyperplasia (high per **PLAY** zee ah)
- hypochondria (high poh **KON** dree ah)
- hypothyroidism (high poh **THIGH** roy dism)
- hysterosalpingography
  (hiss ter oh sal ping **OG** rah fee)
- ice packs
- immunization (im yoo nih **ZAY** shun)
- immunotherapy (im yoo noh **THAIR** ah pee)
- impetigo (im peh **TYE** goh)
- inhalation method (in hah **LAY** shun)
- insomnia (in **SOM** nee ah)
- insulin reaction (**IN** soo lin)
- intensive care unit (ICU)
- intravenous method (in trah **VEE** nus)
- intubation (in too **BAY** shun)
- intussusception (in tus suh **SEP** shun)
- invasive disease (in **VAY** siv dih **ZEEZ**)
- juvenile rheumatoid arthritis
  (**ROO** mah toyd ar **THRY** tis)
- Kaposi's sarcoma (**KAP** oh seez sar **KOH** mah)
- kleptomania (klep toh **MAY** nee ah)
- laser surgery
- lateral recumbent (**LAT** er al ree **KUM** bent)
- lateral view
- lead poisoning
- leukemia (loo **KEE** mee ah)
- leukoplakia (loo koh **PLAY** kee ah)
- lithotomy (lith **OT** oh mee)
- local anesthesia (an ess **THEE** zee ah)
- long-term care facility
- low sex drive
- lower extremity (LE)
- lumbar puncture (**LUM** bar **PUNK** chur)
- lymphangiography (lim fan jee **OG** rah fee)
- lymphoma (lim **FOH** mah)
- magnetic resonance imaging (MRI)
  (mag **NEH** tik **REHZ** oh nance)
- major depression (**MAY** jer dee **PRES** shun)
- malignant (mah **LIG** nant)
- malignant melanoma
  (mah **LIG** nant mel ah **NOH** mah)
- malingering (mah **LING** er ing)
- mammography (mam **OG** rah fee)
- mania (**MAY** nee ah)
- masochism (**MAS** oh kizm)
- massage (mah **SAHZH**)

- measles (rubeola) (roo bee **OH** lah)
- meconium ileus (meh **KOH** nee um **ILL** ee us)
- medulloblastoma (meh dull oh blas **TOH** mah)
- mental retardation
- metastases (mets) (meh **TASS** tah seez)
- metastasis (mets) (meh **TASS** tah sis)
- mobility
- morbidity (mor **BID** ih tee)
- mortality (mor **TAL** ih tee)
- multiple myeloma
  (**MULL** tih pl my eh **LOH** mah)
- multiple personality disorder (**MULL** tih pl per son **AL** ih tee dis **OR** der)
- multiple sclerosis (MS)
  (**MULL** tih pl skleh **ROH** sis)
- mumps
- muscular dystrophy (**MUSS** kew lar **DIS** troh fee)
- mutation (mew **TAY** shun)
- myelogram (**MY** eh loh gram)
- narcissistic personality disorder
  (nar sis **SIST** ik per son **AL** ih tee dis **OR** der)
- near-drowning
- needle biopsy (**BYE** op see)
- neonatologists (nee oh nay **TALL** oh jists)
- neoplasm (**NEE** oh plazm)
- nephrosarcoma (nef roh sar **KOH** mah)
- nerve block
- nerve conduction velocity
- neuroblastoma (noo roh blass **TOH** mah)
- neurosis (noo **ROH** sis)
- non-Hodgkin's lymphoma (NHL)
- nonorganic failure to thrive (NFTT)
- nurse anesthetist (ah **NES** the tist)
- nursing home
- oblique view (oh **BLEEK**)
- obsessive-compulsive disorder
  (ob **SESS** iv kom **PUHL** siv)
- occupational therapy
- oncogenic (ong koh **JEN** ik)
- oncology (ong **KALL** oh jee)
- open wounds
- operative report
- orthotics (or **THOT** iks)
- osteoarthritis (oss tee oh ar **THRY** tis)
- osteoporosis (oss tee oh por **ROH** sis)
- otitis media (oh **TYE** tis **MEE** dee ah)
- PA view
- pain control
- palliative therapy (**PAL** ee ah tiv **THAIR** ah pee)
- panic attacks
- paranoid personality disorder
  (**PAIR** ah noyd per son **AL** ih tee dis **OR** der)
- paraplegia (pair ah **PLEE** jee ah)
- Parkinson's disease (**PARK** in sons dih **ZEEZ**)
- passive aggressive personality
  (**PASS** iv ah **GRESS** iv per son **AL** ih tee)
- passive range of motion
- pathological gambling (path ah **LOJ** ih kal)
- pathologist (path **ALL** oh jist)
- pediatricians (pee dee ah **TRISH** ans)

- pediatrics (pee dee **AT** riks)
- pedophilia (pee doh **FILL** ee ah)
- percussion (per **KUH** shun)
- perioperative (per ee **OP** er ah tiv)
- pertussis (whooping cough) (per **TUH** sis)
- phobias (**FOH** bee ahs)
- phonophoresis (foh noh foh **REE** sis)
- photophobia (foh toh **FOH** bee ah)
- physiatrist (fiz ee **AT** rist)
- physical medicine
- physical therapy
- pneumothorax (new moh **THOH** raks)
- poisoning
- poliomyelitis (poh lee oh my ell **EYE** tis)
- positron emission tomography (PET)
  (**PAHZ** ih tron ee **MISH** un toh **MOG** rah fee)
- postoperative (post **OP** er ah tiv)
- postural drainage with clapping
- premature ejaculation (ee jak yoo **LAY** shun)
- preoperative (pree **OP** er ah tiv)
- pressure sore
- primary site
- probe
- prone (**PROHN**)
- prosthetics (pros **THET** iks)
- protocol (prot) (**PROH** toh kall)
- psychiatric nurses (sigh kee **AT** rik)
- psychiatric social workers (sigh kee **AT** rik)
- psychiatrist (sigh **KIGH** ah trist)
- psychiatry (sigh **KIGH** ah tree)
- psychogenic (sigh koh **JEN** ik)
- psychologist (sigh **KALL** oh jist)
- psychology (sigh **KALL** oh jee)
- psychopathy (sigh **KOP** ah thee)
- psychopharmacology
  (sigh koh far mah **KALL** oh jee)
- psychosis (sigh **KOH** sis)
- psychosomatic (sigh koh soh **MAT** ik)
- psychotherapy (sigh koh **THAIR** ah pee)
- pyromania (pie roh **MAY** nee ah)
- quad cane
- quadriplegia (kwod rih **PLEE** jee ah)
- radiation therapy
  (ray dee **AY** shun **THAIR** ah pee)
- radical surgery
- radioactive (ray dee oh **AK** tiv)
- radioactive implant (ray dee oh **AK** tiv)
- radiography (ray dee **OG** rah fee)
- radioisotope (ray dee oh **EYE** soh tohp)
- radiologist (ray dee **ALL** oh jist)
- radiology (ray dee **ALL** oh jee)
- radiopaque (ray dee oh **PAYK**)
- range of motion
- regional anesthesia (an ess **THEE** zee ah)
- rehabilitation (ree hah bill ih **TAY** shun)
- remission (rih **MISH** un)
- repetitive motion injury
- resection (ree **SEK** shun)
- residency
- respiratory failure (**RES** pih rah tor ee)

- restorative care
- retinoblastoma (ret ih noh blas **TOH** mah)
- Reye's syndrome (**RISE SIN** drohm)
- rheumatoid arthritis (RA) (**ROO** mah toyd ar **THRY** tis)
- roentgen (**RENT** gen)
- roentgen ray (**RENT** gen)
- roentgenologist (rent gen **ALL** oh jist)
- roseola (roh zee **OH** lah)
- sarcoma (sar **KOH** mah)
- scalpel
- scan
- scarlet fever (scarlatina) (**SCAR** let **FEE** ver) (scar lah **TEE** nah)
- scrub nurse
- senile (**SEE** nyl)
- shield
- shock
- shower chair
- sleepwalking
- sonogram (**SON** oh gram)
- speculum (**SPEK** yoo lum)
- spinal cord injury
- sprain
- stabilize
- staging
- staging laparotomy (lap ah **ROT** oh mee)
- strain
- subcutaneous (sub kyoo **TAY** nee us)
- sucking chest wound
- sudden infant death syndrome (SIDS)
- supine (soo **PINE**)
- surgeon (**SER** jen)
- surgery (**SER** jer ee)
- suture material (**SOO** cher)
- syncope (**SIN** koh pee)
- tagging

- tenaculum (teh **NAK** yoo lum)
- tendonitis (ten dun **EYE** tis)
- terminal illness
- therapeutic (thair ah **PEW** tik)
- therapeutic exercise (thair ah **PEW** tik)
- thermograph (**THER** moh graf)
- thermotherapy (ther moh **THAIR** ah pee)
- thoracotomy (thor ah **KOT** oh mee)
- topical anesthesia (**TOP** ih kal an ess **THEE** zee ah)
- topically
- tourniquet (**TOOR** nih ket)
- traction (**TRAK** shun)
- transcutaneous electrical nerve stimulation (TENS) (tranz kyoo **TAY** nee us ee **LEK** trih kl nerve stim yoo **LAY** shun)
- trauma (**TRAW** mah)
- Trendelenburg (**TREN** dee len berg)
- trephine (treh **FINE**)
- triage (tree **AHZH**)
- tumors (**TOO** mors)
- Type 2 diabetes mellitus (dye ah **BEE** teez **MELL** ih tus)
- ultrasound (US) (**ULL** trah sound)
- upper extremity
- uptake
- urinal (**YOO** rih nal)
- vaccination
- venography (vee **NOG** rah fee)
- vital signs (VS)
- voyeurism (**VOY** er izm)
- walker
- well-baby check-ups
- well-child check-ups
- whirlpool
- Wilm's tumor (**VILMZ TOO** mor)
- X-ray

Getting Connected

Multimedia Extension Activities

CD-ROM

Use the CD-ROM enclosed with your textbook to gain additional reinforcement through interactive word building exercises, spelling games, labeling activities, and additional quizzes.

www.prenhall.com/fremgen

Use the above address to access the free, interactive Companion Website created for this textbook. Get hints, instant feedback, and textbook references to chapter-related multiple choice questions, and labeling and matching exercises. In addition, you will find an audio glossary, case studies, Internet exploration exercises, flashcards, and a comprehensive exam.

Answers

CHART NOTE (ONCOLOGY)

1. oncologist—specialist in the treatment of cancer   2. exploratory surgery—surgery performed to determine if cancer is present   3. biopsies—small samples of tissue removed for examination under a microscope   4. malignant—cancerous with a tendency to grow worse   5. neoplasm—new and abnormal growth   6. Grade II—graded to be moderately differentiated   7. encapsulated—enclosed in a sheath of tissue   8. metastases—spreading to another part of the body   9. nephrosarcoma—cancer of the kidney   10. protocol—plan of treatment   11. chemotherapy—use of chemical agents with a specific toxic effect

PRACTICE EXERCISES

A. 1. emergency medical services   2. emergency medical technician   3. cerebrovascular accident   4. myocardial infarction   5. respirations, pulse, blood pressure, skin color, body temperature, pupil reaction   6. epilepsy   7. epistaxis   8. anaphylactic shock

B. 1. myocardial infarction   2. neonatal intensive care unit   3. chest pain   4. immediately   5. shortness of breath   6. complains of   7. cerebrovascular accident   8. gunshot wound   9. fracture   10. surgical intensive care unit   11. cardiac care unit   12. delerium tremens   13. sudden infant death syndrome

C. 1. chronic disease   2. restorative care   3. nursing home   4. ambulate   5. terminal illness

D. 1. activities of daily living   2. eating, toileting, dressing, bathing, mobility, continence of bowels and urine   3. Alzheimer's disease, fractures, arteriosclerosis, arthritis, osteoarthritis, aphasia

E. 1. c   2. d   3. a   4. e   5. b

F. 1. magnetic resonance imaging   2. barium   3. anteroposterior   4. computerized tomography   5. right lateral   6. posteroanterior   7. left lateral   8. positive emission tomography   9. upper gastrointestinal series   10. lower gastrointestinal series

G. 1. uterus and fallopian tubes   2. aorta   3. gallbladder   4. lymphatic vessel   5. breast   6. heart and blood vessels   7. bronchus   8. spinal cord

H. 1. radioisotope   2. X-ray   3. scan   4. diagnostic, therapeutic   5. cyclotron   6. ultrasound or echograph   7. thermograph

I. 1. lymphatic system   2. blood producing organs   3. skin mole   4. brain or spinal cord   5. cartilage   6. kidney   7. skin   8. connective tissue   9. glandular tissue   10. multiple areas, often of the skin

J. 1. h   2. d   3. g   4. j   5. f   6. b   7. i   8. a   9. e   10. c

K. 1. c   2. f   3. i   4. a   5. b   6. h   7. j   8. d   9. g   10. e

L. 1. range of motion   2. cerebrovascular accident   3. herniated nucleus pulposus   4. lower extremity   5. electromyogram   6. transcutaneous electrical nerve stimulation   7. multiple sclerosis   8. spinal cord injury   9. electrical stimulation   10. ultrasound

M. 1. massage   2. debridement   3. hydrotherapy   4. postural drainage with clapping   5. active exercises   6. phonophoresis   7. cryotherapy   8. traction

N. 1. h   2. e   3. j   4. g   5. a   6. i   7. c   8. f   9. b   10. d

O. 1. general anesthesia   2. local anesthesia   3. topical anesthesia   4. regional anesthesia

P. 1. i   2. k   3. h   4. j   5. e   6. f   7. b   8. a   9. d   10. c   11. g

Q. 1. minor tranquilizers   2. humanistic psychotherapy   3. lithium   4. antipsychotic drugs   5. psychoanalysis   6. antidepressant drugs

R. hepatitis B, diphtheria, tetanus, pertussis, Haemophilus influenza type b, polio, measles, mumps, rubella, chickenpox

S. 1. h   2. a   3. d   4. i   5. l   6. b   7. e   8. f   9. k   10. j   11. g   12. c

APPENDIX

ABBREVIATIONS

Abbreviation	Meaning	Abbreviation	Meaning
–	minus/concave	am, AM	morning
@	at	AMI	acute myocardial infarction
+	plus/convex	AML	acute myelogenous leukemia
3x	three times	amt	amount
5-FU	5-fluorouracil	Angio	angiography
–	before	ANS	autonomic nervous system
A&P	ascultation and percussion	ante	before
aa	of each	AP	anteroposterior
AB	abortion	APB	atrial premature beat
Ab	abortion	aq	aqueous (water)
ABG	arterial blood gases	ARC	AIDS-related complex
AC	air conduction	ARDS	adult respiratory distress syndrome
ac	before meals	ARF	acute renal failure
ACAT	automated computerized axial tomography	ARF	acute respiratory failure
Acc	accommodation	ARMD	age-related macular degeneration
ACL	anterior cruciate ligament	AROM	active range of motion
ACLS	advanced cardiac life support	AS	aortic stenosis, arteriosclerosis, left ear
ACTH	adrenocorticotropic hormone	ASCVD	arteriosclerotic cardiovascular disease
AD	right ear	ASD	atrial septal defect
ad lib	as desired	ASHD	arteriosclerotic heart disease
ADD	attention deficit disorder	ASL	American Sign Language
ADH	antidiuretic hormone	Astigm.	astigmatism
ADHD	attention deficit hyperactivity disorder	AU	both ears
ADL	activities of daily living	AV, A-V	atrioventricular
AF	atrial fibrillation	Ba	barium
AGN	acute glomerulonephritis	BaE	barium enema
AH	abdominal hysterectomy	baso	basophil
AI	aortic insufficiency	BBB	bundle branch block (L for left; R for right)
AIDS	acquired immunodeficiency syndrome	BC	bone conduction
AIH	artificial insemination homologous	BE	barium enema
ALL	acute lymphocytic leukemia	bid	twice a day
ALS	amyotropic lateral sclerosis	BM	bowel movement
alt dieb	alternate days	BMR	basal metabolic rate
alt hor	alternate hours	BP	blood pressure
alt noc	alternate nights		

Abbreviation	Meaning	Abbreviation	Meaning
BPD	bipolar disorder	CNS	central nervous system
BPH	benign prostatic hypertrophy	CO_2	carbon dioxide
bpm	beats per minute	COLD	chronic obstructive lung disease
Broncho	bronchoscopy	COPD	chronic obstructive pulmonary disease
BS	breath sounds, bowel sounds	CP	cerebral palsy, chest pain
BUN	blood urea nitrogen	CPD	cephalopelvic disproportion
BX, bx	biopsy	CPR	cardiopulmonary resuscitation
c̄	with	CRF	chronic renal failure
C	100	CS	sputum culture and sensitivity
C&S	culture and sensitivity test	CS, CS-section	cesarean section
c.gl.	correction with glasses	CSD	congenital septal defect
c/o	complains of	CSF	cerebrospinal fluid
C1, C2, etc.	first cervical vertebra, second cervical vertebra, etc.	C-spine	cervical spine film
Ca	calcium, cancer	CT	computerized tomography
CA	cancer, chronological age	CTA	clear to auscultation
CABG	coronary artery bypass graft	CTS	carpal tunnel syndrome
CAD	coronary artery disease	CUC	chronic ulcerative colitis
cap(s)	capsule(s)	CV	cardiovascular
CAPD	continuous ambulatory peritoneal dialysis	CVA	cerebrovascular accident
CAT, CT	computerized axial tomography	CVP	central venous pressure
cath	catheterization	CWP	childbirth without pain
CBC	complete blood count	Cx	cervix
CBD	common bile duct	CXR	chest X-ray
CC	clean-catch urine specimen	cyl	cylindrical lens
cc	cubic centimeter	cysto	cystoscopic exam
CCU	cardiac care unit, coronary care unit	d	day
CD4	protein on T-cell helper lymphocyte	D	diopter (lens strength)
CDH	congenital dislocation of the hip	D & C	dilation and curettage
CGL	chronic granulocytic leukemia	D/C, d/c, DISC	discontinue
CHD	congestive heart disease	dB	decibel
chemo	chemotherapy	DEA	Drug Enforcement Agency
CHF	congestive heart failure	Derm	dermatology
CHO	carbohydrate	DI	diabetes insipidus
chol	cholesterol	diff	differential
Ci	curie	dil	dilute
CIC	coronary intensive care	disp	dispense
CIS	carcinoma in situ	DM	diabetes mellitus
Cl	chloride	DOA	dead on arrival
CLL	chronic lymphocytic leukemia	DOB	date of birth
		DOE	dyspnea on exertion

Abbreviation	Meaning
DPT	diphtheria, pertussis, tetanus
dr	dram
DRE	digital rectal exam
DS	Down syndrome
DSA	digital subtraction angiography
DSM	Diagnostic and Statistical Manual for Mental Disorders
DTR	deep tendon reflex
DT'S	delerium tremens
DUB	dysfunctional uterine bleeding
DVA	distance visual acuity
DVT	deep vein thrombosis
Dx	diagnosis
E. coli	*Escherichia coli*
EAU	exam under anesthesia
EBV	Epstein-Barr virus
ECC	endocervical curettage
ECCE	extracapsular cataract extraction
ECG, EKG	electrocardiogram
ECT	electroconvulsive therapy
EDC	estimated date of confinement
EEG	electroencephalogram, electroencephalography
EENT	eyes, ears, nose, throat
EGD	esophagogastroduodenoscopy
ELISA	enzyme-linked immunosorbent assay
elix	elixir
EM	emmetropia (normal vision)
EMG	electromyogram
EMS	emergency medical services system
EMT	emergency medical technician
EMT-P	paramedic
emul	emulsion
Endo	endoscopy
ENT	ear, nose, and throat
EOM	extraocular movement
eosin	eosinophil
ER	emergency room
ERCP	endoscopic retrograde cholangiopancreatography

Abbreviation	Meaning
ERT	estrogen replacement therapy, external radiation therapy
ERV	expiratory reserve volume
ESR, SR, sed rate	erythrocyte sedimentation rate
EST	electric shock therapy
e-stim	electrical stimulation
ESWL	extracorporeal shock-wave lithotripsy
et	and
ET	endotracheal
ext	extract/external
FBS	fasting blood sugar
FDA	Federal Drug Administration
Fe	iron
FEF	forced expiratory flow
FEKG	fetal electrocardiogram
FEV	forced expiratory volume
FHR	fetal heart rate
FHT	fetal heart tone
fl	fluid
FRC	functional residual capacity
FS	frozen section
FSH	follicle-stimulating hormone
FTND	full-term normal delivery
FTT	failure to thrive
FVC	forced vital capacity
Fx, FX	fracture
Ga	gallium
GA	general anesthesia
gal	gallon
GB	gallbladder
geri-chair	geriatric chair
GH	growth hormone
GI	gastrointestinal
GI, grav I	first pregnancy
GM, gm	gram
gr	grain
GSW	gunshot wound
gt	drop
gtt	drops
GTT	glucose tolerance test

Abbreviation	Meaning	Abbreviation	Meaning
GU	genitourinary	iii	three
GYN, gyn	gynecology	IM	intramuscular
H	hour, hypodermic	inj	injection
H₂O	water	IOL	intraocular lens
HAA	hepatitis-associated antigen	IOP	intraocular pressure
HAV	hepatitis A virus	IPD	intermittent peritoneal dialysis
HBIG	hepatitis B immune globulin	IPPB	intermittent positive pressure breathing
HBOT	hyperberic oxygen therapy	IRDS	infant respiratory distress syndrome
HBV	hepatitis B virus	IRT	internal radiation therapy
HCG	human chorionic gonadotropin	IRV	inspiratory reserve volume
HCT, Hct, crit	hematocrit	IU	international unit
HCV	hepatitis C virus	IUD	intrauterine device
HD	hemodialysis, Hodgkin's disease	IV	intravenous
HDL	high-density lipoproteins	IVC	intravenous cholangiogram
HEENT	head, ears, eyes, nose, throat	IVCD	intraventricular conduction delay
Hgb, Hb	hemoglobin	IVP	intravenous pyelogram
HGH	human growth hormone	IVU	intravenous urogram
HiB	*Haemophilus influenzae* type b	JVP	jugular venous pulse
HIV	human immunodeficiency virus	K	potassium
HMD	hyaline membrane disease	KB	knee bearing
HNP	herniated nucleus pulposus	kg	kilogram
HRT	hormone replacement therapy	KS	Kaposi's sarcoma
hs	hour of sleep	KUB	kidney, ureter, bladder
HSG	hysterosalpingography	kV	kilovolt
HSO	hysterosalpingoophrectomy	kW	kilowatt
HSV	herpes simplex virus	L	left, liter
HTN	hypertension	L&A	light and accommodation
Hz	Hertz	L1, L2, etc.	first lumbar vertebra, second lumbar vertebra, etc.
i	one	LAC	laceration
I & D	incision and drainage	LASIK	laser-assisted in-situ keratomileusis
I & O	intake and output	LAT, lat	lateral
IBD	inflammatory bowel disease	LB	large bowel
IBS	irritable bowel syndrome	LBW	low birth weight
IC	intracardiac	LDL	low-density lipoproteins
ICCE	intracapsular cataract cryoextraction	LE	left eye, lower extremity, lupus erythematosus
ICU	intensive care unit	LGI	lower gastrointestinal series
ID	intradermal	LIF	left iliac fossa
IDDM	insulin-dependent diabetes mellitus	liq	liquid
Ig	immunoglobins (IgA, IgD, IgE, IgG, IgM)		
ii	two		

Abbreviation	Meaning
LK&S	liver, kidney, and spleen
LL	left lateral
LLE	left lower extremity
LLL	left lower lobe
LLQ	left lower quadrant
LMP	last menstrual period
LOM	limitation of motion
LP	lumbar puncture
LUE	left upper extremity
LUL	left upper lobe
LUQ	left upper quadrant
LVAD	left ventricular assist device
Lymph, lymph	lymphocyte
mA	milliampere
MA	mental age
MAO	monoamine oxidase
MBC	maximal breathing capacity
mcg	microgram
mCi	millicurie
mEq	milliequivalent
mets	metastases
mg	milligram
MH	marital history
MI	myocardial infarction, mitral insufficiency
MICU	mobile intensive care unit
mL	milliliter
mm	millimeter
mmHg	millimeters of mercury
MMR	measles, mumps, rubella
Mono, mono	monocyte, mononucleosis
MR	mitral regurgitation
MRI	magnetic resonance imaging
MS	mitral stenosis, multiple sclerosis, musculoskeletal
MSH	melanocyte-stimulating hormone
MTX	methotrexate
MUA	manipulation under anesthesia
MV	minute volume
MVA	motor vehicle accident
MVP	mitral valve prolapse

Abbreviation	Meaning
MVV	maximal voluntary ventilation
MY	myopia
n&v	nausea and vomiting
Na	sodium
NAD	no apparent distress
NB	newborn
NCU	nongonococcal urethritis
NED	no evidence of disease
NFTT	nonorganic failure to thrive
NG	nasogastric (tube)
NGU	nongonococcal urethritis
NHL	non-Hodgkin's lymphoma
NICU	neonatal intensive care
NIDDM	non-insulin-dependent diabetes mellitus
NMR	nuclear magnetic resonance
no sub	no substitute
noc, noct	night
non rep	do not repeat
NPDL	nodular, poorly differentiated lymphocytes
NPH	neutral protamine Hagedorn (insulin)
NPO	nothing by mouth
NS	normal saline
NSAID	non-steroidal anti-inflammatory drug
NSR	normal sinus rhythm
NVA	near visual acuity
O	pint
O&P	ova and parasites
O_2	oxygen
OB	obstetrics
OCD	obsessive-compulsive disorder
OCG	oral cholecystography
od	once a day, daily
OD	overdose, right eye
oint., ung	ointment
om	every morning
OM	otitis media
Ophth.	ophthalmology
OR	operating room
ortho	orthopedics
OS	left eye

Abbreviation	Meaning	Abbreviation	Meaning
OT	occupational therapy	PPD	purified protein derivative (tuberculin test)
OTC	over the counter	preop, pre-op	preoperative
Oto	otology	prep	preparation, prepared
OU	each eye	PRK	photo refractive keratectomy
oz	ounce	prn	as needed
p	after	Pro time	prothrombin time
P	pulse	PROM	passive range of motion
P.O.	per os (by mouth)	prot	protocol
PA	posteroanterior	PSA	prostate specific antigen
PAP	Papanicolaou test, pulmonary arterial pressure	pt	pint
PARR	postanesthetic recovery room	PT	prothrombin time, physical therapy
PAT	paroxysmal atrial tachycardia	PTC	percutaneous transhepatic cholangiography
PBI	protein bound iodine	PTCA	percutaneous transluminal coronary angioplasty
pc	after meals	PTH	parathyroid hormone
PCP	*Pneumocystis carinii* pneumonia	pulv	powder
PCV	packed cell volume	PVC	premature ventricular contraction
PDR	*Physicians Desk Reference*	q	every
PE tube	polyethylene tube placed in the eardrum	qam	every morning
PEG	pneumoencephalogram, percutaneous endoscopic gastrostomy	qd	once a day, every day
per	with	qh	every hour
PERRLA	pupils equal, round, react to light and accommodation	qhs	every night
		qid	four times a day
PET	positive emission tomography	qod	every other day
PFT	pulmonary function test	qs	quantity sufficient
PGH	pituitary growth hormone	R	respiration, right, roentgen
pH	acidity or alkalinity of urine	Ra	radium
PI, para I	first delivery	RA	rheumatoid arthritis
PID	pelvic inflammatory disease	rad	radiation absorbed dose
PKU	phenylketonuria	RAI	radioactive iodine
PM	evening	RAIU	radioactive iodine uptake
PMN, seg, poly	polymorphonuclear neutrophil	RBC	red blood cell
PMP	previous menstrual period	RD	respiratory disease
PMS	premenstrual syndrome	RDA	recommended daily allowance (dietary allowance)
PND	paroxysmal nocturnal dyspnea (also postnasal drip)	RDS	respiratory distress syndrome
PNS	peripheral nervous system	RE	right eye
po	by mouth	REM	rapid eye movement
PO	phone order	RIA	radioimmunoassay
PP	postprandial (after meals)	RIF	right iliac fossa
		RL	right lateral

Abbreviation	Meaning
RLE	right lower extremity
RLL	right lower lobe
RLQ	right lower quadrant
RML	right mediolateral
RML	right middle lobe
ROM	range of motion
RP	retrograde pyelogram
RRT	registered radiologic technologist
RRV	respiratory reserve volume
RUE	right upper extremity
RUL	right upper lobe
RUQ	right upper quadrant
Rx	take
s	without
s.gl.	without correction or glasses
S/R	suture removal
S1	first heart sound
S1, S2, etc.	first sacral vertebra, second sacral vertebra, etc.
S2	second heart sound
SA, S-A	sinoatrial
SBE	subacute bacterial endocarditis
SBFT	small bowel follow-through
SC	subcutaneous
SCI	spinal cord injury
SCLE	subacute cutaneous lupus erythematosus
SEE-2	Signing Exact English
SG	skin graft
SG	specific gravity
SGOT	serum glutamic oxaloacetic transaminase
SICU	surgical intensive care unit
SIDS	sudden infant death syndrome
Sig	label as follows/directions
SK	streptokinase
sl	under the tongue
SLE	systemic lupus erythematosus
SMD	senile macular degeneration
SOB	shortness of breath
sol	solution
SOM	serous otitis media

Abbreviation	Meaning
SPP	suprapubic prostatectomy
ss	one-half
st	stage
ST	skin test
stat, STAT	at once, immediately
STD	skin test done, sexually transmitted disease
STSG	split-thickness skin graft
Subc, SubQ, Subcu, Subq	subcutaneous
subling	sublingual
suppos, supp.	suppository
susp	suspension
SVT	supraventricular tachycardia
syr	syrup
T & A	tonsillectomy and adenoidectomy
T, tbsp	tablespoon
t, tsp	teaspoon
T1, T2, etc.	first thoracic vertebra, second thoracic vertebra, etc.
T_3	triiodothyronine
T_4	thyroxine
T4	T-cell lymphocyte (destroyed by the AIDS virus)
T_7	free thyroxine index
T8	T-cell lymphocyte (cytotoxic or killer cell)
tab	tablet
TAH	total abdominal hysterectomy
TB	tuberculosis
TENS	transcutaneous electrical nerve stimulation
TFT	thyroid function test
THR	total hip replacement
TIA	transient ischemic attack
tid	three times a day
tinc, tr	tincture
TKA	total knee arthroplasty
TKR	total knee replacement
TLC	total lung capacity
TNM	tumor, nodes, metastases
TO	telephone order
top	apply topically

Abbreviation	Meaning	Abbreviation	Meaning
tPA	tissue-type plasminogen activator	ut dict, UD	as directed
TPN	total parenteral nutrition	UT	under the tongue
TPR	temperature, pulse, and respiration	UTI	urinary tract infection
TSH	thyroid-stimulating hormone	UV	ultraviolet
TSS	toxic shock syndrome	VA	visual acuity
TUR	transurethral resection	VC	vital capacity
TURP	transurethral resection of prostate	VD	venereal disease
TV	tidal volume	VDRL	Venereal Disease Research Laboratory
TX, Tx	traction, treatment	VF	visual field
u	unit	VLDL	very low density lipoproteins
U/A, UA	urinalysis	VO	verbal order
UC	uterine contractions	VPB	ventricular premature beat
UC	urine culture	VS	vital signs
UCHD	usual childhood diseases	VSD	ventricular septal defect
UE	upper extremity	WBC	white blood cell
UGI	upper gastrointestinal series	WNL	within normal limits
ung	ointment	WPW	Wolff–Parkinson–White syndrome
URI	upper respiratory infection	wt	weight
US	ultrasound	x4	four times

PREFIX APPENDIX

Prefix	Meaning
a-	without, away from
ab-	away from
ad-	toward
alb-	white
ambi-	both, both sides
an-	without
ante-	before, in front of
antero-	before, in front of
anti-	against
auto-	self
bi-	two
brady-	slow
chlor-	green
circum-	around
con-	with, together
contra-	against
cryo-	cold
cyan-	blue
de-	down
dextro-	on the right
di-	two
dia-	through, across
diplo-	double
dorso-	back
dys-	painful, difficult
ec-	out, out from
endo-	within, inner
epi-	upon, over, above
erythr-	red
eu-	normal, good
ex-	away from or out
exo-	out
hemi-	half
hetero-	different
homo-	same
hydro-	water
hyper-	over, above
hypo-	under, below
im-	not
in-	not, into
infra-	under, beneath, below
inter-	among, between
intra-	within, inside
latero-	side

Prefix	Meaning
leuk-	white
macro-	large
mal-	bad, ill
medi-	middle
melan-	black
meso-	middle
meta-	change, beyond
micro-	small
mid-	middle
mono-	one
multi-	many
myo-	muscle
neo-	new
nulli-	none
pachy-	thick
pan-	all
para-	beside, beyond, near
per-	through
peri-	around or about
poly-	many
post-	behind or after
postero-	after, behind
pre-	before, in front of
pro-	before, in front of
pseudo-	false
quad-	four
re-	again, back
retro-	backward, behind
rube-	red
sclero-	hard
semi-	partial, half
sinistro-	to the left
sub-	below, under
super-	above, excess
supra-	above
sym-	together
syn-	together
tachy-	rapid, fast
trans-	through, across
tri-	three
ultra-	beyond, excess
uni-	one
xanth-	yellow

SUFFIX APPENDIX

Suffix	Meaning
-a	converts a word root to a noun
-ac	pertaining to
-al	pertaining to
-algesia	pain, sensitivity
-algia	pain
-an	pertaining to
-ar	pertaining to
-arche	beginning
-ary	pertaining to
-blast	immature, embryonic
-cele	hernia, protrusion
-centesis	puncture to withdraw fluid
-chalasis	relaxation
-cide	kill
-cise	cut
-clasia	to surgically break
-cle	small
-coccus	berry-shaped
-crine	to secrete
-cusis	hearing
-cyesis	state of pregnancy
-cyte	cell
-cytosis	condition of cells
-derma	skin
-desis	stabilize, fuse
-dipsia	thirst
-dynia	pain
-eal	pertaining to
-ectasis	dilatation
-ectomy	surgical removal
-ectopia	displacement
-emesis	vomit
-emia	blood condition
-er	one who
-esthesia	feeling, sensation
-gen	that which produces
-genesis	produces, generates
-genic	producing
-globulin	protein
-gram	record

Suffix	Meaning
-graph	instrument for recording
-graphy	process of recording
-gravida	pregnancy
-ia	state, condition
-iac	pertaining to
-iasis	abnormal condition
-iatric	medicine, physician
-iatrist	physician
-ic	pertaining to
-ical	pertaining to
-ile	pertaining to
-ine	a substance
-ion	process
-ior	pertaining to
-ism	state of
-ist	one who specializes in
-itis	inflammation
-ium	converts word root into a noun
-ize	to make, to use, take away
-kinesia	movement
-lapse	to slide, sag
-lepsy	seizure
-lith	stone
-logist	one who studies
-logy	study of
-lytic	destruction
-malacia	softening
-mania	excessive excitement
-manometer	instrument to measure pressure
-megaly	enlarged
-meter	instrument for measuring
-metry	process of measuring
-mycosis	fungal infection
-oid	resembling
-ole	small
-ology	study of
-oma	tumor, mass
-opaque	nontransparent
-opia	vision
-ory	pertaining to

Abbreviation	Meaning	Abbreviation	Meaning
-ose	pertaining to	**-rrhage**	excessive, abnormal flow
-osis	abnormal condition	**-rrhaphy**	suture
-ostomy	surgically create an opening	**-rrhea**	discharge, flow
-otomy	incision into	**-rrhexis**	rupture
-ous	pertaining to	**-salpinx**	fallopian tube
-para	to bear	**-sclerosis**	hardening
-paresis	weakness	**-scope**	instrument for viewing
-parous	bearing, give birth	**-scopy**	process of visually examining
-partum	birth, labor	**-sis**	condition
-pathy	disease	**-spasm**	involuntary muscle contraction
-penia	abnormal decrease	**-stalsis**	constriction, contraction
-pepsia	digestion	**-stasis**	standing still
-pexy	surgical fixation	**-stenosis**	narrowing
-phagia	eat, swallow	**-sthenia**	strength
-phasia	speech	**-taxia**	muscular coordination
-phil	to have an attraction for	**-tension**	pressure
-philia	to have an attraction for	**-therapy**	treatment
-phobia	irrational fear	**-tic**	pertaining to
-phoria	feeling, mental state	**-tocia**	labor, childbirth
-physis	to grow	**-tome**	instrument used to cut
-plakia	plate, patch	**-toxic**	poison
-plasia	growth, formation	**-tripsy**	surgical crushing
-plasm	growth, formation	**-trophy**	nourishment, development
-plasty	surgical repair	**-tropia**	to turn
-plegia	paralysis	**-tropic**	stimulate
-pnea	breathing	**-ule**	small
-poiesis	formation	**-um**	converts word root into a noun
-porosis	porous	**-uria**	condition of the urine
-prandial	pertaining to a meal	**-us**	converts word root into a noun
-ptosis	drooping	**-version**	turning of

abdomin/o	abdomen	**blast/o**	primitive cell
acetabul/o	acetabulum	**blephar/o**	eyelid
acous/o	hearing	**brachi/o**	arm
acr/o	extremities	**bronch/i**	bronchus
acu/o	needle, sharp	**bronch/o**	bronchus
aden/o	gland	**bronchi/o**	bronchiole
adenoid/o	adenoids	**bronchiol/o**	bronchiole
adip/o	fat	**bucc/o**	cheek
adren/o	adrenal glands	**burs/o**	sac
adrenal/o	adrenal glands	**calc/i**	calcium
aer/o	air	**calc/o**	calcium
agglutin/o	clumping	**calcane/o**	calcaneus, heel bone
albin/o	white	**carcin/o**	cancer
algesi/o	pain	**cardi/o**	heart
aliment/o	nourish	**carp/o**	wrist
alveol/o	alveolus; air sac	**caud/o**	tail
ambly/o	dull or dim	**caus/o**	burn, burning
amni/o	amnion	**cec/o**	cecum
amnion/o	amnion	**celi/o**	abdomen
amyl/o	starch	**cephal/o**	head
an/o	anus	**cerebell/o**	cerebellum
andr/o	male	**cerebr/o**	cerebrum
angi/o	vessel	**cervic/o**	neck, cervix
ankyl/o	stiff joint	**cervis/o**	cervix, neck
anter/o	front	**cheil/o**	lip
append/o	appendix	**chem/o**	chemical
appendic/o	appendix	**chol/e**	bile, gall
aque/o	water	**chol/o**	bile, gall
arter/o	artery	**cholangi/o**	bile duct
arteri/o	artery	**cholecyst/o**	gallbladder
arthr/o	joint	**choledoch/o**	common bile duct
asthesi/o	sensation, feeling	**chondr/o**	cartilage
ather/o	fatty substance, plaque	**chori/o**	chorion
atri/o	atrium	**chrom/o**	color
audi/o	hearing	**chron/o**	time
audit/o	hearing	**cis/o**	to cut
aur/o	ear	**clavicul/o**	clavicle, collar bone
auricul/o	ear	**cleid/o**	clavicle, collar bone
axill/o	armpit	**coagul/o**	clotting
balan/o	glans penis	**coccyg/o**	coccyx
bas/o	base	**cochle/o**	cochlea
bi/o	life	**col/o**	colon
bil/i	bile, gall	**colon/o**	colon
bilirubin/o	bilirubin	**colp/o**	vagina

comat/o	deep sleep, coma	**erg/o**	work
condyl/o	condyle, bony projection	**erythem/o**	flush
conjunctiv/o	conjunctiva	**erythemat/o**	redness
cor/o	pupil	**erythr/o**	red
corne/o	cornea	**esophag/o**	esophagus
coron/o	heart	**esthesi/o**	feeling
cortic/o	cortex, outer layer	**estr/o**	female
cost/o	rib	**femor/o**	femur, thigh bone
crani/o	head, skull	**fet/i**	fetus
crin/o	secrete	**fet/o**	fetus
cry/o	cold	**fibrin/o**	fibers, fibrous
crypt/o	hidden	**fibul/o**	fibula, smaller outer bone of lower leg
culd/o	cul-de-sac		
cutane/o	skin	**flex/o**	to bend
cyan/o	blue	**fluor/o**	fluorescence, luminous
cycl/o	ciliary muscle	**galact/o**	milk
cyst/o	bladder, cyst, sac	**gangli/o**	ganglion
cyt/o	cell	**ganglion/o**	ganglion
dacry/o	tear; tear duct	**gastr/o**	stomach
dactyl/o	fingers, toes	**gingiv/o**	gums
dent/i	tooth	**glauc/o**	gray
dent/o	tooth	**gli/o**	glue
derm/o	skin	**glomerul/o**	glomerulus
dermat/o	skin	**gloss/o**	tongue
diaphor/o	profuse sweating	**gluc/o**	sugar
diaphragmat/o	diaphragm	**glyc/o**	sugar
dipl/o	double	**glycogen/o**	glycogen
dips/o	thirst	**glycos/o**	sugar, glucose
dist/o	away	**gon/o**	seed
diverticul/o	diverticulum, blind pouch	**gonad/o**	sex glands
dors/o	back of body	**granul/o**	granules
duct/o	duct	**gravid/o**	pregnancy
duoden/o	duodenum	**gynec/o**	woman, female
dur/o	hard	**hem/o**	blood
electr/o	electricity	**hemangi/o**	blood vessel
embol/o	embolus	**hemat/o**	blood
embry/o	embryo	**hemoglobin/o**	hemoglobin
encephal/o	brain	**hepat/o**	liver
enter/o	small intestines	**herni/o**	hernia
eosin/o	red, rosy	**hidr/o**	sweat
epididym/o	epididymis	**hist/o**	tissue
epiglott/o	epiglottis	**histi/o**	tissue
episi/o	vulva	**home/o**	sameness
epitheli/o	epithelium	**hormon/o**	hormone

humer/o	humerus, upper arm bone	mandibul/o	mandible, jaw bone
hydr/o	water	mast/o	breast
hymen/o	hymen	mastoid/o	mastoid process
hypn/o	sleep	maxill/o	maxilla, upper jaw bone
hyster/o	uterus, womb	meat/o	meatus
ichthy/o	scaly, dry	medi/o	middle
ile/o	ileum	mediastin/o	mediastinum
ili/o	ilium	medull/o	medulla
immun/o	immune	melan/o	black
infer/o	below	men/o	menses, menstruation
inguin/o	groin	mening/o	meninges
insulin/o	insulin	meningi/o	meninges
intestin/o	intestine	ment/o	mind
ir/o	iris	metacarp/o	metacarpus, hand bones
irid/o	iris	metatars/o	metatarsals, foot bones
is/o	same	metr/o	uterus
ischi/o	ischium, part of hip bone	mi/o	smaller, less
jejun/o	jejunum	mon/o	one
kal/i	potassium	morph/o	shape
kerat/o	cornea, hard, horny	muc/o	mucus
kyph/o	hump	muscul/o	muscle
labi/o	lip	mut/a	genetic change, mutation
labyrinth/o	labyrinth	my/o	muscle
lacrim/o	tears	myc/o	fungus
lact/o	milk	mydr/o	larger, widen
lamin/o	lamina, part of vertebra	myel/o	spinal cord, bone marrow
lapar/o	abdomen	myring/o	eardrum
laryng/o	larynx	myx/o	mucus
later/o	side	narc/o	numb, stupor
leth/o	death	nas/o	nose
leuk/o	white	nat/i	birth
leukocyt/o	white cell	nat/o	birth
lingu/o	tongue	natr/o	sodium
lip/o	fat	necr/o	death
lith/o	stone	nephr/o	kidney
lob/o	lobe	neur/o	nerve
lord/o	swayback, curve	neutr/o	neutral
lumb/o	loin, lower back	noct/i	night
lymph/o	lymph	norm/o	rule, order
lymphaden/o	lymph node	nucle/o	nucleus
lymphangi/o	lymph vessel	o/o	egg
macul/o	stain, spot	ocul/o	eye
malleol/o	malleolus, ankle process	odont/o	tooth
mamm/o	breast	olecran/o	olecranon, bony projection in elbow

olig/o	scanty	**pharyng/o**	throat
omphal/o	navel, umbilicus	**phas/o**	speech
onc/o	tumor	**phleb/o**	vein
onych/o	nail	**phon/o**	voice
oophor/o	ovary	**phot/o**	light
ophthalm/o	eye	**phren/o**	diaphragm, mind
opt/i	eye, vision	**phys/o**	growing
opt/o	eye, vision	**pil/o**	hair
optic/o	eye	**pituitar/o**	pituitary gland
or/o	mouth	**plas/o**	formation of cells
orch/o	testes	**pleur/o**	pleura, side
orchi/o	testes	**pneum/o**	lung, air
orchid/o	testes	**pneumat/o**	lung, air
orth/o	straight, upright	**pneumon/o**	lung, air
oste/o	bone	**poli/o**	gray matter
ot/o	ear	**polyp/o**	polyp
ov/i	egg	**poster/o**	back
ov/o	egg	**presby/o**	old age
ovari/o	ovary	**proct/o**	anus and rectum
ovul/o	ovary	**prostat/o**	prostate
ox/i	oxygen	**prosth/o**	addition
ox/o	oxygen	**proxim/o**	near
oxy/o	oxygen	**psych/o**	mind
palat/o	palate	**pub/o**	pubis, part of hip bone
palpebr/o	eyelid	**pulmon/o**	lung
pancreat/o	pancreas	**pupill/o**	pupil
papill/o	optic disc	**py/o**	pus
papul/o	pimple	**pyel/o**	renal pelvis
par/o	labor, childbirth	**pylor/o**	pylorus
parathyroid/o	parathyroid gland	**pyret/o**	fever
part/o	labor, childbirth	**radi/o**	radiation, X-ray, radius, lower arm bone
patell/o	patella, kneecap		
path/o	disease	**radicul/o**	nerve root
pector/o	chest	**rect/o**	rectum
ped/o	foot, child	**ren/o**	kidney
pelv/o	pelvis	**reticul/o**	immature, net
pericardi/o	pericardium	**retin/o**	retina
perine/o	perineum	**rhin/o**	nose
peritone/o	peritoneum	**rhytid/o**	wrinkle
phac/o	lens	**roentgen/o**	X-ray
phag/o	eat, swallow	**rrhythm/o**	rhythm
phalang/o	phalanges, bones of fingers and toes	**sacr/o**	sacrum
		salping/o	fallopian tubes, uterine tubes
pharmac/o	drug	**sangui/o**	blood

sarc/o	flesh	**thromb/o**	clot
scapul/o	scapula, shoulder blade	**thrombocyt/o**	platelet
schiz/o	divided	**thym/o**	thymus
scler/o	hard, sclera	**thyr/o**	thyroid gland
scoli/o	vertebra, backbone	**thyroid/o**	thyroid gland
seb/o	sebum, oil	**tibi/o**	tibia, inner bone of lower leg
sect/o	cut	**toc/o**	childbirth
semin/o	semen	**tonsill/o**	tonsils
seps/o	infection	**tox/o**	toxic, poison
sial/o	saliva, salivary gland	**toxic/o**	toxic, poison
sigmoid/o	sigmoid colon	**trache/o**	trachea, windpipe
sinus/o	sinus, cavity	**trich/o**	hair
somat/o	body	**tympan/o**	eardrum, middle ear
somn/o	sleep	**uln/o**	ulna, lower arm
son/o	sound	**umbilic/o**	navel, umbilical
sperm/o	sperm, spermatozoa, aspermia	**ungu/o**	nail
spermat/o	sperm	**ur/o**	urine, urinary tract
spher/o	round	**ureter/o**	ureter, urinary tube
sphygm/o	pulse	**urethr/o**	urethra
spin/o	spine, back bone	**urin/o**	urine
spir/o	breathing	**uter/o**	uterus
splen/o	spleen	**uve/o**	vascular
spondyl/o	vertebrae, backbone	**uvul/o**	uvula
squam/o	scale-like	**vag/o**	vagus nerve
staped/o	stapes	**vagin/o**	vagina
staphyl/o	grape-like clusters	**valv/o**	valve
steat/o	fat	**valvul/o**	valve
ster/o	steroid, solid	**varic/o**	varicose veins
stern/o	sternum, breast bone	**vas/o**	vas deferens
steth/o	chest	**vas/o**	vessel
stomat/o	mouth	**ven/o**	vein
super/o	above	**ventr/o**	belly
system/o	system	**ventricul/o**	ventricle
tars/o	ankle	**venul/o**	venule
ten/o	tendon	**vertebr/o**	vertebra, backbone
tend/o	tendon	**vesic/o**	bladder, blister
tendin/o	tendon	**vesicul/o**	seminal vesicle
tens/o	stretch	**viscer/o**	internal organ
test/o	testes	**vit/o**	blemish
thel/o	nipple	**vitre/o**	glassy
therm/o	heat	**vulv/o**	vulva
thorac/o	chest	**xer/o**	dry

TEXT GLOSSARY

abdominal   Pertaining to the abdomen.

abdominal cavity   The superior portion of the abdominopelvic cavity.

abdominal pain   In an emergency situation this pain is usually acute. Requires immediate evaluation since there may be a need for surgery.

abdominal ultrasonography   Using ultrasound equipment to produce sound waves that create an image of the abdominal organs.

abdominopelvic cavity   A ventral cavity consisting of the abdominal and pelvic cavities. It contains digestive, urinary, and reproductive organs.

abdominoplasty   Surgical repair of the abdomen.

abduction   Directional term meaning to move away from the median or middle line of the body.

abnormal psychology   The study and treatment of behaviors that are outside of normal and are detrimental to the person or society. These maladaptive behaviors range from occasional difficulty coping with stress, to bizarre actions and beliefs, to total withdrawal.

ABO system   The major system of blood typing.

abortion (AB)   Termination of a pregnancy before the fetus reaches a viable point in development.

abrasion   Scraping away a portion of the surface of the skin. Performed to remove acne scars, tattoos, and scar tissue.

abruptio placentae   Emergency condition in which the placenta tears away from the uterine wall before the twentieth week of pregnancy. Requires immediate delivery of the baby.

abscess   Swelling of soft tissues of the jaw as a result of infection.

accessory organs   The accessory organs to the digestive system consists of the organs that are part of the system, but not part of the continuous tube from mouth to anus. The accessory organs are the liver, pancreas, gall bladder, and salivary glands.

accommodation (Acc)   Ability of the eye to adjust to variations in distance.

acetabulum   A cup-shaped cavity formed by the juncture of the ilium, ischium, and pubis. The head of the femur fits into the acetabulum. Also called the hip socket.

achromatopsia   Condition of color blindness; more common in males.

acidosis   Excessive acidity of bodily fluids due to the accumulation of acids, as in diabetic acidosis.

acne   Inflammatory disease of the sebaceous glands and hair follicles that results in papules and pustules.

acne rosacea   Hypertrophy of sebaceous glands causing thickened skin generally on the nose, forehead, and cheeks.

acne vulgaris   A common form of acne occurring in adolescence from an oversecretion of the oil glands. It is characterized by papules, pustules, blackheads, and whiteheads.

acoustic   Pertaining to hearing.

acoustic neuroma   Benign tumor of the eighth cranial nerve sheath, which can cause symptoms from pressure being exerted on tissues.

acquired immunity   The protective response of the body to a specific pathogen.

acquired immunodeficiency syndrome (AIDS)   Disease that involves a defect in the cell-mediated immunity system. A syndrome of opportunistic infections that occur in the final stages of infection with the human immunodeficiency virus (HIV). This virus attacks T4 lymphocytes and destroys them, which reduces the person's ability to fight infection.

acromegaly   Chronic disease of adults that results in an elongation and enlargement of the bones of the head and extremities. There can also be mood changes.

active acquired immunity   Immunity developing after direct exposure to a pathogen.

active exercises   Exercises that a patient performs without assistance.

active range of motion (AROM)   Range of motion for joints that a patient is able to perform without the assistance of someone else.

active-resistive exercises   Exercises in which the patient will work against an artificial resistance applied to a muscle, such as a weight. Used to increase strength.

activities of daily living (ADL)   The activities usually performed in the course of a normal day, such as eating, dressing, and washing.

acute care hospital   Hospitals that typically provide services to diagnose (laboratory, diagnostic imaging) and treat (surgery, medications, therapy) diseases for a short period of time. In addition, they usually provide emergency and obstetrical care. Also called general hospital.

acute glomerulonephritis (AGN)   A form of nephritis that usually follows a streptococcal infection of the upper respiratory tract.

acute illness   Illness that begins suddenly and does not last long.

acute myocardial infarction (AMI)   Occurs when a portion of the heart muscle dies due to the partial or complete closure of the coronary arteries. Also called a heart attack.

adaptive equipment   Equipment used by the elderly that has been structured to aid them in mobility, eating, and managing the other activities of daily living. This equipment includes special walkers and spoons for the stroke patient.

addiction Acquired dependence on a drug.

Addison's disease Disease named for Thomas Addison, a British physician, that results from a deficiency in adrenocortical hormones. There may be an increased pigmentation of the skin, generalized weakness, and weight loss.

adduction Directional term meaning to move toward the median or middle line of the body.

adductor longus A leg muscle named for the direction the fibers pull. This muscle contracts to adduct or pull the leg in toward the midline.

adenocarcinoma Malignant adenoma in a glandular organ.

adenoidectomy Excision of the adenoids.

adenoiditis Inflammation of the adenoid tissue.

adenoids Another term for pharyngeal tonsils. The tonsils are a collection of lymphatic tissue found in the nasopharynx to combat microorganisms entering the body through the nose.

adenoma Neoplasm or tumor of a gland.

adipectomy Surgical removal of fat.

adipose tissue A type of connective tissue. Also called fat. It stores energy and provides protective padding for underlying structures.

adrenal glands A pair of glands in the endocrine system located just above each kidney. This gland is composed of two sections, the cortex and the medulla, that function independently of each other. The cortex secretes steroids, such as aldosterone, cortisol, androgens, estrogens, and progestins. The medulla secretes epinephrine and norepinephrine. The adrenal glands are regulated by adrenocorticotropic hormone, which is secreted by the pituitary gland.

adrenal medulla The inner portion of the adrenal gland. It secretes epinephrine and norepinephrine.

adrenalectomy Excision of the adrenal gland.

adrenaline A hormone produced by the adrenal medulla. Also known as epinephrine. Some of its actions include increasing heart rate and force of contraction, bronchodilation, and relaxation of intestinal muscles.

adrenalitis Inflammation of an adrenal gland.

adrenocorticotropic hormone (ACTH) A hormone secreted by anterior pituitary. It regulates function of the adrenal gland cortex.

adrenomegaly Enlarged adrenal gland.

adrenopathy Adrenal gland disease.

adult respiratory distress syndrome (ARDS) Acute respiratory failure in adults characterized by tachypnea, dyspnea, cyanosis, tachycardia, and hypoxemia.

aerosal Drugs inhaled directly into the nose and mouth.

afferent arteriole Arteriole that carries blood into the glomerulus.

afferent neurons Nerve that carries impulses to the brain and spinal cord from the skin and sense organs. Also called sensory neurons.

agglutinate Clumping together to form small clusters. Platelets agglutinate to start the clotting process.

agglutination Antigen–antibody reaction in which a solid antigen clumps together with a soluble antibody. Often used to refer to the process of clumping together of blood cells.

aging Gradual progressive changes that relate to the passage of time. There is no standard by which everyone ages.

agranulocyte Nongranular leukocyte. This is one of the two types of leukocytes found in plasma that are classified as either monocytes or lymphocytes.

aided exercises Exercises in which the patient has assistance in performing the exercise from someone or something else.

AIDS-related complex (ARC) Early stage of AIDS. There is a positive test for the virus but only mild symptoms of weight loss, fatigue, skin rash, and anorexia.

air contrast barium enema Using both barium and air to visualize the colon.

airway Includes the mouth, pharynx, larynx, trachea, bronchi, and lungs. These must remain patent (open) for respiration to take place.

albino A person not able to produce melanin. An albino person has white hair and skin and the pupils of the eye are red.

albumin A protein that is normally found circulating in the blood stream. It is abnormal for albumin to be in the urine.

aldosterone A hormone produced by the adrenal cortex. It regulates the levels of sodium and potassium in the body and as a side-effect the volume of water lost in urine.

alimentary canal Also known as the gastrointestinal system or digestive system. This system covers the area between the mouth and the anus and includes 30 feet of intestinal tubing. It has a wide range of functions. This system serves to store and digest food, absorb nutrients, and eliminate waste. The major organs of this system are the mouth, pharynx, esophagus, stomach, small intestine, colon, rectum, and anus.

allergen Antigen capable of causing a hypersensitivity or allergy in the body.

allergic reaction Can be life threatening if there is a severe drop in blood pressure and a swelling of the airway as a result of an allergy.

allergy Hypersensitivity to a substance in the environment or a medication.

alopecia Absence or loss of hair, especially of the head.

alveoli The tiny air sacs at the end of each bronchiole. The alveoli are surrounded by a capillary network. Gas exchange takes place as oxygen and carbon dioxide diffuse across the alveolar and capillary walls.

Alzheimer's disease Chronic, organic mental disorder consisting of dementia that is more prevalent in adults between 40 and 60. Involves progressive disorientation, apathy, speech and gait disturbances, and loss of memory.

ambulatory Able to walk.

ambulatory care center A facility that provides services that do not require overnight hospitalization. The services range from simple surgeries, to diagnostic testing, to therapy. Also called a surgical center or an outpatient clinic.

amenorrhea   Absence of menstruation, which can be the result of many factors, including pregnancy, menopause, and dieting.

American Sign Language (ASL)   Nonverbal method of communicating in which the hands and fingers are used to indicate words and concepts. Used by people who are deaf and speech-impaired.

amino acids   An organic substance found in plasma. It is used by cells to build proteins.

ammonia   A waste produce of cell metabolism found in plasma.

amnesia   Loss of memory in which people forget their identity as a result of a head injury or disorder, such as epilepsy, senility, and alcoholism. Can be either temporary or permanent.

amniocentesis   Puncturing of the amniotic sac using a needle and syringe for the purpose of withdrawing amniotic fluid for testing. Can assist in determining fetal maturity, development, and genetic disorders.

amnion   The inner of two membranous sacs surrounding the fetus. The amniotic sac contains amniotic fluid in which the baby floats.

amniorrhea   Discharge of amniotic fluid.

amnioscopy   Procedure to view inside the amniotic sac.

amniotic fluid   The fluid inside the amniotic sac.

amniotomy   Incision into the amniotic sac.

amplification device   Used to increase certain sounds for the hearing impaired person. Also known as hearing aid.

amputation   Partial or complete removal of a limb for a variety of reasons, including tumors, gangrene, intractable pain, crushing injury, or uncontrollable infection.

amyotrophic lateral sclerosis (ALS)   Disease with muscular weakness and atrophy due to degeneration of motor neurons of the spinal cord. Also called Lou Gehrig's disease, after the New York Yankees' baseball player who died from the disease.

anacusis   Total absence of hearing; unable to perceive sound. Also called deafness.

anal sphincter   Ring of muscle that controls anal opening.

analgesia   A reduction in the perception of pain or sensation due to a neurological condition or medication.

analgesic   Relieves pain without the loss of consciousness. May be either narcotic or nonnarcotic. Narcotic drugs are derived from the opium poppy and act on the brain to cause pain relief and drowsiness.

anaphylactic shock   Life-threatening condition resulting from the ingestion of food or medications that produce a severe allergic response. There are circulatory and respiratory problems that occur, including respiratory distress, hypotension, edema, tachycardia, and convulsions.

anaphylaxis   Severe reaction to an antigen.

anastomosis   Creating a passageway or opening between two organs or vessels.

anatomical divisions   System that divides the abdomen into nine regions.

anatomical position   Used to describe the positions and relationships of a structure in the human body. For descriptive purposes the assumption is always that the person is in the anatomical position. The body is standing erect with the arms at the side of the body, the palms of the hands facing forward, and the eyes looking straight ahead. The legs are parallel with the feet and toes pointing forward.

Ancillary Report   Report in a patient's medical record from various treatments and therapies the patient has received, such as rehabilitation, social services, respiratory therapy, or from the dietician.

androgen   A class of steroid hormones secreted by the adrenal cortex. These hormones, such as testosterone, produce a masculinizing effect.

anemia   Reduction in the number of red blood cells (RBCs) or amount of hemoglobin in the blood; results in less oxygen reaching the tissues.

anesthesia   Partial or complete loss of sensation with or without a loss of consciousness as a result of a drug, disease, or injury.

anesthesiologist   A physician who has a specialization in the practice of administering anesthetics.

Anesthesiologist's Report   A medical record document that relates the details regarding the drugs given to a patient and the patient's response to anesthesia and vital signs during surgery.

anesthetic   Produces a lack of feeling that may be of local or general effect, depending on the type of administration.

aneurysm   Weakness in the wall of an artery that results in localized widening of the artery.

aneurysmectomy   Surgical removal of the sac of an aneurysm.

angina pectoris   Severe chest pain with a sensation of constriction around the heart. Caused by a deficiency of oxygen to the heart muscle.

angiocardiography   X-ray of the heart's blood vessels after injecting a radiopaque dye.

angiocarditis   Inflammation of the heart and blood vessels.

angiogram   X-ray of a blood or lymphatic vessel that is taken in rapid sequence after injection of a radiopaque substance into the blood vessel.

angiography   Process of taking an X-ray of blood or lymphatic vessels after injection of a radiopaque substance.

angioma   Tumor, usually benign, consisting of blood vessels.

angioplasty   Surgical repair of blood vessels.

angiorrhaphy   Suturing a vessel.

angioscope   Instrument used to view inside a vessel.

angioscopy   Procedure of viewing the inside of a vessel.

angiospasm   Involuntary muscle contraction of a vessel.

angiostenosis   Narrowing of a vessel.

ankylosis   Stiffening of a joint due to a disease process. Joint may fuse with bony or fibrous tissue.

anorchism   Congenital absence of one or both testes.

anorexia   Loss of appetite that can accompany other conditions such as a gastrointestinal (GI) upset.

anorexia nervosa A type of eating disorder characterized by severe disturbance in body image and marked refusal to eat.

anoxemia Absence of oxygen in the blood.

anoxia Lack of oxygen.

antacid Neutralizes acid in the stomach.

anteflexion While the uterus is normally in this position, an exaggeration of the forward bend of the uterus is abnormal. The forward bend is near the neck of the uterus. The position of the cervix, or opening of the uterus, remains normal.

antepartum Before birth.

anterior Directional term meaning near or on the front or belly side of the body.

anterior cruciate ligament (ACL) reconstruction Replacing a torn ACL with a graft by means of arthroscopy.

anterior lobe The anterior portion of the pituitary gland. It secretes adrenocorticotropic hormone, follicle-stimulating hormone, growth hormone, luteinizing hormone, melanocyte-stimulating hormone, prolactin, and thyroid-stimulating hormone.

anteversion In this position the uterus is actually tipped forward without bending, so that the cervix becomes tipped toward the sacrum and the fundus is tipped toward the pubis.

antianxiety Relieves or reduces anxiety and muscle tension. Used to treat panic disorders, anxiety, and insomnia.

antiarrhythmic Controls cardiac arrhythmias by altering nerve impulses within the heart.

antibiotic Destroys or prohibits the growth of microorganisms. Used to treat bacterial infections. Have not been found to be effective in treating viral infections. To be effective must be taken regularly for a specified period.

antibody Protein material produced in the body as a response to the invasion of a foreign substance.

antibody-mediated immunity The production of antibodies by B cells in response to an antigen. Also called humoral immunity.

anticholinergic Blocks the function of the parasympathetic nervous system. Used to treat intestinal, bladder, and bronchial spasms.

anticoagulant Substance that prevents or delays the clotting or coagulation of blood.

anticonvulsant Prevents or relieves convulsions. Drugs such as phenobarbital reduce excessive stimulation in the brain to control seizures and other symptoms of epilepsy.

antidepressant Prevents or relieves the symptoms of depression. Also used in the prevention of migraine headaches.

antidiabetic Insulin drug that controls diabetes by regulating the level of glucose in the blood and the metabolism of carbohydrates and fat.

antidiarrheal Prevents or relieves diarrhea.

antidiuretic Any substance that reduces the volume of urine.

antidiuretic hormone (ADH) A hormone secreted by the posterior pituitary. It promotes water reabsorption by the kidney tubules.

antidote Substance that will neutralize poisons or their side effects.

antiemetic Controls nausea and vomiting.

antigen Substance that is capable of inducing the formation of an antibody. The antibody then interacts with the antigen in the antigen–antibody reaction.

antigen–antibody reaction Combination of the antigen with its specific antibody to increase susceptibility to phagocytosis and immunity.

antihemorrhagic Substance that prevents or stops hemorrhaging.

antihistamine Acts to control allergic symptoms by counteracting histamine, which exists naturally in the body, and which is released in allergic reactions.

antihypertensive Prevents or controls high blood pressure. Some of these drugs act to block nerve impulses that cause arteries to constrict and thus increase the blood pressure. Other drugs slow the heart rate and decrease its force of contraction. Still others may reduce the amount of the hormone aldosterone in the blood that is causing the blood pressure to rise.

anti-inflammatory Acts to counteract inflammation.

antipyretic Used to reduce fever.

antisocial personality A personality disorder in which the patient engages in behaviors that are illegal or outside of social norms.

antitussive Controls or relieves coughing. Codeine is an ingredient in many prescription cough medicines that acts upon the brain to control coughing.

antrum The tapered distal end of the stomach.

anuria Complete suppression of urine formed by the kidneys and a complete lack of urine excretion.

anus The terminal opening of the digestive tube.

anxiety A feeling of apprehension or worry.

aorta The largest artery in the body. It is located in the mediastinum and carries oxygenated blood away from the left side of the heart.

aortic Pertaining to the aorta.

aortic insufficiency (AI) Failure of the aortic valve to close completely, which allows blood to leak back into the left ventricle.

aortic stenosis Narrowing of the aorta.

aortic valve The semilunar valve between the left ventricle of the heart and the aorta in the heart. It prevents blood from flowing backwards into the ventricle.

aortogram X-ray record of the aorta after a radiopaque dye has been inserted.

aortography Process of taking an X-ray of the aorta after injection of a radiopaque material.

AP view Stands for anteroposterior; positioning the patient so that the X-rays pass through the body from the anterior side to the posterior side.

apex Directional term meaning tip or summit.

aphagia Not eating.

aphasia   Inability to communicate through speech. Often an aftereffect of a stroke (CVA).

apnea   The condition of not breathing.

apocrine gland   Type of sweat gland that open into hair follicles located in the pubic, anal, and mammary areas. These glands secrete a substance that can produce an odor when it comes into contact with bacteria on the skin causing what is commonly referred to as body odor.

appendectomy   Surgical removal of the appendix.

appendicitis   Inflammation of the appendix.

appendicular skeleton   The appendicular skeleton consists of the bones of the upper and lower extremities, shoulder, and pelvis.

appendix   A small outgrowth at the end of the cecum. Its function or purpose is unknown.

aqueous humor   A watery fluid filling the spaces between the cornea and lens.

arachnoid layer   The delicate middle layer of the meninges.

areola   The pigmented area round the nipple of the breast.

arrhythmia   Irregularity in the heartbeat or action.

arterial   Pertaining to the artery.

arterial blood gases (ABG)   Lab test that measures the amount of oxygen, carbon dioxide, and nitrogen in the blood, and the pH.

arterial embolism   Obstruction of an artery by a floating blood clot.

arteries   The blood vessels that carry blood away from the heart.

arteriography   Process of taking an X-ray of arteries after injection of a radiopaque dye.

arterioles   The smallest branches of the arteries. They carry blood to the capillaries.

arteriorrhexis   A ruptured artery.

arteriosclerosis   Condition with thickening, hardening, and loss of elasticity of the walls of the arteries.

arteriosclerotic heart disease (ASHD)   Chronic heart disorder caused by a hardening of the walls of the coronary arteries.

artery graft   Section of a blood vessel that is transplanted from one part of the body to another to repair a defect.

arthralgia   Pain in a joint.

arthritis   Inflammation of a joint that is usually accompanied by pain and swelling. A chronic disease.

arthrocentesis   Removal of synovial fluid with a needle from a joint space, such as in the knee, for examination.

arthroclasia   Surgically breaking loose a stiffened joint.

arthrodesis   Surgical fusion or stiffening of a joint to provide stability. This is sometimes done to relieve the pain of arthritis.

arthrography   Visualization of a joint by radiographic study after injection of a contrast medium into the joint space.

arthroplasty   Surgical reconstruction of a joint.

arthroscopic surgery   Use of an arthroscope to facilitate performing surgery on a joint.

arthroscopy   Examination of the interior of a joint by entering the joint with an arthroscope. The arthroscope contains a small television camera that allows the physician to view the interior of the joint on a monitor during the procedure.

arthrotomy   Surgically cutting into a joint.

articulation   Another term for a joint, the point where two bones meet.

artificial pacemaker   Electrical device that substitutes for the natural pacemaker of the heart. It controls the beating of the heart by a series of rhythmic electrical impulses.

artificial ventilation   Forcing air or oxygen into the lungs when breathing has stopped or is inadequate.

ascending colon   The section of the colon following the cecum. It ascends the right side of the abdomen.

ascites   Collection or accumulation of fluid in the peritoneal cavity.

aspermia   Lack of, or failure to ejaculate, sperm.

asphyxia   Lack of oxygen that can lead to unconsciousness and death if not corrected immediately. Some of the common causes are drowning, foreign body in the respiratory tract, poisoning, and electric shock.

aspirator   A surgical instrument used to suction fluids.

assisted living   Living arrangement in which the person may have his or her own apartment space but joins other residents for meals and other activities.

asthenia   Lack or loss of strength, causing extreme weakness.

asthma   Disease caused by various conditions, such as allergens, and resulting in constriction of the bronchial airways and labored respirations. Can cause violent spasms of the bronchi (bronchospasms) but is generally not a life-threatening condition. Medication can be very effective.

asthmatic attack   Attack of difficulty in breathing (dyspnea) and wheezing due to bronchial constriction.

astigmatism (Astigm)   A condition in which light rays are focused unevenly on the eye, which causes a distorted image due to an abnormal curvature of the cornea.

astringent   Substance that causes tissues to dry up and contract; also may be used to stop bleeding.

astrocyte   Star-shaped cells found in the nervous system that surround and support the neurons. They perform important metabolic functions, but do not participate in conducting electrical impulses.

astrocytoma   Tumor of the brain or spinal cord that is composed of astrocytes.

ataxia   Having a lack of muscle coordination as a result of a disorder or disease.

atelectasis   Condition in which lung tissue collapses, which prevents the respiratory exchange of oxygen and carbon dioxide. Can be caused by a variety of conditions, including pressure upon the lung from a tumor or other object.

atherectomy   Excision of fatty substance.

atherosclerosis   The most common form of arteriosclerosis. Caused by the formation of yellowish plaques of cholesterol buildup on the inner walls of the arteries.

atria   The two upper chambers of the heart. The left atrium receives blood returning from the lungs, and the right atrium receives blood returning from the body.

atrial   Pertaining to the atrium.

atrial natriuretic hormone (ANF)   A hormone secreted by special cells in the heart's atrial wall. This hormone stimulates the kidney tubules to secrete more sodium and in this way lose more water.

atrioventricular defect   Heart defect between the atrium and ventricle.

atrioventricular node   This area at the junction of the right atrium and ventricle receives the stimulus from the sinoatrial node and sends the impulse to the ventricles through the bundle of His.

atrioventricular valve (AV)   The heart valves located between an atria and a ventricle. Includes the tricuspid valve in the right side of the heart and the bicuspid or mitral valve in the left side of the heart.

atrophy   Lack or loss of normal development.

attention deficit disorder   A type of mental disorder diagnosed in childhood characterized by poor attention and inability to control behavior. The child may or may not be hyperactive.

atypical   Abnormal.

audiogram   Chart that shows the faintest sounds a patient can hear during audiometry testing.

audiologist   Medical professional trained to perform hearing tests using equipment such as an audiometer, fit and test hearing aids, and provide auditory rehabilitation.

audiology   Study of hearing.

audiometer   Instrument to measure hearing.

audiometric test   Test of hearing ability by determining the lowest and highest intensity (decibels) and frequencies (hertz) that a person can distinguish. The patient may sit in a soundproof booth and receive sounds through earphones as the technician decreases the sound or lowers the tones.

audiometry   Process of measuring hearing.

auditory canal   The canal that leads from the external opening of the ear to the ear drum.

aural   Pertaining to the ear.

auricle   Also called the pinna. The external ear. It functions to capture sound waves as they go past the outer ear.

auscultation   Listening to the sounds within the body by using a stethoscope.

autism   A type of mental disorder diagnosed in childhood in which the child exhibits an extreme degree of withdrawal from all social contacts.

autohemotherapy   Using a person's own blood in a transfusion by withdrawing and injecting the blood intramuscularly.

autologous transfusion   Procedure for collecting and storing a patient's own blood several weeks prior to the actual need. It can then be used to replace blood lost during a surgical procedure.

autonomic nervous system   The portion of the nervous system that consists of nerves to the internal organs that function involuntarily. It regulates the functions of glands (especially the salivary, gastric, and sweat glands), the adrenal medulla, heart, and smooth muscle tissue. This system is divided into two parts: sympathetic and parasympathetic.

axial skeleton   The axial skeleton includes the bones in the head, spine, chest, and trunk.

axillary   Commonly referred to as the armpit. There is a collection of lymph nodes in this area that drains each arm.

axon   Single projection of a neuron that conducts impulse away from nerve cell body.

azoospermia   Absence of sperm in the semen.

B cells   Common name for B-lymphocytes, responds to foreign antigens by producing protective antibodies.

B lymphocytes   The humoral immunity cells, which respond to foreign antigens by producing protective antibodies. Simply referred to as B cells.

Babinski's reflex   Reflex test to determine lesions and abnormalities in the nervous system. The Babinski reflex is present if the great toe extends instead of flexes when the lateral sole of the foot is stroked. The normal response to this stimulation would be a flexion, or upward movement, of the toe.

bacteria   Primitive, single-celled microorganisms that are present everywhere. Some are capable of causing disease in humans.

bacterium   Single-celled microorganism. In the stomach, one type of bacterium that may cause peptic or stomach ulcers.

balanitis   Inflammation of the skin covering the glans penis.

balanoplasty   Surgical repair of the glans penis.

balanorrhea   Discharge from the glans penis.

ball and socket   A type of freely moving synovial joint. The two main examples in humans are the shoulder and hip joints.

barium (Ba)   Soft metallic element from the earth used as a radiopaque X-ray dye.

barium enema (BE, lower GI series)   Radiographic examination of the small intestine, large intestine, or colon in which an enema containing barium (Ba) is administered to the patient while the X-ray pictures are taken.

barium swallow (upper GI series)   A barium (Ba) mixture swallowed while X-ray pictures are taken of the esophagus, stomach, and duodenum used to visualize the upper gastrointestinal tract (upper GI).

Bartholin's glands   Glands located on either side of the vaginal opening that secrete mucus for vaginal lubrication.

basal cell carcinoma   Tumor of the basal cell layer of the epidermis. A frequent type of skin cancer that rarely metastasizes or spreads. These cancers can arise on sun-exposed skin.

basal layer   The deepest layer of the epidermis. This living layer constantly multiplies and divides to supply cells to replace the cells that are sloughed off the skin surface.

basal metabolic rate (BMR)   Somewhat outdated test to measure the energy used when the body is in a state of rest.

base   Directional term meaning bottom or lower part.

basic life support   Combination of cardiopulmonary resuscitation (CPR) and emergency cardiac care to maintain respiration and circulation of a victim until victim is transported to a medical facility.

basophils   A granulocyte white blood cell that releases histamine and heparin in damaged tissues.

bedside commode   Chairlike portable toilet that can be placed at the side of the bed for people who have difficulty walking.

Bell's palsy   One-sided facial paralysis with an unknown cause. The person cannot control salivation, tearing of the eyes, or expression. The patient will eventually recover.

benign   A tumor that is not cancerous. A benign tumor is generally not progressive or recurring.

benign prostatic hypertrophy (BPH)   Enlargement of the prostate gland commonly seen in males over 50.

biceps   An arm muscle named for the number of attachment points. Bi- means two and biceps have two heads attached to the bone.

bicuspids   Premolar permanent teeth having two cusps or projections that assist in grinding food. Humans have eight bicuspids.

bicuspid valve   A valve between the left atrium and ventricle. It prevents blood from flowing backwards into the atrium. It has two cusps or flaps. It is also called the mitral valve.

bile   Substance produced by the liver and stored in the gallbladder. It is added to the chyme in the duodenum and functions to emulsify fats so they can be digested and absorbed. Cholesterol is essential to bile production.

binocular   Pertaining to two eyes.

biopsy (BX, bx)   A piece of tissue is removed by syringe and needle, knife, punch, or brush to examine under a microscope. Used to aid in diagnosis.

bipolar disorder   A mental disorder in which the patient has alternating periods of depression and mania.

bite or sting   Puncture wound of the skin made by humans, animals, insects, ticks, bees, hornets, or wasps. There is a danger of infection. An emergency situation arises if the person is allergic to venom in stings.

bite-wing X-ray   X-ray taken with part of the film holder held between the teeth, and the film held parallel to the teeth.

bladder neck obstruction   Blockage of the bladder outlet into the urethra.

bleeding time   Test to measure the amount of time needed for the blood to coagulate.

blepharitis   Inflammatory condition of the eyelash follicles and glands of the eyelids that results in swelling, redness, and crusts of dried mucus on the lids. Can be the result of allergy or infection.

blepharochalasis   In this condition the upper eyelid increases in size due to a loss of elasticity, which is followed by swelling and recurrent edema of the lids. The skin may droop over the edges of the eyes when the eyes are open.

blepharoplasty   Surgical repair of the eyelid.

blepharoptosis   Drooping eyelid.

blood   The major component of the hematic system. It consists of watery plasma, red blood cells, and white blood cells.

blood pressure (BP)   Measurement of the pressure that is exerted by blood against the walls of a blood vessel.

blood serum test   Blood test to measure the level of substances such as calcium, electrolytes, testosterone, insulin, and glucose. Used to assist in determining the function of various endocrine glands.

blood typing   The blood of one person is different from another's due to the presence of antigens on the surface of the erythrocytes. The major method of typing blood is the ABO system and includes types A, B, O, and AB. The other major method of typing blood is the Rh factor, consisting of the two types, Rh+ and Rh-.

blood urea nitrogen (BUN)   Blood test to measure kidney function by the level of nitrogenous waste, or urea, that is in the blood.

blood vessels   The closed system of tubes that conducts blood throughout the body. It consists of arteries, veins, and capillaries.

body   The main portion of the stomach.

body mechanics   Use of good posture and position while performing activities of daily living to prevent injury and stress on body parts.

boil   Acute inflammation of subcutaneous layer of skin, gland, or hair follicle. Also called a furuncle.

bolus   Chewed up morsel of food ready to be swallowed.

bone   A type of connective tissue and an organ of the musculoskeletal system. They provide support for the body and serve as sites of muscle attachments.

bone graft   Piece of bone taken from the patient and used to replace a removed bone or a bony defect at another site.

bone marrow aspiration   Removing a sample of bone marrow by syringe for microscopic examination. Useful for diagnosing such diseases as leukemia. For example, a proliferation (massive increase) of white blood cells could confirm the diagnosis of acute leukemia.

bone marrow biopsy   Removal of a small amount of bone marrow for microscopic examination to determine the presence of malignant tumor cells.

bone scan   Patient is given a radioactive dye and then scanning equipment is used to visualize bones. It is especially useful in observing the progress of treatment for osteomyelitis and cancer metastases to the bone.

Bowman's capsule   Also called the glomerular capsule. Part of the renal corpuscle. It is a double-walled cuplike structure that encircles the glomerulus. In the filtration stage of urine production, waste products filtered from the blood enter Bowman's capsule as the glomerular filtrate.

bradycardia   Abnormally slow heart rate, below 60 bpm.

bradykinesia Slow movement, commonly seen with the rigidity of Parkinson's disease.

bradypepsia Slow digestion rate.

brain The brain is one of the largest organs in the body and coordinates most body activities. It is the center for all thought, memory, judgment, and emotion. Each part of the brain is responsible for controlling different body functions, such as temperature regulation and breathing. The four sections to the brain are the cerebrum, cerebellum, diencephalon, and brain stem.

brain scan Injection of radioactive isotopes into the circulation to determine the function and abnormality of the brain.

brain stem This area of the brain has three components: medulla oblongata, pons, and the mid-brain. The brain stem is a pathway for impulses to be conducted between the brain and the spinal cord. It also contains the centers that control respiration, heart rate, and blood pressure. In addition, the twelve pairs of cranial nerves begin in the brain stem.

brain tumor Intracranial mass, either benign or malignant. A benign tumor of the brain can be fatal since it will grow and cause pressure on normal brain tissue. The most malignant brain tumors in children are gliomas.

brand name The name a pharmaceutical company chooses as the trademark or market name for its drug. Also called proprietary or trade name.

breasts Milk-producing glands to provide nutrition for newborn. Also called mammary glands.

breech presentation Placement of the fetus in which the buttocks or feet are presented first for delivery rather than the head.

bridge Dental appliance that is attached to adjacent teeth for support to replace missing teeth.

broad spectrum Ability of a drug to be effective against a wide range of microorganisms.

bronchi The plural of bronchus.

bronchial tree Term referring to the branched bronchial tube system throughout the lungs.

bronchial tubes An organ of the respiratory system that carries air into each lung.

bronchiectasis Results from a dilation of a bronchus or the bronchi that can be the result of infection. This abnormal stretching can be irreversible and result in destruction of the bronchial walls. The major symptom is a large amount of purulent (pus-filled) sputum. Rales (bubbling chest sound) and hemoptysis may be present.

bronchioles The narrowest air tubes in the lungs. Each bronchiole terminates in tiny air sacs called alveoli.

bronchitis An acute or chronic inflammation of the lower respiratory tract that often occurs after other childhood infections such as measles.

bronchodilator Dilates or opens the bronchi (airways in the lungs) to improve breathing.

bronchogenic carcinoma Malignant lung tumor that originates in the bronchi. Usually associated with a history of cigarette smoking.

bronchogram An X-ray record of the lungs and bronchial tubes.

bronchography Process of taking an X-ray of the lung after a radiopaque substance has been placed into the trachea or bronchial tree.

bronchoplasty Surgical repair of a bronchial defect.

bronchoscope An instrument to view inside a bronchus.

bronchoscopy (Broncho) Using the bronchoscope to visualize the bronchi. The instrument can also be used to obtain tissue for biopsy and to remove foreign objects.

bronchospasm An involuntary muscle spasm in the bronchi.

bronchotomy Surgical incision of a bronchus, larynx, or trachea.

bronchus The distal end of the trachea splits into a left and right main bronchi as it enters each lung. Each main bronchus is subdivided into smaller branches. The smallest bronchi are the bronchioles. Each bronchiole ends in tiny air sacs called alveoli.

bruit Term used interchangeably with the word murmur. A gentle, blowing sound that is heard during auscultation.

buccal Drugs that are placed under the lip or between the cheek and gum.

bulbourethral gland Also called Cowper's gland. These two small male reproductive system glands are located on either side of the urethra just distal to the prostate. The secretion from these glands neutralizes the acidity in the urethra and the vagina.

bulimia Eating disorder that is characterized by recurrent binge eating and then purging of the food with laxatives and vomiting.

bundle of His The bundle of His is located in the interventricular septum. It receives the electrical impulse from the atrioventricular node and distributes it through the ventricular walls causing them to contract simultaneously.

bunion Inflammation of the bursa of the great toe.

bunionectomy Removal of the bursa at the joint of the great toe.

Burkitt's lymphoma Tumor of the lymph tissue that involves sites other than lymph nodes. Commonly found in the jaw and is more common in Central Africa.

burn A full-thickness burn exists when all the layers are burned; also called a third-degree burn. A partial thickness burn exists when the first layer of skin, the epidermis, is burned, and the second layer of skin, dermis, is damaged; also called a second-degree burn.

bursa A saclike connective tissue structure found in some joints. It protects moving parts from friction. Some common bursa locations are the elbow, knee, and shoulder joints.

bursectomy Excision of a bursa.

bursitis Inflammation of a bursa between bony prominences and muscles or tendons. Common in the shoulder and knee.

bursolith A stone in a bursa.

calcitonin   A hormone secreted by the thyroid gland. It stimulates deposition of calcium into bone.

calcium   An inorganic substance found in plasma. It is important for bones, muscles, and nerves.

calculus   A stone formed within an organ by an accumulation of mineral salts. Found in the kidney, renal pelvis, ureters, bladder, or urethra. Plural is calculi.

calyx   A duct that connects the renal papilla to the renal pelvis. Urine flows from the collecting tubule through the calyx and into the renal pelvis.

cancellous bone   The bony tissue found inside a bone. It contains cavities that hold red bone marrow. Also called spongy bone.

cancer (Ca)   Malignant tumors are the leading cause of death in children between the ages of three and fifteen years of age.

candidiasis   Yeastlike infection of the skin and mucous membranes that can result in white plaques on the tongue and vagina.

canines   Also called the cuspid teeth or eyeteeth. Permanent teeth located between the incisors and the bicuspids that assist in biting and cutting food. Humans have four canine teeth.

capillaries   The smallest blood or lymphatic vessels. Blood capillaries are very thin to allow gas, nutrient, and waste exchange between the blood and the tissues. Lymph capillaries collect lymph fluid from the tissues and carry it to the larger lymph vessels.

carbon dioxide   A waste produce of cellular energy production. It is removed from the cells by the blood and eliminated from the body by the lungs.

carbuncle   Inflammation and infection of the skin and hair follicle that may result from several untreated boils. Most commonly found on neck, upper back, or head.

carcinogen   Substance or chemical agent that produces cancer or increases the risk of developing it. For example, cigarette smoke and insecticides are considered to be carcinogens.

carcinoma   New growth or malignant tumor that occurs in epithelial tissue. Can spread to other organs through the blood or direct extension from the organ.

carcinoma in situ (CIS)   Malignant tumor that has not extended beyond the original site.

carcinoma of the testes   Cancer of one or both testicles.

cardiac   Pertaining to the heart.

cardiac arrest   When the heart stops beating and circulation ceases.

cardiac catheterization   Passage of a thin tube (catheter) through an arm vein and the blood vessels leading into the heart. Done to detect abnormalities, to collect cardiac blood samples, and to determine the pressure within the cardiac area.

cardiac enzymes   Complex protein molecules found only in heart muscle. Cardiac enzymes are taken by blood sample to determine the amount of heart disease or damage.

cardiac magnetic resonance imaging (MRI)   Noninvasive imaging procedure in which images of the heart and blood vessels are recorded for examination to determine defects.

cardiac muscle   The involuntary muscle found in the heart.

cardiac sphincter   Also called the lower esophageal sphincter. Prevents food and gastric juices from backing up into the esophagus.

cardiodynia   Heart pain.

cardiologist   A physician specializing in treating diseases and conditions of the cardiovascular system.

cardiology   The branch of medicine specializing in conditions of the cardiovascular system.

cardiolysis   Surgical procedure to separate bands of scar tissue, called adhesions, that have formed between the pericardium and chest cavity wall.

cardiomegaly   Abnormally enlarged heart.

cardiomyopathy   General term for a disease of the myocardium that may be caused by alcohol abuse, parasites, viral infection, and congestive heart failure.

cardiopulmonary resuscitation (CPR)   Emergency treatment provided by persons trained in CPR and given to patients when their respirations and heart stop. CPR provides oxygen to the brain, heart, and other vital organs until medical treatment can restore a normal heart and pulmonary function.

cardiorrhaphy   Surgical suturing of the heart.

cardiotomy   Making an incision into the heart.

cardiotonic   Strengthens the heart muscle.

cardiovascular system (CV)   System that transports blood to all areas of the body. Organs of the cardiovascular system include the heart and blood vessels (arteries, veins, and capillaries). Also called the circulatory system.

cardioversion   A procedure that converts serious irregular heart beats, such as fibrillation, by giving electric shocks to the heart.

cardioverter   Instrument that uses electrodes placed externally over the heart to provide an electric shock for the purpose of converting an arrhythmia to normal sinus rhythm.

caries   Gradual decay and disintegration of teeth that can result in inflamed tissue and abscessed teeth.

carotid endarterectomy   Surgical procedure for removing an obstruction within the carotid artery, a major artery in the neck that carries oxygenated blood to the brain. Developed to prevent strokes but found to be useful only in severe stenosis with TIA.

carpal tunnel release   Surgical cutting of the ligament in the wrist to relieve nerve pressure caused by carpal tunnel disease, which can be caused by repetitive motion such as typing.

carpal tunnel syndrome   A painful disorder of the wrist and hand, induced by compression of the median nerve as it passes under ligaments on the palm side of the wrist. Symptoms include weakness, pain, burning, tingling, and aching in the forearm, wrist, and hand.

carpals   The wrist bones in the upper extremity.

cartilage   Strong flexible connective tissue found in several locations in the body, such as covering the ends of bones in a synovial joint, nasal septum, external ear, eustachian tube, larynx, trachea, bronchi, and the intervertebral discs.

cartilaginous joint   A joint that allows slight movement but holds bones firmly in place by a solid piece of cartilage. The pubic symphysis is an example of a cartilaginous joint.

cartilaginous tissue   Strong but flexible connective tissue. The fetal skeleton is composed of cartilaginous tissue.

cast   Application of a solid material to immobilize an extremity or portion of the body as a result of a fracture, dislocation, or severe injury. It is most often made of plaster of paris.

castration   Excision of the testicles in the male or the ovaries in the female.

cataract   Diminished vision resulting from the lens of the eye becoming opaque or cloudy. Treatment is usually surgical removal of the cataract.

cathartic   Causes bowel movements to occur.

catheterization   Insertion of a tube through the urethra and into the urinary bladder for the purpose of withdrawing urine or inserting dye.

caudal   Directional term meaning toward the feet or tail, or below.

cauterization   Destruction of tissue using an electric current, a caustic product, or a hot iron, or by freezing.

cecum   First portion of the colon. It is a blind pouch off the beginning of the large intestine. The appendix grows out of the end of the cecum.

celiac disease   The chronic inability to tolerate foods containing gluten (wheat). Symptoms include distended abdomen, diarrhea, vomiting, muscle wasting, and lethargy.

celiotomy   Incision into the abdomen.

cell   The basic unit of all living things. All tissues and organs in the body are composed of cells. They perform survival functions such as reproduction, respiration, metabolism, and excretion. Some cells are also able to carry on specialized functions, such as contraction by muscle cells and electrical impulse transmission by nerve cells.

cell body   The portion of the nerve cell that includes the nucleus.

cell-mediated immunity   Immunity that results from the activation of sensitized T lymphocytes. The immune response causes antigens to be destroyed by the direct action of cells. Also called cellular immunity.

cellular immunity   Also called cell-mediated immunity. This process results in the production of T cells and natural killer, NK, cells that directly attach to foreign cells. This immune response fights invasion by viruses, bacteria, fungi, and cancer.

cellulitis   Inflammation of the cellular or connective tissues.

central nervous system   The portion of the nervous system that consists of the brain and spinal cord. It receives impulses from all over the body, processes this information, and then responds with an action. It consists of both gray matter and white matter.

cephalalgia   A headache.

cephalic   Directional term meaning toward the head, or above.

cerebellar   Pertaining to the cerebellum.

cerebellitis   Inflammation of the cerebellum.

cerebellum   The second largest portion of the brain, it is located beneath the posterior portion of the cerebrum. This part of the brain aids in coordinating voluntary body movements and maintaining balance and equilibrium. It is attached to the brain stem by the pons. The cerebellum refines the muscular movement that is initiated in the cerebrum.

cerebral   Pertaining to the cerebrum.

cerebral angiography   X-ray of the blood vessels of the brain after the injection of a radiopaque dye.

cerebral cortex   The outer layer of the cerebrum. It is composed of folds of gray matter called gyri, which are separated by sulci.

cerebral palsy (CP)   A group of disabilities caused by injury to the brain either before or during birth or very early in infancy. This is the most common permanent disability in childhood.

cerebrospinal   Pertaining to the cerebrum and spine.

cerebrospinal fluid   Watery clear fluid found in the ventricles of the brain. It provides protection from shock or sudden motion to the brain.

cerebrospinal fluid (CSF) analysis   Laboratory examination of the clear, watery, colorless fluid from within the brain and spinal cord. Infections and the abnormal presence of blood can be detected in this test.

cerebrospinal fluid shunts   A surgical procedure in which a bypass is created to drain cerebrospinal fluid. It is used to treat hydrocephalus by draining the excess cerebrospinal fluid from the brain and diverting it to the abdominal cavity.

cerebrovascular accident (CVA)   Also called a stroke. The development of an infarct due to loss in the blood supply to an area of the brain. Blood flow can be interrupted by a ruptured blood vessel (hemorrhage), a floating clot (embolus), a stationary clot (thrombosis), or compression. The extent of damage depends on the size and location of the infarct and often includes speech problems and muscle paralysis.

cerebrum   The largest section of the brain. It is located in the upper portion and is the area that possesses our thoughts, judgment, memory, and association skills, and the ability to discriminate between items. The outer layer of the cerebrum is the cerebral cortex, which is composed of folds of gray matter. The elevated portions of the cerebrum, or convolutions, are called gyri and are separated by fissures or sulci. The cerebrum has both a left and right division or hemisphere. Each hemisphere has four lobes: frontal, parietal, occipital, and temporal.

cerumen   Also called ear wax. A thick waxy substance produced by oil glands in the auditory canal. This wax helps to protect and lubricate the ear.

cervical   Pertaining to the neck.

cervical biopsy   Taking a sample of tissue from the cervix to test for the presence of cancer cells.

cervical cancer   Malignant growth in the cervix. An especially difficult type of cancer to treat, it causes 5 percent of the cancer deaths in women. PAP tests have helped to detect early cervical cancer.

cervical polyps   Fibrous or mucous tumor or growth found in the cervix. These are removed surgically if there is a danger that they will become malignant.

cervical vertebrae   The seven vertebrae in the neck region.

cervicectomy   Excision of the cervix.

cervicitis   Inflammation of the cervix.

cervix   The narrow, distal portion of the uterus that joins to the vagina.

cesarean section (CS, C-section)   Surgical delivery of a baby through an incision into the abdominal and uterine walls. Legend has it that the Roman emperor Julius Caesar was the first person born by this method.

chalazion   Small hard tumor or mass, similar to a sebaceous cyst, developing on the eyelids. May require incision and drainage (I & D).

chancroid   Highly infectious nonsyphilitic venereal ulcer.

chart   Documents the details of a patient's hospital stay. Each health care professional that has contact with the patient in any capacity completes the appropriate report of that contact and adds it to the medical chart. This results in a permanent physical record of the patient's day-to-day condition, when and what services he or she receives and the response to treatment. Also called the medical record.

cheilorrhaphy   Suture of the lip.

chemical name   The name for a drug based on its chemical formula or molecular structure.

chemobrasion   Abrasion using chemicals. Also called a chemical peel.

chemotherapy (chemo)   Treating disease by using chemicals that have a toxic effect upon the body, especially cancerous tissue.

chest X-ray (CXR)   Taking a radiographic picture of the lungs and heart from the back and sides.

Cheyne–Stokes respiration   Abnormal breathing pattern in which there are long periods (10 to 60 seconds) of apnea followed by deeper, more rapid breathing.

chickenpox   A contagious infection caused by a *Herpes* virus. It is characterized by a raised rash that turns into blisters and finally scabs over. Also called varicella.

chiropodist   Specialist in treating disorders of the feet. More modern term is podiatrist.

chiropractic   Practice of treating patients using manipulation of the vertebral column.

chlamydial infection   Parasitic microorganism causing genital infections in males and females. Can lead to pelvic inflammatory disease in females and eventual infertility.

choking   Obstruction within the respiratory passage that interferes with breathing and circulation.

cholangiogram   X-ray picture of the bile ducts.

cholecystectomy   Surgical excision of the gallbladder. Removal of the gallbladder through the laparoscope is a newer procedure with fewer complications than the more invasive abdominal surgery. The laparoscope requires a small incision into the abdominal cavity.

cholecystitis   Inflammation of the gallbladder.

cholecystogram   Dye given orally to the patient is absorbed and enters the gallbladder. An X-ray is then taken.

choledocholithotomy   Removal of a gallstone through an incision into the bile duct.

choledocholithotripsy   Crushing of a gallstone in the common bile duct.

cholelithiasis   Formation or presence of stones or calculi in the gallbladder or common bile duct.

cholesterol   An organic substance found in plasma. It is used by cells to build cell membranes and by the liver to produce bile. Too much cholesterol is associated with blocked arteries.

chondrectomy   Excision of cartilage.

chondromalacia   Softening of cartilage.

chondroplasty   Surgical repair of cartilage.

chondrosarcoma   Sarcoma of cartilage tissue.

chorea   Involuntary nervous disorder that results in muscular twitching of the limbs or facial muscles.

choriocarcinoma   Rare type of cancer of the uterus. May occur following a normal pregnancy or abortion.

chorion   The outer of two membranous sacs surrounding the fetus. It helps to form the placenta.

choroid   The middle layer of the eyeball. This layer provides the blood supply for the eye.

chromosomes   The genetic material carried by each cell.

chronic disease   Illness that comes on slowly and can be long-lasting.

chronic obstructive pulmonary disease (COPD)   Progressive, chronic, and usually irreversible condition in which the lungs have a diminished capacity for inspiration (inhalation) and expiration (exhalation). The person may have difficulty breathing upon exertion (dyspnea) and a cough. Also called chronic obstructive lung disease (COLD).

chyme   Semisoft mixture of food and digestive fluids that pass from the stomach into the small intestines.

cicatrix   A scar.

cilia   A term for eyelashes that protect the eye from foreign particles or for nasal hairs that help filter dust and bacteria out of inhaled air.

ciliary body   The intraocular eye muscles that change the shape of the lens.

circulating nurse   Nurse who assists the surgeon and scrub nurse by providing needed materials during the procedure and by handling the surgical specimen. This person does not wear sterile clothing and may enter and leave the operating room during the procedure.

circulatory system   System that transports blood to all areas of the body. The organs of the circulatory system include the heart and blood vessels (arteries, veins, and capillaries). Also called the cardiovascular system.

circumcision   Surgical removal of the end of the prepuce or foreskin of the penis. Generally performed on the newborn male at the request of the parents. The primary reason is for ease of hygiene. Circumcision is also a ritual practice in some religions.

circumduction   Movement in a circular direction from a central point.

cirrhosis   Chronic disease of the liver.

cisterna chyli   A pouch-like sac at the beginning of the thoracic duct.

clamp   A surgical instrument used to grasp tissue and control bleeding.

clavicle   Also called the collar bone. A bone of the pectoral girdle.

clean catch specimen (CC)   Urine sample obtained after cleaning off the urinary opening and catching or collecting a sample in midstream (halfway through the urination process) to minimize contamination from the genitalia.

cleft lip   Congenital anomaly in which the upper lip fails to come together. Often seen along with a cleft palate. Corrected with surgery.

cleft palate   Congenital anomaly in which the roof of the mouth has a split or fissure. Corrected with surgery.

clinical divisions   System that divides the abdomen into four regions.

clinical psychologist   A specialist in evaluating and treating persons with mental and emotional disorders.

clitoris   A small organ containing erectile tissue that is covered by the labia minora. It contains sensitive tissue that is aroused during sexual stimulation and is similar to the penis in the male.

closed fracture   A simple fracture with no open skin or wound.

coarctation of the aorta   Severe congenital narrowing of the aorta.

coccygeal   Pertaining to the coccyx or tail bone.

coccyx   The tail bone, the four small fused vertebrae at the distal end of the vertebral column.

cochlea   A portion of the labyrinth associated with hearing. It is rolled in the shape of a snail shell. The organs of Corti line the cochlea.

cochlear   Pertaining to the cochlea.

cochlear implant   Mechanical device that is surgically placed under the skin behind the outer ear (pinna). It converts sound signals into magnetic impulses to stimulate the auditory nerve. Can be beneficial for those with profound sensorineural hearing loss.

cochlear nerve   The branch of the vestibulocochlear nerve that carries hearing information to the brain.

coitus   Term for sexual intercourse.

colectomy   Surgical removal of the colon.

collagen   An insoluble fibrous protein present in connective tissue that forms a flexible mat to protect the skin and other parts of the body.

collecting tubule   A portion of the renal tubule.

Colles' fracture   A specific type of wrist fracture.

colon   Also called the large intestines. Functions to reabsorb most of the fluid in the digested food. The material that remains after water reabsorption is the feces. The sections of the colon are the cecum, ascending colon, transverse colon, descending colon, and sigmoid colon.

colonoscope   Instrument to view inside the colon.

colonoscopy   A flexible fiberscope passed through the anus, rectum, and colon is used to examine the upper portion of the colon. Polyps and small growths can be removed during this procedure.

color vision tests   Use of polychromic (multi-colored) charts to determine the ability of the patient to recognize color.

colostomy   Surgical creation of an opening in some portion of the colon through the abdominal wall to the outside surface. The fecal material (stool) drains into a bag worn on the abdomen.

colposcope   Instrument to view inside the vagina.

colposcopy   Visual examination of the cervix and vagina using a colposcope or instrument with a magnifying lens.

coma   Abnormal deep sleep or stupor resulting from an illness or injury.

combining form   The word root plus the combining vowel. It is always written with a / between the word root and the combining vowel. For example, in the combining form cardi/o, cardi is the word root and /o is the combining vowel.

combining vowel   A vowel inserted between word parts that makes it possible to pronounce long medical terms. It is usually the vowel *o*.

comedo   Medical term for a blackhead. It is an accumulation of sebum in a sebaceous gland that has become blackened.

comminuted fracture   A fracture in which the bone is shattered, splintered, or crushed into many pieces or fragments. The fracture is completely through the bone.

commissurotomy   Surgical incision to change the size of an opening. For example, in mitral commissurotomy, a stenosis or narrowing is treated by cutting away at the adhesions around the mitral opening (orifice).

common bile duct   A duct that carries bile from the gallbladder to the duodenum.

compact bone   The hard exterior surface bone. Also called cortical bone.

complete blood count (CBC)   Blood test that consists of five tests: red blood cell count (RBC), white blood count (WBC), hemoglobin (Hg), hematocrit (Hct), and white blood cell differential.

complete fracture   A fracture in which the bone is completely broken through with neither fragment connected to the other.

compound fracture   An open fracture in which the skin has been broken through by the fracture.

computerized axial tomography (CT)   Computer-assisted X-ray used to detect tumors and fractures. Also referred to as a CAT or CT scan.

concussion   Injury to the brain that results from a blow or impact from an object. Can result in unconsciousness, dizziness, vomiting, unequal pupil size, and shock.

conductive hearing loss   Loss of hearing as a result of the blocking of sound transmission in the middle ear and outer ear.

condyle   Refers to the rounded portion at the end of a bone.

condyloma   Wartlike growth on the external genitalia.

cones   The sensory receptors of the retina that are active in bright light and see in color.

congenital anomaly   Any abnormality present at birth. A birth defect.

congenital heart anomaly   Heart defect that is present at birth.

congenital hip dysplasia   An orthopedic condition in which the head of the femur does not articulate with the acetabulum. The hip dislocation can be partial or complete.

congenital septal defect (CSD)   Defect, present at birth, in the wall separating two chambers of the heart. Results in a mixture of oxygenated and deoxygenated blood being carried to the surrounding tissues. There can be an atrial septal defect (ASD) and a ventricular septal defect (VSD).

congestive heart failure (CHF)   Pathological condition of the heart in which there is a reduced outflow of blood from the left side of the heart. Results in weakness, breathlessness, and edema.

conization   Surgical removal of a core of cervical tissue. Also refers to partial removal of the cervix.

conjunctiva   A protective mucous membrane lining on the underside of each eyelid and across the anterior surface of each eyeball.

conjunctivitis   Also referred to as pinkeye or an inflammation of the conjunctiva.

connective tissue   The supporting and protecting tissue in body structures. Examples are fat or adipose tissue, cartilage, and bone.

connective tissue membrane   A membrane that contains only a single layer of connective tissue. It does not have an epithelial layer. The most common type of connective tissue membrane is the synovial membrane that lines synovial joints.

conscious   Condition of being awake and aware of surroundings.

constipation   Experiencing difficulty in defecation or infrequent defecation.

Consultation Report   Document in a patient's medical record. They are the reports given by specialists who the physician has requested to evaluate the patient.

contraception   Prevention of a pregnancy using artificial means such as an intrauterine device (IUD) or medication (birth control pills).

contraceptive   Used to prevent conception.

contraction   Contraction of the muscles of the uterus to forcibly expel the fetus.

contraindication   Condition in which a particular drug should not be used.

Controlled Substance Act of 1970   Law that regulates the manufacture and distribution of drugs that are capable of causing dependence.

controlled substances   Drugs that have a potential for being addictive (habit-forming) or can be abused.

convergence   The moving inward of the eyes to see an object close to the face.

conversion reaction   A somatoform disorder in which the patient unconsciously substitutes physical signs or symptoms for anxiety. The most common physical signs or symptoms are blindness, deafness, and paralysis.

convulsion   Severe involuntary muscle contractions and relaxations. These have a variety of causes, such as epilepsy, fever, and toxic conditions.

Cooley's anemia   Condition in which a rare form of anemia or a reduction of red blood cells is found in some people of Mediterranean origin.

copulation   Term for sexual intercourse.

cor pulmonale   Hypertrophy of the right ventricle of the heart as a result of lung disease.

cordectomy   Removal of part of the spinal cord.

corium   The living layer of skin located between the epidermis and the subcutaneous tissue. Also referred to as the dermis, it contains hair follicles, sweat glands, sebaceous glands, blood vessels, lymph vessels, nerve fibers, and muscle fibers.

cornea   A portion of the sclera that is clear and transparent and allows light to enter the interior of the eye. It also plays a role in bending light rays.

coronal plane   A vertical plane that divides the body into front (anterior or ventral) and back (posterior or dorsal) sections. Also called the frontal plane.

coronary   Pertaining to the heart.

coronary artery   A group of three arteries that branch off the aorta and carry blood to the myocardium.

coronary artery bypass graft (CABG)   Open-heart surgery in which a blood vessel is grafted to route blood around the point of constriction in a diseased coronary artery.

coronary care unit (CCU)   Specialized hospital unit equipped to care for and monitor patients who have suffered a heart attack.

coronary ischemia   Insufficient blood supply to the heart muscle due to an obstruction.

coronary thrombosis   Blood clot in a coronary vessel of the heart causing the vessel to close completely or partially.

corpus   The body or central portion of the uterus.

cortex   The outer layer of an organ. In the endocrine system, it refers to the outer layer of the adrenal glands.

cortical   Pertaining to the cortex.

cortical bone   The hard exterior surface bone. Also called compact bone.

corticosteroids   General term for the group of hormones secreted by the adrenal cortex. They include mineralocorticoid hormones, glucocorticoid hormones, and steroid sex hormones.

cortisol   A steroid hormone secreted by the adrenal cortex. It regulates carbohydrate metabolism.

Cowper's gland   Also called bulbourethral gland. These two small male reproductive system glands are located on either side of the urethra just distal to the prostate. The secretion from these glands neutralizes the acidity in the urethra and the vagina.

cranial   Pertaining to the skull.

cranial cavity   A dorsal body cavity. It is within the skull and contains the brain.

cranial nerves   Nerves that arise from the brain.

craniocele   Protrusion of the brain from within the skull.

cranioplasty   Surgical repair of the skull.

craniotomy   Incision into the skull.

cranium   The skull; bones that form a protective covering over the brain.

crash cart   Emergency cart on wheels that contains medications and equipment needed in emergency situations. The cart can be moved to the patient's bedside or from one office to another.

creatinine   A waste product of muscle metabolism.

crepitation   Sound of broken bones rubbing together.

cretinism   Congenital condition due to a lack of thyroid that may result in arrested physical and mental development.

Crohn's disease   Form of chronic inflammatory bowel disease affecting the ileum and/or colon. Also called regional ileitis.

croup   Acute viral respiratory infection common in infants and young children and characterized by a hoarse cough.

crown   Portion of a tooth that is covered by enamel. Also an artificial covering for the tooth created to replace the original enamel.

crowning   When the head of the baby is visible through the vaginal opening. A sign that birth is imminent.

cryoextraction   Procedure in which cataract is lifted from the lens with an extremely cold probe.

cryoretinopexy   Surgical fixation of the retina by using extreme cold.

cryosurgery   Exposing tissues to extreme cold in order to destroy them. Used in treating malignant tumors, and to control pain and bleeding.

cryotherapy   Using cold for therapeutic purposes.

cryptorchidism   Failure of the testes to descend into the scrotal sac before birth. Generally, the testes will descend before the boy is one year old. A surgical procedure called orchidopexy may be required to bring the testes down into the scrotum permanently. Failure of the testes to descend could result in sterility in the male.

CT scan (CAT)   Use of computerized tomography to diagnose disorders of the lymphoid organs.

culdoscopy   Examination of the female pelvic cavity by introducing an endoscope through the wall of the vagina.

culture and sensitivity (C&S)   A laboratory test in which a colony of pathogens that have been removed from an infected area are grown to identify the pathogen and then determine its sensitivity to a variety of antibiotics.

cumulative action   Action that occurs in the body when a drug is allowed to accumulate or stay in the body.

curettage   Removal of superficial skin lesions with a curette (surgical instrument shaped like a spoon) or scraper.

curette   A surgical instrument used to scrape and remove tissue.

Current Procedural Terminology (CPT)   A coding system developed by the American Medical Association. Providers use this system to report the procedures it provides to a patient.

Cushing's syndrome   Set of symptoms named after Harvey Cushing, an American neurosurgeon that result from hypersecretion of the adrenal cortex. This may be the result of a tumor of the adrenal glands. The syndrome may present symptoms of weakness, edema, excess hair growth, skin discoloration, and osteoporosis.

cuspids   Permanent teeth located between the incisors and the bicuspids that assist in biting and cutting food. Humans have four cuspids. Also called canine teeth or eyeteeth.

cusps   The leaflets or flaps of a heart valve.

cutaneous membrane   This is another term for the skin.

cuticle   The thin skin-like layer overlapping the base of a nail.

cyanosis   Slightly bluish color of the skin due to a deficiency of oxygen and an excess of carbon dioxide in the blood. It is caused by a variety of disorders, ranging from chronic lung disease to congenital and chronic heart problems.

cyclotron   Equipment consisting of a particle accelerator in which the particles are rotated between magnets.

cyst   Fluid-filled sac under the skin.

cystalgia   Bladder pain.

cystectomy   Excision of the bladder.

cystic fibrosis   Hereditary condition causing the exocrine glands to malfunction. The patient produces very thick mucous that causes severe congestion within the lungs and digestive system. Through more advanced treatment, many children are now living into adulthood with this disease.

cystitis   Inflammation of the bladder.

cystocele   Hernia or outpouching of the bladder that protrudes into the vagina. This may cause urinary frequency and urgency.

cystography   Process of instilling a contrast material or dye into the bladder by catheter to visualize the urinary bladder on X-ray.

cystolith   Bladder stone.

cystoplasty   Surgical repair of the bladder.

cystorrhagia   Rapid bleeding from the bladder.

cystoscopy   Visual examination of the urinary bladder using an instrument called a cystoscope.

cystostomy   Creation of an opening through the body wall and into the bladder.

cystotomy   Incision into the bladder.

cytologic testing   Examination of cells to determine their structure and origin. PAP smears are considered a form of cytologic testing.

cytopenia   A decrease in the number of circulating cells—erythrocytes, leukocytes, platelets—in the blood.

cytotoxic   Pertaining to poisoning cells.

cytotoxic cells   T cells that are destructive to cells and can kill foreign invasion cells. Also called T8 cells.

dacryocystitis   Inflammation of tear sac.

day surgery   A type of outpatient surgery in which the patient is discharged on the same day he or she is admitted; also called ambulatory surgery.

deafness   The inability to hear or having some degree of hearing impairment.

debridement   Removal of foreign material and dead or damaged tissue from a wound.

decibel (dB) Measures the intensity or loudness of a sound. Zero dB is the quietest sound measured and 120 dB is the loudest sound commonly measured.

deciduous teeth The twenty teeth that begin to erupt around the age of six months. Eventually pushed out by the permanent teeth.

decongestant Reduces nasal congestion and swelling.

decubitus ulcers Bedsores or pressure sores caused by pressure over bony prominences on the body. They are caused by a lack of blood flow.

deep Directional term meaning away from the surface of the body.

defibrillation A procedure that converts serious irregular heart beats, such as fibrillation, by giving electric shocks to the heart.

defibrillator Equipment that sends an electrical charge through a person's body in an attempt to enable the heart to start beating in a normal manner.

delirium State of mental confusion with a lack of orientation to time and place.

delusions A false belief held with conviction even in the face of strong evidence to the contrary.

dementia Progressive impairment of intellectual function that interferes with performing the activities of daily living. Patients have little awareness of their condition. Found in disorders such as Alzheimer's.

dendrites Branched processes off a neuron that receives impulses and carries them to the cell body.

dental Pertaining to teeth.

dentin The main bulk of the tooth. It is covered by enamel.

dentist Person who is authorized, based on education, training, and licensure, to practice dentistry.

denture Partial or complete set of artificial teeth that are set in plastic materials. Substitute for the natural teeth and related structures.

deoxygenated Blood in the veins that is low in oxygen content.

depigmentation Loss of normal skin color or pigment.

dermabrasion Abrasion or rubbing using wire brushes or sandpaper.

dermatitis Inflammation of the skin.

dermatofibroma Fibrous tumor of the skin. It is painless, round, firm, red, and generally found on the extremities.

dermatographia Skin writing. Wheals develop on the skin of some people as a result of tracing on the skin with an instrument or fingernail.

dermatologist A physician specialized in the diagnosis and treatment of diseases of the integumentary system.

dermatology The branch of medicine specializing in conditions of the integumentary system.

dermatome Instrument for cutting the skin or thin transplants of skin.

dermatopathy General term for skin disease.

dermatoplasty The surgical repair of the skin.

dermis The living layer of skin located between the epidermis and the subcutaneous tissue. It is also referred to as the corium or the *true skin*. It contains hair follicles, sweat glands, sebaceous glands, blood vessels, lymph vessels, nerve fibers, and muscle fibers.

descending colon The section of the colon that descends the left side of the abdomen.

developmental disabilities A disorder that interferes with the normal growth and development of a child. This condition may affect muscles or mental abilities.

diabetes insipidus (DI) Disorder caused by the inadequate secretion of a hormone by the posterior lobe of the pituitary gland. There may be polyuria and polydipsia. This is more common in the young.

diabetes mellitus A serious disease in which the pancreas fails to produce insulin or the insulin does not work properly. Consequently, the patient has very high blood sugar. The kidney will attempt to lower the high blood sugar level by excreting excess sugar in the urine.

diabetic coma Abnormal deep stupor occurring as a result of lack of insulin. The person will have a sweet breath, from acidosis.

diabetic retinopathy Secondary complication of diabetes that affects the blood vessels of the retina, resulting in visual changes and even blindness.

Diagnosis Related Groups (DRG) A method of classification placing patients into groups based on their primary and secondary diagnoses that was developed for Medicare. Each diagnostic group is assigned a dollar figure based on an estimate of the cost of caring for patients with this diagnosis. Providers receive this reimbursement regardless of the actual expenses incurred. This is referred to as a prospective payment system.

diagnostic Procedure to determine the cause and nature of a person's illness.

Diagnostic Reports Found in a patient's medical record. It consists of the results of all diagnostic tests performed on the patient, principally from the lab and medical imaging (for example, X-rays and ultrasound).

diaphoresis Excessive or profuse sweating.

diaphragm The major muscle of inspiration. It separates the thoracic from the abdominal cavity.

diaphragmatic breathing The correct style of breathing for singers and public speakers. With this type of breathing, the abdomen expands during inspiration and contracts during expiration. The shoulders remain motionless.

diaphragmatocele A protrusion of the stomach through the diaphragm into the chest cavity. Also called a hiatal hernia.

diaphysis The shaft portion of a long bone.

diarrhea Passing of frequent, watery bowel movements. Usually accompanies gastrointestinal (GI) disorders.

diastolic pressure The lower pressure within blood vessels during the relaxation phase of the heart beat.

diencephalon The portion of the brain that contains two of the most critical areas of the brain, the thalamus and the hypothalamus.

differential Blood test to determine the number of each variety of leukocytes.

digestive system   System that digests food and absorbs nutrients. Organs include the mouth, pharynx, esophagus, stomach, small and large intestines, liver, gallbladder, and anus. Also called the gastrointestinal system.

digital rectal exam (DRE)   Manual examination for an enlarged prostate gland performed by palpating (feeling) the prostate gland through the wall of the rectum.

dilation and curettage (D & C)   Surgical procedure in which the opening of the cervix is dilated and the uterus is scrapped or suctioned of its lining or tissue. Often performed after a spontaneous abortion and to stop excessive bleeding from other causes.

dilation stage   The first stage of labor. It begins with uterine contractions that press the fetus against the cervix causing it to dilate to 10 cm and become thin. The thinning of the cervix is called effacement.

dilator   A surgical instrument used to enlarge an opening by stretching.

dilute   To weaken the strength of a substance by adding something else.

diphtheria   A bacterial infection of the respiratory system characterized by severe inflammation that can form a membrane coating in the upper respiratory tract that can cause marked difficulty breathing.

diplopia   Double vision.

discharge planning   Preparation made by the caregivers and family for a patient upon discharge from a hospital or nursing home.

Discharge Summary   Part of a patient's medical record. It is a comprehensive outline of the patient's entire hospital stay. It includes condition at time of admission, admitting diagnosis, test results, treatments and patient's response, final diagnosis, and follow-up plans.

dissection   The surgical cutting of parts for separation and study.

distal   Directional term meaning located farthest from the point of attachment to the body.

distal convoluted tubule   A portion of the renal tubule.

diuresis   Abnormal secretion of large amounts of urine.

diuretic   Increases the excretion of urine, which promotes the loss of water and salt from the body. Can assist in lowering blood pressure; therefore, these drugs are used to treat hypertension. Potassium in the body may be depleted with continued use of diuretics. Potassium-rich foods such as bananas, kiwi, and orange juice can help correct this deficiency.

diverticulectomy   Surgical removal of a diverticulum.

diverticulitis   Inflammation of a diverticulum or sac in the intestinal tract, especially in the colon.

diverticulosis   Condition of having blind pouches off the colon or small intestines.

dominant   If a person has one dominant and one recessive gene for a trait, the dominant gene will mask the recessive gene, allowing the dominant trait to be displayed.

Doppler ultrasonography   Measurement of sound-wave echos as they bounce off tissues and organs to produce an image. Can assist in determining heart and blood vessel damage.

Doppler ultrasound   Using an instrument placed externally over the uterus to examine the fetal heart.

dorsal   Directional term meaning near or on the back or spinal cord side of the body.

dorsiflexion   Backward bending, as of hand or foot.

Down syndrome   Disorder that produces moderate-to-severe mental retardation and multiple defects. The physical characteristics of a child with this disorder are a sloping forehead, flat nose or absent bridge to the nose, low-set eyes, and a general dwarfed physical growth. The disorder occurs more commonly when the mother is over 40.

draping   Process of covering the patient with sterile cloths that allow only the operative site to be exposed to the surgeon.

drowning   Asphyxiation due to an immersion in water or a liquid.

Drug Enforcement Agency (DEA)   The government agency that enforces regulation of controlled substances.

drug tolerance   Decrease in susceptibility to a drug after continued use of the drug.

Duchenne muscular dystrophy   Muscular disorder in which there is progressive wasting away of various muscles, including leg, pelvic, and shoulder muscles. Children with this disorder have difficulty climbing stairs and running and may eventually be confined to a wheelchair. Other complications relating to the heart and respiratory system can be present. It is caused by a recessive gene and is more common in males. Often results in a shortened life-span.

ductus deferens   Also called vas deferens. The ductus deferens is a long, straight tube that carries sperm from the epididymis up into the pelvic cavity, where it continues around the bladder and empties into the urethra. It is one of the components, along with nerves and blood vessels, of the spermatic cord.

duodenum   The first section of small intestines. Digestion is completed in the duodenum after the chyme mixes with digestive juices from the pancreas and gallbladder.

dura mater   The term means tough mother. It is the fibrous outermost meninges layer that forms a tough protective layer.

dwarfism   Condition of being abnormally small. It may be the result of a hereditary condition or an endocrine dysfunction.

dyskinesia   Difficult or painful movement.

dysmenorrhea   Painful cramping that is associated with menstruation.

dyspepsia   Indigestion.

dysphagia   Having difficulty eating.

dysphasia   Impairment of speech as a result of a brain lesion.

dyspnea   Difficult, labored breathing.

dystocia   Abnormal or difficult labor and childbirth.

dystrophy   Abnormal or poor development.

dysuria   Painful or difficult urination. This is a symptom in many disorders, such as cystitis, urethritis, enlarged prostate in the male, and prolapsed uterus in the female.

ear   The sensory organ for hearing.

ear drops   Placed directly into the ear canal for the purpose of relieving pain or treating infection.

ecchymosis   Skin discoloration or bruise caused by blood collecting under the skin.

echocardiogram   Noninvasive diagnostic method using ultrasound to visualize internal cardiac structures, especially the cardiac valves.

echoencephalogram   Recording of the ultrasonic echos of the brain. Useful in determining abnormal patterns of shifting in the brain.

eclampsia   Convulsive seizures and coma that can occur in a woman between the twentieth week of pregnancy and the first week of postpartum. Often associated with hypertension.

ectopic pregnancy   Fetus that becomes abnormally implanted outside the uterine cavity. This is a condition requiring immediate surgery.

ectropion   Term referring to eversion (turning outward) of the eyelid.

eczema   Superficial dermatitis accompanied by papules, vesicles, and crusting.

edema   Condition in which the body tissues contain excessive amounts of fluid.

effacement   The thinning of the cervix during labor.

efferent arteriole   Arteriole that carries blood away from the glomerulus.

efferent neurons   Nerves that carry impulses away from the brain and spinal cord to the muscles and glands. Also called motor neurons.

ejaculation   The impulse of forcing seminal fluid from the male urethra.

elder abuse   Mistreatment of the elderly.

electrocardiogram (ECG, EKG)   Record of the electrical activity of the heart. Useful in the diagnosis of abnormal cardiac rhythm and heart muscle (myocardium) damage.

electrocardiography   Process of recording the electrical activity of the heart.

electrocautery   To destroy tissue with an electric current.

electroconvulsive therapy (ECT)   A procedure occasionally used for cases of prolonged major depression in which an electrode is placed on one or both sides of the patient's head and current is turned on briefly causing a convulsive seizure. A low level of voltage is used in modern ECT and the patient is administered a muscle relaxant and an anesthesia. Advocates of this treatment state that it is a more effective way to treat severe depression than with the use of drugs. It is not effective with disorders other than depression, such as schizophrenia and alcoholism.

electroencephalogram   A record of the brain's electrical activity.

electroencephalograph   Instrument used to record the brain's electrical activity.

electroencephalography (EEG)   Recording the electrical activity of the brain by placing electrodes at various positions on the scalp. Also used in sleep studies to determine if there is a normal pattern of activity during sleep.

electrolyte   Chemical compound that separates into charged particles, or ionizes, in a solution. Sodium chloride (NaCl) and potassium (K) are examples of electrolytes.

electromyography   Recording of the electrical patterns of a muscle in order to diagnose diseases.

electron   Minute particle with a negative electrical charge that is emitted from radioactive substances. These are called *rays*.

elephantiasis   Inflammation, obstruction, and destruction of the lymph vessels that results in enlarged tissues due to edema.

ELISA (enzyme-linked immunosorbent assay)   A blood test for an antibody to the AIDS virus. A positive test means that the person has been exposed to the virus. In the case of a false-positive reading, the Western blot test would be used to verify the results.

embolectomy   Surgical removal of an embolus or clot from a blood vessel.

embolism   Obstruction of a blood vessel by a blood clot or foreign substance, such as air or fat.

embolus   Obstruction of a blood vessel by a blood clot that moves from another area.

embryo   The term to describe the developing infant from fertilization until the end of the eighth week.

emergency care   A level of patient care that is reserved for life threatening illnesses that probably require hospitalization, such as a heart attack.

emergency childbirth   Childbirth that happens quickly before the mother and assistants are prepared. The signs and symptoms of an impending delivery are: a bloody show of mucus; a feeling and desire of the mother to bear down or push with the contractions; strong uterine contractions that become close together; the baby's head *crowning* or appearing at the vaginal opening; and the visible bulging of the baby's head against the bag of waters (if it has not broken.)

emergency medical technician (EMT)   Person trained in techniques of administering emergency care.

emergency medicine   The branch of medicine specializing in emergency care of the acutely ill and injured.

emergency room   Area of a hospital or a free-standing unit that is prepared to care for the severely ill and injured.

emesis   Vomiting, usually with some force.

emetic   Induces vomiting.

emmetropia (EM)   State of normal vision.

emphysema   Pulmonary condition that can occur as a result of long-term heavy smoking. Air pollution also worsens this disease. The patient may not be able to breathe except in a sitting or standing position.

empyema   Pus within the pleural space, usually the result of infection.

enamel   The hardest substance in the body. Covers the outer surface of teeth.

encapsulated   Growth enclosed in a sheath of tissue that prevents tumor cells from invading surrounding tissue.

encephalitis Inflammation of the brain due to disease factors such as rabies, influenza, measles, or smallpox.

encephalocele Protrusion of the brain through the cranial cavity.

encephalomalacia Brain softening.

encephalosclerosis Condition of hardening of the brain.

endarterectomy Removal of the inside layer of an artery.

endocarditis Inflammation of the inner lining layer of the heart. May be due to microorganisms or to an abnormal immunological response.

endocardium The inner layer of the heart, which is very smooth and lines the chambers of the heart.

endocervicitis Inflammation of the inner aspect of the cervix.

endocrine glands A glandular system that secretes hormones directly into the bloodstream rather than into a duct. Endocrine glands are frequently referred to as ductless glands. The endocrine system includes the thyroid gland, adrenal glands, parathyroid glands, pituitary gland, pancreas (islets of Langerhans), testes, ovaries, and thymus gland.

endocrine system The body system that consists of glands that secrete hormones directly into the blood stream. The endocrine glands include the adrenal glands, parathyroid glands, pancreas, pituitary gland, testes, ovaries, thymus gland, and thyroid gland.

endocrinologist Physician who specializes in the treatment of endocrine glands, including diabetes.

endocrinology The branch of medicine specializing in conditions of the endocrine system.

endocrinopathy A disease of the endocrine system.

endometrial biopsy Taking a sample of tissue from the lining of the uterus to test for abnormalities.

endometrial cancer Cancer of the endometrial lining of the uterus.

endometriosis Abnormal condition of endometrium tissue appearing throughout the pelvis or on the abdominal wall. This tissue is usually found within the uterus.

endometritis Inflammation of the endometrial lining of the uterus.

endometrium The inner lining of the uterus. It contains a rich blood supply and reacts to hormonal changes every month, which results in menstruation. During a pregnancy, the lining of the uterus does not leave the body but remains to nourish the unborn child.

endophthalmitis Inflammation within the eye.

endoscope Instrument to view inside a tubular or hollow organ.

endoscopic retrograde cholangiopancreatography (ERCP) Using an endoscope to X-ray the bile and pancreatic ducts.

endoscopic surgery Use of a lighted instrument to examine the interior of a cavity.

endoscopy A general term for a procedure to visually examine the inside of a body cavity or a hollow organ using an instrument called an endoscope. Specific examples of endoscopy relating to the digestive system include colonoscopy, esophagoscopy, gastrointestinal endoscopy, and gastroscopy.

endotracheal Pertaining to inside the trachea.

endotracheal intubation Placing a tube through the mouth to create an airway.

enteritis Inflammation of only the small intestine.

enterorrhaphy Suture small intestines.

entropion Term referring to inversion (turning inward) of the eyelid.

enuresis Involuntary discharge of urine after the age by which bladder control should have been established. This usually occurs by the age of five. Also called bed-wetting at night.

eosinophils A granulocyte white blood cell that destroy parasites and increase during allergic reactions.

epicardium The outer layer of the heart. It forms part of the pericardium.

epicondyle A projection located above or on a condyle.

epidermal Pertaining to upon the skin.

epidermis The superficial layer of skin. It is composed of squamous epithelium cells. These are flat scale-like cells that are arranged in layers, called stratified squamous epithelium. The many layers of the epidermis create a barrier to infection. The epidermis does not have a blood supply, so it is dependent on the deeper layers of skin for nourishment. However, the deepest epidermis layer is called the basal layer. These cells are alive and constantly dividing. Older cells are pushed out toward the surface by new cells forming beneath. During this process, they shrink and die, becoming filled with a protein called keratin. The keratin-filled cells are sloughed off as dead cells.

epidermoid cyst Cyst in the skull and phalanges of the fingers.

epididymectomy Surgical excision of the epididymis.

epididymis The epididymis is a coiled tubule that lies on top of the testes within the scrotum. This tube stores sperm as they are produced and turns into the vas deferens.

epididymitis Inflammation of the epididymis that causes pain and swelling in the inguinal area.

epidural hematoma Mass of blood in the space outside the dura mater of the brain and spinal cord.

epigastric Pertaining to above the stomach. An anatomical division of the abdomen, the middle section of the upper row.

epiglottis A flap of cartilage that covers the larynx when a person swallows. This prevents food and drink from entering the larynx and trachea.

epiglottitis Swelling of the epiglottis, causing an airway obstruction. A potentially life-threatening condition that can be caused by bacterial infection.

epilepsy Recurrent disorder of the brain in which convulsive seizures and loss of consciousness occur.

epinephrine A hormone produced by the adrenal medulla. Also known as adrenaline. Some of its actions include increased heart rate and force of contraction, bronchodilation, and relaxation of intestinal muscles.

epiphysis The wide ends of a long bone.

episiorrhaphy   Suture the perineum.

episiotomy   Surgical incision of the perineum to facilitate the delivery process. Can prevent an irregular tearing of tissue during birth.

epispadias   Congenital opening of the urethra on the dorsal surface of the penis.

epistaxis   Nosebleed.

epithelial   Pertaining to the epithelium.

epithelial membrane   Membranes that contain two layers of tissue: a superficial layer or epithelial tissue and an underlying connective tissue layer. The three common types of epithelial membranes are cutaneous, serous, and mucous membranes.

epithelial tissue   Tissue found throughout the body as the skin, the outer covering of organs, and the inner lining for tubular or hollow structures.

Epstein-Barr virus   Virus that is believed to be the cause of infectious mononucleosis, was discovered by Anthony Epstein, a British virologist, and Yvonne Barr, a French physician.

equilibrium   The sense of balance.

erectile tissue   Tissue with numerous blood vessels and nerve endings. It becomes filled with blood and enlarges in size in response to sexual stimulation.

ergonomics   The study of human work including how the requirements for performing work and the work environment affect the musculoskeletal and nervous system.

erythema   Redness or flushing of the skin.

erythroblastosis fetalis   Condition in which antibodies enter the fetus's blood and cause anemia, jaundice, edema, and enlargement of the liver and spleen. Also called hemolytic disease of the newborn.

erythrocyte   Also called red blood cells or RBCs. Cells that contain hemoglobin, an iron-containing pigment that binds oxygen in order to transport it to the cells of the body.

erythrocyte sedimentation rate (ESR)   Blood test to determine the rate at which mature red blood cells settle out of the blood after the addition of an anticoagulant. An indicator of the presence of an inflammatory disease.

erythroderma   Red skin.

erythropoiesis   The process of forming erythrocytes.

Escherichia coli **(E. coli)**   Normal bacteria found in the intestinal track; the most common cause of lower urinary track infections due to improper hygiene after bowel movements.

esophageal stricture   Narrowing of the esophagus, which makes the flow of fluids and food difficult.

esophagogastrostomy   Surgical creation of an opening between the esophagus and the stomach.

esophagoscopy and biopsy   The esophagus is visualized by passing an instrument down the esophagus. A tissue sample for biopsy may be taken.

esophagostomy   Surgical creation of an opening into the esophagus.

esophagus   The tube that carries food from the pharynx to the stomach.

esotropia   Inward turning of the eye. An example of a form of strabismus (muscle weakness of the eye).

estimated date of confinement (EDC)   Estimation date when the baby will be born based on a calculation from the last menstrual period of the mother.

estrogen   One of the hormones produced by the ovaries. It works with progesterone to control the menstrual cycle and it is responsible for producing the secondary sexual characteristics.

ethmoid bone   A cranial bone.

eupnea   Normal breathing.

eustachian tube   Tube or canal that connects the middle ear with the nasopharynx and allows for a balance of pressure between the outer and middle ear. Infection can travel via the mucous membranes of the eustachian tube, resulting in middle ear infections.

euthyroid   Normal thyroid.

eversion   Directional term meaning turning outward.

Ewing's sarcoma   Malignant growth found in the shaft of long bones that spreads through the periosteum. Removal is treatment of choice, as this tumor will metastasize or spread to other organs.

excretory urography   Injection of dye into the bloodstream followed by taking an X-ray to trace the action of the kidney as it excretes the dye.

exfoliative cytology   Scraping cells from tissue and then examining them under a microscope.

exhalation   To breath air out of the lungs. Also called expiration.

exocrine glands   Glands that secrete substances into a duct. Tears and tear ducts are examples of an exocrine gland.

exophthalmic   Pertaining to outward turning eyes.

exophthalmos   Condition in which the eyeballs protrude, such as in Graves' disease. This is generally caused by an overproduction of thyroid hormone.

exotropia   Outward turning of the eye. Also an example of strabismus (muscle weakness of the eye).

expectorant   Assists in the removal of secretions from the bronchopulmonary membranes.

expiration   To breath air out of the lungs. Also called exhalation.

exploratory laparotomy   Abdominal operation for the purpose of examining the abdominal organs and tissues for signs of disease or other abnormalities.

exploratory surgery   Surgery performed for the purpose of determining if there is cancer present or if a known cancer has spread. Biopsies are generally performed.

explosive disorder   An impulse control disorder in which the patient is unable to control violent rages.

extension   Movement that brings limb into or toward a straight condition.

external   Being on the outside or outer surface.

external ear   The outermost portion of the ear. It consists of the auricle, auditory canal, and ear drum.

extracellular fluid   Water found outside the cells; also called interstitial fluid.

extracorporeal shockwave lithotripsy (ESWL) Use of ultrasound waves to break up stones. Process does not require surgery.

eye The sensory organs for vision.

eye drops Placed into the eye to control eye pressure in glaucoma. Also used during eye examinations to dilate the pupil of the eye for better examination of the interior of the eye.

eye muscles There are six muscles that connect the eyeball to the orbit cavity. These muscles allow for rotation of the eyeball.

eye socket The cavity in the front of the skull containing the eyeball. It is formed from several bones and has a soft fatty tissue lining.

eyeball The eye by itself, without any appendages such as the eye muscles or tear ducts.

eyelids An upper and lower fold of skin that provides protection from foreign particles, injury from the sun and intense light, and trauma. Both the upper and lower edges of the eyelids have small hairs or cilia. In addition, sebaceous or oil glands are located in the eyelids. These secrete a lubricating oil.

falling test Test used to observe balance and equilibrium. The patient is observed balancing on one foot, then with one foot in front of the other, and then walking forward with eyes open. The same test is conducted with the patient's eyes closed. Swaying and falling with the eyes closed can indicate an ear and equilibrium malfunction.

fallopian tubes Organ in the female reproductive system that transports eggs from the ovary to the uterus.

fascia Connective tissue that wraps muscles. It tapers at each end of a skeletal muscle to form tendons.

fasciectomy Surgical removal of the fascia, which is the fibrous membrane covering and supporting muscles.

fasting blood sugar (FBS) Blood test to measure the amount of sugar circulating throughout the body after a twelve-hour fast.

febrile convulsions Convulsions brought on by an elevated temperature.

feces Food that cannot be digested becomes a waste product and is expelled or defecated as feces.

Federal Food and Drug Administration (FDA) A department of the Federal Department of Health and Human Services that regulates drug sales and distribution.

Federal Food, Drug, and Cosmetic Act of 1938 Law that stipulates the actual control of drugs. This act was initiated to ensure the safety of food, drugs, and cosmetics that are sold within U.S. borders.

femur Also called the thigh bone. It is a lower extremity bone.

fertilization Also called impregnation. The fusion of an ova and sperm to produce an embryo.

fetal heart rate (FHR) The heart rate of the fetus can be monitored with an electronic device during labor to detect signs of fetal distress. The normal heart rate of the fetus is rapid, ranging from 120 to 160 beats per minute.

fetal heart tone (FHT) Listening for the fetal heart sound to determine strength and general condition of the fetus. This is also done during the labor process.

fetal monitoring Using electronic equipment placed on the mother's abdomen to check the baby's heart rate and strength during labor.

fetus The term to describe the developing newborn from the end of the eighth week until birth.

fibrillation Abnormal quivering or contractions of heart fibers. When this occurs within the fibers of the ventricle of the heart, arrest and death can occur. Emergency equipment to defibrillate, or convert the heart to a normal beat, is necessary.

fibrin Whitish protein formed by the action of thrombin and fibrinogen, which is the basis for the clotting of blood.

fibrinogen Blood protein that is essential for clotting to take place.

fibroid tumor Benign tumor or growth that contains fiberlike tissue. Uterine fibroid tumors are the most common tumors in women.

fibrosarcoma Tumor containing connective tissue that occurs in bone marrow. It is found most frequently in the femur, humerus, and jaw bone.

fibrous joint A joint that has almost no movement because the ends of the bones are joined together by thick fibrous tissue. The sutures of the skull are an example of a fibrous joint.

fibula One of the lower leg bones in the lower extremity.

film Thin sheet of cellulose material coated with a light-sensitive substance that is used in taking photographs. There is a special photographic film that is sensitive to X-rays.

film badge Badge containing film that is sensitive to X-rays. This is worn by all personnel in radiology to measure the amount of X-rays to which they are exposed.

fimbriae The fingerlike extensions on the end of the fallopian tubes. The fimbriae drape over each ovary in order to direct the ovum into the fallopian tube after it is expelled by the ovary.

fine motor skills The use of precise and coordinated movements in such activities as writing, buttoning, and cutting.

fingerspelling Using various hand and finger shapes and positions to represent the written alphabet. These positions can be strung together to form words.

first aid Providing emergency care to the injured or disabled before the physician arrives or the patient can be transported to a hospital.

fissure A deep groove or slit-type opening.

fissured fracture An incomplete longitudinal fracture.

fissures Also called sulci. The grooves that separate the gyri of the cerebral cortex.

fistula Abnormal tubelike passage from one body cavity to another.

fistulectomy Excision of a fistula.

flat bone A type of bone with a thin flattened shape. Examples include the scapula, ribs, and pelvic bones.

flexion   Act of bending or being bent.

fluid and electrolyte imbalance   Serious secondary development in young children with another illness or infection, particularly those with high fever, vomiting, and diarrhea.

fluorescein angiography   Process of injecting a dye (fluorescein) to observe the movement of blood for detecting lesions in the macular area of the retina. Used to determine if there is a detachment of the retina.

fluoroscopy   Use of a fluoroscope to picture the shadows of objects. Also referred to as X-rays.

Foley catheter   Indwelling, thin, sterile tubing placed into the urinary bladder to withdraw urine continuously.

follicle-stimulating hormone (FSH)   A hormone secreted by anterior pituitary gland. It stimulates growth of eggs in females and sperm in males.

foramen   A passage or opening through a bone for nerves and blood vessels.

forceps   A surgical instrument used to grasp tissues.

foreign bodies   Slivers, cinders, dirt, or small objects that lodge in the eyes, ears, nose, or skin, or internally.

forensic dentistry   Using dental records to identify unknown deceased persons.

foreskin   Also called the prepuce. A protective covering over the glans penis. It is this covering of skin that is removed during circumcision.

formed elements   The solid, cellular portion of blood. It consists of erythrocytes, leukocytes, and platelets.

fossa   A shallow cavity or depression within or on the surface of a bone.

fovea centralis   The area of the retina that has the sharpest vision.

Fowler position   Surgical position in which the patient is sitting with back positioned at a 45° angle.

fracture   An injury to a bone that causes it to break. Fractures are named to describe the type of damage to the bone.

fracture pan   Small bedpan with a flat edge that will go under the person who is bedridden.

frequency   A greater than normal occurrence in the urge to urinate, without an increase in the total daily volume of urine. Frequency is an indication of inflammation of the bladder or urethra.

frontal bone   A cranial bone.

frontal lobe   One of the four cerebral hemisphere lobes. It controls motor functions.

frontal plane   A vertical plane that divides the body into front (anterior or ventral) and back (posterior or dorsal) sections. Also called the coronal plane.

frostbite   Freezing or the effect of freezing a part of the body. Exposed areas such as ears, nose, cheeks, fingers, and toes are generally affected.

frozen section (FS)   A thin piece of tissue is cut from a frozen specimen for rapid examination under a microscope.

fundus   The domed upper portion of an organ such as the stomach or uterus.

fungal scrapings   Scrapings, taken with a curette or scraper, of tissue from lesions are placed on a growth medium and examined under a microscope to identify fungal growth.

fungi   Organisms found in the Kingdom Fungi. Some are capable of causing disease in humans, such as yeast infections or histoplasmosis.

furuncle   Staphylococcal skin abscess with redness, pain, and swelling. Also called a boil.

gait   Manner of walking.

gallbladder   This small organ is located just under the liver. It functions to store the bile produced by the liver. The gallbladder releases bile into the duodenum through the common bile duct.

gallstones   Stones that form in the gallbladder, usually from excess cholesterol.

gamma globulin   Protein component of blood containing antibodies that help to resist infection.

ganglion   Knotlike mass of nerve tissue located outside the brain and spinal cord.

ganglion cyst   Benign cyst at the end of long bones.

gangrene   Necrosis of the skin usually due to deficient blood supply.

gastrectomy   Surgical removal of the stomach.

gastric glands   Glands in the lining of the stomach that secrete acid and digestive enzymes. They are regulated by the autonomic nervous system.

gastritis   Inflammation of the stomach that can result in pain, tenderness, nausea, and vomiting.

gastrodynia   Stomach pain.

gastroenteritis   Inflammation of the stomach and small intestines.

gastroenterologist   A physician specialized in treating diseases and conditions of the gastrointestinal tract.

gastroenterology   Branch of medicine specializing in conditions of the gastrointestinal system.

gastrointestinal endoscopy   A flexible instrument or scope is passed either through the mouth or anus to facilitate visualization of the gastrointestinal (GI) tract.

gastrointestinal system (GI)   System that digests food and absorbs nutrients. Organs include the mouth, pharynx, esophagus, stomach, small and large intestines, liver, gallbladder, and anus. Also called the digestive system.

gastromalacia   Softening of the stomach.

gastroscope   Instrument to view inside the stomach.

gastrostomy   Surgical creation of a gastric fistula or opening through the abdominal wall. The opening is used to place food into the stomach when the esophagus is not entirely open (esophageal stricture).

gastrostomy tube   Thin tubing placed into the stomach for liquid feedings.

Geiger counter   Instrument used for detecting radiation.

general anesthesia   General anesthesia produces a loss of consciousness including an absence of pain sensation. It is administered to a patient by either an intravenous or inhalation method. The patient's vital signs are carefully monitored when using a general anesthetic.

general hospital Hospitals that typically provide services to diagnose (laboratory, diagnostic imaging) and treat (surgery, medications, therapy) diseases for a short period of time. In addition, they usually provide emergency and obstetrical care. Also called an acute care hospital.

generic name The recognized and accepted official name for a drug. Each drug has only one generic name. This name is not subject to trademark, so any pharmaceutical manufacturer may use it. Also called nonproprietary name.

genes The basic unit of heredity that occupies a specific location on a chromosome. Each chromosome contains many genes. Each gene controls a specific body trait.

genetics The study of heredity and the influence of chemicals on the genes.

genital herpes Creeping skin disease that can appear like a blister or vesicle, caused by a sexually transmitted virus.

genital tract Referring to the female or male sexual organs.

genital warts Growths and elevations of warts on the genitalia of both males and females that can lead to cancer of the cervix in females.

genitalia The male and female reproductive organs.

genitourinary Referring to the organs of the urinary system and the female or male sexual organs.

geriatric chair (geri-chair) Wheeled chair that reclines and has a tray for meals. Provides security for a confused person because he or she is unable to get up from the chair without assistance.

German measles A contagious viral disease that resembles measles (rubeola) but has a shorter course of infection and little fever. Also called rubella.

gerontology The scientific study of the effects of aging and age-related diseases.

gestation Length of time from conception to birth, generally nine months. Calculated from the first day of the last menstrual period, with a range of from 259 days to 280 days.

gestational period The length of time of pregnancy, approximately forty weeks.

giant cell tumor Benign tumor that appears at the epiphysis but does not interfere with joint movement. May become malignant or return after removal.

gigantism Excessive development of the body due to the overproduction of the growth hormone by the pituitary gland. The opposite of dwarfism.

gingivectomy Excision of the gums.

gingivitis Inflammation of the gums characterized by swelling, redness, and a tendency to bleed.

glands The organs of the body that release secretions. Exocrine glands, like sweat glands, release their secretions into ducts. Endocrine glands, such as the thyroid gland, release their hormones directly into the blood stream.

glans penis The larger and softer tip of the penis. It is protected by a covering called the prepuce or foreskin.

glaucoma Increase in intraocular pressure, which, if untreated, may result in atrophy (wasting away) of the optic nerve and blindness. Glaucoma is treated with medication and surgery. There is an increased risk of developing glaucoma in persons over sixty years of age, people of African ancestry, persons who have sustained a serious eye injury, and anyone with a family history of diabetes or glaucoma.

glioblastoma Neurological tumor.

glioma Sarcoma of neurological origin.

glomerular capsule Also called Bowman's capsule. Part of the renal corpuscle. It is a double-walled cuplike structure that encircles the glomerulus. In the filtration stage of urine production, waste products filtered from the blood enter Bowman's capsule as the glomerular filtrate.

glomerular filtrate The product of the filtration stage of urine production. Water, electrolytes, nutrients, wastes, and toxins that are filtered from blood passing through the glomerulus. The filtrate enters Bowman's capsule.

glomerulonephritis Inflammation of the kidney (primarily of the glomerulus). Since the glomerular membrane is inflamed, it becomes more permeable and will allow protein and blood cells to enter the filtrate. Results in protein in the urine (proteinuria) and hematuria.

glomerulus Ball of capillaries encased by Bowman's capsule. In the filtration stage of urine production, wastes filtered from the blood leave the glomerulus capillaries and enter Bowman's capsule.

glossectomy Complete or partial removal of the tongue.

glottis The opening between the vocal cords. Air passes through the glottis as it moves through the larynx. Changing the tension of the vocal cords changes the size of the opening.

glucagon A hormone secreted by pancreas. It stimulates the liver to release glucose into the blood.

glucocorticoid A group of hormones secreted by the adrenal cortex. They regulate carbohydrate levels in the body. Cortisol is an example of a glucocorticoid.

glucose The form of sugar used by the cells of the body to make energy. It is transported to the cells in the blood.

glucose tolerance test (GTT) Test to determine the blood sugar level. A measured dose of glucose is given to a patient either orally or intravenously. Blood samples are then drawn at certain intervals to determine the ability of the patient to utilize glucose. Used for diabetic patients to determine their insulin response to glucose.

gluteus maximus A muscle named for its size and location: gluteus means *rump area* and maximus means *large*.

glycosuria Presence of an excess of sugar in the urine.

goiter Enlargement of the thyroid gland.

gonads The organs responsible for producing sex cells. The female gonads are the ovaries and they produce ova. The male gonads are the testes and they produce sperm.

gonioscopy Use of an instrument called a gonioscope to examine the anterior chamber of the eye to determine ocular motility and rotation.

gonorrhea Sexually transmitted inflammation of the mucous membranes of either sex. Can be passed on to an infant during the birth process.

gout Inflammation of the joints caused by excessive uric acid.

grade A tumor can be graded from grade I through grade IV. The grade is based on the microscopic appearance of the tumor cells. A grade I tumor is well differentiated and is easier to treat than the more advanced grades.

grand mal A type of severe epilepsy seizure characterized by a loss of consciousness and convulsions. It is also called a tonic-clonic seizure, indicating that the seizure alternates between strong continuous muscle spasms (tonic) and rhythmic muscle contraction and relaxation (clonic).

granulocytes Granular polymorphonuclear leukocyte. There are three types: neutrophil, eosinophil, and basophil.

Grave's disease Condition, named for Robert Graves, an Irish physician, that results in overactivity of the thyroid gland and can result in a crisis situation. Also called hyperthyroidism.

gravida A pregnant woman.

gray matter Tissue within the central nervous system. It consists of unsheathed or uncovered nerve cell bodies and dendrites.

greenstick fracture Fracture in which there is an incomplete break; one side of the bone is broken and the other side is bent. This type of fracture is commonly found in children due to their softer and more pliable bone structure.

gross motor skills The use of large muscle groups that coordinate body movements such as walking, running, jumping, and balance.

growth hormone A hormone secreted by the anterior pituitary that stimulates growth of the body.

gum disease Inflammation of the gums, leading to tooth loss, which is generally due to poor dental hygiene.

gynecologist A physician specialized in treating conditions and diseases of the female reproductive system.

gynecology Branch of medicine specializing in conditions of the female reproductive system.

gyri The convoluted, elevated portions of the cerebral cortex. They are separated by fissures or sulci.

habituation Development of an emotional dependence on a drug due to repeated use.

hair A structure in the integumentary system.

hair follicle Cavities in the dermis that contain the hair root. Hair grows longer from the root.

halitosis Bad or offensive breath, which can often be a sign of disease.

hallucinations The perception of an object that is not there or event that has not happened. Hallucinations may be visual, auditory, olfactory, gustatory, or tactile.

Hashimoto's disease Chronic form of thyroiditis, named for a Japanese surgeon.

head The large ball-shaped end of a bone. It may be separated from the shaft of the bone by an area called the neck.

head injury Blunt trauma to the skull causing bleeding and edema resulting in damage to the brain. Symptoms may include paralysis and mental difficulties. Symptoms may

be permanent or temporary depending on the severity of the injury.

health maintenance organization (HMO) An organization that contracts with a group of physicians and other health care workers to provide care exclusively for its members. The HMO pays the health care workers a prepaid fixed amount per member whether that member requires medical attention or not.

hearing aid Apparatus or mechanical device used by persons with impaired hearing to amplify sound. Same as amplification device.

hearing impairment Loss of hearing sufficient to interfere with a person's ability to communicate.

hearing level Audiometer reading in decibels (dB) that corresponds to the listener's hearing threshold ratio, which is the softest sound the listener can hear, expressed in decibels (dB).

heart Organ of the cardiovascular system that contracts to pump blood through the blood vessels.

heart transplantation Replacement of a diseased or malfunctioning heart with a donor's heart.

heart valve prolapse The cusps or flaps of the heart valve are too loose and fail to shut tightly, allowing blood to flow backwards through the valve when the heart chamber contracts. Most commonly occurs in the mitral valve, but may affect any of the heart valves.

heart valve stenosis The cusps or flaps of the heart valve are too stiff. Therefore, they are unable to open fully, making it difficult for blood to flow through, or to shut tightly, allowing blood to flow backwards. This condition may affect any of the heart valves.

heat application Applying either dry or moist warmth to a body part to produce the slight dilitation of blood vessels in the skin. Causes muscle relaxation in the deeper regions of the body and increases circulation, which aids healing.

heat hydrotherapy Application of warm water as a therapeutic treatment. Can be done in baths, swimming pools, and whirlpools.

Heimlich maneuver Technique for removing a foreign body or food from the trachea or pharynx when it is choking a person. The maneuver consists of applying pressure just under the diaphragm to pop the obstruction out.

hemangioma Common benign, vascular tumor usually located on the skull or vertebral body.

hematemesis To vomit blood from the gastrointestinal tract, often looks like coffee grounds.

hematocrit (HCT, Hct, crit) Blood test to measure the volume of red blood cells (erythrocytes) within the total volume of blood.

hematocytopenia Condition of too few blood cells in the circulation.

hematologist A physician who specializes in treating diseases and conditions of the blood.

hematology Branch of medicine specializing in conditions of the hematic system.

hematoma Swelling or mass of blood caused by a break in a vessel in an organ or tissue, or beneath the skin.

hematopoiesis   The process of forming blood.

hematosalpinx   Condition of having blood in the fallopian tubes.

hematuria   Condition of blood in the urine.

hemianopia   Loss of vision in half of the visual field. A stroke patient may suffer from this disorder.

hemiparesis   Weakness or loss of motion on one side of the body.

hemiplegia   Paralysis on only one side of the body.

hemisphere   The left and right halves of the cerebral cortex. Each hemisphere is divided into four lobes: frontal, parietal, occipital, and temporal.

hemodialysis (HD)   Use of an artificial kidney machine that filters the blood of a person to remove waste products. Use of this technique in patients who have defective kidneys is lifesaving.

hemoglobin (Hg)   Iron-containing pigment of red blood cells that carries oxygen from the lungs to the tissue.

hemolysis   The destruction of blood cells.

hemolytic disease of the newborn   Condition in which antibodies in the mother's blood enter the fetus's blood and cause anemia, jaundice, edema, and enlargement of the liver and spleen. Also called erythroblastosis fetalis.

hemophilia   Hereditary blood disease in which there is a prolonged blood clotting time. It is transmitted by a sex-linked trait from females to males. It appears almost exclusively in males.

hemoptysis   Coughing up blood or blood-stained sputum.

hemorrhage   Blood flow, the escape of blood from a blood vessel.

hemorrhoidectomy   Surgical excision of hemorrhoids from the anorectal area.

hemorrhoids   Varicose veins in the rectum.

hemostasis   To stop bleeding or the stagnation of the circulating blood.

hemostat   A surgical instrument used to grasp blood vessels to control bleeding.

hemostatic   Any drug, medicine, or clotting protein from blood that stops bleeding, such as vitamin K or factor VIII (the clotting factor missing in hemophiliacs).

hemothorax   Condition of having blood in the chest cavity.

hepatic lobectomy   Surgical removal of a lobe of the liver.

hepatitis   Infectious, inflammatory disease of the liver. Hepatitis B and C types are spread by contact with blood and bodily fluids of an infected person.

hepatitis B   Serious, inflammatory disease of the liver caused by the hepatitis B virus. It is spread through contact with blood and body fluids. There is a vaccine that provides protection.

hepatoma   Liver tumor.

herniated nucleus pulposus (HNP)   A rupture of the fibrocartilage disk between two vertebrae. This results in pressure on a spinal nerve and causes pain, weakness, and nerve damage. Also called a slipped disk.

herniorrhaphy   Suture a hernia.

hertz (Hz)   Measurement of the frequency or pitch of sound. The lowest pitch on an audiogram is 250 Hz. The measurement can go as high as 8000 Hz, which is the highest pitch measured.

hesitancy   A decrease in the force of the urine stream, often with difficulty initiating the flow. It is often a symptom of a blockage along the urethra, such as an enlarged prostate gland.

hilum   Center of the concave side of the kidney which is an important landmark on the kidney. It is the site where the renal artery enters, the renal vein leaves, the ureter leaves, and nerves enter and leave the kidney.

hirsutism   Excessive hair growth over the body.

histology   The study of tissues.

histoplasmosis   Pulmonary disease caused by a fungus found in dust in the droppings of pigeons and chickens.

History and Physical   Medical record document written by the admitting physician. It details the patient's history, results of the physician's examination, initial diagnoses, and physician's plan of treatment.

Hodgkin's disease   Also called Hodgkin's lymphoma. Cancer of the lymphatic cells found in concentration in the lymph nodes.

Holter monitor   Portable ECG monitor worn by the patient for a period of a few hours to a few days to assess the heart and pulse activity as the person goes through the activities of daily living.

home health care   Agencies that provide nursing, therapy, personal care, or housekeeping services in the patient's own home.

homeostasis   Steady state or state of balance within the body. The kidneys assist in maintaining this regulatory, steady state.

homologous transfusion   Replacement of blood by transfusion of blood received from another person.

hordeolum   Refers to a stye (or *sty*), a small purulent inflammatory infection of a sebaceous gland of the eye, treated with hot compresses and surgical incision.

horizontal plane   A horizontal plane that divides the body into upper (superior) and lower (inferior) sections. Also called the transverse plane.

hormone   A chemical substance secreted by an endocrine gland. It enters the blood stream and is carried to target tissue. Hormones work to control the functioning of the target tissue. Given to replace the loss of natural hormones or to treat disease by stimulating hormonal effects.

hormone therapy   Treatment of cancer with natural hormones or with chemicals that produce hormone-like effects.

horny cells   Describes keratin-filled epidermal cells. Keratin is the hard protein found in nails and hair.

hospices   An organized group of health care workers that provide supportive treatment to dying patients and their families.

Hospital Formulary   A resource for drug information. It contains up-to-date information about drugs and their use.

hospitalization   Admission to a hospital for diagnostic tests, surgery, or treatment.

hot moist compresses Applying moist heat with wet pads.

human immunodeficiency virus (HIV) Virus that causes AIDS; also known as a retrovirus.

humerus The upper arm bone in the upper extremity.

humoral immunity Immunity that responds to antigens, such as bacteria and foreign agents, by producing antibodies. Also called antibody-mediated immunity.

Huntington's chorea Rare condition characterized by bizarre involuntary movements called chorea. The patient may have progressive mental and physical disturbances that generally begin around 40.

hyaline membrane disease (HMD) Condition seen in premature infants whose lungs have not had time to develop properly. The lungs are not able to expand fully and a membrane (hyaline membrane) actually forms that causes extreme difficulty in breathing and may result in death. Also known as infant respiratory distress syndrome (IRDS).

hydrocele Accumulation of fluid within the testes.

hydrocephalus Accumulation of cerebrospinal fluid within the ventricles of the brain, causing the head to be enlarged. It is treated by creating an artificial shunt for the fluid to leave the brain.

hydrochloric acid Acid secreted by the stomach lining. Aids in digestion.

hydronephrosis Distention of the pelvis due to urine collecting in the kidney resulting from an obstruction.

hydrosalpinx Condition of having water in the fallopian tubes.

hydrotherapy Using water for treatment purposes.

hymen A thin membranous tissue that covers the external vaginal opening or orifice. This membrane is broken during the first sexual encounter of the female. It can also be broken prematurely by the use of tampons or during some sports activities.

hymenectomy Surgical removal of the hymen. Performed when the hymen tissue is particularly tough.

hyoid bone A single, U-shaped bone suspended in the neck between the mandible and larynx. It is a point of attachment for swallowing and speech muscles.

hyperbaric oxygen therapy Use of oxygen under greater than normal pressure to treat cases of smoke inhalation, carbon monoxide poisoning, and other conditions. In some cases the patient is placed in a hyperbaric oxygen chamber for this treatment.

hypercalcemia Condition of having an excessive amount of calcium in the blood.

hyperemia Redness of the skin caused by increased blood flow to the skin.

hyperesthesia Having excessive sensation.

hyperglycemia Having an excessive amount of glucose (sugar) in the blood.

hyperkalemia Condition of having an excessive amount of potassium in the blood.

hyperkinesia An excessive amount of movement.

hypernephroma Renal or kidney cell carcinoma.

hyperopia With this condition a person can see things in the distance but has trouble reading material at close vision. Also known as farsightedness.

hyperpigmentation Abnormal amount of pigmentation in the skin, which is seen in diseases such as acromegaly and adrenal insufficiency.

hyperplasia Excessive development of normal cells within an organ.

hyperpnea Excessive deep breathing.

hypertension High blood pressure.

hypertensive heart disease Heart disease as a result of persistently high blood pressure, which damages the blood vessels and ultimately the heart.

hyperthyroidism Condition resulting from overactivity of the thyroid gland that can result in a crisis situation. Also called Graves' disease.

hypertrophy An increase in the bulk or size of a tissue or structure.

hypnotic Used to produce sleep or hypnosis.

hypocalcemia Condition of having a low calcium level in the blood.

hypochondria A somatoform disorder involving a preoccupation with health concerns.

hypodermic Pertaining to under the skin.

hypogastric Pertaining to below the stomach. An anatomical division of the abdomen, the middle section of the bottom row.

hypoglycemia Condition of having a low sugar level in the blood.

hypoglycemic Lowers blood glucose level.

hyponatremia Condition of having a low sodium level in the blood.

hypopnea Insufficient or shallow breathing.

hypospadias Congenital opening of the male urethra on the underside of the penis.

hypotension Low blood pressure.

hypothalamus The hypothalamus is a portion of the diencephalon that lies just below the thalamus. It controls body temperature, appetite, sleep, sexual desire, and emotions such as fear. It also regulates the release of hormones from the pituitary gland and regulates the parasympathetic and sympathetic nervous systems.

hypothyroidism Result of a deficiency in secretion by the thyroid gland. This results in a lowered basal metabolism rate with obesity, dry skin, slow pulse, low blood pressure, sluggishness, and goiter. Treatment is replacement with synthetic thyroid hormone.

hypoxemia Deficiency of oxygen in the blood.

hypoxia Absence of oxygen in the tissues.

hysterectomy Removal of the uterus.

hysteropexy Surgical fixation of the uterus.

hysterorrhexis Rupture of the uterus.

hysterosalpingography Process of taking an X-ray of the uterus and oviducts after a radiopaque material is injected into the organs.

hysteroscopy Inspection of the uterus using a special endoscope instrument.

ice packs Using ice in a bag or container to treat localized conditions.

idiopathic When something occurs without a known cause.

idiosyncrasy Unusual or abnormal response to a drug or food.

ileitis Inflammation of the ileum.

ileocecal valve Sphincter between the ileum and the cecum.

ileostomy Surgical creation of a passage through the abdominal wall into the ileum.

ileum The third portion of the small intestines. Joins the colon at the cecum. The ileum and cecum are separated by the ileocecal valve.

ilium One of three bones that form the os coxae or innominate bone of the pelvis.

immune response Ability of lymphocytes to respond to specific antigens.

immunization Providing protection against communicable diseases by stimulating the immune system to produce antibodies against that disease. Children can now be immunized for the following diseases: hepatitis B, diphtheria, tetanus, pertussis, tetanus, *Haemophilus influenza* type b, polio, measles, mumps, rubella, and chickenpox. Also called vaccination.

immunoglobulins Antibodies secreted by the B cells. All antibodies are immunoglobulins. They assist in protecting the body and its surfaces from the invasion of bacteria. For example, the immunoglobulin IgA in colostrum, the first milk from the mother, helps to protect the newborn from infection.

immunologist A physician who specializes in treating infectious diseases and other disorders of the immune system.

immunology Branch of medicine specializing in conditions of the lymphatic and immune systems.

immunosuppressive Suppresses the body's natural immune response to an antigen. This is used to control autoimmune diseases such as multiple sclerosis and rheumatoid arthritis.

immunotherapy The production or strengthening of a patient's immune system in order to treat a disease.

impacted fracture Fracture in which bone fragments are pushed into each other.

impacted wisdom tooth Wisdom tooth that is tightly wedged into the jawbone so that it is unable to erupt.

impetigo A highly contagious staphylococcal skin infection, most commonly occurring on the faces of children. It begins as blisters that then rupture and dry into a thick, yellow crust.

implant Prosthetic device placed in the jaw to which a tooth or denture may be anchored.

impotent Inability to copulate due to inability to maintain an erection.

impregnation Also called fertilization. The fusion of an ova and sperm to produce an embryo.

impulse Wave of sudden excitement; refers to the movement of an electrical current along a nerve.

incision and drainage (I&D) Making an incision to create an opening for the drainage of material such as pus.

incisors Biting teeth in the very front of the mouth that function to cut food into smaller pieces. Humans have eight incisors.

incomplete fracture Fracture in which the line of fracture does not include the entire bone.

incus One of the three ossicles of the middle ear. Also called the anvil.

infarct Area of tissue within an organ that undergoes necrosis (death) following the loss of blood supply.

inferior Directional term meaning toward the feet or tail, or below.

inferior venae cavae The branch of the venae cavae that drains blood from the abdomen and lower body.

inflammatory bowel disease (IBD) Ulceration of the mucous membranes of the colon of unknown origin. Also known as ulcerative colitis.

inflammatory process Nonspecific immune response that occurs as a reaction to any type of bodily injury. The signs are redness, heat, swelling, and pain.

Informed Consent A medical record document, voluntarily signed by the patient or a responsible party, that clearly describes the purpose, methods, procedures, benefits, and risks of a diagnostic or treatment procedure.

inguinal Commonly referred to as the groin. There is a collection of lymph nodes in this region that drain each leg.

inguinal hernia Hernia or outpouching of intestines into the inguinal region of the body.

inhalation To breath air into the lungs. Also called inspiration.

inhalation method Breathing in drugs in vapor form.

innate immunity Immunity that is not specific to a particular disease and does not require prior exposure to the pathogen. Also called natural immunity.

inner ear The innermost section of the ear. It contains the cochlea, semicircular canals, saccule, and utricle.

innominate bone Also called the os coxae or hip bone. It is the pelvis portion of the lower extremity. It consists of the ilium, ischium, and pubis and unites with the sacrum and coccyx to form the pelvis.

insomnia A sleeping disorder characterized by a marked inability to fall asleep.

inspiration To breath air into the lungs. Also called inhalation.

insulin The hormone secreted by the pancreas. It regulates the level of sugar in the blood stream. The more insulin present in the blood, the lower the blood sugar will be.

insulin reaction Reaction that occurs when a diabetic patient receives too much insulin. Glucose in the form of juice or candy is administered if the patient is conscious.

integumentary system The skin and its appendages including sweat glands, oil glands, hair, and nails. Sense organs that allow us to respond to changes in temperature, pain, touch, and pressure are located in the skin. It is the largest organ in the body.

intensive care unit (ICU) Specialized hospital unit equipped to care for and monitor patients who have suffered severe injuries and illnesses and require constant supervision and lifesaving measures.

interatrial Pertaining to between the atria.

interatrial septum The wall or septum that divides the left and right atria.

intercostal muscles Muscles between the ribs. When they contract they raise the ribs, which helps to enlarge the thoracic cavity.

intermittent positive pressure breathing (IPPB) Method for assisting patients to breath using a mask connected to a machine that produces an increased pressure.

intermuscular Pertaining to between the muscles.

internal medicine Branch of medicine specializing in conditions of the internal organs.

International Classification of Diseases 9th Revision Clinical Modification (ICD-9-CM) An official list of diseases was developed by the World Health Organization. The ICD-9-CM number consists of three to five digits that conveys general and specific information regarding a diagnoses.

internist A physician specialized in treating diseases and conditions of internal organs such as the respiratory system.

interpreter Person with training in areas such as sign language, fingerspelling, and speech, who can transmit verbal or written messages to the hearing-impaired person.

interstitial cystitis Disease of unknown cause in which there is inflammation and irritation of the bladder. Most commonly seen in middle-aged women.

interventricular Pertaining to between the ventricles.

interventricular septum The wall or septum that divides the left and right ventricles.

intervertebral Pertaining to between vertebrae.

intracavitary Injection into a body cavity such as the peritoneal and chest cavity.

intracoronary artery stent Placing a stent within a coronary artery to treat coronary ischemia due to atherosclerosis.

intracranial Pertaining to inside the skull.

intradermal Pertaining to within the skin.

intramuscular Pertaining to within the muscle.

intraocular Pertaining to within the eye.

intrathecal Injection into the meninges space surrounding the brain and spinal cord.

intrauterine device (IUD) Devise that is inserted into the uterus by a physician for the purpose of contraception.

intravascular thrombolytic therapy Drugs, such as streptokinase or tissue-type plasminogen activator (tPA), are injected into a blood vessel to dissolve clots and restore blood flow.

intravenous (IV) Injection into the veins. This route can be set up so that there is a continuous administration of medication.

intravenous cholangiogram (IVC) A dye is administered intravenously to the patient that allows for X-ray visualization of the bile vessels.

intravenous cholecystography A dye is administered intravenously to the patient that allows for X-ray visualization of the gallbladder.

intravenous method Drugs injected into a vein.

intravenous pyelogram (IVP) Injecting a contrast medium into a vein and then taking an X-ray to visualize the renal pelvis.

intubation Insertion of a tube into the larynx or trachea through the glottis to allow for air to enter the lungs.

intussusception An intestinal condition in which one portion of the intestine telescopes into an adjacent portion causing an obstruction, and gangrene if untreated.

invasive disease Tendency of a malignant tumor to spread to immediately surrounding tissue and organs.

inversion Directional term meaning turning inward or inside out.

involuntary muscle tissue Muscles that are not under voluntary control. Includes cardiac muscle (in the heart) and smooth muscle (in internal organs like the digestive system).

iodine A mineral required by the thyroid to produce its hormones.

iridectomy Excision of the iris.

iridoplegia Paralysis of the iris.

iridosclerotomy Incision into the iris and sclera.

iris The colored portion of the eye. It can dilate or constrict to change the size of the pupil and control the amount of light entering the interior of the eye.

iritis Inflammation of the iris.

irregular bones A type of bone having an irregular shape. Vertebrae are irregular bones.

irritable bowel syndrome (IBS) Disturbance in the functions of the intestine from unknown causes. Symptoms generally include abdominal discomfort and an alteration in bowel activity.

ischemia Localized and temporary deficiency of blood supply due to an obstruction of the circulation.

ischium One of the three bones that form the os coxae or innominate bone of the pelvis.

islets of Langerhans The regions within the pancreas that secretes insulin and glucagon.

jaundice Yellow cast to the skin, mucous membranes, and the whites of the eyes caused by the deposit of bile pigment from too much bilirubin in the blood. Bilirubin is a waste product produced when worn out red blood cells are broken down. May be a symptom of disorders such as gallstones blocking the common bile duct or carcinoma of the liver.

jejunoileostomy Formation of a passage between the jejunum and the ileum.

jejunostomy Surgical creation of a permanent opening into the jejunum.

jejunum The middle portion of the small intestines. Site of nutrient absorption.

joints The point at which two bones meet. It provides flexibility.

juvenile rheumatoid arthritis A form of rheumatoid arthritis that usually affects the larger joints of children under the age of sixteen years.

Kaposi's sarcoma Form of skin cancer frequently seen in acquired immunodeficiency syndrome (AIDS) patients. Consists of brownish-purple papules that spread from the skin and metastasize to internal organs.

Kegel exercises   Exercises to strengthen female pubic muscles. The exercises are useful in treating incontinence and as an aid in the childbirth process.

keloid   Formation of a scar after an injury or surgery that results in a raised, thickened red area.

keratin   A hard protein substance produced by the body. It is found in hair and nails, and filling the inside of epidermal cells.

keratitis   Inflammation of the cornea.

keratoplasty   Surgical repair of the cornea (corneal transplant).

keratosis   Overgrowth and thickening of the epithelium.

ketoacidosis   Acidosis due to an excess of ketone bodies (waste products). A serious condition that requires immediate treatment and can result in death for the diabetic patient if not reversed.

kidney   The two kidneys are located in the lumbar region of the back behind the parietal peritoneum. They are under the muscles of the back, just a little above the waist. The kidneys have a concave or depressed area that gives them a bean-shaped appearance. The center of this concavity is called the hilum.

kleptomania   An impulse control disorder in which the patient is unable to refrain from stealing. The items are often trivial and unneeded.

kyphosis   Abnormal increase in the outward curvature of the thoracic spine. Also known as hunchback or humpback.

labia majora   A fold of skin that serves as protection for the female external genitalia and urethral meatus.

labia minora   A fold of skin that serves as protection for the female external genitalia and urethral meatus.

labor   The period of time beginning with uterine contractions and ending with the birth of the baby. There are three stages: the cervical dilation stage, the period of forceful expulsion of the infant, and the stage of placental delivery.

labyrinth   The term that refers to the inner ear. It is several fluid-filled cavities within the temporal bone. The labyrinth consists of the cochlea, vestibule, and three semicircular canals. Hair cells called the organs of Corti line the inner ear. These hair cells change the sound vibrations to electrical impulses and send the impulses to the brain via the vestibulocochlear nerve.

labyrinthectomy   Excision of the labyrinth.

labyrinthitis   Labyrinth inflammation.

lacrimal   Pertaining to tears.

lacrimal bone   A facial bone.

lacrimal ducts   Tear ducts located in the inner corner of the eye socket. They collect the tears and drain them into the lacrimal sac.

lacrimal gland   A gland located in the outer corner of each eyelid. It washes the anterior surface of the eye with fluid called tears.

lacrimal sac   Lacrimal sacs receive tears from the lacrimal ducts and carry them to the nasal cavity.

lactation   The function of secreting milk after childbirth from the breasts or mammary glands.

lactic   Pertaining to milk.

lactorrhea   Discharge of milk.

laminectomy   Removal of a portion of a vertebra in order to relieve pressure on the spinal nerve.

laparoscope   Instrument to view inside the abdomen.

laparoscopy   An instrument or scope is passed into the abdominal wall through a small incision. The abdominal cavity is then examined for tumors and other conditions with this lighted instrument. Also called peritoneoscopy.

laparotomy   Incision into the abdomen.

laryngectomy   Surgical removal of the larynx. This procedure is most frequently performed for excision of cancer.

laryngitis   Inflammation of the larynx causing difficulty in speaking.

laryngopharynx   The inferior section of the pharynx. It lies at the same level in the neck as the larynx. Air has already entered the larynx, therefore the laryngopharynx carries food and drink to the esophagus.

laryngoplasty   Surgical repair of the larynx.

laryngoscope   An instrument to view voice box.

laryngoscopy   Examination of the interior of the larynx with a lighted instrument.

laryngostomy   Surgical creation of an opening into the voice box.

larynx   Also called the voice box. Respiratory system organ responsible for producing speech. It is located just below the pharynx.

laser   Device that emits intense, small beams of light capable of destroying or fixing tissue in place.

laser-assisted in-situ keratomileusis (LASIK)   Correction of myopia using laser surgery to remove corneal tissue.

laser surgery   Use of a controlled beam of light for cutting, hemostasis, or tissue destruction.

laser therapy   Removal of skin lesions and birthmarks using a laser beam that emits intense heat and power at a close range. The laser converts frequencies of light into one small, powerful beam.

last menstrual period (LMP)   Date when the last menstrual period started.

lateral (lat)   Directional term meaning to the side.

lateral recumbent   Lying on either the left or right side.

lateral view   Positioning the patient so that the side of the body faces the X-ray machine.

laxative   A mild cathartic.

lead poisoning   Poisoning that occurs in children who ingest lead, often from paint chips.

left hypochondriac   An anatomical division of the abdomen, the left side of the upper row.

left iliac   An anatomical division of the abdomen, the left side of the bottom row. Also called left inguinal.

left inguinal   An anatomical division of the abdomen, the left side of the bottom row. Also called left iliac.

left lower quadrant (LLQ)   A clinical division of the abdomen. It contains portions of small and large intestines, left ovary and fallopian tube, and left ureter.

left lumbar   An anatomical division of the abdomen, the left side of the middle row.

left subclavian vein The circulatory system vein that receives lymph from the thoracic duct.

left upper quadrant (LUQ) A clinical division of the abdomen. It contains the left lobe of the liver, spleen, stomach, portion of the pancreas, and portion of small and large intestines.

Legionnaire's disease Severe, often fatal disease characterized by pneumonia and gastrointestinal symptoms. Caused by a gram-negative bacillus and named after people who came down with it at an American Legion convention in 1976.

lens The transparent structure behind the pupil and iris. It functions to bend light rays so they land on the retina.

lethargy Condition of sluggishness or stupor.

leukemia Cancer of the WBC-forming bone marrow; results in a large number of abnormal WBCs circulating in the blood.

leukocytes Also called white blood cells or WBCs. A group of several different types of cells that provide protection against the invasion of bacteria and other foreign material. They are able to leave the blood stream and search out the foreign invaders (bacteria, virus, and toxins), where they perform phagocytosis.

leukoderma Disappearance of pigment from the skin in patches, causing a milk-white appearance. Also called vitiligo.

leukoplakia Formation of white patches or spots on the mucous membranes of the cheek or tongue. These lesions may become malignant.

ligaments Very strong bands of connective tissue that bind bones together at a joint.

lingual tonsils Tonsils located on the very posterior section of the tongue as it joins with the pharynx.

lipectomy Surgical removal of fat.

lipocytes Medical term for cells that contain fat molecules.

lipoma Fatty tumor that generally does not metastasize.

liposuction Removal of fat beneath the skin by means of suction.

lithotomy Surgical incision to remove kidney stones.

lithotomy position Lying face up with hips and knees bent at 90° angles.

lithotripsy Destroying or crushing kidney stones in the bladder or urethra with a device called a lithotriptor.

liver A large organ located in the right upper quadrant of the abdomen. It serves many functions in the body. Its digestive system role includes producing bile, processing the absorbed nutrients, and detoxifying harmful substances.

liver biopsy Excision of a small piece of liver tissue for microscopic examination. Generally used to determine if cancer is present.

liver scan A radioactive substance is administered to the patient by an intravenous (IV) route. When the substance enters the liver cells, the organ can be visualized. This is used to detect tumors, abscesses, and other pathologies that result in hepatomegaly (an enlarged liver).

lobectomy Surgical removal of a lobe of the lung. Often the treatment of choice for lung cancer.

local anesthesia Local anesthesia produces a loss of sensation in one localized part of the body. The patient remains conscious when this type of anesthetic is used. It is administered either topically or via a subcutaneous route.

long bone A type of bone that is longer than it is wide. Examples include the femur, humerus, and phalanges.

long-term care facility A facility that provides long-term care for patients who need extra time to recover from an illness or accident before they return home or for persons who can no longer care for themselves. Also called a nursing home.

loop of Henle A portion of the renal tubule.

lordosis Abnormal increase in the forward curvature of the lumbar spine. Also known as swayback.

low birth weight (LBW) Abnormally low weight in a newborn. It is usually considered to be less than 5.5 pounds.

low sex drive A sexual disorder characterized by having a decreased interest in sexual intimacy.

lower esophageal sphincter Also called the cardiac sphincter. Prevents food and gastric juices from backing up into the esophagus.

lower extremity (LE) The leg.

lumbar Pertaining to the five low back vertebrae.

lumbar puncture (LP) Puncture with a needle into the lumbar area (usually the fourth intervertebral space) to withdraw fluid for examination and for the injection of anesthesia. Also called spinal puncture or spinal tap.

lumbar vertebrae The five vertebrae in the low back region.

lumen The space, cavity, or channel within a tube or tubular organ or structure in the body.

lungs The major organs of respiration. The lungs consists of air passageways, the bronchi and bronchioles, and the air sacs, alveoli. Gas exchange takes place within the alveoli.

lunula The lighter colored, half-moon region at the base of a nail.

luteinizing hormone A hormone secreted by the anterior pituitary. It regulates function of male and female gonads and plays a role in releasing ova in females.

lymph Clear, transparent, colorless fluid found in the lymphatic vessels and the cisterna chyli.

lymph ducts The two largest vessels in the lymphatic system, the lymphatic duct and the thoracic duct.

lymph nodes Small organs in the lymphatic system that filter bacteria and other foreign organisms from the body fluids.

lymph vessels Vessels in the lymphatic system that carry lymph fluid throughout the body.

lymphadenectomy Excision of a lymph node. This is usually done to test for malignancy.

lymphadenitis Inflammation of the lymph glands. Referred to as swollen glands.

lymphadenography X-ray image of lymph nodes following injection of a radiopaque dye.

lymphadenopathy Disease of the lymph nodes.

lymphangiogram X-ray taken of the lymph vessels after the injection of dye. The lymph flow through the chest is traced.

lymphangiography   Process of taking an X-ray of the lymph vessels after the injection of a radiopaque material.

lymphangioma   Benign mass of lymphatic vessels.

lymphatic   Pertaining to lymph.

lymphatic duct   One of the two largest lymphatic vessels. It drains the right arm, chest walls, and both lungs. It empties the lymph into the right subclavian vein.

lymphatic system   System that helps the body fight infection. Organs include the spleen, lymph vessels, and lymph nodes.

lymphocytes   An agranulocyte white blood cells that provides protection through the immune response.

lymphoidectomy   Surgical excision of lymphoid tissue.

lymphoma   A tumor of lymphatic tissue.

macrophage   Phagocytic cells that are found in large quantities in the lymph nodes. They engulf foreign particles.

macula lutea   Images are projected onto the area of the retina.

macular degeneration   Deterioration of the macular area of the retina of the eye. May be treated with laser surgery to destroy the blood vessels beneath the macula.

macule   Flat, discolored area that is flush with the skin surface. An example would be a freckle or a birthmark.

magnetic resonance imaging (MRI)   Medical imaging that uses radio-frequency radiation as its source of energy. It does not require the injection of contrast medium or exposure to ionizing radiation. The technique is useful for visualizing large blood vessels, the heart, the brain, and soft tissues.

major depression   A mood disorder characterized by a marked loss of interest in usually enjoyable activities, disturbances in sleep and eating patterns, fatigue, suicidal thoughts, and feelings of hopelessness, worthlessness, and guilt.

malabsorption syndrome   Inadequate absorption of nutrients from the intestinal tract. May be caused by a variety of diseases and disorders, such as infections and pancreatic deficiency.

male pattern baldness   Genetically determined pattern of progressive hair loss. It begins with a receding hairline at the forehead and eventually leads to loss of hair on the top of the head.

malignant   A tumor that is cancerous. Malignant tumors are generally progressive and recurring.

malignant lymphoma   Cancerous tumor of lymphatic tissue; most commonly occurs in lymph nodes, the spleen, or other body sites containing large amounts of lymphatic cells.

malignant melanoma   Malignant, darkly pigmented tumor or mole of the skin.

malingering   A type of factitious disorder in which the patient intentionally feigns illness for attention or secondary gain.

malleus   One of the three ossicles of the middle ear. Also called the hammer.

mammary glands   The breasts; milk-producing glands to provide nutrition for newborn.

mammogram   X-ray record of the breast.

mammography   Process of X-raying the breast.

mammoplasty   Surgical repair of the breast.

managed care   A systematic approach to delivering high quality, comprehensive health care while controlling costs, mainly by eliminating duplicate and unwarranted facilities and services.

mandible   The lower jawbone.

mania   A mood disorder characterized by extreme elation and euphoria. The patient displays rapid speech, flight of ideas, decreased sleep, distractibility, grandiosity, and poor judgment.

marsupialization   Creating a pouch to promote drainage by surgically opening a closed area such as a cyst.

masochism   A sexual disorder characterized by receiving sexual gratification from being hurt or abused.

massage   Kneading or applying pressure by hands to a part of the patient's body to promote muscle relaxation and reduce tension.

mastalgia   Breast pain.

mastectomy   Excision of the breast.

mastitis   Inflammation of the breast, which is common during lactation but can occur at any age.

mastoid antrotomy   Surgical opening made in the cavity within the mastoid process to alleviate pressure from infection and allow for drainage.

mastoid process   The bony process of the skull felt just behind the ear.

mastoid X-ray   X-ray taken of the mastoid bone to determine the presence of an infection, which can be an extension of a middle ear infection.

mastoidectomy   Excision of the mastoid bone.

mastoiditis   Inflammation of the mastoid bone.

mastoidotomy   Incision into the mastoid bone.

maxilla   The upper jawbone.

measles   A highly contagious viral disease characterized by fever, malaise, lung congestion, and rash. Also called seven-day measles, red measles, or rubeola.

meatotomy   Surgical enlargement of the urinary opening (meatus).

meconium ileus   An obstruction of the small intestine of a newborn infant caused by an impaction of thick meconium, a substance that collects in the intestines of a fetus and becomes the first stool of a newborn.

medial   Directional term meaning to the middle or near the middle of the body or the structure.

mediastinal   There is a collection of lymph nodes located in the mediastinum (central chest area) that drain the chest.

mediastinum   The central region of the chest cavity. It contains the organs between the lungs, including the heart, aorta, esophagus, and trachea.

medical record   Documents the details of a patient's hospital stay. Each health care professional that has contact with the patient in any capacity completes the appropriate report of that contact and adds it to the medical chart. This results in a permanent physical record of the patient's day-to-day condition, when and what services he or she receives, and the response to treatment. Also called a chart.

medulla   The central area of an organ. In the endocrine system it refers to the adrenal medulla.

medulla oblongata   A portion of the brain stem that connects the spinal cord with the brain. It contains the respiratory, cardiac, and blood pressure control centers.

medulloblastoma   Soft malignant tumor of the brain.

melanin   The black color pigment in the skin. It helps to prevent the sun's ultraviolet rays from entering the body.

melanocytes   Special cells in the basal layer of the epidermis. They contain the black pigment melanin that gives skin its color and protects against the ultraviolet rays of the sun.

melanocyte-stimulating hormone   A hormone secreted by the anterior pituitary. It stimulates pigment production in the skin.

melanoma   Also called malignant melanoma. A dangerous form of skin cancer caused by an overgrowth of melanin in a melanocyte. It may metastasize or spread. Exposure to ultraviolet light is a risk factor for developing melanoma.

membrane   Thin structures that cover and protect the body surface, line body cavities, and line some of the internal organs, such as the digestive and respiratory passages. Membranes also secrete lubricating fluids to reduce friction during some processes, such as respiration, and serve to anchor organs and bones. There are two major types of membranes, epithelial and connective tissue.

menarche   The first menstrual period.

Ménière's disease   Abnormal condition within the labyrinth of the inner ear that can lead to a progressive loss of hearing. The symptoms are dizziness or vertigo, hearing loss, and tinnitus (ringing in the ears).

meninges   Three connective tissue membrane layers that surround the brain and spinal cord. The three layers are dura mater, arachnoid layer, pia mater. The dura mater and arachnoid layer are separated by the subdural space. The arachnoid layer and pia mater are separated by the subarachnoid space.

meningioma   Slow-growing tumor in the meninges of the brain.

meningitis   Inflammation of the membranes of the spinal cord and brain that is caused by a microorganism.

meningocele   Congenital hernia in which the meninges, or membranes, protrude through an opening in the spinal column or brain.

meniscectomy   Removal of the knee cartilage (meniscus).

menopause   Cessation or ending of menstrual activity. This is generally between the ages of forty and fifty-five.

menorrhagia   Excessive bleeding during the menstrual period. Can be either in the total number of days or the amount of blood or both.

menstruation   The loss of blood and tissue as the endometrium is shed by the uterus. The flow exits the body through the cervix and vagina. The flow occurs approximately every twenty-eight days.

mental retardation   A disorder characterized by a diminished ability to process intellectual functions.

metabolism   The sum of all the chemical processes taking place in the body.

metacarpals   The hand bones in the upper extremity.

metastases   The spreading of a cancerous tumor from its original site to different locations of the body. Singular is metastasis.

metastasis (mets)   Movement and spread of cancer cells from one part of the body to another. Metastases is plural.

metastasized   When cancerous cells migrate away from a tumor site. They commonly move through the lymphatic system and become trapped in lymph nodes.

metatarsals   The ankle bones in the lower extremity.

metrorrhea   Discharge from the uterus.

microorganisms   A microscopic organism that is capable of invading the body and possibly causing disease.

micturition   Another term for urination.

midbrain   A portion of the brain stem.

middle ear   The middle section of the ear. It contains the ossicles.

midsagittal plane   A vertical plane that divides the body into equal left and right halves.

mineralocorticoid   A group of hormones secreted by the adrenal cortex. They regulate electrolytes and fluid volume in the body. Aldosterone is an example of a mineralocorticoid.

miotic   Any substance that causes the pupil to constrict.

miscarriage   The unplanned loss of a fetus. Also called a spontaneous abortion.

mitral stenosis (MS)   Narrowing of the opening (orifice) of the mitral valve, which causes an obstruction in the flow of blood from the atrium to the ventricle.

mitral valve   A valve between the left atrium and ventricle in the heart. It prevents blood from flowing backwards into the atrium. It is also called the bicuspid valve because it has two cusps or flaps.

mitral valve prolapse (MVP)   Common and serious condition in which the cusp of the mitral valve drops down (prolapses) into the left atrium during systole.

mobility   State of having normal movement of all body parts.

molars   Large somewhat flat-topped back teeth. Function to grind food. Humans have up to twelve molars.

monocytes   An agranulocyte white blood cell that is important for phagocytosis.

mononucleosis   Acute infectious disease with a large number of atypical lymphocytes. Caused by the Epstein–Barr virus. There may be abnormal liver function.

monoparesis   Weakness of one extremity.

monoplegia   Paralysis of one extremity.

Monospot   Test for infectious mononucleosis in which there is a nonspecific antibody called heterophile antibody.

morbidity   Number that represents the number of sick persons in a particular population.

mortality   Number that represents the number of deaths in a particular population.

mouth   The external opening of the alimentary canal. It contains the teeth and tongue for biting and chewing food.

mucosa   The lining of the stomach and intestines.

mucous membrane   These membranes line body passages that open directly to the exterior of the body, such as the mouth and reproductive tract, and secrete a thick substance, or mucus.

multigravida   Woman who has had more than one pregnancy.

multipara   Woman who has given birth to more than one child.

multiple myeloma   Neoplasm that infiltrates the bone and bone marrow and eventually forms multiple tumor masses. A progressive and highly lethal disease.

multiple personality disorder   A type of dissociative disorder in which the person displays two or more distinct conscious personalities that alternate in controlling the body. The alternate personalities may or may not be aware of each other.

multiple sclerosis (MS)   Inflammatory disease of the central nervous system. Rare in children. Generally strikes adults between the ages of twenty and forty. There is progressive weakness and numbness.

mumps   A contagious viral disease characterized by high fever and inflammation and swelling of the parotid salivary glands.

murmur   An abnormal heart sound such as a soft blowing sound or a harsh click. They may be soft and heard only with a stethoscope, or so loud they can be heard several feet away.

muscle biopsy   Removal of muscle tissue for pathological examination.

muscle relaxant   Produces the relaxation of skeletal muscle.

muscle tissue   Tissue that is able to contract and shorten its length, thereby producing movement. Muscle tissue may be under voluntary control (attached to the bones) or involuntary control (heart and digestive organs).

muscles   Muscles are bundles of parallel muscle tissue fibers. As these fibers contract (shorten in length) they pull whatever they are attached to closer together. This may move two bones closer together or make an opening more narrow. A muscle contraction occurs when a message is transmitted from the brain through the nervous system to the muscles.

muscular   Pertaining to muscles.

muscular dystrophy   Inherited disease causing a progressive muscle weakness and atrophy.

musculoskeletal system (MS)   System that provides support for the body and produces movement. Organs of the musculoskeletal system includes muscles, tendons, bones, joints, and cartilage.

mutation   Change or transformation from the original.

myasthenia   Lack of muscle strength.

myasthenia gravis   Disorder causing loss of muscle strength and paralysis. This is an autoimmune disease.

mydriatic   Any substance that causes the pupil to dilate.

myelin   Tissue that wraps around many of the nerve fibers. It is composed of fatty material and functions as an insulator.

myelinated   Nerve fibers covered with a layer of myelin.

myelogram   X-ray record of the spinal cord following injection of meninges with radiopaque dye.

myelography   Injection of a radiopaque dye into the spinal canal. An X-ray is then taken to examine the normal and abnormal outlines made by the dye.

myeloma   Malignant neoplasm originating in plasma cells in the bone.

myelomalacia   Spinal cord softening.

myelomeningocele   A hernia composed of meninges and spinal cord.

myocardial   Pertaining to heart muscle.

myocardial infarction (MI)   Condition caused by the partial or complete occlusion or closing of one or more of the coronary arteries. Symptoms include severe chest pain or heavy pressure in the middle of the chest. A delay in treatment could result in death. Also referred to as MI or heart attack.

myocarditis   Inflammation of heart muscle.

myocardium   The middle layer of the muscle. It is thick and composed of cardiac muscle. This layer produces the heart contraction.

myopathy   Any disease of muscles.

myopia (MY)   With this condition a person can see things that are close up but distance vision is blurred. Also known as nearsightedness.

myoplasty   Surgical repair of muscle.

myorrhaphy   Suture a muscle.

myringitis   Ear drum inflammation.

myringoplasty   Surgical reconstruction of the eardrum. Also called tympanoplasty.

myringotomy   Surgical puncture of the eardrum with removal of fluid and pus from the middle ear, to eliminate a persistent ear infection and excessive pressure on the tympanic membrane. A polyethylene tube is placed in the tympanic membrane to allow for drainage of the middle ear cavity.

myxedema   Condition resulting from a hypofunction of the thyroid gland. Symptoms can include anemia, slow speech, enlarged tongue and facial features, edematous skin, drowsiness, and mental apathy.

nails   A structure in the integumentary system.

narcissistic personality   A personality disorder characterized by an abnormal sense of self-importance.

narcolepsy   Chronic disorder in which there is an extreme uncontrollable desire to sleep.

narcotic   Produces sleep or stupor. In moderate doses this drug will depress the central nervous system and relieve pain. In excessive doses it will cause stupor, coma, and even death. Can become habit forming (addictive).

nasal bone   A facial bone.

nasal cavity   Large cavity just behind the external nose that receives the outside air. It is covered with mucous membrane to cleanse the air. The nasal septum divides the nasal cavity into left and right halves.

nasal septum   A flexible cartilage wall that divides the nasal cavity into left and right halves. It is covered by mucous membrane.

nasogastric   Pertaining to the nose and stomach.

nasopharynx   The superior section of the pharynx that receives air from the nose.

natural immunity   Immunity that is not specific to a particular disease and does not require prior exposure to the pathogen. Also called innate immunity.

natural killer (NK) cells   T cells that can kill by entrapping foreign cells, tumor cells, and bacteria. Also called T8 cells.

near-drowning   When a person lives after being underwater for a period of time that could have resulted in drowning. The person may require resuscitation to bring back a heartbeat or pulse.

necrosis   Dead tissue.

needle biopsy   Using a sterile needle to remove tissue for examination under a microscope.

neonate   Term used to describe the newborn infant during the first four weeks of life.

neonatologists   Physicians specialized in the care of newborn infants.

neonatology   Study of the newborn.

neoplasm   An abnormal growth of tissue that may be benign or malignant. Also called a tumor.

nephrectomy   Excision of a kidney.

nephritis   Inflammation of the kidney.

nephrography   Process of X-raying the kidney after injecting radiopaque dye.

nephrolithiasis   The presence of calculi in the kidney.

nephrologist   A physician specialized in the diagnosis and treatment of diseases of the kidney and urinary system.

nephrology   Branch of medicine specializing in conditions of the urinary system.

nephroma   Kidney tumor.

nephromalacia   Softening of the kidney.

nephromegaly   Enlarged kidney.

nephron   The functional or working unit of the kidney that filters the blood and produces the urine. There are more than one million nephrons in an adult kidney. Each nephron consists of a renal corpuscle and the renal tubules.

nephropathy   Kidney disease.

nephropexy   Surgical fixation of a kidney.

nephroptosis   Drooping kidney.

nephrorrhaphy   Suturing a kidney.

nephrosarcoma   Cancer of the kidney. Also called Wilm's tumor, it occurs mainly in children.

nephrosclerosis   Hardening of the kidney.

nephrosis   Abnormal condition (degeneration) of the kidney.

nephrostomy   Create a new opening across the body wall into the kidney.

nephrotomy   Incision into a kidney.

nerve block   Also referred to as regional anesthesia. This anesthetic interrupts a patient's pain sensation in a particular region of the body. The anesthetic is injected near the nerve that will be blocked from sensation. The patient usually remains conscious.

nerve conduction velocity   A test to determine if nerves have been damaged by recording the rate at which an electrical impulse travels along a nerve. If the nerve is damaged, the velocity will be decreased.

nerves   Structures in the nervous system that conduct electrical impulses from the brain and spinal cord to muscles and other organs.

nervous system   System that coordinates all the conscious and subconscious activities of the body. Organs include the brain, spinal cord, and nerves.

nervous tissue   Nervous tissue conducts electrical impulses to and from the brain and the rest of the body.

neural   Pertaining to nerves.

neuralgia   Nerve pain.

neurasthenia   Lack of nerve strength.

neurectomy   Excision of a nerve.

neuritis   Inflammation of a nerve or nerves, causing pain.

neuroblastoma   Malignant hemorrhagic tumor arising out of the sympathetic system, especially the adrenal medulla. This is found primarily in infants and children.

neurologist   Physician who specializes in disorders of the nervous system.

neurology   Branch of medicine specializing in conditions of the nervous system.

neurolysis   Nerve destruction.

neuroma   Nerve tumor.

neuron   The name for an individual nerve cell. Neurons group together to form nerves and other nervous tissue.

neuroplasty   Surgical repair of nerves.

neurorrhaphy   Suture a nerve.

neurosis   Mental disorder in which there are symptoms such as depression and anxiety.

neurosurgeon   A physician specializing in treating conditions and diseases of the nervous systems by surgical means.

neurosurgery   Branch of medicine specializing in surgery on the nervous system.

neurotomy   Incision into a nerve.

neutrophils   A granulocyte white blood cell that is important for phagocytosis. It is also the most numerous of the leukocytes.

nevus   Pigmented (colored) congenital skin blemish, birthmark or mole. Usually benign but may become cancerous.

newborn (NB)   Interchangeable with the term *neonate*, meaning infants less than one month old.

nitrogenous wastes   Waste products that contain nitrogen. These products, such as ammonia and urea, are produced during protein metabolism.

nocturia   Excessive urination during the night. May or may not be abnormal.

nodule   Solid, raised group of cells.

non-Hodgkin's lymphoma (NHL)   Cancer of the lymphatic tissues other than Hodgkin's lymphoma.

nonorganic failure to thrive (NFTT)   A condition in infants in which the weight remains below the fifth percentile of weight for children of the same age, not associated with a particular disease.

nonprescription drug   Drugs that are accessible in drugstores without a prescription. Also called over-the-counter (OTC) drugs.

nonproprietary name   The recognized and accepted official name for a drug. Each drug has only one generic name, which is not subject to trademark, so any pharmaceutical manufacturer may use it. Also called generic name.

norepinephrine   A hormone secreted by the adrenal medulla. It is a strong vasoconstrictor.

nose   Outside air enters the respiratory system through the nose. The nose includes the external nasal opening and the nasal cavity.

nucleus   The cell organelle that contains the chromosomes. Mature red blood cells have lost their nuclei.

nulligravida   Woman who has never been pregnant.

nullipara   Woman who has never produced a viable baby.

nurse   To breastfeed a baby.

nurse anesthetist   A registered nurse who has received additional training and education in the administration of anesthetic medications.

Nurse's Notes   Medical record document that records the patient's care throughout the day. It includes vital signs, treatment specifics, patient's response to treatment, and patient's condition.

nursing home   A facility that provides long-term care for patients who need extra time to recover from an illness or accident before they return home or for persons who can no longer care for themselves. Also called a long-term care facility.

nystagmus   Jerky-appearing involuntary eye movement.

obesity   Having an abnormal amount of fat in the body.

oblique fracture   Fracture at an angle to the bone.

oblique muscle   Oblique means slanted. Two of the eye muscles are oblique muscles.

oblique view   Positioning the patient so that the X-rays pass through the body on an angle.

obsessive-compulsive behavior   A type of anxiety disorder in which the person performs repetitive rituals in order to reduce anxiety.

obstetrician   A physician specialized in providing care for pregnant women and delivering infants.

obstetrics (OB)   Branch of medicine that treats women during pregnancy and childbirth, and immediately after childbirth.

occipital bone   A cranial bone.

occipital lobe   One of the four cerebral hemisphere lobes. It controls eyesight.

occult blood test   Self-administered test on the feces to determine if blood is present.

occupational therapy (OT)   Assists patients to regain, develop, and improve skills that are important for independent functioning. Occupational therapy personnel work with people who, because of illness, injury, developmental, or psychological impairments, require specialized training in skills that will enable them to lead independent, productive, and satisfying lives. Occupational therapists instruct patients in the use of adaptive equipment and techniques, body mechanics, and energy conservation. They also employ modalities such as heat, cold, and therapeutic exercise.

oculomycosis   Condition of eye fungus.

olecranon process   A process off the ulna that is part of the elbow joint. It is commonly referred to as the funny bone.

oligomenorrhea   Scanty menstrual flow.

oligospermia   Condition of having few sperm.

oliguria   Condition of scanty amount of urine.

oncogenic   Cancer causing.

oncology   The branch of medicine dealing with tumors.

onychectomy   Excision of a nail.

onychia   Infected nailbed.

onychomalacia   Softening of nails.

onychomycosis   Abnormal condition of nail fungus.

onychophagia   Nail biting.

oophorectomy   Removal of an ovary.

oophoritis   Inflammation of an ovary.

open fracture   Fracture in which the skin has been broken through to the fracture.

open heart surgery   Surgery that involves incision of the heart, coronary arteries, or the heart valves.

open wounds   A wound that has penetrated the skin. Deep wounds due to abrasion, incision, laceration, and puncture may require emergency care and suturing.

Operative Report   A medical record report from the surgeon detailing an operation. It includes a pre- and post-operative diagnosis, specific details of the surgical procedure itself, and how the patient tolerated the procedure.

ophthalmalgia   Eye pain.

ophthalmic   Pertaining to the eyes.

ophthalmic artery   The artery that supplies blood to the eyeball.

ophthalmologist   A physician specialized in treating conditions and diseases of the eye.

ophthalmology   Branch of medicine specializing in conditions of the eye.

ophthalmoplegia   Paralysis of the eye.

ophthalmorrhagia   Rapid bleeding from the eye.

ophthalmoscope   Instrument to view inside the eye.

ophthalmoscopy   Examination of the interior of the eyes using an instrument called an ophthalmoscope. The physician will dilate the pupil in order to see the cornea, lens, and retina. Identifies abnormalities in the blood vessels of the eye and some systemic diseases.

opportunistic infections   Infectious diseases that are associated with AIDS since they occur as a result of the lowered immune system and resistance of the body to infections and parasites.

opposition   Moves thumb away from palm; the ability to move the thumb into contact with the other fingers.

optic   Pertaining to the eye.

optic disk   The area of the retina associated with the optic nerve. Also called the blind spot.

optic nerve   The second cranial nerve that carries impulses from the retinas to the brain.

optician   Specialist in grinding corrective lenses.

optometer   Instrument to measure vision.

optometrist   A doctor of optometry specializes in testing visual acuity and prescribing corrective lenses.

optometry   Process of measuring vision.

oral   Pertaining to the mouth.

oral cholecystography   The patient swallows a radiopaque dye so that X-ray pictures can be taken that allow visualization of the gallbladder and its components.

oral hypoglycemic agent   Medication taken by mouth that causes a decrease in blood sugar. This is not used for insulin-dependent patients. There is no proof that this medication will prevent the long-term complications of diabetes mellitus.

oral surgeon   Dentist specializing in surgical treatment of the teeth and surrounding tissues.

orbit   Also called the eye socket. The cavity in the front of the skull containing the eyeball. It is formed from several bones and has a soft fatty tissue lining.

orchidectomy   Excision of the testes.

orchidopexy   Surgical fixation to move undescended testes into the scrotum and attaching to prevent retraction.

orchiectomy   Surgical removal of the testes.

orchioplasty   Surgical repair of the testes.

orchiotomy   Incision into the testes.

organ of Corti   The sensory receptor hair cells lining the cochlea. These cells change the sound vibrations to electrical impulses and send the impulses to the brain via the vestibulocochlear nerve.

organism   A whole, living individual. The sum of all the cells, tissues, organs, and systems working together to sustain life.

organs   Groups of different types of tissue coming together to perform special functions. For example, the heart contains muscular fibers, nerve tissue, and blood vessels.

oropharynx   The middle section of the pharynx that receives food and drink from the mouth.

orthodontics   The dental specialty concerned with straightening teeth.

orthodontist   Dentist who is an expert in orthodontia, which is straightening teeth.

orthopedics   Branch of medicine specializing in the diagnosis and treatment of conditions of the musculoskeletal system.

orthopedist   Physician who specializes in treatment of conditions of the musculoskeletal system.

orthopnea   Term to describe a patient who needs to sit up straight in order to breath comfortably.

orthotics   The use of equipment, such as splints and braces, to support a paralyzed muscle, promote a specific motion, or correct musculoskeletal deformities.

orthotist   Person skilled in orthotics.

os coxae   Also called the innominate bone or hip bone. It is the pelvis portion of the lower extremity. It consists of the ilium, ischium, and pubis and unites with the sacrum and coccyx to form the pelvis.

osmosis   Diffusion of water through a permeable membrane that allows the passage of the water (the solvent) but does not permit the solute to pass.

osseous tissue   Bony tissue. One of the hardest tissues in the body.

ossicles   The three small bones in the middle ear. The bones are the incus, malleus, and stapes. The ossicles amplify and conduct the sound waves to the inner ear.

ossification   The process of bone formation.

osteoarthritis   Noninflammatory type of arthritis resulting in degeneration of the bones and joints, especially those bearing weight.

osteoblast   An embryonic bone cell.

osteoblastoma   Benign lesion or tumor generally found on the spine, where it may cause paralysis.

osteocarcinoma   Cancer of the bone.

osteochondroma   Tumor composed of both cartilage and bony substance.

osteoclasia   Intentional breaking of a bone in order to correct a deformity.

osteocyte   Mature bone cells.

osteoid osteoma   Painful tumor usually found in the lower extremities.

osteomalacia   Softening of the bones caused by a deficiency of phosphorus or calcium. It is thought that in children the cause is insufficient sunlight and vitamin D.

osteomyelitis   Inflammation of the bone and bone marrow due to infection; can be difficult to treat.

osteopath   Physician who specializes in osteopathy. This physician would use the initials D.O.

osteopathy   Form of medicine that places great emphasis on the musculoskeletal system and the body system as a whole. Manipulation is also used as part of the treatment.

osteoporosis   Decrease in bone mass that results in a thinning and weakening of the bone with resulting fractures. The bone becomes more porous, especially in the spine and pelvis.

osteotome   An instrument to cut bone.

osteotomy   Incision into a bone.

otalgia   Ear pain.

otic   Pertaining to the ear.

otitis   Ear inflammation.

otitis media (OM)   Commonly referred to as middle ear infection; seen frequently in children. Often preceded by an upper respiratory infection.

otolaryngology   Branch of medicine specializing in conditions of the ear, nose and throat.

otologist   A physician specialized in the diagnosis and treatment of diseases of the ear.

otology   Study of ear.

otomycosis   Fungal infection of the ear, usually in the auditory canal.

otoplasty Corrective surgery to change the size of the external ear or pinna. The surgery can either enlarge or lessen the size of the pinna.

otopyorrhea Pus discharge from the ear.

otorhinolaryngologist A physician who specializes in the treatment of diseases of the ear, nose, and throat.

otorhinolaryngology Branch of medicine that treats diseases of the ears, nose, and throat. Also referred to as ENT.

otosclerosis Progressive hearing loss caused by immobility of the stapes bone.

otoscope Instrument to view inside the ear.

otoscopy Examination of the ear canal, eardrum, and outer ear using the otoscope. Foreign material can be removed from the ear canal with this procedure.

outpatient clinic A facility that provides services that do not require overnight hospitalization. The services range from simple surgeries to diagnostic testing to therapy. Also called an ambulatory care center or a surgical center.

ova The female sex cell or gamete produced in the ovary. An ovum fuses with a sperm to produce an embryo. Singular is ovum.

ova and parasites Laboratory examination of feces with a microscope for the presence of parasites or their eggs.

oval window The division between the middle and inner ear.

ovarian carcinoma Cancer of the ovary.

ovarian cyst Sac that develops within the ovary.

ovaries The female gonads. These two glands are located on either side of the lower abdominopelvic region of the female. They are responsible for the production of the sex cells, ova, and the hormones estrogen and progesterone.

over-the-counter Drugs that are accessible in drugstores without a prescription. Also called nonprescription drugs.

ovulation The release of an ovum from the ovary.

ovum The female sex cell or gamete. It is produced in the ovary. An ovum fuses with a sperm to produce an embryo. Plural is ova.

oxygen Gaseous element absorbed by the blood from the air sacs in the lungs. It is necessary for cells to make energy.

oxygenated Term for blood with a high oxygen level.

oxytocin A hormone secreted by the posterior pituitary. It stimulates uterine contractions during labor and delivery.

PA view Stands for posteroanterior; positioning the patient so that the X-rays pass through the body from the posterior side to the anterior side.

pacemaker Another name for the sinoatrial node of the heart; also, a surgically implanted device to artificially initiate a heart contraction.

pachyderma Thickening of the skin.

Paget's disease A fairly common metabolic disease of the bone from unknown causes. It usually attacks middle-aged and elderly people and is characterized by bone destruction and deformity.

pain control Managing pain through the use of a variety of means, including medications, biofeedback, and mechanical devices.

palate The roof of the mouth. The anterior portion is hard or bony, and the posterior portion is soft or flexible.

palatine bone A facial bone.

palatine tonsils Tonsils located in the lateral wall of the pharynx close to the mouth.

palliative therapy Treatment designed to reduce the intensity of painful symptoms, but not to produce a cure.

palsy Temporary or permanent loss of the ability to control movement.

pancreas Organ in the digestive system that produces digestive enzymes. Also a gland in the endocrine system that produces two hormones, insulin and glucagon.

pancreatic Pertaining to the pancreas.

pancreatic enzymes Digestive enzymes produced by the pancreas and added to the chyme in the duodenum.

pancreatitis Inflammation of the pancreas.

panhysterectomy Excision of the entire uterus, including the cervix.

panhysterosalpingo-oophorectomy Removal of the entire uterus, cervix, ovaries, and fallopian tubes. A total hysterectomy.

panic attacks A type of anxiety disorder characterized by a sudden onset of intense apprehension, fear, terror, or impending doom often accompanied by a racing heart rate.

panplegia Paralysis of all four extremities.

pansinusitis Inflammation of all the sinuses.

PAP (Papanicolaou) smear Test for the early detection of cancer of the cervix named after the developer of the test, George Papanicolaou, a Greek physician. A scraping of cells is removed from the cervix for examination under a microscope.

papilla The tip of each renal pyramid. It points toward the hilum. Each papilla is connected to a calyx, which is a duct that joins the renal pelvis.

papillae Raised projections on the surface of the tongue that contain taste buds. Taste buds are sensory receptors that can distinguish among bitter, sweet, sour, and salty flavors.

papule Small, solid, circular raised spot on the surface of the skin, often as a result of an inflammation in an oil gland.

paralysis Temporary or permanent loss of function or voluntary movement.

paranoid personality A personality disorder characterized by exaggerated feelings of persecution.

paraplegia Paralysis of the lower portion of the body and both legs.

parasites An organism that lives in or on another organism in order to derive nourishment.

parasympathetic A branch of the autonomic nervous system. This system serves as a counterbalance for the sympathetic nerves. Therefore, it causes the heart rate to slow down, lower the blood pressure, constrict eye pupils, and increase digestion.

parathyroid glands Four small glands located on the back surface of the thyroid gland. The parathyroid hormone secreted by these glands regulates the amount of calcium in the blood.

parathyroid hormone   The hormone secreted by the parathyroid glands. The more hormone, the higher the calcium level in the blood and the lower the level stored in bone. A low hormone level will cause tetany.

parathyroidectomy   Excision of one or more of the parathyroid glands. This is performed to halt the progress of hyperparathyroidism.

parathyroidoma   A parathyroid gland tumor.

parenteral   A route for introducing medication other than through the gastrointestinal tract; most commonly involves injection into the body through a needle and syringe.

parietal   Term meaning the outermost layer.

parietal bone   A cranial bone.

parietal layer   The outer pleural layer around the lungs. It lines the inside of the chest cavity.

parietal lobe   One of the four cerebral hemisphere lobes. It receives and interprets nerve impulses from sensory receptors.

parietal pericardium   The outer layer of the pericardium surrounding the heart.

parietal peritoneum   The outer layer of the serous membrane sac lining the abdominopelvic cavity.

parietal pleura   The outer layer of the serous membrane sac lining the thoracic cavity.

Parkinson's disease   Chronic disorder of the nervous system with fine tremors, muscular weakness, rigidity, and a shuffling gait.

paronychia   Infection around a nail.

parotid glands   A pair of salivary glands located in front of the ears.

paroxysmal nocturnal dyspnea (PND)   Attacks of shortness of breath (SOB) that occur only at night and awaken the patient.

passive acquired immunity   Immunity that results when a person receives protective substances produced by another human or animal. This may take the form of maternal antibodies crossing the placenta to a baby or an anti-toxin injection.

passive aggressive personality   A personality disorder in which the person expresses feelings or anger or hostility through indirect or covert actions.

passive range of motion (PROM)   Therapist putting a patient's joints through a full range of motion without assistance from the patient.

patella   Also called the knee cap. It is a lower extremity bone.

patent   Open or unblocked, such as a patent airway.

patent ductus arteriosus   Congenital heart anomaly in which the opening between the pulmonary artery and the aorta fails to close at birth. This condition requires surgery.

pathogenic   Microscopic organisms, such as bacteria, that are capable of causing disease.

pathogens   Disease-bearing organisms.

pathologic fracture   Fracture caused by diseased or weakened bone.

pathological gambling   An impulse control disorder in which the patient is unable to control the urge to gamble.

pathologist   A physician who specializes in evaluating specimens removed from living or dead patients.

Pathologist's Report   A medical record report given by a pathologist who studies tissue removed from the patient (for example: bone marrow, blood, or tissue biopsy).

pediatricians   Physicians who are involved in the prevention and treatment of childhood diseases.

pediatrics   The branch of medicine specialized in caring for children.

pediculosis   Infestation with lice.

pedophilia   A sexual disorder characterized by having sexual interest in children.

pelvic   Pertaining to the pelvis.

pelvic cavity   The inferior portion of the abdominopelvic cavity.

pelvic examination   Physical examination of the vagina and adjacent organs performed by a physician placing the fingers of one hand into the vagina. A visual examination is performed using a speculum.

pelvic inflammatory disease (PID)   Any inflammation of the female reproductive organs, generally bacterial in nature.

pelvic ultrasonography   Use of ultrasound waves to produce an image or photograph of an organ, such as the uterus, ovaries, or fetus.

pelvimetry   Measurement of the pelvic area, which helps in determining if the fetus can be delivered vaginally.

pemphigus vulgaris   Blisters forming in the skin and mucous membranes.

penis   The penis is the male sex organ. It is composed of erectile tissue that becomes erect during sexual stimulation, allowing it to be placed within the female vagina for ejaculation of semen. The larger, soft tip is referred to as the glans penis.

peptic ulcer   Ulcer occurring in the lower portion of the esophagus, stomach, and duodenum and thought to be caused by the acid of gastric juices.

percussion   Use of the fingertips to tap the body lightly and sharply. Aids in determining the size, position, and consistency of the underlying body part.

percutaneous transhepatic cholangiography (PTC)   A contrast medium is injected directly into the liver to visualize the bile ducts. Used to detect obstructions.

percutaneous transluminal coronary angioplasty (PTCA)   Method for treating localized coronary artery narrowing. A balloon catheter is inserted through the skin into the coronary artery and inflated to dilate the narrow blood vessel.

pericardial cavity   Cavity formed by the serous membrane sac surrounding the heart.

pericardiectomy   Surgical excision of part of the pericardium.

pericarditis   Inflammatory process or disease of the pericardium.

pericardium   The double-walled outer sac around the heart. The inner layer of the pericardium is called the epicardium, the outer layer is the heart itself. This sac contains pericardial fluid that reduces friction caused by the heart beating.

perimetritis   Inflammation around the uterus.

perineum   In the male, the external region between the scrotum and anus. In the female, the external region between the vagina and anus.

periodontal disease   Disease of the supporting structures of the teeth, including the gums and bones.

perioperative   The period of time that includes before, during, and after a surgical procedure.

periosteum   The membrane that covers most bones. It contains numerous nerves and lymphatic vessels.

peripheral nervous system   The portion of the nervous system that contains the cranial nerves and spinal nerves. These nerves are mainly responsible for voluntary muscle movement, smell, taste, sight, and hearing.

peristalsis   The wave-like muscular movements in the wall of the digestive system tube—esophagus, stomach, small intestines, and colon—that functions to move food along the tube.

peristaltic waves   The wave-like contractions of the muscles in a tubular organ, such as the ureters, that propel forward any substance inside the tube.

peritoneal dialysis   Removal of toxic waste substances from the body by placing warm chemically balanced solutions into the peritoneal cavity. Used in treating renal failure and certain poisonings.

peritoneum   Membranous sac that lines the abdominal cavity and encases the abdominopelvic organs. The kidneys are an exception since they lay outside the peritoneum and alongside the vertebral column.

peritonsillar abscess   Infection of the tissues between the tonsils and the pharynx. Also called a quinsy sore throat.

permanent teeth   The thirty-two permanent teeth begin to erupt at about the age of six. Generally complete by the age of sixteen.

pertussis   A contagious bacterial infection of the larynx, trachea, and bronchi characterized by coughing attacks that end with a whooping sound. Also called whopping cough.

petechiae   Flat, pinpoint, purplish spots from bleeding under the skin.

petit mal   A type of epilepsy seizure that lasts only a few seconds to half a minute, characterized by a loss of awareness and an absence of activity. It is also called an absence seizure.

pH   A number between 1 and 14 that indicates how acidic or basic a substance is. A solution with a pH of 1 is very acidic, 7 is neutral, and 14 is very basic.

phacoemulsification   Use of high-frequency sound waves to emulsify (liquefy) a lens with a cataract, which is then aspirated (removed by suction) with a needle.

phagocyte   Neutrophil component of the blood; has the ability to ingest and destroy bacteria.

phagocytic cells   Having the ability to engulf. Phagocytic white blood cells are able to engulf bacteria and other invading pathogens.

phagocytosis   The process of engulfing or ingesting material. Several types of white blood cells function by engulfing bacteria.

phalanges   The finger bones in the upper extremities and the toe bones in the lower extremities.

pharmaceutical   Related to medication or pharmacies.

pharmacist   One who is licensed to prepare and dispense drugs.

pharmacology   Study of the origins, nature, properties, and effects of drugs on the living organism.

pharyngeal tonsils   Another term for adenoids. The tonsils are a collection of lymphatic tissue found in the nasopharynx to combat microorganisms entering the body through the nose.

pharyngitis   Inflammation of the mucous membrane of the pharynx, usually caused by a viral or bacterial infection. Commonly called a sore throat.

pharynx   Medical term for the throat. The passageway that conducts air from the nasal cavity to the trachea, and also carries food and drink from the mouth to the esophagus. The pharynx is divided into three sections: the nasopharynx, oropharynx, and laryngopharynx.

phimosis   Narrowing of the foreskin over the glans penis that results in difficulty with hygiene. This condition can lead to infection or difficulty with urination. It is treated with circumcision, the surgical removal of the foreskin.

phlebitis   Inflammation of a vein.

phleborrhaphy   Suturing a vein.

phlebotomy   Creating an opening into a vein to withdraw blood.

phlegm   Thick mucus secreted by the membranes that line the respiratory tract. When phlegm is coughed through the mouth, it is called *sputum*. Phlegm is examined for color, odor, and consistency.

phobias   A type of anxiety disorder in which a person has irrational fears. An example is photophobia, the fear of light.

phonophoresis   The use of ultrasound waves to introduce medication across the skin into the subcutaneous tissues.

photorefractive keratectomy (PRK)   Use of a laser to reshape the cornea to correct errors of refraction.

photon absorptiometry   Measurement of bone density using an instrument for the purpose of detecting osteoporosis.

photophobia   Fear of light.

photosensitivity   Condition in which the skin reacts abnormally when exposed to light such as the ultraviolet rays of the sun.

physiatrist   Physician specializing in rehabilitation or physical medicine.

physical medicine   Use of natural methods, including physical therapy, to cure diseases and disorders.

physical therapy (PT)   Treating disorders using physical means and methods. Physical therapy personnel assess joint motion, muscle strength and endurance, function of heart and lungs, and performance of activities required in daily living, along with other responsibilities. Physical therapy treatment includes gait training, therapeutic exercise, massage, joint and soft tissue mobilization, thermal and cryotherapy, electrical stimulation, ultrasound, and

hydrotherapy. These methods strengthen muscles, improve motion and circulation, reduce pain, and increase function.

Physician's Desk Reference   A resource for drug information. It is an easy-to-use resource and should be in every physician's office or medical facility.

Physician's Orders   Medical record document that contains a complete list of the care, medications, tests, and treatments the physician orders for the patient.

Physician's Progress Notes   Part of a patient's medical record. It is the physician's daily record of the patient's condition, results of the physician's examinations, summary of test results, updated assessment and diagnoses, and further plans for the patient's care.

physicians' offices   Individual or groups of physicians providing diagnostic and treatment services in a private office setting rather than a hospital.

pia mater   The term means soft mother. This thin innermost meninges layer is applied directly to the surface of the brain.

pica   Eating disorder in which there is a craving for material that is not food, such as clay, grass, wood, paper, soap, and plaster.

pilonidal cyst   Cyst in the sacrococcygeal region due to tissue being trapped below the skin.

pineal gland   A gland in the endocrine system that produces a hormone called melatonin.

pinna   Also called the auricle. The external ear, which functions to capture sound waves as they go past the outer ear.

pituitary gland   An endocrine gland located behind the optic nerve in the brain. It is also called the master gland since it controls the functions of many other endocrine glands. It is divided into two lobes: anterior and posterior. The anterior pituitary gland secretes hormones that aid in controlling growth and stimulating the thyroid gland, sexual glands, and adrenal cortex. The posterior pituitary is responsible for the antidiuretic hormone and oxytocin.

placebo   Inactive, harmless substance used to satisfy a patient's desire for medication. It is also given to control groups of patients in research studies in which another group receives a drug. The effect of the placebo versus the drug is then observed.

placenta   Also called afterbirth. An organ attached to the uterine wall that is composed of maternal and fetal tissues. Oxygen, nutrients, carbon dioxide, and wastes are exchanged between the mother and baby through the placenta. The baby is attached to the placenta by way of the umbilical cord.

placenta previa   Occurs when the placenta is in the lower portion of the uterus and thus blocks the birth canal.

placental stage   The third stage of labor, which takes place after delivery of the infant. The uterus resumes strong contractions and the placenta detaches from the uterine wall and is delivered through the vagina.

plantar flexion   Bend sole of foot; point toes downward.

plaque   Gummy mass of microorganisms that grows on the crowns of teeth and spreads along the roots. It is colorless and transparent.

plasma   The liquid portion of blood containing 90% water. The remaining 10% consists of plasma proteins (serum albumin, serum globulin, fibrinogen, and prothrombin), inorganic substances (calcium, potassium, and sodium), organic components (glucose, amino acids, cholesterol), and waste products (urea, uric acid, ammonia, and creatinine).

plasma proteins   Proteins that are found in plasma. Includes serum albumin, serum globulin, fibrinogen, and prothrombin.

platelets   Cells responsible for the coagulation of blood. These are also called thrombocytes and contain no hemoglobin.

pleura   A protective double layer of serous membrane around the lungs. The parietal membrane is the outer layer and the visceral layer is the inner membrane. It secretes a thin, watery fluid to reduce friction associated with lung movement.

pleural cavity   Cavity formed by the serous membrane sac surrounding the lungs.

pleural effusion   Abnormal presence of fluid or gas in the pleural cavity. Physicians can detect the presence of fluid by tapping the chest (percussion) or listening with a stethoscope (auscultation).

pleural rub   Grating sound made when two surfaces, such as the pleura surfaces, rub together during respiration. It is caused when one of the surfaces becomes thicker as a result of inflammation or other disease conditions. This rub can be felt through the fingertips when they are placed on the chest wall or heard through the stethoscope.

pleurisy   Inflammation of the pleura.

pleurocentesis   A puncture of the pleura to withdraw fluid from the thoracic cavity in order to diagnose disease.

pleuropexy   Surgical fixation of the pleura.

plication   Taking tucks surgically in a structure to shorten it.

pneumoconiosis   Condition resulting from inhaling environmental particles that become toxic, such as coal dust (anthracosis), or asbestos (asbestosis).

Pneumocystis carinii **pneumonia (PCP)**   Pneumonia with a nonproductive cough, very little fever, and dyspnea. Seen in persons with weakened immune systems, such as patients with AIDS.

pneumoencephalography (PEG)   X-ray examination of the brain following withdrawal of cerebrospinal fluid and injection of air or gas via spinal puncture.

pneumonectomy   Surgical removal of lung tissue.

pneumonia   Inflammatory condition of the lung, which can be caused by bacterial and viral infections, diseases, and chemicals.

pneumonomycosis   Disease of the lungs caused by a fungus.

pneumothorax   Collection of air or gas in the pleural cavity, which can result in the collapse of a lung.

podiatrist   Specialist in treating disorders of the feet.

poisoning   Ingestion of harmful or toxic material into the body.

poliomyelitis   Acute viral disease that causes an inflammation of the gray matter of the spinal cord, resulting in paralysis in some cases. Has been brought under almost total control through vaccinations.

polyarteritis   Inflammation of many arteries.

polycythemia   Many cells in the blood.

polycythemia vera   Production of too many red blood cells in the bone marrow.

polydipsia   Condition of having an excessive amount of thirst, such as in diabetes.

polyethylene tube (PE tube)   Small tube surgically placed in a child's ear to assist in drainage of infection.

polymyositis   Disease involving muscle inflammation and weakness from an unknown cause.

polyneuritis   Inflammation of many nerves.

polyp   Small tumor with a pedicle or stem attachment. They are commonly found in vascular organs such as the nose, uterus, and rectum.

polypectomy   Surgical removal of a polyp.

polyphagia   To eat excessively.

polyposis   Small tumors that contain a pedicle or footlike attachment in the mucous membranes of the large intestine (colon).

polyuria   Condition of having excessive urine production. This can be a symptom of disease conditions such as diabetes.

pons   This portion of the brain stem forms a bridge between the cerebellum and cerebrum. It is also where nerve fibers cross from one side of the brain to control functions and movement on the other side of the brain.

pore   Opening for a sweat gland duct on the surface of the skin.

positron emission tomography (PET)   Use of positive radionuclides to reconstruct brain sections. Measurements can be taken of oxygen and glucose uptake, cerebral blood flow, and blood volume.

posterior   Directional term meaning near or on the back or spinal cord side of the body.

posterior lobe   The posterior portion of the pituitary gland. It secretes antidiuretic hormone and oxytocin.

posteroanterior (PA) and lateral of the chest   Routine X-ray of the heart and lungs.

postnasal   Pertaining to behind the nose.

postoperative   The period of time immediately following the surgery.

postpartum   Period immediately after delivery or childbirth.

postprandial   Pertaining to after a meal.

postural drainage   Draining secretions from the bronchi by placing the patient in a position that uses gravity to promote drainage. Used for the treatment of cystic fibrosis and bronchiectasis, and before lobectomy surgery.

postural drainage with clapping   Drainage of secretions from the bronchi or a lung cavity by having the patient lies so that gravity allows drainage to occur. Clapping is using the hand in a cupped position to perform percussion on the chest. Assists in loosening secretions and mucus.

potassium   An inorganic substance found in plasma. It is important for bones and muscles.

preeclampsia   Toxemia of pregnancy that, if untreated, can result in true eclampsia. Symptoms include hypertension, headaches, albumin in the urine, and edema.

preferred provider organization (PPO)   A PPO enters into contracts with individual medical professionals who agree to provide services to the PPO members at a reduced rate.

prefix   A word part added in front of the word root. It frequently gives information about the location of the organ, the number of parts or the time (frequency). Not all medical terms have a prefix.

pregnancy   The time from fertilization of an ovum to the birth of the newborn.

pregnancy test   Chemical test that can determine a pregnancy during the first few weeks. Can be performed in a physician's office or with a home-testing kit.

premature   Early.

premature birth   Delivery in which the infant (neonate) is born before the thirty-seventh week of gestation (pregnancy).

premature ejaculation   A sexual disorder characterized by rapid sexual climax and ejaculation.

premenstrual syndrome (PMS)   Symptoms that develop just prior to the onset of a menstrual period, which can include irritability, headache, tender breasts, and anxiety.

premolar   Another term for the bicuspid teeth.

prenatal visits   Appointments with a physician or nurse practitioner for the purpose of monitoring the mother's pregnancy.

preoperative (preop, pre-op)   The period of time preceding surgery.

prepatellar bursitis   Inflammation of the bursa located between the patella and the knee joint. Also called housemaid's knee.

prepuce   Also called the foreskin. A protective covering over the glans penis. It is this covering of the skin that is removed during circumcision.

presbycusis   Loss of hearing that can accompany the aging process.

presbyopia   Visual loss due to old age, resulting in difficulty in focusing for near vision (such as reading).

prescription   A written explanation to the pharmacist regarding the name of the medication, the dosage, and the times of administration.

prescription drug   A drug that can only be ordered by a licensed physician, dentist, or veterinarian.

pressure sore   Open sore caused by excessive rubbing on the skin or lying too long in the same position. Also called a decubitus ulcer.

preventative care   Level of patient care that emphasizes immunizations, check-ups, and patient education to prevent disease.

primary care   Providers, such as family practice physicians or nurse practitioners, who treat routine medical problems and make referrals to specialists when indicated.

primary site   Desigantes where a malignant tumor first appeared.

primigravida   Woman who has been pregnant once.

primipara   Woman who has given birth once.

probe   A surgical instrument used to explore tissue.

process   A projection from the surface of a bone.

proctology Branch of medicine specializing in conditions of the lower gastrointestinal system.

proctoplasty Plastic surgery of the anus and rectum.

proctoptosis Drooping rectum.

proctoscopy Examination of the anus and rectum with an endoscope inserted through the rectum.

progesterone One of the hormones produced by the ovaries. It works with estrogen to control the menstrual cycle.

prolactin A hormone secreted by the anterior pituitary. It stimulates mild production.

prolapsed umbilical cord When the umbilical cord of the baby is expelled first during delivery and is squeezed between the baby's head and the vaginal wall. This presents an emergency situation since the baby's circulation is compromised.

prolapsed uterus Fallen uterus that can cause the cervix to protrude through the vaginal opening. Generally caused by weakened muscles from vaginal delivery or as the result of pelvic tumors pressing down.

pronation To turn downward or backward, as with the hand or foot.

prone Directional term meaning lying horizontally facing downward.

prophylactic Procedure performed to prevent something else from happening. For example, even if the appendix is normal, it is sometimes removed during abdominal operations to prevent a future attack of appendicitis.

prophylaxis Prevention of disease. For example, an antibiotic can be used to prevent the occurrence of a disease.

proprietary name The name a pharmaceutical company chooses as the trademark or market name for its drug. Also called brand or trade name.

prospective payment system A payment system in which providers receive a preset reimbursement, regardless of the actual expenses incurred.

prostate cancer Slow-growing cancer that affects a large number of males after age fifty. The PSA (prostate-specific antigen) test is used to assist in early detection of this disease.

prostate gland A gland in the male reproductive system that produces fluids that nourish the sperm.

prostate-specific antigen (PSA) A blood test to screen for prostate cancer. Elevated blood levels of PSA are associated with prostate cancer.

prostatectomy Surgical removal of the prostate gland.

prostatic hyperplasia Abnormal cell growth within the prostate.

prostatitis Inflamed condition of the prostate gland that may be a result of an infection.

prostatocystitis Inflammation of the prostate and bladder.

prostatolith Prostate stone.

prostatolithotomy Incision into the prostate in order to remove a stone.

prostatorrhea Discharge from the prostate gland.

prosthesis Artificial device used as a substitute for a body part that is either congenitally missing or absent as a result of accident or disease; for instance, an artificial leg or hip prosthesis.

prosthetist Person who fabricates and fits prostheses.

protein-bound iodine test (PBI) Blood test to measure the concentration of thyroxine (T_4) circulating in the bloodstream. The iodine becomes bound to the protein in the blood and can be measured. Useful in establishing thyroid function.

prothrombin Protein element within the blood that interacts with calcium salts to form thrombin.

prothrombin time (Pro time) Measurement of the time it takes for a sample of blood to coagulate.

protocol The actual plan of care, including the medications, surgeries, and treatments for the care of a patient. Often, the entire health care team, including the physician, oncologist, radiologist, nurse, and patient, will assist in designing the treatment plan.

protozoa A single-celled member of the Kingdom Protozoa; some cause disease in man.

proximal Directional term meaning located closest to the point of attachment to the body.

proximal convoluted tubule A portion of the renal tubule.

pruritus Severe itching.

pseudocyesis False pregnancy.

psoriasis Chronic inflammatory condition consisting of crusty papules forming patches with circular borders.

psychedelic Drug such as lysergic acid diethylamide (LSD) that can produce visual hallucinations.

psychiatric nurse A nurse with additional training in the care of patients with mental, emotional, and behavioral disorders.

psychiatric social worker A social worker with additional training in the care of patients with mental, emotional, or behavioral disorders.

psychiatrist Physician who specializes in the treatment and prevention of mental disorders.

psychiatry The branch of medicine that deals with the diagnosis, treatment, and prevention of mental disorders.

psychogenic Caused by the mind.

psychologist Specialist trained in the study of psychological analysis, therapy, and research.

psychology The study of human behavior and thought process. This behavioral science is primarily concerned with understanding how human beings interact with their physical environment and with each other.

psychopathy Disease of the mind.

psychopharmacology The study of the effects of drugs on the mind and particularly the use of drugs in treating mental disorders. The main classes of drugs for the treatment of mental disorders are antipsychotic drugs, antidepressant drugs, minor tranquilizers, and lithium.

psychosis Severe mental disorder with symptoms such as depression and anxiety. The patient is not in touch with reality and may withdraw into an inner world, as in schizophrenia, or become severely emotionally impaired, as in mania.

psychosomatic Pertaining to the relationship between the mind and the body. Relates to physical disorders that are thought to originate in the emotional state of the patient.

psychotherapy A method of treating mental disorders by mental rather than chemical or physical means. It includes psychoanalysis, humanistic therapies, and family and group therapy.

puberty Beginning of menstruation and the ability to reproduce. Usually occurs around sixteen years of age.

pubic symphysis The point where the left and right pubic bones meet and are held together by a thick piece of cartilage, making it a cartilaginous joint.

pubis One of the three bones that form the os coxae or innominate bone.

puerperium Term used when discussing the mother's first three to six weeks after childbirth.

pulmonary angiography Injecting dye into a blood vessel for the purpose of taking an X-ray of the arteries and veins of the lungs.

pulmonary artery The large artery that carries deoxygenated blood from the right ventricle to the lung.

pulmonary circulation The pulmonary circulation transports deoxygenated blood from the right side of the heart to the lungs where oxygen and carbon dioxide are exchanged. Then it carries oxygenated blood back to the left side of the heart.

pulmonary edema Condition in which lung tissue retain an excessive amount of fluid. Results in labored breathing.

pulmonary embolism Blood clot or air bubble in the pulmonary artery or one of its branches.

pulmonary function test (PFT) Breathing equipment used to determine respiratory function and measure lung volumes and gas exchange.

pulmonary medicine The study of diseases of the respiratory system. Also called thoracic medicine.

pulmonary valve The semilunar valve between the right ventricle and pulmonary artery in the heart. It prevents blood from flowing backwards into the ventricle.

pulmonary vein Large vein that returns oxygenated blood from the lungs to the left atrium.

pulmonologist A physician specialized in treating diseases and disorders of the respiratory system.

pulmonology Branch of medicine specializing in conditions of the respiratory system.

pulse Expansion and contraction produced by blood as it moves through an artery. The pulse can be taken at several pulse points throughout the body where an artery is close to the surface.

pupil The hole in the center of the iris. The size of the pupil is changed by the iris dilating or constricting.

purgative A cathartic.

purpura Hemorrhages into the skin and mucous membranes.

purulent Pus-filled sputum, which can be the result of infection.

pustule Raised spot on the skin containing pus.

pyelitis Inflammation of the renal pelvis.

pyelogram X-ray record of the renal pelvis after injection of a radiopaque dye.

pyelonephritis Inflammation of the renal pelvis and the kidney. One of the most common types of kidney disease. It may be the result of a lower urinary tract infection that moved up to the kidney by way of the ureters. There may be large quantities of white blood cells and bacteria in the urine, and blood (hematuria) may even be present in the urine in this condition. Can occur with any untreated or persistent case of cystitis.

pyeloplasty Surgical repair of the renal pelvis.

pyloric sphincter Sphincter at the distal end of the stomach. Controls the passage of food into the duodenum.

pyloric stenosis Condition in which the pyloric sphincter becomes abnormally narrow. Food is not able to pass from the stomach into the small intestines. The main symptom is emesis or vomiting.

pyogenic Pus-forming.

pyorrhea Discharge of purulent material from dental tissue.

pyosalpinx Condition of having pus in the fallopian tubes.

pyothorax Condition of having pus in the chest cavity.

pyramids Triangular or wedge-shaped structures found in the medulla of the kidney. The tip, called the papilla, of each pyramid points toward the hilum. They consist of parallel loops of Henle and collecting tubules.

pyromania An impulse control disorder in which the patient is unable to control the impulse to start fires.

pyuria Presence of pus in the urine.

quad cane Walking cane with four prongs at the base to provide steady support.

quadriplegia Paralysis of all four extremities. Same as tetraplegia.

radiation therapy Use of X-rays to treat disease, especially cancer.

radical surgery Extensive surgery to remove as much tissue associated with a tumor as possible.

radiculitis Nerve root inflammation.

radioactive Substance capable of emitting or sending out radiant energy.

radioactive implant Embedding a radioactive source directly into tissue to provide a highly localized radiation dosage to damage nearby cancerous cells. Also called brachytherapy.

radioactive iodine uptake test (RAIU) Test in which radioactive iodine is taken orally (PO) or intravenously (IV) and the amount that is eventually taken into the thyroid gland (the uptake) is measured to assist in determining thyroid function.

radiography Making of X-ray pictures.

radioimmunoassay (RIA) Test used to measure the levels of hormones in the plasma of the blood.

radioisotope Radioactive form of an element.

radiologist Physician who practices diagnosis and treatment by the use of radiant energy. He or she is responsible for interpreting X-ray films.

radiology The branch of medicine that uses radioactive substances such as X-rays, isotopes, and radiation to prevent, diagnose, and treat diseases.

radiopaque Structures that are impenetrable to X-rays, appearing as a light area on the radiograph (X-ray).

radius One of the forearm bones in the upper extremity.

rales Abnormal crackling sound made during inspiration. Usually indicates the presence of moisture and can indicate a pneumonia condition.

range of motion The range of movement of a joint, from maximum flexion through maximum extension. It is measured as degrees of a circle.

Raynaud's phenomenon Periodic ischemic attacks affecting the extremities of the body, especially the fingers, toes, ears, and nose. The affected extremities become cyanotic and very painful. These attacks are brought on by arterial constriction due to extreme cold or emotional stress.

recessive A person must have two recessive genes in order for the recessive trait to be displayed.

rectal Introduced directly into the rectal cavity in the form of suppositories or solution. Drugs may have to be administered by this route if the patient is unable to take them by mouth due to nausea, vomiting, and surgery.

rectum An area at the end of the digestive tube for storage of feces that leads to the anus.

rectus abdominis A muscle named for its location and the direction of its fibers: rectus means straight and abdominis means abdominal.

rectus muscle Rectus means straight. Four of the eye muscles are rectus muscles.

red blood cells Also called erythrocytes or RBCs. Cells that contain hemoglobin, and iron-containing pigment that binds oxygen in order to transport it to the cells of the body.

red blood count (RBC) Blood test to determine the number of erythrocytes in a volume of blood. A decrease in the red blood cells may indicate anemia; an increase may indicate polycythemia.

red bone marrow Tissue that manufactures most of the blood cells. It is found in cancellous bone cavities.

reduction Correcting a fracture by realigning the bone fragments. Closed reduction is doing this without entering the body. Open reduction is making a surgical incision at the site of the fracture to do the reduction, often necessary where there are bony fragments to be removed.

reflux esophagitis Acid from the stomach backs up into the esophagus causing inflammation and pain.

refraction Eye examination performed by a physician to determine and correct refractive errors in the eye.

refractive error Defect in the ability of the eye to focus accurately on the image hitting it. Occurs in farsightedness and nearsightedness.

regional anesthesia Regional anesthesia is also referred to as a nerve block. This anesthetic interrupts a patient's pain sensation in a particular region of the body. The anesthetic is injected near the nerve that will be blocked from sensation. The patient usually remains conscious.

regurgitation Return of fluids and solids from the stomach into the mouth. Similar to *emesis* but without the force.

rehabilitation Process of treatment and exercise that can help a disabled person attain maximum function and well-being.

rehabilitation centers Facilities that provide intensive physical and occupational therapy. They include inpatient and outpatient treatment.

remission Period during which the symptoms of a disease or disorder leave. Can be temporary.

renal artery Artery that originates from the abdominal aorta and carries blood to the nephrons of the kidney.

renal colic Pain caused by a kidney stone, which can be an excruciating and generally requires medical treatment.

renal corpuscle Part of a nephron. It is a double-walled cuplike structure called the glomerular capsule or Bowman's capsule and contains a capillary network called the glomerulus. An afferent arteriole carries blood to the glomerulus and an efferent arteriole carries blood away from the glomerulus. The filtration stage of urine production occurs in the renal corpuscle as wastes are filtered from the blood in the glomerulus and enter Bowman's capsule.

renal pelvis Large collecting site for urine within the kidney. Collects urine from each calyx. Urine leaves the renal pelvis via the ureter.

renal transplant Surgical replacement of a donor kidney.

renal tubule Network of tubes found in a nephron. It consists of the proximal convoluted tubule, the loop of Henle, the distal tubule, and the collecting tubule. The reabsorption and secretion stages of urine production occur within the renal tubule. As the glomerular filtrate passes through the renal tubule, most of the water and some of the dissolved substances, such as amino acids and electrolytes, are reabsorbed. At the same time, substances that are too large to filter into Bowman's capsule, such as urea, are secreted directly from the blood stream into the renal tubule. The filtrate that reaches the collecting tubule becomes urine.

renal vein Vein that carries blood away from the kidneys.

repetitive motion injury Musculoskeletal system damage that results from simple motions being repeated many times within a given period of time. Often associated with assembly line work in which the worker performs one specialized task over and over.

reproductive system System in both males and females that produces eggs and sperm and provides a place for conception and the growth of the fetus. Female organs include the ovaries, fallopian tubes, uterus, vagina, and mammary glands. Male organs include the testes, vas deferens, urethra, prostate gland, and penis.

resection To surgically cut out; excision.

residency Time spent by a physician in training after the internship.

residual hearing Amount of hearing that is still present after damage has occurred to the auditory mechanism.

respiratory failure Failure of the respiratory system to maintain adequate gas exchange in the lungs to sustain life.

respiratory system   System that brings oxygen into the lungs and expels carbon dioxide. Organs include the nose, pharynx, larynx, trachea, bronchial tubes, and lungs.

restorative care   Care focused on assisting the individual to attain the highest level of physical and mental ability possible.

reticulocyte   Red blood cell containing granules or filaments in an immature stage of development.

retina   The innermost layer of the eye. It contains the visual receptors called rods and cones. The rods and cones receive the light impulses and transmit them to the brain via the optic nerve.

retinal   Pertaining to the retina.

retinal blood vessels   The blood vessels that supply oxygen to the rods and cones of the retina.

retinal detachment   Occurs when the retina becomes separated from the choroids layer. This separation seriously damages blood vessels and nerves resulting in blindness.

retinitis pigmentosa   Progressive disease of the eye that results in the retina becoming hard (sclerosed), pigmented (colored), and atrophied (wasting away). There is no known cure for this condition.

retinoblastoma   Malignant glioma of the retina.

retinopathy   Retinal disease.

retroflexion   In this position the uterus is bent back (retro-) upon itself. However, the cervix remains in its normal position.

retrograde pyelogram   A diagnostic X-ray in which dye is inserted through the urethra to outline the bladder, ureters, and renal pelvis.

retroperitoneal   Pertaining to behind the peritoneum. Used to describe the position of the kidneys, which is outside of the peritoneal sac alongside the spine.

retrosternal   Pertaining to behind the sternum.

retroversion   The uterus is turned backward with the cervix in an exaggerated direction of the pubis.

retrovirus   Virus, such as HIV, in which the virus copies itself using the host's DNA.

Reye's syndrome   A brain inflammation that occurs in children following a viral infection, usually the flu or chickenpox. It is characterized by vomiting and lethargy and may lead to coma and death.

Rh factor   An antigen marker found on erythrocytes of persons with Rh+ blood.

rheumatic heart disease   Valvular heart disease as a result of having had rheumatic fever.

rheumatoid arthritis (RA)   Chronic form of arthritis with inflammation of the joints, swelling, stiffness, pain, and changes in the cartilage that can result in crippling deformities.

rhinitis   Inflammation of the nose.

rhinomycosis   Condition of having a fungal infection in the nose.

rhinoplasty   Plastic surgery of the nose.

rhinorrhagia   Rapid and excessive flow of blood from the nose.

rhinorrhea   Watery discharge from the nose, especially with allergies or a cold, runny nose.

Rh-negative   A person with Rh– blood type. The person's RBCs do not have the Rh marker and will make antibodies against Rh+ blood.

Rh-positive   A person with RH+ blood type. The person's RBCs have the Rh marker.

rhonchi   Somewhat musical sound during expiration, often found in asthma or infection, and caused by spasms of the bronchial tubes. Also called wheezing.

rhytidectomy   Surgical removal of excess skin to eliminate wrinkles. Commonly referred to as a facelift.

rhytidoplasty   Excision of wrinkles.

rib cage   Also called the chest cavity. It is the cavity formed by the curved ribs extending from the vertebral column around the sides and attaching to the sternum. The ribs are part of the axial skeleton.

rickets   Deficiency in calcium and vitamin D found in early childhood that results in bone deformities, especially bowed legs.

right hypochondriac   An anatomical division of the abdomen; the right upper row.

right iliac   An anatomical division of the abdomen; the right lower row. Also called the right inguinal.

right inguinal   An anatomical division of the abdomen; the right lower row. Also called the right iliac.

right lower quadrant (RLQ)   A clinical division of the abdomen. It contains portions of small and large intestines, right ovary and fallopian tube, appendix, right ureter.

right lumbar   An anatomical division of the abdomen, the right middle row.

right subclavian vein   The circulatory system vein that receives lymph from the right lymphatic duct.

right upper quadrant (RUQ)   A clinical division of the abdomen. It contains the right lobe of the liver, the gallbladder, a portion of the pancreas, and portions of small and large intestine.

rigor mortis   Stiffness of skeletal muscles that is seen in death.

Rinne and Weber tuning-fork tests   The physician holds a tuning fork, an instrument that produces a constant pitch when it is struck against or near the bones on the side of the head. These tests assess both nerve and bone conduction of sound.

rods   The sensory receptors of the retina that are active in dim light and do not perceive color.

roentgen   Unit for describing an exposure dose of radiation.

roentgen ray   The preferred term is X-ray.

roentgenologist   Physician who is skilled in X-ray diagnosis and treatment. The preferred term is radiologist.

Romberg's test   Test used to establish neurological function in which the person is asked to close his or her eyes and place their feet together. This best for body balance is positive if the patient sways when the eyes are closed.

root canal Dental treatment involving the pulp cavity of the root of a tooth. Procedure is used to save a tooth that is badly infected or abscessed.

roseola A viral infection with a rosy red rash.

rotation Moving around a central axis.

rugae The prominent folds in the mucosa of the stomach. They smooth out and almost disappear allowing the stomach to expand when it is full of food.

ruptured intervertebral disk Herniation or outpouching of a disk between two vertebrae—also called herniated disk. May require surgery.

saccule Found in the inner ear. It plays a role in equilibrium.

sacral Pertaining to the sacrum.

sacrum The five fused vertebrae that form a large flat bone in the upper buttock region.

sagittal plane A vertical plane that divides the body into left and right sections.

salivary glands Exocrine glands with ducts that open into the mouth. They produce saliva, which makes the bolus of food easier to swallow and begins the digestive process. There are three pairs of salivary glands: parotid, submandibular, and sublingual.

salpingitis Inflammation of the fallopian tube or tubes.

salpingocyesis Tubal pregnancy.

salpingo-oophorectomy Removal of a fallopian tube and ovary.

salpingostomy The creation of an artificial opening in a fallopian tube.

sanguinous Pertaining to blood.

sarcoidosis Inflammatory disease of the lymph system in which lesions may appear in the liver, skin, lungs, lymph nodes, spleen, eyes, and small bones of the hands and feet.

sarcoma Cancer arising from the connective tissue, such as muscle or bone. May affect the kidneys, bladder, bones, liver, lungs, and spleen.

scabies Contagious skin disease caused by an egg-laying mite that causes intense itching; often seen in children.

scalpel A surgical instrument used to cut and separate tissue.

scan Recording the emission of radioactive waves on a photographic plate after a substance has been injected into the body.

scapula Also called the shoulder blade. An upper extremity bone.

scarlet fever A streptococcal infection characterized by fever and a dense bright red rash that is followed by peeling. Also called scarlatina.

sclera The tough protective outer layer of the eyeball. It is commonly referred to as the white of the eye.

scleral buckling Placing a band of silicone around the outside of the sclera to stabilize a detaching retina.

scleroderma Disorder in which the skin becomes taut, thick, and leatherlike.

scleromalacia Softening of the sclera.

sclerotomy Incision into the sclera.

scoliosis Abnormal lateral curvature of the spine.

scrotum A sac that serves as a container for the testes. This sac, which is divided by a septum, supports the testicles and lies between the legs and behind the penis.

scrub nurse Surgical assistant who hands instruments to the surgeon. This person wears sterile clothing and maintains the sterile operative field.

sebaceous cyst Sac under the skin filled with sebum or oil from a sebaceous gland. This can grow to a large size and may need to be excised.

sebaceous gland Also called oil glands. They produce a substance called sebum that lubricates the skin surface.

seborrhea Excessive discharge of sebum.

sebum Thick oily substance secreted by sebaceous glands that lubricates the skin to prevent drying out. When sebum accumulates, it can cause congestion in the sebaceous glands and whiteheads or pimples may form. When the sebum becomes dark it is referred to as a comedo or blackhead.

sedative Produces relaxation without causing sleep.

seizure Sudden attack of severe muscular contractions associated with a loss of consciousness. This is seen in grand mal epilepsy.

semen Semen contains sperm and fluids secreted by male reproductive system glands. It leaves the body through the urethra.

semen analysis This procedure is used when performing a fertility workup to determine if the male is able to produce sperm. Semen is collected by the patient after abstaining from sexual intercourse for a period of three to five days. The sperm in the semen are analyzed for number, swimming strength, and shape. This is also used to determine if a vasectomy has been successful. After a period of six weeks, no sperm should be present in a sample from the patient.

semicircular Pertaining to a half circle.

semicircular canals A portion of the labyrinth associated with balance and equilibrium.

semilunar valve The heart valves located between the ventricles and the great arteries leaving the heart. The pulmonary valve is located between the right ventricle, and the pulmonary artery and the aortic valve is located between the left ventricle and the aorta.

seminal vesicles Two male reproductive system glands located at the base of the bladder. They secrete a fluid that nourishes the sperm into the vas deferens. This fluid plus the sperm constitutes much of the semen.

seminiferous tubules Network of coiled tubes that make up the bulk of the testes. Sperm development takes place in the walls of the tubules and the mature sperm are released into the tubule in order to leave the testes.

senile Mental weakness associated with old age in some people.

sensorineural hearing loss Type of hearing loss in which the sound is conducted normally through the external and middle ear but there is a defect in the inner ear or with the cochlear nerve, resulting in the inability to hear. A hearing aid may help.

sensory receptors   Nerve fibers that are located directly under the surface of the skin. These receptors detect temperature, pain, touch, and pressure. The messages for these sensations are conveyed to the brain and spinal cord from the nerve endings in the skin.

septoplasty   Surgical repair of the septum.

serous   Watery secretion of serous membranes.

serous membrane   These membranes are found lining body cavities and secrete a thin, watery fluid that acts as a lubricant as organs rub against one another.

serum   Clear, sticky fluid that remains after the blood has clotted.

serum albumin   One of the proteins in blood serum.

serum electrolyte level   A laboratory test to measure the amount of sodium, potassium, and chloride ions in the blood.

serum globulin   Proteins in the blood.

serum glucose tests   Blood test performed to assist in determining insulin levels and useful for adjusting medication dosage.

serum lipoprotein level   A laboratory test to measure the amount of cholesterol and triglycerides in the blood.

sexual intercourse   Process of sexual relations or coitus.

shield   Protective device used to protect against radiation.

shingles   Eruption of vesicles along a nerve, causing a rash and pain. Caused by the same virus as chickenpox.

shock   Situation in which not enough blood is flowing to the heart for normal function. The symptoms of shock are paleness, staring eyes, dilated pupils, weak and rapid pulse, increased shallow respirations, and decreased blood pressure.

short bone   A type of bone that is roughly cube-shaped. The carpals are short bones.

shortness of breath (SOB)   Term used to indicate that a patient is having some difficulty breathing. The causes can range from mild SOB after exercise to SOB associated with heart disease.

shower chair   Waterproof chair that is placed inside the shower stall so that a weak person may sit during showering.

shunt   Abnormal connection between two cavities or organs. In a cardiovascular shunt there is an abnormal connection between the cavities of the heart.

sialolith   A salivary gland stone.

sickle cell anemia   Severe, chronic, incurable disorder that results in anemia and causes joint pain, chronic weakness, and infections. It is more common in people of Mediterranean and African heritage. The actual blood cell is crescent-shaped.

side effect   Response to a drug other than the effect desired.

sigmoid colon   The final section of colon. It follows an S-shaped path and terminates in the rectum.

Signing Exact English (SEE-2)   Translation of English into signs. American Sign Language (ASL) is used in combination with other sign languages and fingerspelling to correspond exactly to the spoken English.

silicosis   Form of respiratory disease resulting from the inhalation of silica (quartz) dust. Considered an occupational disease.

simple fracture   Fracture with no open skin or wound.

sinoatrial node (SA)   Also called the pacemaker of the heart. It is an area of the right atria that initiates the electrical pulse that causes the heart to contract.

sinus   A hollow cavity within a bone.

sinus X-ray   Taking an X-ray view of the sinus cavity from the front of the head.

sinuses   Air-filled cavities within the facial bones. They are lined with mucous membrane and play a role in sound production.

skeletal muscle   A voluntary muscle that is attached to bones by a tendon.

skin   The major organ of the integumentary system. It forms a barrier between the external and internal environments.

skin graft   The transfer of skin from a normal area to cover another site. Used to treat burn victims and after some surgical procedures.

skin tests (ST)   Test to determine the patient's reaction to a suspected allergen by injecting a small amount under the skin (interdermal) with a needle. The reaction of the patient to this material is then read to indicate any allergy. Examples of such tests are the tuberculin (TB) test, Mantoux (PPD) test, patch test, and Schick test.

sleep disorder   Any condition that interferes with sleep other than environmental noises. Can include difficulty sleeping (insomnia), nightmares, night terrors, sleepwalking, and apnea.

sleep walking   A sleeping disorder in which the patient performs complex activities while asleep.

slit lamp microscope   Instrument used in ophthalmology for examining the posterior surface of the cornea.

small intestine   The portion of the digestive tube between the stomach and colon, and the major site of nutrient absorption. There are three sections: duodenum, jejunum, and ileum.

smooth muscle   An involuntary muscle found in internal organs such as the digestive organs or blood vessels.

Snellen's chart   Chart used for testing distance vision. It contains letters of varying size and is administered from a distance of 20 feet. A person who can read at 20 feet what the average person can read at that distance is said to have 20/20 vision.

sodium   An inorganic substance found in plasma.

sonogram   The image produced by ultrasound waves bouncing off internal body structures.

sound   Metal rod curved at one end with a handle at the other end, used to treat a stricture or an obstruction in the urethra. A physician passes the sound up the urethra.

special sense organs   The special sense organs perceive environmental conditions. The eyes, ears, nose, and tongue contain special sense organs.

specialty care   Providers, such as orthopedists or surgeons, who see patients who have been referred by the primary care provider for problems known to require the services of a specialist.

specialty care hospitals Hospitals that provide care for very specific types of disease. A good example is a psychiatric hospital.

speculum A surgical instrument used to spread apart walls of a cavity.

speech pathologist Medical professional trained to evaluate and train the person who is hearing impaired in using any one, or all, of the following: speech, sign language, fingerspelling, and residual hearing.

speechreading Ability to watch a person's mouth and word formation during speaking to interpret what they are saying. Also referred to as lipreading.

sperm Also called spermatozoon (plural is spermatozoa). The male sex cell. One sperm fuses with the ova to produce a new being.

spermatic cord The term for the cord-like collection of structures that include the vas deferens, arteries, veins, nerves, and lymph vessels. The spermatic cord suspends the testes within the scrotum.

spermatogenesis Formation of mature sperm.

spermatolysis Destruction of sperm.

spermatolytic Destruction of spermatozoa.

spermatozoa Also called sperm, the singular is spermatozoon. The male sex cell. One sperm fuses with the ova to produce a new being.

spermatozoon Also called sperm, the plural is spermatozoa. The male sex cell. One sperm fuses with the ova to produce a new being.

sphenoid bone A cranial bone.

sphincter A ring of muscle around a tubular organ. It can contract to control the opening of the tube.

sphygmomanometer Instrument for measuring blood pressure. Also referred to as a blood pressure cuff.

spina bifida Congenital defect in the walls of the spinal canal in which the laminae of the vertebra do not meet or close. Results in membranes of the spinal cord being pushed through the opening. Can also result in other defects, such as hydrocephalus.

spinal Pertaining to the spine.

spinal canal The canal that extends through the vertebrae and contains the spinal cord.

spinal cavity A dorsal body cavity within the spinal column that contains the spinal cord.

spinal cord The spinal cord provides a pathway for impulses traveling to and from the brain. It is a column of nerve fibers that extends from the medulla oblongata of the brain down to the level of the second lumbar vertebra.

spinal cord injury (SCI) Bruising or severing of the spinal cord from a blow to the vertebral column resulting in muscle paralysis and sensory impairment below the injury level.

spinal fusion Surgical immobilization of adjacent vertebrae. This may be done for several reasons, including correction for a herniated disk.

spinal nerves The nerves that arise from the spinal cord.

spinal puncture Puncture with a needle into the spinal cord area to withdraw fluid for examination or for the injection of anesthesia. Also called a lumbar puncture.

spinal stenosis Narrowing of the spinal canal causing pressure on the cord and nerves.

spiral fracture Fracture in an "S" shaped spiral. It can be caused by a twisting injury.

spirometer Instrument consisting of a container into which a patient can exhale for the purpose of measuring the air capacity of the lungs.

spirometry Using a devise to measure the breathing capacity of the lungs.

spleen Organ in the lymphatic system that filters microorganisms and old red blood cells from the blood.

spleen scan A radioactive material injected into the patient through an intravenous (IV) route enters the spleen for visualization of this organ. Used to detect tumors, cysts, abscesses, and other splenomegaly.

splenectomy Excision of the spleen.

splenomegaly Enlargement of the spleen.

splenopexy Artificial fixation of a movable spleen.

spongy bone The bony tissue found inside a bone. It contains cavities that hold red bone marrow. Also called cancellous bone.

spontaneous abortion Loss of a fetus without any artificial aid. Also called a miscarriage.

sprain Pain and disability caused by trauma to a joint. A ligament may be torn in severe sprains.

sputum Mucus or phlegm that is coughed up from the lining of the respiratory tract. Tested to determine what type of bacteria or virus is present as an aid in selecting the proper antibiotic treatment.

sputum culture and sensitivity (CS) Testing sputum by placing it on a culture medium and observing any bacterial growth. The specimen is then tested to determine antibiotic effectiveness.

sputum cytology Testing for malignant cells in sputum.

squamous cell carcinoma Epidermal cancer that may go into deeper tissue but does not generally metastasize.

stabilize Maintaining a victim's condition without allowing it to worsen. In most cases the vital signs remain unchanged when a patient is stabilized.

staging The process of classifying tumors based on their degree of tissue invasion and the potential response to therapy. The TNM staging system is frequently used. The T refers to the tumor's size and invasion, the N refers to lymph node involvement, and the M refers to the presence of metastases of the tumor cells.

staging laparotomy Surgical procedure in which the abdomen is entered to determine the extent and staging of a tumor.

stapedectomy Removal of the stapes bone to treat otosclerosis (hardening of the bone). A prosthesis or artificial stapes may be implanted.

stapes One of the three ossicles of the middle ear. It is attached to the oval window leading to the inner ear. Also called the stirrup.

stent A stainless steel tube placed within a blood vessel or a duct to widen the lumen.

sterilization   Process of rendering a male or female sterile or unable to conceive children.

sternum   Also called the breast bone. It is part of the axial skeleton and the anterior attachment for ribs.

steroid sex hormones   A class of hormones secreted by the adrenal cortex. It includes aldosterone, cortisol, androgens, estrogens, and progestins.

stethoscope   Instrument for listening to body sounds, such as the chest, heart, or intestines.

stillbirth   Birth in which a viable-aged fetus dies before or at the time of delivery.

stimulant   Speeds up the heart and respiratory system. Used to increase alertness.

stimulus   Something that activates or excites the nerve and results in an impulse.

stomach   A J-shaped muscular organ that acts as a sac to collect, churn, digest, and store food. It is composed of three parts: the fundus, body, and antrum. Hydrochloric acid is secreted by glands in the mucous membrane lining of the stomach. Food mixes with other gastric juices and the hydrochloric acid to form a semisoft mixture called chyme, which then passes into the duodenum.

strabismus   An eye muscle weakness resulting in each eye looking in a different direction at the same time. May be corrected with glasses, eye exercises, and/or surgery. Also called lazy eye or crossed eyes.

strabotomy   Incision into the eye muscles in order to correct strabismus.

strain   Trauma to muscle from excessive stretching or pulling.

stratified squamous epithelial   Describes the layers of flat or scale-like cells found in the epidermis. Stratified means multiple layers and squamous means flat.

stress/exercise testing   Method for evaluating cardiovascular fitness. The patient is placed on a treadmill or a bicycle and then subjected to steadily increasing levels of work. An EKG and oxygen levels are taken while the patient exercises.

stricture   Narrowing of a passageway in the urinary system.

stridor   Harsh, high-pitched, noisy breathing sound that is made when there is an obstruction of the bronchus or larynx. Found in conditions such as croup in children.

subarachnoid space   The space located between the arachnoid layer and pia mater. It contains cerebrospinal fluid.

subcutaneous   Pertaining to under the skin.

subcutaneous layer   This is the deepest layer of the skin where fat is formed. This layer of fatty tissue protects the deeper tissues of the body and acts as an insulation for heat and cold.

subdural   Pertaining to under the dura mater.

subdural hematoma   Mass of blood forming beneath the dura mater of the brain.

subdural space   The space located between the dura mater and the arachnoid layer.

sublingual   Pertaining to under the tongue.

sublingual glands   A pair of salivary glands in the floor of the mouth.

submandibular glands   A pair of salivary glands in the floor of the mouth.

subscapular   Pertaining to under the shoulder blade.

substernal   Pertaining to below the sternum.

sucking chest wound   Open wound in the chest that draws outside air into the chest cavity.

sudden infant death syndrome (SIDS)   The sudden, unexplained death of an infant in which a postmortem examination fails to determine the cause of death.

suffix   A word part attached to the end of a word. It frequently indicates a condition, disease, or procedure. Almost all medical terms have a suffix.

sulci   Also called fissures. The grooves that separate the gyri of the cerebral cortex.

superficial   Directional term meaning toward the surface of the body.

superior   Directional term meaning toward the head, or above.

superior venae cavae   The branch of the vena cavae that drains blood from the chest and upper body.

supernumerary bone   Extra bone, generally a finger or toe, found in newborns.

supination   Turn the palm or foot upward.

supine   Directional term meaning lying horizontally and facing upward.

suppositories   A method for administering medication by placing it in a substance that will melt after being placed in a body cavity, usually rectally, and release the medication.

suprasternal   Pertaining to above the sternum.

surgeon   A physician who has completed additional training of five years or more in a surgical specialty area. The specialty areas include orthopedics, neurosurgery, gynecology, ophthalmology, urology, and thoracic, vascular, cardiac, plastic, and general surgery.

surgery   The branch of medicine dealing with operative procedures to correct deformities and defects, repair injuries, and diagnose and cure diseases.

surgical center   A facility that provides services that range from simple surgeries to diagnostic testing to therapy and do not require overnight hospitalization. Also called an ambulatory care center or an outpatient clinic.

suture material   Used to close a wound or incision. Examples are catgut, silk thread, or staples. They may or may not be removed when the wound heals, depending on the type of material that is used.

sutures   The fibrous joints formed between the cranial bones.

sweat glands   Glands that produce sweat, which assists the body in maintaining its internal temperature by creating a cooling effect when it evaporates.

sweat test   Test performed on sweat to determine the level of chloride. There is an increase in skin chloride in the disease cystic fibrosis.

sympathectomy   Excision of a portion of the sympathetic nervous system. Could include a nerve or a ganglion.

sympathetic   A branch of the autonomic nervous system. This system stimulates the body in times of stress and crisis by increasing heart rate, dilating airways to allow for more oxygen, increasing blood pressure, inhibiting digestion, and stimulating the production of adrenaline during a crisis.

syncope   Fainting.

syndrome   Group of symptoms and signs that when combined present a clinical picture of a disease or condition.

synovial fluid   The fluid secreted by a synovial membrane in a synovial joint. It lubricates the joint and reduces friction.

synovial joint   A freely moving joint that is lubricated by synovial fluid.

synovial membrane   The membrane that lines a synovial joint. It secretes a lubricating fluid called synovial fluid.

syphilis   Infectious, chronic, venereal disease that can involve any organ. May exist for years without symptoms. Treated with the antibiotic penicillin.

systemic   Pertaining to a system.

systemic circulation   The systematic circulation transports oxygenated blood from the left side of the heart to the cells of the body and then back to the right side of the heart.

systemic lupus erythematosus (SLE)   Chronic disease of the connective tissue that injures the skin, joints, kidneys, nervous system, and mucous membranes. May produce a characteristic butterfly rash across the cheeks and nose.

systems   A system is composed of several organs working in a compatible manner to perform a complex function or functions. Examples include the digestive system, the cardiovascular system, and the respiratory system.

systolic pressure   The maximum pressure within blood vessels during a heart contraction.

T₃   Abbreviation for triiodothyronine, a thyroid hormone.

T₄   Abbreviation for thyroxine, a thyroid hormone.

T cells   A lymphocyte active in cellular immunity.

T lymphocytes   A type of lymphocyte involved with producing cells that physically attack and destroy pathogens.

tachycardia   Abnormally fast heart rate, over 100 bpm.

tachypnea   Rapid breathing rate.

tagging   Attachment of a radioactive material to a chemical and tracing it as it moves through the body.

talipes   Congenital deformity of the foot. Also referred to as a clubfoot.

talipes equinus   Only the front of the foot touches the ground, causing the person to walk on the toes.

talipes planus   The arch is broken, causing the entire foot to be flat on the ground.

talipes valgus   The foot is everted, with the inner side of the foot resting on the ground.

talipes varus   The foot is inverted, and the outer side of the foot touches the ground.

tarsals   The ankle bones in the lower extremity.

Tay–Sachs disease   Disorder caused by a deficiency of an enzyme, which can result in mental and physical retardation and blindness. It is transferred by a recessive trait and is most commonly found in families of Eastern European Jewish decent. Death generally occurs before the age of four.

temporal bone   A cranial bone.

temporal lobe   One of the four cerebral hemisphere lobes. It controls hearing and smell.

tenaculum   A long-handled clamp surgical instrument.

tendon   The strong connective tissue cords that attach skeletal muscles to bones.

tendonitis   Inflammation of a tendon.

tenodynia   Pain in a tendon.

tenorrhaphy   Suture a tendon.

terminal illness   Illness from which one will not recover.

testes   The male gonads. The testes are oval glands located in the scrotum that produce sperm and the male hormone, testosterone.

testicles   Also called testes (singular is testis). These oval shaped organs are responsible for the development of sperm within the seminiferous tubules. The testes must be maintained at the proper temperature for the sperm to survive. This lower temperature level is controlled by the placement of the scrotum outside the body. The hormone testosterone, which is responsible for the growth and development of the male reproductive organs, is also produced by the testes.

testosterone   Male hormone produced in the testes. It is responsible for the growth and development of the male reproductive organs.

tetany   A condition that results from a calcium deficiency in the blood. It is characterized by muscle twitches, cramps, and spasms.

tetralogy of Fallot   Combination of four congenital anomalies: pulmonary stenosis, an interventricular septal defect, abnormal blood supply to the aorta, and hypertrophy of the right ventricle. Needs immediate surgery to correct.

tetraplegia   Paralysis of all four limbs. Same as quadriplegia.

thalamus   The thalamus is a portion of the diencephalon. It is composed of gray matter and acts as a center for relaying impulses from the eyes, ears, and skin to the cerebrum. Pain perception is also controlled by the thalamus.

T-helper cells   T cells that help the B cells to recognize the antigens. Also called T4 cells.

therapeutic   Treatment of disease by applying specified remedies.

therapeutic exercise   Exercise planned and carried out to achieve a specific physical benefit, such as improved range of motion, muscle strength, or cardiovascular function.

thermograph   Technique that detects and records surface temperatures of the body. The hot and cold spots on the body are revealed, which assists in disease detection. Used to detect cancer of the breast and blood flow in the limbs.

thermotherapy   Applying heat to the body for therapeutic purposes.

thoracalgia   Chest pain.

thoracentesis Surgical puncture of the chest wall for the removal of fluids.

thoracic Pertaining to the chest.

thoracic cavity A ventral body cavity in the chest area that contains the lungs and heart.

thoracic duct The largest lymph vessel. It drains the entire body except for the right arm, chest wall, and both lungs. It empties lymph into the left subclavian vein.

thoracic medicine The study of the respiratory system.

thoracic surgeon A physician specialized in treating conditions and diseases of the respiratory system by surgical teams.

thoracic surgery Branch of medicine specializing in surgery on the respiratory system and thoracic cavity.

thoracic vertebrae The twelve vertebrae in the chest region.

thoracostomy Insertion of a tube into the chest for the purpose of draining off fluid or air.

thoracotomy Incision into the chest.

throat culture Removing a small sample of tissue or material from the pharynx and placing it upon a culture medium to determine bacterial growth.

thrombectomy Surgical removal of a thrombus or blood clot from a blood vessel.

thrombin A clotting enzyme that converts fibrinogen to fibrin.

thrombocytes Also called platelets. Platelets play a critical part in the blood-clotting process by agglutinating into small clusters and releasing thrombokinase.

thrombokinase An enzyme released by platelets in the clotting process. It reacts with prothrombin to form thrombin.

thrombolysis Procedure to dissolve a clot.

thrombophlebitis Inflammation of a vein that results in the formation of blood clots within the vein.

thrombus A blood clot.

thymectomy Removal of the thymus gland.

thymoma Malignant tumor of the thymus gland.

thymosin Hormone secreted by thymus gland. It causes lymphocytes to change into T-lymphocytes.

thymus gland An endocrine gland located in the upper mediastinum that assists the body with the immune function and the development of antibodies. As part of the immune response it secretes a hormone, thymosin, that changes lymphocytes to T cells.

thyroid cartilage A piece of cartilage associated with the larynx. It is also commonly called the Adam's apple and is larger in males.

thyroid echogram Ultrasound examination of the thyroid that can assist in distinguishing a thyroid nodule from a cyst.

thyroid function tests (TFT) Blood tests used to measure the levels of T_3, T_4, and TSH in the bloodstream to assist in determining thyroid function.

thyroid gland This endocrine gland is located on either side of the trachea. Its shape resembles a butterfly with a large left and right lobe connected by a narrow isthmus. This gland produces the hormones thyroxine (also known as T_4) and triiodothyronine (also known as T_3).

thyroid scan Test in which a radioactive element is administered that localizes in the thyroid gland. The gland can then be visualized with a scanning device to detect pathology such as tumors.

thyroidectomy Removal of the entire thyroid or a portion (partial thyroidectomy) to treat a variety of conditions, including nodes, cancer, and hyperthyroidism.

thyroidotomy Incision into the thyroid gland.

thyroid-stimulating hormone A hormone secreted by the anterior pituitary. It regulates function of the thyroid gland.

thyromegaly Enlarged thyroid.

thyroparathyroidectomy Surgical removal (excision) of the thyroid and parathyroid glands.

thyrotoxicosis Condition that results from overproduction of the thyroid glands. Symptoms include a rapid heart action, tremors, enlarged thyroid gland, exophthalmos, and weight loss.

thyroxine (T_4) A hormone produced by the thyroid gland. It is also known as T_4 and requires iodine for its production. This hormone regulates the level of cell metabolism. The greater the level of hormone in the blood stream, the higher cell metabolism will be.

tibia Also called the shin bone. It is a lower extremity bone.

tic Spasmodic, involuntary muscular contraction involving the head, face, mouth, eyes, neck, and shoulders.

tic douloureux Painful condition in which the trigeminal nerve is affected by pressure or degeneration. The pain is of a severe stabbing nature and radiates from the jaw and along the face.

tinea Fungal skin disease resulting in itching, scaling lesions.

tinnitus Ringing in the ears.

tissues Tissues are formed when cells of the same type are grouped together to perform one activity. For example, nerve cells combine to form nerve fibers. There are four types of tissue: nerve, muscle, epithelial, and connective.

tolerance Development of a capacity for withstanding a large amount of a substance, such as foods, drugs, or poison, without any adverse effect. A decreased sensitivity to further doses will develop.

tongue A muscular organ in the floor of the mouth. Works to move food around inside the mouth and is also necessary for speech.

tonometry Measurement of the intraocular pressure of the eye using a tonometer to check for the condition of glaucoma. After a local anesthetic is applied, the physician places the tonometer lightly upon the eyeball and a pressure measurement is taken. Generally part of a normal eye exam for adults.

tonsillectomy Surgical removal of the tonsils.

tonsillitis Inflammation of the tonsils.

tonsils The collections of lymphatic tissue located in the pharynx to combat microorganisms entering the body through the nose or mouth. The tonsils are the pharyngeal tonsils, the palatine tonsils, and the lingual tonsils.

topical   Applied directly to the skin or mucous membranes. They are distributed in ointment, cream, or lotion form. Used to treat skin infections and eruptions.

topical anesthesia   Topical anesthesia is applied using either a liquid or gel placed directly onto a specific area. The patient remains conscious. This type of anesthetic is used on the skin, the cornea, and mucous membranes in dental work.

topically   Medication applied to the surface of the skin.

torsion   Twisting.

total calcium   Blood test to measure the total amount of calcium to assist in detecting parathyroid and bone disorders.

total hip replacement (THR)   Surgical reconstruction of a hip by implanting a prosthetic or artificial hip joint.

tourniquet   Device to restrict blood flow to and from an extremity. Used carefully when hemorrhage is present to prevent further bleeding.

toxic shock syndrome (TSS)   Rare and sometimes fatal staphylococcus infection that generally occurs in menstruating women.

toxicity   Extent or degree to which a substance is poisonous.

toxins   Substances poisonous to the body. Many are filtered out of the blood by the kidney.

trachea   Also called the windpipe. It conducts air from the larynx down to the main bronchi in the chest.

tracheostenosis   Narrowing and stenosis of the lumen or opening into the trachea.

tracheostomy   Surgical procedure used to make an opening in the trachea to create an airway. A tracheostomy tube can be inserted to keep the opening patent.

tracheotomy   Surgical incision into the trachea to provide an airway.

trachoma   Chronic infectious disease of the conjunctiva and cornea caused by bacteria. Occurs more commonly in people living in hot, dry climates. Untreated, it may lead to blindness when the scarring invades the cornea. Trachoma can be treated with antibiotics.

tract   A bundle of fibers located within the central nervous system.

traction   Process of pulling or drawing, usually with a mechanical device. Used in treating orthopedic (bone and joint) problems and injuries.

trade name   The name a pharmaceutical company chooses as the trademark or market name for its drug. Also called proprietary or brand name.

traits   The characteristics controlled by genes, such as eye color.

tranquilizer   Used to reduce mental anxiety and tensions.

transcutaneous electrical nerve stimulation (TENS) Application of a mild electrical stimulation to skin via electrodes placed over a painful area, causing interference with the transmission of the painful stimuli. Can be used in pain management to interfere with the normal pain mechanism.

transfusion   Artificial transfer of blood into the bloodstream.

transient ischemic attack (TIA)   Temporary interference with blood supply to the brain, causing neurological symptoms such as dizziness, numbness, and hemiparesis. May lead eventually to a full-blown stroke (CVA).

transurethral   Pertaining to across the urethra.

transurethral resection of the prostate (TUR)   Surgical removal of the prostate gland by inserting a device through the urethra and removing prostate tissue.

transverse colon   The section of colon that cross the upper abdomen from the right side of the body to the left.

transverse fracture   Complete fracture that is straight across the bone at right angles to the long axis of the bone.

transverse plane   A horizontal plane that divides the body into upper (superior) and lower (inferior) sections. Also called the horizontal plane.

trauma   Physical wound or injury caused by an external force or violence.

treadmill test   Method for evaluating cardiovascular fitness. The patient is placed on a treadmill and then subjected to steadily increasing levels of work. An EKG and oxygen levels are taken while the patient exercises. Also called a *stress test.*

tremor   Involuntary quivering movement of a part of the body.

Trendelenburg position   A surgical position in which the patient is lying face up and on an incline with the head lower than the legs.

trephination   Process of cutting out a piece of bone in the skull to gain entry into the brain or relieve pressure.

trephine   A surgical saw used to remove the disc-shaped piece of tissue.

triage   Quick screening and classification of sick, wounded, or injured persons during a disaster or war. Priorities are determined for the efficient use of medical personnel, equipment, and facilities.

trichomoniasis   Genitourinary infection that is usually without symptoms (asymptomatic) in both males and females. In women the disease can produce itching and/or burning and a foul-smelling discharge, and can result in vaginitis.

trichomycosis   Abnormal condition of hair fungus.

tricuspid   Having three cusps or points.

tricuspid valve   A valve between the right atrium and ventricle of the heart. It prevents blood from flowing backwards into the atrium. A tricuspid valve has three cusps or flaps.

triiodothyronine (T_3)   A hormone produced by the thyroid gland known as T_3 that requires iodine for its production. This hormone regulates the level of cell metabolism. The greater the level of hormone in the blood stream, the higher cell metabolism will be.

trochanter   The large blunt process that provides the attachment for tendons and muscles.

tubal ligation   Surgical tying off of the fallopian tubes to prevent conception from taking place. Results in sterilization of the female.

tubal pregnancy   Implantation of a fetus within the fallopian tube instead of the uterus. Requires immediate surgery.

tubercle   A small, rounded process that provides the attachment for tendons and muscles.

tuberculin skin tests (TB test) Applying a chemical agent (Tine or Mantoux tests) under the surface of the skin to determine if the patient has been exposed to tuberculosis.

tuberculosis (TB) Infectious disease caused by the tubercle bacillus, *Myocobacterium tuberculosis*. Most commonly affects the respiratory system and causes inflammation and calcification of the system. Tuberculosis is again on the uprise and is seen in many patients who have AIDS.

tuberosity A large, rounded process that provides the attachment of tendons and muscles.

tumor Abnormal growth of tissue that may be benign or malignant. Also called a neoplasm.

two-hour postprandial glucose tolerance test Blood test to assist in evaluating glucose metabolism. The patient eats a high-carbohydrate diet and fasts overnight before the test. A blood sample is then taken two hours after a meal.

tympanic Pertaining to the ear drum.

tympanic membrane Also called the ear drum. As sound moves along the auditory canal, it strikes the tympanic membrane causing it to vibrate. This conducts the sound wave into the middle ear.

tympanitis Ear drum inflammation.

tympanometer Instrument to measure the ear drum.

tympanometry Measurement of the movement of the tympanic membrane. Can indicate the presence of pressure in the middle ear.

tympanoplasty Another term for the surgical reconstruction of the eardrum. Also called myringoplasty.

tympanorrhexis Ruptured ear drum.

Type I diabetes mellitus Also called insulin-dependent diabetes mellitus (IDDM). It develops early in life when the pancreas stops insulin production. Therefore, persons with IDDM must take daily insulin injections.

Type II diabetes mellitus Also called non–insulin-dependent diabetes mellitus (NIDDM). It develops later in life when the pancreas produces insufficient insulin. Persons may take oral hypoglycemics to stimulate insulin secretion, or may eventually have to take insulin.

Type A One of the ABO blood types. A person with type A markers on his or her RBCs. Type A blood will make anti-B antibodies.

Type AB One of the ABO blood types. A person with both type A and type B markers on his or her RBCs. Since it has both markers, it will not make antibodies against either A or B blood.

Type B One of the ABO blood types. A person with type B markers on his or her RBCs. Type B blood will make anti-A antibodies.

Type O One of the ABO blood types. A person with no markers on his or her RBCs. Type O blood will not react with anti-A or anti-B antibodies. Therefore, it is considered the universal donor.

ulcer Open sore or lesion in skin or mucous membrane.

ulcerative colitis Ulceration of unknown origin of the mucous membranes of the colon. Also known as inflammatory bowel disease (IBD).

ulna One of the forearm bones in the upper extremity.

ultrasound (US) The use of high-frequency sound waves to create heat in soft tissues under the skin. It is particularly useful for treating injuries to muscles, tendons, and ligaments, as well as muscle spasms. In radiology, ultrasound waves can be used to outline shapes of tissues, organs, and the fetus.

umbilical An anatomical division of the abdomen; the middle section of the middle row.

umbilical cord A cord extending from the baby's umbilicus (navel) to the placenta. It contains blood vessels that carry oxygen and nutrients from the mother to the baby and carbon dioxide and wastes from the baby to the mother.

unconscious Condition or state of being unaware of surroundings, with the inability to respond to stimuli.

ungual Pertaining to the nails.

unit dose Drug dosage system that provides prepackaged, prelabeled, individual medications that are ready for immediate use by the patient.

United States Pharmacopeia-National Formulary A resource for drug information that lists all the official drugs authorized for use in the United States.

universal donor Type O blood is considered the universal donor. Since it has no markers on the RBC surface, it will not trigger a reaction with anti-A or anti-B antibodies.

upper extremity (UE) The arm.

upper gastrointestinal (UGI) series Administering a barium contrast material orally and then taking an X-ray to visualize the esophagus, stomach, and duodenum.

uptake Absorption of radioactive material and medicines into an organ or tissue.

urea A waste product of protein metabolism. It diffuses through the tissues in lymph and is returned to the circulatory system for transport to the kidneys.

uremia An excess of urea and other nitrogenous waste in the blood.

ureterectasis Dilation of the ureter.

ureterolith A calculus in the ureter.

ureterostenosis Narrowing of the ureter.

ureters Organs in the urinary system that transport urine from the kidney to the bladder.

urethra The tube that leads from the urinary bladder to the outside of the body. In the male it is also used by the reproductive system to release semen.

urethralgia Urethral pain.

urethritis Inflammation of the urethra.

urethrorrhagia Rapid bleeding from the urethra.

urethroscope Instrument to view inside the urethra.

urethrostenosis Narrowing of the urethra.

urgency Feeling the need to urinate immediately.

urgent care Level of patient care for those who need immediate attention, but whose condition is not life threatening and does not require hospitalization. A small child with an ear infection or a teenager with a simple fracture are good examples.

uric acid   A waste product from metabolism found in plasma. High levels of uric acid are associated with gout.

urinal   Urine container for males.

urinalysis (U/A, UA)   Laboratory test that consists of the physical, chemical, and microscopic examination of urine.

urinary bladder   Organ in the urinary system that stores urine.

urinary incontinence   Involuntary release of urine. In some patients an indwelling catheter is inserted into the bladder for continuous urine drainage.

urinary meatus   The external opening of the urethra.

urinary retention   An inability to fully empty the bladder, often indicates a blockage in the urethra.

urinary system   System that filters wastes from the blood and excretes the waste products in the form of urine. Organs include the kidneys, ureters, urinary bladder, and urethra.

urine   It is the fluid that remains in the urinary system following the three stages of urine production: filtration, reabsorption, and secretion.

urography   Use of a contrast medium to provide an X-ray of the urinary tract.

urologist   A physician specialized in treating conditions and diseases of the urinary system and male reproductive system.

urology   Branch of medicine specializing in conditions of the urinary system and male reproductive system.

urticaria   Hives, a skin eruption of pale reddish wheals (circular elevations of the skin) with severe itching. Usually associated with food allergy, stress, or drug reactions.

uterus   Also called the womb. An internal organ of the female reproductive system. This hollow, pear-shaped organ is located in the lower pelvic cavity between the urinary bladder and rectum. The uterus receives the fertilized ovum and it becomes implanted in the uterine wall, which provides nourishment and protection for the developing fetus. The uterus is divided into three regions: fundus, corpus, and cervix.

utricle   Found in the inner ear. It plays a role in equilibrium.

vaccination   Providing protection against communicable diseases by stimulating the immune system to produce antibodies against that disease. Children can now be immunized for the following diseases: hepatitis B, diphtheria, tetanus, pertussis, tetanus, *Haemophilus influenza* type b, polio, measles, mumps, rubella, and chickenpox. Also called immunization.

vaccine   Given to promote resistance to infectious diseases.

vagina   Organ in the female reproductive system that receives the penis and semen.

vaginal   Tablets and suppositories inserted vaginally and used to treat vaginal yeast infections and other irritations.

vaginal orifice   The external vaginal opening. It may be covered by a hymen.

vaginitis   Inflammation of the vagina, generally caused by a microorganism.

vagotomy   Surgical resection of the vagus nerve in an attempt to decrease the amount of acid secretion into the stomach. Used as a method of treatment for patients with ulcers.

valve replacement   Excision of a diseased heart valve and replacement with an artificial valve.

valves   A flap-like structure found within the tubular organs such as lymph vessels, veins, and the heart. They function to prevent the backflow of fluid.

valvulitis   Inflammation of a valve.

varicocele   Enlargement of the veins of the spermatic cord, which commonly occurs on the left side of adolescent males. Seldom needs treatment.

varicose veins   Swollen and distended veins, usually in the legs.

vas deferens   Also called ductus deferens. The vas deferens is a long straight tube that carries sperm from the epididymis up into the pelvic cavity, where it continues around the bladder and empties into the urethra. It is one of the components, along with nerves and blood vessels, of the spermatic cord.

vasectomy   Removal of a segment or all of the vas deferens to prevent sperm from leaving the male body. Used for contraception purposes.

vasodilator   Produces a relaxation of blood vessels to lower blood pressure.

vasopressor   Produces the contraction of muscles in the capillaries and arteries that elevates the blood pressure.

vasovasostomy   Creation of a new opening between two sections of vas deferens. Used to reverse a vasectomy.

veins   Blood vessels of the cardiovascular system that carry blood toward the heart.

venae cavae   The very large vein that returns deoxygenated blood from the body to the right side of the heart. It has a superior and an inferior branch.

venereal disease (VD)   Disease usually acquired as the result of heterosexual or homosexual intercourse.

venipuncture   Puncture into a vein to withdraw fluids or to insert medication and fluids.

venography   Process of taking an X-ray tracing of a vein.

venotomy   Surgical incision into a vein.

venous   Pertaining to a vein.

ventral   Directional term meaning near or on the front or belly side of the body.

ventricles   The two lower chambers of the heart that receive blood from the atria and pump it back out of the heart. The left ventricle pumps blood to the body, and the right ventricle pumps blood to the lungs. Also fluid-filled spaces within the cerebrum. These contain cerebrospinal fluid, which is the watery, clear fluid that provides a protection from shock or sudden motion to the brain.

ventricular   Pertaining to a ventricle.

venule   The smallest veins. Venules receive deoxygenated blood leaving the capillaries.

verruca   Warts; a benign neoplasm (tumor) caused by a virus. Has a rough surface that is removed by chemicals and/or laser therapy.

vertebra   The bones of the spinal column that surround and protect the spinal cord.

vertebral canal   The bony canal through the vertebrae that contains the spinal cord.

vertebral column   The vertebral column is part of the axial skeleton. It is a column of twenty-six vertebra that forms the backbone and protects the spinal cord. It is divided into five sections: cervical vertebrae, thoracic vertebrae, lumbar vertebrae, sacrum, and coccyx. Also called spinal column.

vertigo   Dizziness.

vesicle   Small, fluid-filled raised spot on the skin.

vestibular apparatus   Part of the inner ear responsible for equilibrium. Conditions resulting in loss of balance may arise from this area.

vestibular nerve   The branch of the vestibulocochlear nerve responsible for sending equilibrium information to the brain.

vestibulocochlear nerve   The eighth cranial nerve. It is responsible for hearing and balance.

viable   A fetus developed sufficiently to live outside the uterus.

viruses   A group of infectious particles that cause disease.

viscera   The name for the internal organs of the body, such as the lungs, stomach, and liver.

visceral   Pertaining to the viscera or internal organs.

visceral layer   The inner pleural layer. It adheres to the surface of the lung.

visceral pericardium   The inner layer of the pericardium surrounding the heart.

visceral peritoneum   The inner layer of the serous membrane sac encasing the abdominopelvic viscera.

visceral pleura   The inner layer of the serous membrane sac encasing the thoracic viscera.

visual acuity (VA)   Measurement of the sharpness of a patient's vision. Usually, a Snellen's chart is used for this test and the patient identifies letters from a distance of twenty feet.

vital signs (VS)   Respiration, pulse, temperature, skin color, blood pressure, and reaction of pupils. These are signs of the condition of body functions.

vitamin   Organic substance found naturally in foods that is essential for normal metabolism. Most have been produced synthetically to be taken in pill form.

vitiligo   Disappearance of pigment from the skin in patches, causing a milk-white appearance. Also called leukoderma.

vitrectomy   Surgical procedure for replacing the contents of the vitreous chamber of the eye.

vitreous humor   The transparent jelly-like substance inside the eyeball.

vocal cords   The structures within the larynx that vibrate to produce sound and speech.

voluntary muscle tissue   Muscles under voluntary control such as the striated muscles attached to the skeleton.

volvulus   Condition in which the bowel twists upon itself and causes a painful obstruction that requires immediate surgery.

vomer bone   A facial bone.

von Recklinghausen's disease   Excessive production of parathyroid hormone, which results in degeneration of the bones. Named for Friedrich von Recklinghausen, a German histologist.

voyeurism   A sexual disorder characterized by receiving sexual gratification from observing others engaged in sexual acts.

vulva   A general term meaning the external female genitalia. It consists of the Bartholin's glands, labia major, labia minora, and clitoris.

walker   Aluminum device with our without wheels to provide support for someone who is having difficulty walking.

well-baby check-up/well-child check-up   Preventative visits to the doctor's office. The physician will assess the child's growth and development, look for early signs of disease or abnormalities, and administer routine immunization or vaccination. Parents also receive education in topics such as nutrition and child development.

Western blot   Test used as a backup to the ELISA blood test to detect the presence of the antibody to HIV (AIDS virus) in the blood.

wheal   Small, round, raised area on the skin that may be accompanied by itching.

whiplash   Injury to the bones in the cervical spine as a result of a sudden movement forward and backward of the head and neck. Can occur as a result of a rear-end auto collision.

whirlpool   Bath in which there are continuous jets of hot water reaching the body surfaces.

white blood cells   Blood cells that provide protection against the invasion of bacteria and other foreign material.

white blood count (WBC)   Blood test to measure the number of leukocytes in a volume of blood. An increase may indicate the presence of infection or a disease such as leukemia. A decrease in WBCs is caused by X-ray therapy and chemotherapy.

white matter   Tissue in the central nervous system. It consists of myelinated nerve fibers.

Wilm's tumor   Malignant kidney tumor found most often in children.

word root   The foundation of a medical term that provides the basic meaning of the word. In general, the word root will indicate the body system or part of the body that is being discussed. A word may have more than one word root.

xanthoderma   Yellow skin.

xeroderma   Dry skin.

X-ray   High-energy wave that can penetrate most solid matter and present the image on photographic film.

yellow bone marrow   Yellow bone marrow is located mainly in the center of the diaphysis of long bones. It contains mainly fat cells.

zygomatic bone   A facial bone.

INDEX

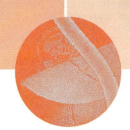

Glossary terms appear in bold.

Antacid, 462, 465, 467, 556
Anteflexion, 337, 556
Antepartum, 556
Anterior, 42, 556
Anterior cruciate ligament (ACL) reconstruction, 123, 556
Anterior lobe, 144, 556
Anteversion, 337, 556
Antianxiety, 465, 467, 556
Antiarrhythmic, 465, 467, 556
Antibiotic, 465, 467, 556
Antibody, 205, 207, 556
Antibody-mediated immunity, 205, 556
Anticholinergic, 465, 468, 556
Anticoagulant, 217, 465, 468, 556
Anticonvulsant, 465, 468, 556
Antidepressant, 465, 468, 524, 556
Antidiabetic, 465, 468, 556
Antidiarrheal, 465, 468, 556
Antidiuretic, 314, 556
Antidiuretic hormone (ADH), 145, 308, 556
Antidote, 463, 465, 556
Antiemetic, 465, 468, 556
Antigen, 205, 207, 556
Antigen–antibody reaction, 207, 556
Antihemorrhagic, 217, 556
Antihistamine, 465, 468, 556
Antihypertensive, 465, 468, 556
Anti-inflammatory, 465, 468, 556
Antipsychotic drugs, 524
Antipyretic, 465, 468, 556
Antisocial personality, 523, 556
Antitussive, 465, 468, 556
Antrum, 276, 556
Anuria, 318, 556
Anus, 280, 556
Anxiety, 494, 523, 556
Anxiety disorders, 523
Aorta, 45, 170, 173, 313, 556
Aortic, 179, 556
Aortic insufficiency (AI), 179, 556
Aortic stenosis, 179, 556
Aortic valve, 169, 556
Aortogram, 556
Aortography, 499, 556
AP view, 497, 556
Apex, 43, 165, 556
Aphagia, 556
Aphasia, 395, 494, 557
Apnea, 488, 557
Apocrine gland, 66, 557
Appendectomy, 292, 557
Appendicitis, 280, 557
Appendicular skeleton, 93, 96, 97, 100–102, 103–104, 557
Appendix, 280, 557
Aqueous humor, 424, 557
Arachnoid layer, 391, 557
Areola, 344, 557
Arrhythmia, 557
Arterial, 557
Arterial blood gases (ABG), 182, 253, 557
Arterial embolism, 179, 557
Arterial system, 174
Arteries, 34, 173, 557
Arteriography, 182, 499, 557
Arterioles, 173, 557
Arteriorrhexis, 557
Arteriosclerosis, 179, 495, 557
Arteriosclerotic heart disease (ASHD), 179, 557
Artery graft, 183, 557
Arthralgia, 557
Arthritis, 116, 118, 495, 512, 557
Arthrocentesis, 122, 557
Arthroclasia, 557

Arthrodesis, 123, 557
Arthrography, 122, 557
Arthroplasty, 123, 557
Arthroscopic, 123
Arthroscopic surgery, 557
Arthroscopy, 122, 124, 557
Arthrotomy, 123, 557
Articulation, 106, 557
Artificial pacemaker, 183, 557
Artificial ventilation, 487, 557
Ascending colon, 280, 557
Ascites, 284, 557
Aspermia, 366, 557
Asphyxia, 248, 488, 557
Aspirator, 518, 557
Assistants, 50
Assisted living, 494, 557
Asthenia, 395, 557
Asthma, 250, 527, 557
Asthmatic attack, 488, 557
Astigmatism (Astigm), 428, 557
Astringent, 465, 557
Astrocyte, 395, 557
Astrocytoma, 397, 505, 557
Ataxia, 395, 557
Atelectasis, 250, 557
Atherectomy, 557
Atherosclerosis, 179, 557
Atria, 168, 557
Atrial, 558
Atrial natriuretic hormone (ANF), 314, 558
Atrioventricular defect, 180, 558
Atrioventricular node, 172, 558
Atrioventricular valve (AV), 169, 558
Atrophy, 558
Attention deficit disorder (ADD), 523, 528, 558
Atypical, 207, 558
Audiogram, 448, 558
Audiologist, 445, 450, 558
Audiology, 558
Audiometer, 448, 558
Audiometric test, 448, 558
Audiometry, 558
Auditory canal, 440, 558
Aural, 558
Auricle, 440, 558
Auscultation, 178, 179, 248, 558
Autism, 523, 558
Autohemotherapy, 221, 558
Autologous transfusion, 221, 558
Autonomic nervous system, 172, 383, 392–393, 558
Axial skeleton, 93, 95, 97–100, 558
Axillary, 202, 558
Axon, 384, 558
Azoospermia, 366, 558

B

B cells, 205, 558
B lymphocytes, 205, 558
Babinski, Joseph, 402
Babinski's reflex, 402, 558
Back, 47–48
Bacteria, 203, 558
Bacterium, 271, 558
Balanitis, 366, 558
Balanoplasty, 558
Balanorrhea, 558
Baldness. See Alopecia
Ball and socket, 107, 558
Balloon angioplasty, 184
Barium (Ba), 497, 558
Barium enema (BE, lower GI series), 290, 292, 499, 558
Barium swallow (upper GI series), 291, 292, 558

Barr, Yvonne, 209
Bartholin's glands, 335, 339, 558
Basal cell carcinoma, 77, 505, 558
Basal layer, 61, 558
Basal metabolic rate (BMR), 153, 558
Base, 43, 559
Basic life support, 487, 559
Basophils, 214, 559
Bedside commode, 495, 559
Bell, Sir Charles, 397
Bell's palsy, 397, 559
Benign, 503, 559
Benign bone tumors, 121
Benign prostatic hypertrophy (BPH), 366, 559
Benign skin neoplasms, 75–76
Biceps, 113, 559
Bicuspid valve, 169, 559
Bicuspids, 273, 274, 559
Bilateral, 7
Bile, 281, 559
Bilirubin, 285
Billing codes, procedural and diagnostic, 17
Binocular, 559
Biopsy (BX, bx), 78, 506, 559
Bipolar disease, 523, 559
Bite, 488, 559
Bite-wing X-ray, 291, 559
Blackhead. See Comedo
Bladder. See Urinary bladder
Bladder neck obstruction, 320, 559
Bleeding time, 218, 559
Blepharitis, 428, 559
Blepharochalasis, 428, 559
Blepharoplasty, 559
Blepharoptosis, 559
Blood, 35,
  circulation of, 170–171, 176
  drawing, 219–221
  formed elements, 213–214
  kidneys and, 313
  plasma, 212–213
  urine and, 315
  See also Hematic system
Blood clot, 181
Blood groupings, 215
Blood pressure (BP), 171, 178, 487, 559
Blood pressure cuff. See Sphygmomanometer
Blood serum test, 153, 559
Blood transfusion, 221
Blood typing, 215, 559
Blood urea nitrogen (BUN), 321, 559
Blood vessels, 34, 173–176, 559
Body, 276, 559
Body cavities, 44–47
Body fluids, 222
Body mechanics, 511, 559
Body membranes, 60
Body organization. See Body structure
Body planes, 40–41
Body structure
  abbreviations relating to, 51
  anatomical position, 38–40
  back, 47–48
  body cavities, 44–47
  body planes, 40–41
  cells, 29–30
  combining forms relating to, 28
  directional and positional terms, 42–43
  key terms, 51–52
  organs and body systems, 32–38
  physicians and assistants, 50
  prefixes relating to, 28
  tissues, 30–31
  word building relating to, 49
Body systems, 29, 32–38
Boil, 74, 559

aden/o	cholecyst/o
Combining Form	Combining Form
angi/o	chondr/o
Combining Form	Combining Form
arteri/o	col/o; colon/o
Combining Form	Combining Form
arthr/o	colp/o; vagin/o
Combining Form	Combining Form
balan/o	conjunctiv/o
Combining Form	Combining Form
bronch/o; bronch/i	cutane/o; dermat/o
Combining Form	Combining Form
carcin/o	cyst/o
Combining Form	Combining Form
cardi/o; coron/o	dent/o; odont/o
Combining Form	Combining Form
cerebr/o	embry/o
Combining Form	Combining Form
cervic/o	encephal/o
Combining Form	Combining Form

gall bladder	gland
Meaning	Meaning
cartilage	vessel
Meaning	Meaning
colon	artery
Meaning	Meaning
vagina	joint
Meaning	Meaning
conjunctiva	glans penis
Meaning	Meaning
skin	bronchus
Meaning	Meaning
bladder	cancer
Meaning	Meaning
teeth	heart
Meaning	Meaning
embryo	cerebrum
Meaning	Meaning
brain	neck
Meaning	Meaning

enter/o	lymph/o
Combining Form	Combining Form
epididym/o	mamm/o; mast/o
Combining Form	Combining Form
esophag/o	men/o
Combining Form	Combining Form
fet/o; fet/i	muscul/o; my/o
Combining Form	Combining Form
gastr/o	myel/o
Combining Form	Combining Form
hemat/o; hem/o	myring/o; tympan/o
Combining Form	Combining Form
hepat/o	nas/o; rhin/o
Combining Form	Combining Form
hyster/o; metr/o, uter/o	nephr/o; ren/o
Combining Form	Combining Form
kerat/o	neur/o
Combining Form	Combining Form
laryng/o	ocul/o; ophthalm/o; opt/o
Combining Form	Combining Form

lymph	small intestines
Meaning	Meaning
breast	epididymis
Meaning	Meaning
menses,menstruation	esophagus
Meaning	Meaning
muscle	fetus
Meaning	Meaning
spinal cord, red bone marrow	stomach
Meaning	Meaning
eardrum	blood
Meaning	Meaning
nose	liver
Meaning	Meaning
kidney	uterus
Meaning	Meaning
nerve	cornea, hard, horny
Meaning	Meaning
eye	larynx
Meaning	Meaning

onych/o; ungu/o	pneum/o; pulmon/o
Combining Form	Combining Form
oophor/o; ovari/o	proct/o
Combining Form	Combining Form
or/o; stomat/o	prostat/o
Combining Form	Combining Form
orch/o; orchid/o; test/o	py/o
Combining Form	Combining Form
oste/o	pyel/o
Combining Form	Combining Form
ot/o	retin/o
Combining Form	Combining Form
pancreat/o	salping/o
Combining Form	Combining Form
phak/o	scler/o
Combining Form	Combining Form
pharyng/o	splen/o
Combining Form	Combining Form
phleb/o; ven/o	tendin/o
Combining Form	Combining Form

lung	nail
Meaning	Meaning
rectum	ovary
Meaning	Meaning
prostate	mouth
Meaning	Meaning
pus	testes
Meaning	Meaning
renal pelvis	bone
Meaning	Meaning
retina	ear
Meaning	Meaning
fallopian tube	pancreas
Meaning	Meaning
sclera, hard	lens
Meaning	Meaning
spleen	throat
Meaning	Meaning
tendon	vein
Meaning	Meaning

thorac/o	dys-
Combining Form	Prefix

thromb/o	epi-
Combining Form	Prefix

trache/o	erythro-
Combining Form	Prefix

ureter/o	eu-
Combining Form	Prefix

urethr/o	hyper-
Combining Form	Prefix

vas/o	hypo-
Combining Form	Prefix

vertebr/o	inter-
Combining Form	Prefix

a-; an-	intra-
Prefix	Prefix

bi-	leuko-
Prefix	Prefix

brady-	macro-
Prefix	Prefix

painful, difficult	chest
Meaning	*Meaning*
upon, over	clot
Meaning	*Meaning*
red	trachea
Meaning	*Meaning*
normal, good	ureter
Meaning	*Meaning*
over, above	urethra
Meaning	*Meaning*
under, below	vas deferens
Meaning	*Meaning*
among, between	vertebra, backbone
Meaning	*Meaning*
within, inside	without
Meaning	*Meaning*
white	two
Meaning	*Meaning*
large	slow
Meaning	*Meaning*

melano-	–centesis
Prefix	Suffix

micro-	–ectasis
Prefix	Suffix

neo-	–ectomy
Prefix	Suffix

peri-	–emia
Prefix	Suffix

poly-	–gram
Prefix	Suffix

retro-	–graph
Prefix	Suffix

sub-	–graphy
Prefix	Suffix

tachy-	–itis
Prefix	Suffix

–algia	–logist
Suffix	Suffix

–cele	–logy
Suffix	Suffix

puncture to withdraw fluid	black
Meaning	Meaning
dilatation	small
Meaning	Meaning
surgical removal	new
Meaning	Meaning
blood condition	around
Meaning	Meaning
record, picture	many
Meaning	Meaning
instrument for recording	backward, behind
Meaning	Meaning
process of recording	below, under
Meaning	Meaning
inflammation	rapid, fast
Meaning	Meaning
one who studies	pain
Meaning	Meaning
study of	hernia, protrusion
Meaning	Meaning

–malacia	–plasty
Suffix	Suffix
–megaly	–rrhed
Suffix	Suffix
–meter	–rrhage
Suffix	Suffix
–metry	–rrhaphy
Suffix	Suffix
–oma	–rrhexis
Suffix	Suffix
–osis	–sclerosis
Suffix	Suffix
–ostomy	–scope
Suffix	Suffix
–otomy	–scopy
Suffix	Suffix
–pathy	–stenosis
Suffix	Suffix
–pexy	–uria
Suffix	Suffix

surgical repair	abnormal softening
Meaning	Meaning
discharge, flow	enlargement, large
Meaning	Meaning
excessive flow	instrument for measuring
Meaning	Meaning
suture	process of measuring
Meaning	Meaning
rupture	tumor, mass
Meaning	Meaning
hardening	abnormal condition
Meaning	Meaning
instrument for viewing	surgically create an opening
Meaning	Meaning
process of viewing	cutting into
Meaning	Meaning
narrowing	disease
Meaning	Meaning
in the urine	surgical fixation
Meaning	Meaning